ASCP QUICK COMPENDIUM
OF
CLINICAL PATHOLOGY

Dedication

I dedicate this book to our four children:
Sarah, Diana, and the Davids.

ASCP

QUICK COMPENDIUM

OF CLINICAL PATHOLOGY

Daniel D Mais, MD

Medical Director of Hematopathology,
Surgical Pathologist, Department of Pathology
St Joseph's Mercy Hospital and Warde Medical Laboratory
Ann Arbor

2ND EDITION

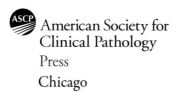
American Society for
Clinical Pathology
Press
Chicago

Publishing Team
Ted Moon and Erik Tanck (design)
Erik Tanck (production)
Joshua Weikersheimer (publishing direction)

Notice
Trade names for equipment and supplies described herein are included as suggestions only. In no way does their inclusion constitute an endorsement or preference by the American Society for Clinical Pathology. The ASCP did not test the equipment, supplies, or procedures and therefore urges all readers to read and follow all manufacturers' instructions and package insert warnings concerning the proper and safe use of products.

12 11 10 09 08   5 4 3 2 1

Printed in Hong Kong

Acknowledgments

My mentor, Dr James L Kelley, taught me to be diagnostician and a doctor. Through his example I saw the way to gain the esteem of clinical colleagues: be prepared, be honest, and, above all, be available. I am grateful to my publisher, Joshua Weikersheimer, who saw the value in this idea and assisted me through to its completion. I am indebted to Dr David F Keren for his teaching and encouragement. I thank Emily for her assistance, friendship, and love.

Preface

This book was written to serve as a concise yet comprehensive source for the review of clinical pathology. It is best suited for those who are familiar with the basics and desire either a guidebook to board preparation. The topics are organized according to the traditional clinical pathology sections. Within each topic I have included, as best I could judge, what it is essential to know for both practical and test preparation purposes.

The typical experience in laboratory medicine training is long, fractured, and uneven, such that much is forgotten and much more is never actually learned. As long as there have been pathology boards, senior residents have sequestered themselves with collections of papers, books, and notes that they hoped to memorize. While I believe that there is merit in this once-over review of everything, there can be much wasted effort without guidance and focus. I wrote this guidebook hoping improve this process, such that it retains its merit and perhaps loses some of its burden.

Thus, shortly after taking the boards in 1998, I organized my papers, books, and notes into a manuscript that became the first edition, published finally in 2005. This was well received, especially by appreciative pathology residents. In addition to gratitude, I was the beneficiary of much constructive criticism, on the basis of which I have made many improvements. All sections have been updated according to the literature published since the first edition. Furthermore, what wisdom I have gained from ten years of taking questions from clinical colleagues, dealing with problems, and committing mistakes has been integrated where applicable. This edition also incorporates the now significantly matured field of diagnostic molecular pathology. The focus has remained on providing a distilled review of clinical pathology, but a greater emphasis has been placed upon practical points when appropriate. Thus, I hope this book will carry the reader beyond the boards and ultimately serve as a useful desktop reference.

— D Mais, MD

Table of

Contents

Chapter 2
Blood Banking & Transfusion
Daniel D Mais & Emily E Volk

Chapter 3
Microbiology

Chapter 4
Hematopathology

Chapter 7
Molecular Methods

Chapter 8
Laboratory Statistics and Quality Control

Index

Chapter 1

Clinical Chemistry

Enzymes

Methods

- **Measurement of enzyme activity** is based upon Michaelis-Menton kinetics which holds, in brief, that the rate of enzyme activity varies linearly with substrate concentration up to the substrate concentration when the enzyme is fully saturated with substrate. At this saturation point, the enzyme is working as fast as it can (V_{max}), and the rate of reaction, all things being equal, **varies only with the enzyme concentration.** Thus, by using an excess of substrate, the enzyme concentration can be determined. The other requirement is a way to measure that the reaction has taken place. Some reaction products can themselves be measured. In other instances, NADH or NAD is utilized in the reaction. Since *NADH absorbs light at 340 nm* (and NAD does not) the formation or disappearance of NADH can be measured. If this is not the case, a reaction that does utilize NAD/NADH can be coupled to the reaction (coupled enzyme assay).

- For example, AST, which converts aspartate (Asp) and α-ketoglutarate (αKG) to oxaloacetate (OAA) and glutamate, does not utilize NADH. So in addition to an excess of NADH and α-ketoglutarate, malate dehydrogenase (MD) is added to the mix. The following reactions occur, the first catalyzed by AST and the second by MD:

  Asp + αKG → AA + glutamate + NADH → malate + NAD

  Thus, the disappearance of NADH (absorbance at 340nm) can be used as a reflection of the activity of AST. This is a coupled enzyme assay.

- An assay that does not utilize NADH/NAD is that used to measure alkaline phosphatase. When an excess of p-nitrophenyl phosphate is added at pH 10, the following reaction is catalyzed by alkaline phosphatase:

  p-nitrophenyl phosphate → p-nitrophenol + phosphate

  P-nitrophenyl phosphate has little absorbance at 405 nm, where p-nitrophenol has its peak absorbance. The absorbance of p-nitrophenol at 405 nm is measured as a reflection of alkaline phosphatase activity. Note that if this same assay is run at pH 5.0, acid phosphatase is measured.

- **Measurements of enzyme antigen** concentration, usually by immunoassay, are routinely employed for a wide range of enzymes. For the most part, the quantity of enzyme determined by immunoassay corresponds with the enzyme activity. Discordance between these two measurements usually takes the form of the immunoassay result overestimating the activity. This effect may be seen in the presence of serum enzyme inhibitors, in a deficiency of a necessary cofactor, macroenzymes, defective enzyme, and proteolytically inactivated enzymes.

  □ Cofactors are substances that bind to an enzyme and enhance their activity. There are inorganic cofactors (zinc, calcium, magnesium, iron, etc) and organic cofactors (also called coenzymes). Coenzymes include NAD, protein S (a cofactor for protein C), pyridoxine (vitamin B_6), etc.

  □ Macroenzymes are ordinary enzymes bound to antibodies. Being bound to an antibody has two effects upon an enzyme: it usually makes it incapable of functioning, and it prevents it from being cleared from the blood.

  □ Defective enzymes may still be antigenically active but enzymatically inactive.

Types of enzyme inhibition F1.1

- **Uninhibited enzyme.** When a plot of V (enzyme velocity) versus [S] (substrate concentration) is made for a given amount of enzyme, an asymptotic curve results which approaches, but never reaches, V_{max} and from which K_m can only be estimated. However, if 1/V is plotted against 1/[S], a straight line results. This is called a Lineweaver-Burke plot, where the y-intercept equals $1/V_{max}$, and the x-intercept is equal to $-1/K_m$.

- **Noncompetitive inhibition** is caused by an inhibitor that binds to the enzyme away from the substrate-binding site. It cannot be overcome by increasing substrate concentration. On the Lineweaver-Burke plot, the y-intercept, which equals $1/V_{max}$, is changed, and the x-intercept is unchanged.

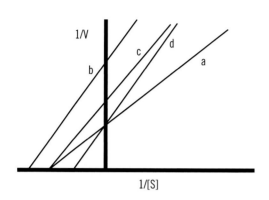

F1.1 Lineweaver-Burke Plots. Y-axis is 1/v=1/rate. X-axis is 1/S=1/substrate concentration. a. uninhibited enzyme, b. uncompetitive inhibition, c. noncompetitive inhibition, d. competitive inhibition

- **Competitive inhibition** is caused when the enzyme's substrate and the inhibitor compete for the same binding site. This type of inhibition can be overcome by increasing substrate concentration. On the Lineweaver-Burke plot, the y-intercept, which equals $1/V_{max}$, is unchanged while the slope, which equals K_m, is decreased.

- **Uncompetitive inhibition** is caused by a substance that binds the enzyme-substrate (ES) complex and stabilizes it. An uncompetitive inhibitor alters both the K_m and the V_{max}.

Units for expressing enzyme activity

- **International unit (IU).** 1 IU = the amount of enzyme that catalyzes the conversion of 1 micromole of substrate per minute.

- **Katal.** 1 katal = the amount of enzyme that catalyzes the conversion of 1 mole of substrate per second.

- 1 IU = 16.7 nanokatals.

Hepatic Enzymes and Other Liver Function Tests

Aspartate aminotransferase (AST/SGOT) and alanine aminotransferase (ALT/SGPT)

- Together, AST and ALT are referred to as the 'liver transaminases.'

- AST is present in cardiac muscle, liver, skeletal muscle, kidney, brain, lung & pancreas (in decreasing order of concentration).

- ALT is more specific for liver, confined mainly to liver and kidney.

- AST is found both within cytoplasm (about 20%) and mitochondria (about 80%).

- ALT is located entirely within the cytoplasm.

- In children, the AST activity is slightly higher than the ALT, with this pattern reversing by age 20. In adults, AST activity tends to be a little lower than ALT. This ratio may again reverse in old age. The ratio of AST:ALT is called the deRitis ratio.

- Both AST and ALT activities are higher in adult males than adult females, and both are higher in African-Americans. While hemolysis raises both, the effect is not as profound as that seen in LDH.

- Intra-individual variation is more significant for ALT than AST, with marked diurnal variation (highest in the afternoon) and day-to-day variation of up to 30%.

- Both AST and ALT may be elevated in heparin therapy to around 3× baseline.

- In renal failure, AST and ALT are significantly lower than in healthy individuals.

Lactate dehydrogenase (LDH)

- LDH is present in numerous tissues and is traditionally separable into 5 isoenzymes by electrophoresis.

- The fastest-moving isoenzymes, LD1 and LD2, are found in greatest abundance in heart, red blood cells, and kidney, with a significantly greater proportion of LD1 than LD2.

3

- The slowest isozymes, LD4 and LD5, are found in liver and skeletal muscle.

- LD3 is found in lung, spleen, lymphocytes, and pancreas.

- The 'sixth' LD, LD6, is sometimes seen migrating cathodal to LD5. Its presence is thought to be a dire finding, indicative of hepatic vascular insufficiency (usually in the setting of cardiovascular collapse).

- The comparative concentrations found in normal serum are LD2>LD1>LD3>LD4>LD5.

- When LD1 is elevated, particularly when there is a 'flipped LD ratio' such that LD1>LD2, three possibilities exist: acute myocardial infarction, hemolysis, and renal infarction.

- Elevated LD4 & LD5 suggests liver damage, but other possibilities include skeletal muscle insults.

- Elevated LD1 & LD5 can be explained by:

  □ acute myocardial infarction which has been complicated by liver congestion or

  □ chronic alcoholism that has been complicated by liver damage and megaloblastic anemia.

- The comparative concentrations in normal cerebrospinal fluid are: LD1>LD2>LD3>LD4>LD5.

Alkaline phosphatase

- There are two types of phosphatases: alkaline (pH optimum is 9) and acid (pH optimum is 5). Acid phosphatases (ACP) are found in greatest concentrations in prostate, red cells, and bone. Traditionally, red cell acid phosphatase was distinguished from other ACPs by its susceptibility to inhibition by 2% formaldehyde and resistance to inhibition by tartrate. This is the same tartrate-resistant acid phosphatase (TRAP) that is found in hairy cell leukemia. Furthermore, a type of non-TRAP acid phosphatase (prostatic acid phosphatase) has been used as a serum marker for prostatic adenocarcinoma. It has been largely replaced in this role by other markers (see below).

- Alkaline phosphatase is produced by bone, bile ducts, intestine, and placenta; likewise, elevated alkaline phosphatase is seen in biliary disease, bone disease, bone growth (children), and pregnancy.

T1.1
Characteristics of Alkaline Phosphatase Isoenzymes

Source	Heat/Urea Inhibition	L-phe Inhibition	Anodal Mobility
Biliary	+	−	1
Bone	+++	−	2
Placenta	−	+++	3
Intestinal	+	+++	4
Regan	− −	+++	3

- Decreased levels are seen in hypophosphatasia (an inborn deficiency) and malnutrition.

- Separate reference ranges are required for children and pregnant women.

- Discovering the source of elevated alkaline phosphatase is a time-honored exercise **T1.1**. By electrophoresis, alkaline phosphatase can be resolved into 4 isoenzymes, each of which displays characteristic degrees of inactivation with heating, urea incubation, and l-phenylalanine. Note especially that heating produces significant (90%) inactivation of bone alkaline phosphatase ("bone burns"), 50% inactivation of biliary alkaline phosphatase, and 0% inactivation of placental alkaline phosphatase. Sensitivity to urea incubation parallels heating.

- Biliary alkaline phosphatase is the most sensitive marker of hepatic metastases.

- Bone alkaline phosphatase is produced by osteoblasts (not osteoclasts) and reflects bone-forming activity. Some of the highest alkaline phosphatase levels are seen in Paget disease of bone. A specific immunoassay for bone alkaline phosphatase is now available.

- The Regan isoenzyme is observed in about 5% of individuals with carcinoma. It appears to be identical to placental alkaline phosphatase.

- Intestinal alkaline phosphatase can be the cause of factitious elevations in nonfasting individuals, particularly in Lewis positive type B or O secretors. Ingesting a meal can elevate the alkaline phosphatase by 30% for 2-12 hours. A repeat fasting alkaline phosphatase may be indicated.

- A minor elevation in alkaline phosphatase—usually a result between 104 and 121 IU/L—is a common clinical problem. Alkaline phosphatase is usually a little higher in men than women (but rises in women beyond middle age) and higher in African-American women than in white women. Many advocate a threshold of 1.5 times the upper limit of normal as an indication for further investigation, particularly if this threshold is breached on 2 separate occasions >6 months apart. Common clinical situations associated with a mildly elevated alkaline phosphatase activity include unrecognized pregnancy, congestive heart failure, hyperthyroidism, and exposure to certain drugs (ibuprofen, acetaminophen). Alkaline phosphatase is a sensitive indicator of hepatic metastases. In women approaching middle age, investigation should include assay for anti-mitochondrial antibodies. In the absence of a concomitant elevation in GGT or 5' nucleotidase, bone origin should be suspected. While it is reasonable to exclude osteomalacia and hyperparathyroidism, one of the most common causes of a raised bone alkaline phosphatase in older people is Page disease.

Gamma-glutamyl transferase (GGT)

- GGT is perhaps the best test to confirm that an elevated alkaline phosphatase is from the biliary tree.

- GGT is found in the biliary epithelial cell, particularly those that line the small interlobular bile ducts and bile ductules. Thus, it is exquisitely sensitive to biliary injury.

- GGT may also be elevated in steatosis, diabetes, hyperthyroidism, rheumatoid arthritis, acute myocardial infarction, and chronic obstructive pulmonary disease.

- Furthermore, GGT is present within the smooth endoplasmic reticulum of hepatocytes, and whenever there is induction due to an excess toxin, GGT levels increase. Thus, GGT is increased in patients exposed to warfarin, barbiturates, dilantin, valproate, methotrexate, and alcohol. GGT is found to be around 2-3×s the upper limit of normal in heavy drinkers. It returns to normal in about 3 weeks with abstinence, and can then be followed as a marker of alcohol consumption.

- GGT is considerably lower in women than men, and considerably higher in African-Americans.

5′-Nucleotidase

- Biliary epithelium is the main source of 5'-nucleotidase, and levels are highest in cholestatic conditions.

- Due to this specificity, it is another test to confirm that an elevated alkaline phosphatase is due to hepatobiliary disease. Its relatively low sensitivity has kept its utility below that of GGT.

Ammonia

- Hyperammonemia is nearly always due to liver failure. However, particularly in children, it should raise suspicion for an inborn error of metabolism (especially urea cycle enzyme deficiencies).

- The sources of ammonia in the body are: skeletal muscle and gut. Bacteria in the gastrointestinal tract break down protein and release ammonia. The normally functioning liver removes this ammonia from the portal circulation and discards it in the form of urea, which is excreted in the urine.

- When there is significant hepatocyte dysfunction, too much collateral circulation, or excess protein in the gut (for example, excess hemoglobin in a variceal bleed), blood ammonia can become disastrously high. These three conditions are likely to be met in a cirrhotic patient, and ammonia is eminently neurotoxic.

- Ammonia measurement requires a fresh specimen which has been chilled during transport and has undergone no hemolysis. Furthermore, a patient who smokes should abstain for several hours preceding the blood draw.

Bilirubin

- Unconjugated (indirect) bilirubin is the water-insoluble form that is produced in the breakdown of heme. It is taken to the liver, tightly bound to albumin where it undergoes glucuronidation to produce the water-soluble conjugated (direct) bilirubin. Conjugated bilirubin is then excreted in the bile, and intestinal bacteria convert this to urobilinogen. While much urobilinogen ends up in the feces, some is reabsorbed and excreted in the urine. Furthermore, some urobilinogen is converted by colonic bacteria into brown pigments (complete biliary obstruction results in white-yellow acholic stool—so-called silver stool of Thompson).

- Note that unconjugated bilirubin, even when quite elevated, does not appear in urine; thus, *bilirubinuria indicates conjugated hyperbilirubinemia.*

- Methods

  - The **diazo-colorimetric methods** rely on the formation of a colored dye through the reaction of bilirubin with a diazo compound. Without the addition of an accelerator (such as an alcohol), mainly conjugated bilirubin is measured (direct reaction). Addition of accelerators permits unconjugated bilirubin to react also, giving a measurement of total bilirubin. The difference between total and direct bilirubin is an estimate of the unconjugated (indirect) bilirubin.

  - **Direct spectrophotometry** can determine the bilirubin concentration by measuring absorbance at 455 nm; potential interference by hemoglobin is corrected for by subtracting the absorbance at 575 nm (hemoglobin's other absorbance peak). This method is only capable of measuring total bilirubin.

- Jaundice can be classified according to the type of bilirubin that is being retained T1.2, T1.3. Unconjugated hyperbilirubinemia is caused by increased production (hemolysis) or a hepatic defect that prevents conjugation. Conjugated hyperbilirubinemia is caused by an excretory defect of already-conjugated bilirubin.

T1.2
Pathophysiologic Differential Diagnosis of Hyperbilirubinemia

Step	Pathologic Processes	Type
Heme conversion to unconjugated bilirubin	Hemolysis (extravascular)	Unconjugated hyperbilirubinemia
Delivery of unconjugated bilirubin to liver	Blood shunting (cirrhosis), Right heart failure	
Uptake of unconjugated bilirubin into hepatocyte	Gilbert syndrome, Drugs: rifampin	
Conjugation of bilirubin in hepatocyte	Crigler-Najjar syndrome Hypothyroidism	
Transmembrane secretion of conjugated bilirubin into canaliculus (hepatocellular jaundice) T1.3	Dubin-Johnson syndrome Hepatitis Endotoxin (sepsis) Pregnancy (estrogen) Drugs: estrogen, cyclosporine	Conjugated hyperbilirubinemia
Flow of conjugated bilirubin through canaliculi and bile ducts (cholestatic jaundice) T1.3	Mechanical obstruction: PBC, PSC, tumor, stricture, stone	

T1.3
Differential Diagnosis of Conjugated Hyperbilirubinemia

	Hepatocellular Jaundice	Cholestatic Jaundice
Alkaline Phosphatase	<3× upper limit of normal	>3× upper limit of normal
Transaminases	>3× upper limit of normal	<3× upper limit of normal
Serum Cholestrol	Normal	Increased
Pruritus	Absent	Present

- If conjugated hyperbilirubinemia is prolonged, conjugated bilirubin can become covalently linked to serum albumin, resulting in a moiety known as δ-bilirubin. Both the liver and kidney are incapable of excreting δ-bilirubin; thus, even after resolution of the underlying cause, conjugated hyperbilirubinemia (in the form of δ-bilirubin) may persist for some time.

Additional tests of hepatic function

- **Protime (PT).** Most coagulation factors are synthesized in hepatocytes and have short half-lives, particularly factor VII with a T ½ of 12 hours. The PT is a sensitive marker of impaired hepatic synthetic function. It is important to note that impaired bile secretion can lead to vitamin K deficiency, since bile salts are required for vitamin K absorption. A prolonged PT due to cholestasis or other causes of impaired vitamin K absorption can be distinguished from a prolonged PT due to hepatocyte injury by administering parenteral vitamin K. In absorptive defects, the protime will shorten in response to parenteral vitamin K.

- **Gamma globulins.** The brisk infiltrate of lymphocytes and plasma cells that histologically characterizes autoimmune hepatitis is reflected in serum hypergammaglobulinemia. In autoimmune hepatitis, there is a marked polyclonal increase in IgG, and in primary biliary cirrhosis, there is a polyclonal increase in IgM. Furthermore, the combination of impaired hepatic synthesis and enhanced immunoglobulin synthesis results in a decreased albumin:globulin (A/G) ratio; an A/G<1.0 is usually the result of liver disease.

T1.4
Causes of Neonatal Hyperbilirubinemia

Unconjugated	Conjugated
Physiologic jaundice	Biliary obstruction (extrahepatic biliary atresia)
Breast milk jaundice	Sepsis or TORCH infection
Polycythemia	Neonatal hepatitis (idiopathic, Wilson disease, α₁-antitrypsin deficiency)
Hemolysis (HDN, hemoglobinopathies, inherited membrane or enzyme defects)	Metabolic disorders (galactosemia, hereditary fructose intolerance, glycogen storage disease)
Bowel obstruction (Hirschsprung disease, cystic fibrosis, ileal atresia)	Inherited disorders of bilirubin transport (Dubin-Johnson syndrome, Rotor syndrome)
Inherited disorders of bilirubin metabolism (Gilbert syndrome, Crigler-Najjar syndrome)	Parenteral alimentation

Neonatal jaundice T1.4

- Most cases of neonatal jaundice are entirely benign—so-called physiologic jaundice—and result from hepatic enzymes that are not yet at full capacity, leading to a build-up of unconjugated bilirubin. Physiologic jaundice has the following characteristics:

  □ Usually noted between days 2-3 of neonatal life and rarely rises at a rate greater than 5 mg/dL/day.

  □ Usually peaks by day 4-5 and rarely exceeds 5-6 mg/dL.

- In some cases, however, bilirubin levels become very high. The most common causes of severe hyperbilirubinemia in neonates are hemolytic disease of the newborn (HDN) and sepsis. The poorly developed blood-brain barrier permits unconjugated bilirubin to cause damage to the central nervous system (kernicterus). The pathologic correlates of kernicterus include yellow staining of the subthalamic nucleus, hippocampus, thalamus, globus pallidus, putamen, cerebellar nuclei, and cranial nerve nuclei.

- So the problem facing the clinician is when to worry about neonatal jaundice. Features suggesting that hyperbilirubinemia is not due to benign physiologic jaundice include:

  □ Appearance of jaundice within the first 24 hours of life

  □ A rising bilirubin beyond 1 week

  □ Persistence of jaundice past 10 days.

  □ A total bilirubin that exceeds 12 mg/dL.

  □ A single-day increase of >5 mg/dL.

  □ A conjugated (direct-reacting) bilirubin that exceeds 2 mg/dL.

- In the healthy term infant, phototherapy should be considered when bilirubin exceeds 10 mg/dL before 12 hours of age, 12 mg/dL before 18 hours of age, and 14 mg/dL before 24 hours of age. Exchange transfusions are considered when the bilirubin exceeds 20 mg/dL. Phototherapy converts unconjugated bilirubin into a molecule that can be excreted without conjugation; phototherapy is not useful for conjugated hyperbilirubinemia.

- The differential diagnosis for neonatal hyperbilirubinemia depends upon the predominant type of bilirubin—conjugated or unconjugated—and the time of onset. Jaundice appearing in the 1st 24 hours suggests erythroblastosis fetalis, a concealed hemorrhage, sepsis, or TORCH infection. Jaundice appearing between the 3rd and 7th day suggests bacterial sepsis, particularly of urinary tract origin. Jaundice arising after the 1st week suggests breast milk jaundice, sepsis, extrahepatic biliary atresia, cystic fibrosis, congenital paucity of bile ducts (Alagille syndrome), neonatal hepatitis, galactosemia, or inherited forms of hemolytic anemia (eg, PK deficiency, hereditary spherocytosis, G6PD deficiency).

- Transcutaneous bilirubin. Since it has become common to discharge newborns after 24 hours in hospital, a means of predicting which neonates will benefit from pre-discharge phototherapy has been sought. Transcutaneous bilirubin measurements can detect hyperbilirubinemia before jaundice is visible, and they have been shown to correlate reasonably well with serum bilirubin measurements. They can be used to screen otherwise healthy term infants to determine which may benefit from a serum bilirubin assay, thus sparing the great majority of infants a venipuncture. While transcutaneous bilirubin screening has not been shown to decrease the utilization of serum bilirubin testing, it appears capable of decreasing the number of readmissions for hyperbilirubinemia.

Laboratory evaluation of acute hepatic injury

- Acute hepatic injury may manifest with constitutional symptoms, jaundice, and/or elevated transaminases. It may be due to acute viral hepatitis (HAV, HBV, HCV), autoimmune hepatitis, toxin, drug, ischemia, or Wilson disease.

- Hepatitis serologies, ANA, ceruloplasmin, and clinical history often point to the specific etiology. With regard to drug history, most hepatic injury occurs within the first 4 months of drug administration. The pattern of changes in liver function tests—particularly transaminases, bilirubin, and protime—may be useful to suggest an etiology and to estimate the degree of hepatic injury.

- Acute viral hepatitis due to HAV or HBV most often leads to complete recovery; however, acute HCV hepatitis goes on to chronic hepatitis in >80% of cases. Serologic testing for HAV and HBV (IgM anti-HAV, IgM anti-HBc, HBsAg) are very dependable for diagnosing acute infection. However, the anti-HCV antibody test has only about 60% sensitivity in acute infection. HCV RNA testing has about 90%-95% sensitivity.

- Transaminases

    □ Acute hepatic injury due to ischemic or toxic insults produce the most profound elevations in transaminases—often >100 times the upper limit of normal (ULN). Such elevations are rare in acute viral hepatitis.

    □ When the AST is greater than 3,000 U/L, the etiology is a toxin in >90% of cases.

    □ AST is over ten times the upper limit of normal (ULN) in >50% of patients with acute viral hepatitis; however, it reaches this level only rarely in alcoholic hepatitis.

    □ The AST:ALT ratio is over 2 in 80% of patients with toxic, ischemic, and alcoholic hepatitis. It is usually <1 in viral hepatitis.

    □ Unlike the PT and Bili, the degree of transaminase elevation poorly reflects the degree of hepatic injury.

- Bilirubin

    □ Jaundice occurs in 70% of patients with alcoholic hepatitis and acute hepatitis A.

    □ Jaundice is present in only about 20-30% of acute hepatitis B and acute hepatitis C.

    □ Jaundice is rare in children with acute viral hepatitis, and it is rare in toxic or ischemic hepatic injury.

    □ The distribution of bilirubin (direct vs. total) in acute hepatic injury and obstructive jaundice is similar: usually >50% direct.

    □ The aminotransferases begin to fall before the bilirubin peaks in all forms of acute hepatic injury.

    □ Bilirubin > 15 mg/dL is indicative of severe liver injury and an unfavorable prognosis.

- The protime (PT) is probably the best indicator of prognosis in acute hepatic injury. PT prolongation >4.0 seconds indicates severe liver injury and an unfavorable prognosis.

Pancreatic Enzymes

Amylase

- Serum amylase consists primarily of salivary and pancreatic isoenzymes. Typically, when serum amylase is subjected to electrophoresis, 6 bands result. The first three are salivary, while the slowest three are pancreatic. Amylase isoenzymes can also be differentiated by inhibition tests: salivary amylase is sensitive to inhibition by the wheat germ lectin, *triticum vulgaris*. Lastly, assays based on monoclonal antibodies directed against specific isoenzymes are very accurate.

- Serum amylase rises within 2-24 hours of the onset of acute pancreatitis and returns to normal in 2-3 days. Higher levels do not correlate with severity, but higher levels are more specific for the diagnosis of acute pancreatitis. Persistence of elevated serum amylase suggests a complication such as a pseudocyst.

- Nearly all patients have concomitant increases in urine amylase. Amylase is primarily cleared by glomerular filtration; thus renal insufficiency spuriously elevates the serum amylase. The specificity of amylase can be improved by calculating the fractional excretion of amylase. Fractional excretion (FE) of any substance (x) is the ratio of the renal clearance of x (Cl_x) divided by the glomerular filtration rate (GFR); in other words, the clearance of x divided by the clearance of creatinine (Cl_x/Cl_{Cr}). The clearance of any substance (x) refers to the volume of plasma cleared of that substance over a certain time (eg, 24 hours) by the kidneys and is determined by measuring a certain urine volume (V_u), urine concentration of x (U_x), and plasma concentration of x (P_x).

Fractional excretion of a compound (x) = FE_x

- The sensitivity of serum amylase for acute pancreatitis is 90%-98%, while the specificity is only around 70%-75%. The specificity of urine amylase and $FE_{amylase}$ is higher.

- Up to 10% of cases of acute pancreatitis are associated with normal levels of amylase; this finding is most common in people with hypertriglyceridemia-associated acute pancreatitis, since triglycerides competitively interfere with the amylase assay.

- There are numerous non-pancreatic causes of hyper-amylasemia: diabetic ketoacidosis, peptic ulcer disease, acute cholecystitis, ectopic pregnancy, salpingitis, bowel ischemia, intestinal obstruction, macroamylasemia, and renal insufficiency. Amylase may also be raised somewhat by the administration of opioid analgesics, due presumably to contracture of the sphincter of Oddi. In all of these instances, the degree of elevation tends to be lower than that seen in acute pancreatitis, but with substantial overlap: pancreatitis causes amylase in the range of 250-1000 Somogyi units; other conditions, 200-500.

- Macroamylasemia has an incidence of about 1%. It is an acquired condition in which apparently healthy individuals have markedly elevated serum amylase (low urine amylase) due to Ig-amylase complexes.

Lipase

- Unlike amylase, lipase is essentially specific for the pancreas.

- Its rise parallels that of amylase, but it remains elevated for up to 14 days.

- It is less reliant on renal clearance than amylase, requiring greater renal impairment to produce a false positive.

- For these reasons it is often considered superior to amylase in the diagnosis of acute pancreatitis.

Laboratory Evaluation of Acute Pancreatitis

- **Confirming acute pancreatitis.** Amylase has limited sensitivity and specificity, for the reasons described above. In particular, it is important to recall that hypertriglyceridemia, one of the more common causes of acute pancreatitis, competitively interferes with the amylase assay. Moreover, there are numerous causes of an elevated serum amylase, including other intra-abdominal inflammatory conditions (eg, bowel infarction, salpingitis), salivary gland pathology, renal insufficiency, and macroamylasemia. At the often-applied cut-off of 3 X the upper limit of normal, the specificity is 95%, and the sensitivity is 60-80%. Lipase remains elevated for longer than amylase (up to 14 days), giving greater sensitivity in patients with a delayed presentation. Like amylase, lipase may be elevated in other intra-abdominal diseases and in renal insufficiency, but hypertriglyceridemia does not interfere with lipase measurement. At a cut-off activity of 600 IU/L, specificity is 95% and sensitivity between 55% and 100%. Other markers of acute pancreatitis include the serum and urinary trypsinogen-2 and elastase-1. While not at the moment widely available, these have shown excellent performance, and a negative urinary trypsinogen-2 has a negative predictive value of 99%.

T1.5
Ranson Criteria

Criterion	Value	At
Age	>55 yrs	Admission
WBC Count	>16 × 10^9/L	Admission
Glucose	>11 mmol/L	Admission
AST	>250 U/L	Admission
LDH	>350 U/L	Admission
Urea	>1.8 mmol/L increase	48 hours
Calcium	<2 mmol/L	48 hours
PaO$_2$	<60 mmHg	48 hours
Base deficit	>4	48 hours
Fluid sequestration	>6 L	48 hours
Hematocrit	>10 decrease	48 hours

- **Prognosis.** Aggressive management—ICU admission, parenteral feeding, and systemic antibiotics—is undertaken in those patients felt to be at risk for fulminant pancreatitis and death. To help identify patients at risk for this outome, several indices have been developed. For example, the Ranson criteria T1.5 provide a specificity of 90%; however these criteria predict severe disease in only 50% of those who subsequently develop it. Furthermore, a Ranson score cannot be assigned until 48 hours after admission. Despite these limitations, better laboratory markers of disease severity have not been identified. Serum amylase and lipase levels are poor predictors of severity.

- **Etiology.** Detecting stone disease early is clinically important, since ERCP can significantly improve outcome. An ultrasound has only 50% sensitivity. An ALT >150 IU/L has a specificity of >95% for gallstone pancreatitis, but the sensitivity is only about 50%. A lipase:amylase ratio >5 is suggestive of alcohol-induced pancreatitis, but has a sensitivity of only 50%. Tests for additional causes of acute pancreatitis include triglycerides, serum calcium, paired viral serology titers (mumps, coxsackievirus, cytomegalovirus, varicella zoster virus, herpes simplex virus, hepatitis B viruses, and HIV). Inherited diseases may underlie a small but significant minority of cases, particularly when there is a history of recurrent episodes of pancreatitis beginning in childhood. Mutations in cationic trypsinogen (*PRSS-1*), pancreatic secretory trypsin inhibitor (*PSTI*), and cystic fibrosis transmembrane conductance regulator (*CFTR*) have been identified in some patients with familial recurrent acute pancreatitis.

Tests of pancreatic exocrine function include the secretin-cholecystokinin (secretin-CCK, secretin-pancreozymin) test, fecal elastase-1, and fecal fat.

- In the secretin-CCK test, an endoscope is introduced and the duodenal concentrations of pancreatic exocrine products (bicarbonate, amylase, lipase, trypsin) are measured after the intravenous administration of secretin and CCK.

- Non-invasive 'tubeless' tests include fecal fat, fecal chymotrypsin (bentiromide), and fecal elastase-1. Fecal fat tests include a fecal oil-red-O stain and 72-hour fecal fat quantitation. The direct stain has a sensitivity of only about 70%. The latter, obviously somewhat cumbersome, test is considered quite ensitive for pancreatic insufficiency. Severe ileal diseases (eg, Crohn disease) or ileal resection can also produce a positive fecal fat test. The sensitivity and specificity of elastase-1 appears superior to that of chymotrypsin. Note that the D-xylose test is a measure of small bowel mucosal absorptive capacity and not a test of pancreatic exocrine function.

Laboratory evaluation of pancreatic cysts T1.6

Myocardial Enzymes and Other Markers of Myocardial Injury

Creatine kinase (CK)

- CK has three isoenzymes distinguishable by electrophoresis: CK-MM, CK-MB, CK-BB. The fastest migrating is BB (CK1), followed by MB (CK2), then MM (CK3) F1.2.

  □ CK-BB (CK1) is found primarily in the **brain,** with lesser amounts in bladder, stomach, and prostate. Of the three, it is the most widely distributed, nearly all tissues in the body having some percentage of their CK comprised of BB. It is the fastest migrating CK on electrophoresis.

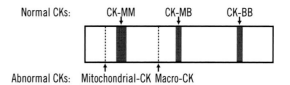

F1.2 Creatine phosphokinase electrophoresis

T1.6

Pancreatic Cyst Evaluation

Cyst Type	Clinical Findings	Cyst Aspirate	
		Cytology	Chemistry
Pseudocyst	Associated with pancreatitis, ovoid unilocular lesion with thick wall adjacent to pancreas	Amorphous material, inflammatory cells; no epithelium	↑ Amylase ↓ CEA ↑ CA 19-9
Serous cystadenoma	Elderly female, microcystic lesion within pancreas	Bland cuboidal epithelial cells	↓ Amylase ↓ CEA ↓ CA 19-9
Mucinous cystadenoma (mucinous cystic neoplasm)	Middle-aged female, macrocystic lesion within pancreas	Bland mucinous epithelial cells	↓ Amylase ↑ CEA nl-↑CA 19-9
Intraductal papillary mucinous tumor	Elderly male or female, variable appearance, dilated duct	Bland to atypical mucinous epithelial cells	↑ Amylase ↑ CEA nl-↑CA 19-9
Solid-cystic (solid-pseudopapillary tumor)	Adult female, solid and cystic lesion	Bland, neuroendocrine-like cells, myxoid stroma	↓ Amylase ↓ CEA ↓ CA 19-9

□ CK-MM (CK3) is found in skeletal and cardiac muscle. Skeletal muscle is about 99% MM, cardiac about 70% MM. In normal subjects serum CK is composed of about 100% MM isoenzyme, mostly from skeletal muscle. MM is the slowest migrating fraction.

□ CK-MB (CK2) is found in cardiac and skeletal muscle. Cardiac muscle is about 30% MB, skeletal about 1% MB. Skeletal muscle is the source of nearly all MB circulating in the serum of normal individuals. MB migrates between MM and BB on electrophoresis.

■ Although electrophoresis is the traditional means to detect CK-MB, immunoassays (CK-MB 'mass assay') are now widely used for this purpose. Immunoassays provide much faster results and better accuracy, particularly in the low (clinical decision-making) range. Total CK is usually measured by an enzymatic assay. The ratio of CK-MB to total CK (the 'relative index') adds to the ability of either assay alone to distinguish myocardial infarction. A relative index of about 2% is often the chosen cut-off. Some types of CK-MB immunoassays—immunoinhibition assays—are susceptible to falsely elevated CK-MB due to hemolysis, the presence of CK-BB (in stroke), and macro-CK.

■ Abnormal CK types

□ **Macro-CK** is a CK-Ig complex. On electrophoresis, it migrates between MM and MB. It is found in completely healthy elderly women.

□ **Mitochondrial CK** migrates very close to MM, usually slower than MM. It is seen in patients with advanced, often disseminated, malignancies and is associated with a poor prognosis.

■ CK isoforms (CK subforms) are metabolic breakdown products of CK. In serum, CK released from damaged myocardial cells undergoes enzymatic cleavage. It takes several (>4) hours for cleavage to begin. With the advent of high-resolution electrophoresis, it was found that CK-MB actually resolves into two bands, and CK-MM resolves into 3 bands. The forms initially released from myocardium are CK-MB2 (CK-MB1 being the cleaved type) and CK-MM3 (CKMM1 and 2 being cleavage products). Thus, persons with an elevated ratio of CK-MB2/CK-MB1 or CK-MM3/CK-MM1 are likely to have had a recent enzyme leak. These CKCK

isoform ratios provide about 90-100% sensitivity for AMI when tested within 4-6 hours after onset. They perform comparably with CK-MB. Assays for CK isoforms are not widely available, and published reports do not appear to display significant advantages over CK-MB.

Troponin I

■ Troponins are a group of enzymes consisting of troponin T (TnT), troponin I (TnI) and troponin C (TnC) that are involved in mediating the actin-myosin interactions that result in muscle contraction. While the same gene encodes cardiac and skeletal muscle TnC, separate genes encode TnI and TnT in cardiac and skeletal muscle. Immunoassays can distinguish cardiac troponins (cTnI and cTnT) from skeletal muscle troponins.

■ While a small proportion of cardiac muscle troponin is free in the cytoplasm, the vast majority of it is bound to actin and myosin. Thus, there is both an immediate release of cytoplasmic troponin by infarcted cardiac muscle (within 4-8 hours) and a sustained release of bound troponin over the next 10-14 days.

■ Only cardiac troponin I (cTnI) is currently widely available for use in clinical diagnosis. TnI and TnT are similar in many respects, including their kinetics following myocardial infarction. However, cTnT is marginally less cardio-specific than cTnI, being elevated occasionally in skeletal muscle disease and renal failure. Studies have consistently shown the exceptional cardiospecificity of cTnI. Unlike CK-MB and myoglobin, it is not elevated in skeletal muscle injury or in vigorous exercise. However, it may be elevated in non-ischemic forms of cardiac injury—cardiac contusion, myocarditis—albeit at lower levels.

Myoglobin (Mgb) is the most sensitive of the cardiac markers and is the earliest marker of acute myocardial infarction. For practical purposes, myoglobin should be elevated as soon as an infarcting patient presents to the emergency department. It is, however, the least cardiospecific of the cardiac markers.

Ischemia-modified albumin (IMA)

- Under normal conditions, albumin is capable of rapidly and tightly binding cobalt. This occurs at the protein's N-terminus. This amino-terminal binding site is altered when albumin circulates through microenvironments with conditions—such as acidosis, hypoxemia, free radicals, altered calcium—that occur during ischemia. The altered form of albumin has reduced cobalt-binding capacity.

- In the Altered Cobalt Binding (ACB) assay, a measured quantity of cobalt is added to patient plasma, and the amount of unbound cobalt is measured. The quantity of unbound cobalt is a measure of so-called ischemia-modified albumin (IMA).

- Ischemia-modified albumin rises within minutes of myocardial ischemia and returns to baseline within 6 hours due to rapid hepatic clearance. It thus shows promise as a marker of transient ischemia.

Unbound free fatty acid (u-FFA) is elevated in reversible and irreversible cardiac ischemia, usually very early.

B-type natriuretic peptide (BNP)

- Natriuretic peptides cause vasodilation and natriuresis (sodium excretion in urine). There are three types of natriuretic peptide:

  - Atrial (A-type) natriuretic peptide (ANP) is stored in granules within atrial myocytes. It is affected by both atrial filling pressure and ventricular wall tension.

  - Brain (B-type) natriuretic peptide (BNP) is synthesized within ventricular myocytes. It correlates directly with ventricular wall tension. It is usually rapidly degraded following production. The N-terminal peptide fragment (N-terminal pro-BNP), which is cleaved from pro-BNP to make the active hormone BNP, is more stable and provides more longitudinal information.

  - C-type natriuretic peptide (CNP). Much less is known about this peptide.

- Plasma natriuretic peptide levels are elevated in patients with heart failure. The BNP appears to correlate most responsively with recent changes in fluid status.

- BNP has been shown to be useful in distinguishing cardiac from noncardiac causes of dyspnea. BNP has proven to be excellent marker for congestive heart failure (CHF).

- BNP provides prognostic information in patients with congestive heart failure and in patients with acute coronary syndromes.

Acute Coronary Syndrome (ACS)

- ACS is a term that is meant to encompass several clinical situations having myocardial ischemia in common: stable angina, unstable angina, acute myocardial infarction (AMI), and sudden cardiac death (SCD). While laboratory assays are very good at diagnosing acute myocardial infarction, they are quite poor, overall, in the diagnosis of other acute coronary syndromes.

- Non-acute myocardial infarction acute coronary syndromes (non-AMI ACS) include angina, unstable angina, ventricular arrhythmia, and other manifestations of transient ischemia without infarction. *Unstable angina* is perhaps the most difficult of these to conceptualize. Broadly defined, it refers to angina whose pattern is changing within an affected patient; thus, this refers to new-onset angina, worsening angina, angina refractory to previously effective treatment, or angina at rest. Unstable angina has long been thought to herald a major cardiac event and has been called pre-infarction angina, crescendo angina, and pre-occlusive syndrome. A particular episode of unstable angina may be very difficult to distinguish from an acute myocardial infarction, and the term is often applied retrospectively to a presentation in which acute myocardial infarction has been ruled-out. The anatomic basis for unstable angina is thought to be an unstable plaque; that is, a plaque complicated by rupture, super-imposed thrombus, or vasospasm. Vasospasm is particularly implicated in so-called variant (Prinzmetal) angina. To date, there has not been much progress in finding biochemical markers of transient myocardial ischemia. The usual markers of myocardial necrosis, such as CK-MB, myoglobin, and troponin, are overall poor markers of non-AMI ACS.

  - Troponins. Elevated troponins in non-AMI ACS somewhat blur the boundary with AMI and serve to indicate which patients with non-AMI ACS are in serious danger. In some studies, up to a third of those diagnosed with unstable angina have elevation in troponin, and mortality in these patients approaches that of traditionally-defined AMI. Additional studies suggest that the likelihood of progression to clear-cut AMI and the mortality in these patients (those with non-AMI ACS having elevated troponin) can, like AMI, be reduced with aggressive intervention.

  - CK-MB and myoglobin have little or no demonstrated role in the diagnosis of non-AMI ACS.

  - BNP in non-AMI ACS is predictive of both recurrence and a higher likelihood of sudden cardiac death.

  - C-reactive protein (CRP) and high-sensitivity CRP (hsCRP) appear to be strong predictors for the development of ACS in healthy individuals, and to predict short-term prognosis following non-AMI ACS. HS-CRP values >10 mg/L within 6-24 hours after symptom onset indicates an increased risk for recurrent cardiac events within 30 days to 1 year. Further, in patients with unstable angina, HS-CRP values >10 mg/L may predict a higher rate of myocardial infarction or mortality than in patients with HS-CRP <10 mg/L.

 □ Ischemia-modified albumin (IMA) has been shown to be a sensitive marker of transient ischemia induced artificially in the setting of percutaneous transluminal coronary angioplasty (PTCA).

■ *Acute myocardial infarction.* The current definition of acute myocardial infarction is as follows: a typical rise and fall of the CK-MB or troponin with ischemic symptoms, ECG changes, or interventionally demonstrated coronary artery abnormality.

 □ **Troponins.** A single positive troponin is highly specific for AMI. A single negative troponin has unacceptably low sensitivity, however. Serial measurements markedly improve the sensitivity of troponin for AMI; the sensitivity of a single troponin test at 4 hours after onset of symptoms is about 50%, a single test at 6 hours has sensitivity of about 75%, and two tests at 6 and 12 hours have a combined sensitivity of approaching 100%. However, for patients presenting several days after onset of symptoms, a single negative troponin can be expected to exclude AMI. This is because cTnI remains elevated for up to 2 weeks following acute myocardial infarction. On the other hand, the cTnI is not useful to determine where the patient is, temporally, with respect to their MI. Whenever a patient has elevated cTnI, therefore, it is still important to measure serial CK-MBs to determine:
(1) whether the MB is going up or down; that is, whether the infarct is acute or resolving, and
(2) whether the MB comes down appropriately; that is, whether there is a complication of MI such as extension of the infarct

 □ **CK-MB.** Increased serum CK is detectable within 3-6 hours of an AMI, with a peak at 20 to 24 hours. Assuming there is not ongoing injury, CK returns to normal within 72 hours. Like troponin, the sensitivity of CK increases with serial measurements, eventually approaching 100%. However, the specificity of CK-MB cannot equal that of troponin, and false-positives are possible with non-ischemic cardiac injury (pericarditis, myocarditis) and skeletal muscle disease (rhabdomyolysis, muscular dystrophy, exercise). In certain individuals (little old ladies), total CK will be normal, but the MB fraction elevation permits diagnosis of MI.

 □ Myoglobin is rapidly and consistently released from damaged muscle, providing an early indicator of myocardial necrosis. In the appropriate time-frame, a normal myoglobin can exclude AMI. We cannot, however, currently isolate myocardial myoglobin from skeletal muscle myoglobin, and myoglobin may be elevated in non-muscle disease (eg, elevated in renal failure and severe systemic illnesses). The negative predictive value of a normal myoglobin at 2 hours following onset of symptoms approaches 100%; however, this gives a great deal of weight to accurate history.

 □ BNP has little utility in the diagnosis of AMI; however, its elevation is very useful to predict the development of post-MI congestive heart failure.

 □ Ischemia-modified albumin (IMA) has a sensitivity of 83%, specificity of 69%, negative predictive value (NPV) of 96%, and a positive predictive value (PPV) of 33% for AMI.

■ **Cardiac reperfusion.** An indication of successful reperfusion following thrombolysis is the so-called washout phenomenon. In successful reperfusion, all of the cardiac markers peak earlier than normal; although, their sequence of peaks parallels that of normal MI. In addition, their peak concentrations may be higher than they would have been with unreperfused MI.

Serum Proteins

Laboratory Methods

Protein quantitation

■ Nitrogen content (the Kjeldahl technique) is the gold standard and involves acid digestion of proteins to release ammonium ions which are then quantified. The assumption made to then calculate protein concentration is that, overall, serum proteins are 16% nitrogen by mass. For various reasons, not the least of which is complexity, this test is not in common usage.

■ Methods that exploit the capacity of solutes to alter light transmitted through a solvent, such as refractometry, suffer from many potential interferences, such as when there is hyperlipidemia, hemoglobinuria, or hyperbilirubinemia.

- Colorimetry (by the Biuret technique) is the recommended routine method for determining total protein. In an alkaline medium copper salts form a purple complex with proteins. The absorbance of the resulting chelate at 540 nm is proportional to total protein concentration.

- Colorimetry (using copper salts in an acid medium instead of the alkaline medium of the Biuret method) can also be used to specifically measure globulins. Albumin can then be calculated by subtracting globulins from the total protein.

- Dye binding techniques (Folin-Ciocalteu, Coomassie brilliant blue, bromcresol green (BCG), purple (BCP) or blue (BCB)) have been applied to the measurement of total protein, particularly for urine and CSF. These techniques suffer from selectivity for some proteins over others. This limitation is capitalized upon, however, for the selective measurement of albumin in serum.

- Spectrophotometry. Proteins absorb ultraviolet light at peaks of 210 and 280 nm. Absorbance at these wavelengths is proportional to protein content.

Protein separation

- Precipitation (salting out) was once used to separate albumin from globulins. Albumin remains in the supernatant and can be measured by any of the above techniques. In addition, precipitation is still used in isolating a single minor protein of interest. Lastly, precipitation is needed to quantify protein in such low-protein fluids as urine and cerebrospinal fluid. In urine, trichloroacetic acid (TCA) is used to precipitate proteins.

- Electrophoresis is the movement of proteins due to an electrical potential.

  □ In this technique, a charge is applied across a medium that is composed of a solid support and a fluid buffer. This charge creates an electromotive force.

  □ The solid support has a slight negative charge and is drawn towards the positive pole (anode), but, being a solid support, it cannot move. There is instead a compensatory flow of the fluid buffer towards the negative pole (cathode). This buffer flow is called endosmosis and has the capacity to carry with it substances suspended within the medium.

  □ If proteins are added to the medium and the charge is applied, two forces act on each protein: electromotive and endosmotic. Since most proteins bear a net negative charge, electromotive force tends to pull them towards the anode (positive pole); whereas, endosmosis pulls them towards the cathode. In the case of gamma globulins, which have a weak net negative charge, the endosmotic force displaces the proteins towards the cathode.
  In the case of most other proteins, the electromotive force exceeds the endosmotic force, and they move to variable extents towards the anode.

- □ Serum protein electrophoresis (SPEP): When electrophoresis is carried out on serum at pH 8.6 on an agarose gel, fixed, and stained, five distinct bands can be seen. The fastest moving band is albumin, followed by the two α bands (α_1 and α_2), the β band, and finally the γ band. The γ band consists of proteins that move very slowly or actually move towards the cathode.

- □ Through manipulations in the gel, buffer, etc, proteins can be resolved into several more bands F1.3. Use of such high-resolution protein electrophoresis is the current standard of practice.

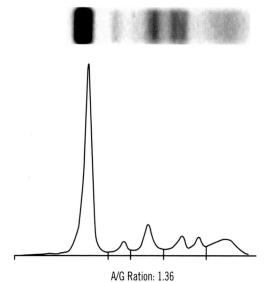

A/G Ration: 1.36
T.P.: 6.6

Fractions	%	Ref. %	g/dL	Ref. g/dL
Albumin	57.6	52.9-66.9	3.8	3.7-4.9
Alpha 1	4.5	3.0-5.8	0.3	0.2-0.4
Alpha 2	12.0	7.5-13.4	0.8	0.5-0.9
Beta	13.4	8.5-13.7	0.9	0.6-1.0
Gamma	12.5	8.8-19.2	0.8	0.6-1.4

F1.3 Normal high-resolution serum protein electrophoresis (HR-SPFP)

▫ Increasing the endosmosis is used to separate gamma globulins into oligoclonal bands in CSF electrophoresis.

▫ Capillary electrophoresis is similar in many respects to gel electrophoresis. Instead of occurring in a gel that contains buffer, however, capillary electrophoresis occurs in a narrow-bore capillary tube that contains buffer. The sample is introduced by immersing the end of the capillary tube into the sample. Voltage is applied, and depending upon molecular size and charge molecules elute from the tube at various times. Rather than staining the gel, absorbance measurements note the elution time and quantity of the different protein fractions. The tracings produced, however, are similar to those seen with high-resolution gel electrophoresis. A form of this technique known as capillary zone electrophoresis (CZE) has supplanted gel elec-trophoresis in some labs. The advantages include small sample size, the ability to automate the procedure, and speed. In addition, CZE appears to be slightly more sensitive than high-resolution gel electrophoresis for the detection of M proteins.

Immunofixation and Immunotyping

■ Immunofixation electrophoresis (IFE), immunotyping, and immunoelectrophoresis (IEP) are methods for characterizing a suspected monoclonal band observed on SPEP or UPEP.

■ IEP **F1.4** is not commonly used any more. The procedure is performed by first placing patient serum in every other of a series of wells that are arranged alongside troughs in an agarose gel. In the remaining wells is placed an aliquot of normal serum. The gel is then subjected to electrophoresis. After electrophoresis, antiserum is added to each trough. After a period of time, precipitation arcs form between the antisera in the troughs and the electrophoresed proteins in the gel. Interpretation depends on visual comparison of the arcs formed with patient serum and the arcs formed with normal serum. The arcs should be symmetrical and in the same location (mirror images).

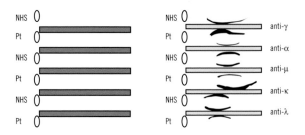

F1.4 Immunoelectrophoresis. On the left are uninoculated wells. On the right is a gel following electrophoresis, diffusion, fixation, and staining. It demonstrates an IgG κ monoclonal protein.

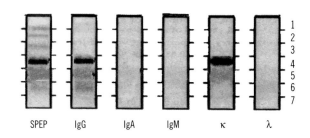

F1.5 Immunofixation electrophoresis (IFE). This study demonstrates an IgG κ monoclonal protein.

■ IFE **F1.5** is much simpler to interpret than IEP. The procedure involves placing patient serum into each of six wells in an agarose gel. The gel is then subjected to electrophoresis. Finally, five different monospecific antisera are applied to the gel: anti-IgG, IgA, IgM, κ, and λ. The entire gel is then stained. Interpretation is relatively straightforward.

■ Immunotyping (IT, immunosubtraction) **F1.6** is often used in conjunction with capillary electrophoresis to identify the M protein. The serum sample is incubated with different solid-phase sepharose beads attached to antibodies against γ, α, μ, κ, or λ. After incubation, the supernatants are subjected to electrophoresis to deter-mine which reagents removed the abnormal spike.

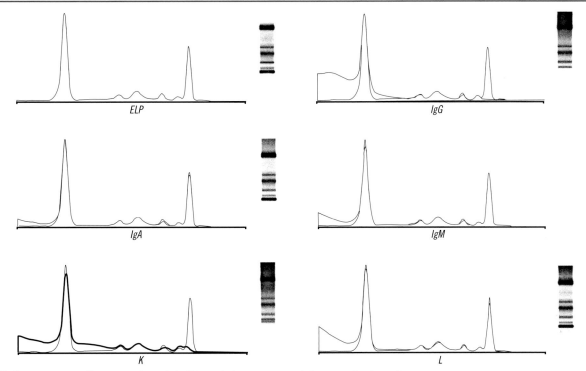

F1.6 Immunotyping (IT, immunosubtraction). This study demonstrates an IgG κ monoclonal protein.

Major Serum Proteins (T1.7)

Albumin is the most abundant protein in human plasma, constituting about 2/3 of total plasma protein. Albumin has many functions, one of which results from its abundance and relates to maintaining serum osmotic pressure. It also functions to carry multiple substances. α-fetoprotein is the albumin equivalent in fetal blood (if present in serum, however, it migrates in α₁). Interestingly, the congenital absence of albumin (analbuminemia) is not a serious problem, only resulting in mild edema and hyperlipidemia. There are several allotypes of albumin, the most common of which is Albumin A. When a variant allotype is present, it may electrophorese at a slightly different rate than albumin A, leading to bisalbuminemia, a benign condition in which two peaks are seen in the albumin band. Albumin's clinical utility resides in the assessment of nutritional status, hepatic synthetic function, and diabetic control. In assessing nutritional status, it is important to know that the half-life of albumin is 17 days. Hepatic synthetic function is somewhat poorly reflected in the albumin, since only in end-stage liver disease is serum albumin noticeably decreased. In fact, the greatest decrements in serum albumin are seen in protein-losing conditions such as protein-losing enteropathy and nephrotic syndrome. In non-diabetic individuals, up to 8% of albumin is normally glycosylated nonenzymatically in the serum; whereas, in diabetics with poor control, up to 25% becomes glycosylated. Albumin is a negative acute phase reactant **T1.8**; that is, in inflammatory conditions, albumin decreases.

Prealbumin is the fastest migrating protein on SPEP. Due to its sparseness, however, it is not normally seen on traditional SPEP and seen only faintly on high-resolution SPEP. It has two main functions: it binds T4 and T3 (hence it is also called transthyretin [TTR] and thyroxine-binding prealbumin [TBPA]), and it binds and carries the retinol-binding protein:vitamin A complex. There is a rare variant prealbumin whose very high affinity for thyroxine leads to elevated total T4 in a euthyroid individual. In addition, prealbumin (transthyretin) is the amyloid precursor protein in senile cardiac amyloidosis, and mutant versions of transthyretin are responsible for familial forms of amyloidosis (eg, familial amyloid polyneuropathy). Its clinical utility resides mainly in the assessment of nutritional

T1.7
High Resolution Serum Protein Electrophoresis

Band	Major Constituent(s)	Notes
Pre-albumin	Prealbumin	Excellent indicator of nutritional status binds thyroid hormones Binds retinol-binding protein Negative acute phase reactant
Albumin	Albumin	Good Indicatior of nutritional status Binds numerous substances Maintains serum oncotic pressure Negative acute phase reactant
Albumin-α_1 interface	α_1-lipoprotein	Constituent of HDL
α_1	$\alpha_{1\text{-antitrypsin}}$	Positive acute phase reactant α_1 antitrypsin deficiency detectable with SPEP
α_1-α_2	Gc globulins α_1 antichymotrypsin	Gc globulin binds vitamin D
α_2	$\alpha_{2\text{-macroglobulin}}$	α_2-macroglobulin relatively elevated in nephrotic syndrome
	haptoglobin	Haptoglobin is a positive acute phase reactant
	ceruloplasmin	Ceruloplasmin binds copper. Low ceruloplasmin not detectable with SPEP
α_2-β interface	Usually empty	Hemoglobin, usually absent from serum, may be present here when there is a hemolysis—a possible pseudo-M-spike
β_1	Transferrin	Transferrin may be high in iron deficiency-a possible pseudo-M-spike
β_1.β_2 interface	β-lipoprotein	Constituent of LDL
β_2	IgA CRP Complements	Fibrinogen, usually absent from serum, may be present here when there is incomplete clotting-a possible pseudo-M-spike
γ_1	γ globulins	Positive acute phase reactants
γ_2	CRP	Positive acute phase reactant

status. In this regard, its short half life of 48 hours makes it particularly useful. Prealbumin crosses the blood-brain barrier and is actively secreted into the cerebrospinal fluid (CSF) by the choroid plexus. Thus, it is a relatively prominent component of CSF protein and a sharp prealbumin band is a hallmark of CSF protein electrophoresis. In heparinized patients, a prominent "prealbumin" band, resulting from an alteration in β-lipoprotein such that it migrates in the prealbumin range, is often seen. True elevations in prealbumin are seen in chronic alcoholics and in corticosteroid therapy. Like albumin, prealbumin is a negative acute phase reactant.

α₁-antitrypsin (AAT) is the major component of the α_1 band. Its main function is to inactivate various proteases such as trypsin and elastase. The SPEP can be used to screen for AAT deficiency, in which the serum will display a markedly diminished α_1 band. AAT is a markedly positive acute phase reactant.

α₁-acid glycoprotein (orosomucoid), also a briskly positive acute phase reactant, is a minor component of the

T1.8
Acute Phase Reactants (APR)

	Protein	Acute Inflammation	Chronic Inflammation
	Pre-Albumin	↓	↓
	Albumin	↓	↓
α_1	α-acid glycoprotein	↑	↑
	α-AT	↑	↑
α_2	Haptoglobin	↑	↑
	Ceruloplasmin	↑	↑
β	Complement (C_3)	↑	↑
	Transferrin	↓	↑
	Fibrinogen	↑	↑
γ	Ig	→↓	↑
	CRP	↑	↑

α_1 band normally but a major component of the increased α_1 band seen in acute inflammation. It may have a useful role in monitoring the activity of chronic inflammatory conditions such as ulcerative colitis.

α_2-macroglobulin is a protease inhibitor whose serum concentration is elevated in liver and renal disease. In particular, its large size prevents its loss in nephrotic syndrome, leading to a relative 10-fold rise in concentration.

Ceruloplasmin, another α_2 protein, functions in copper transport. Although a decreased serum ceruloplasmin is an important marker for Wilson disease, the differential diagnosis of a decreased serum ceruloplasmin also includes: hepatic failure, malnutrition, and Menke syndrome. A falsely normal or elevated ceruloplasmin may be seen in inflammatory states, because ceruloplasmin is an acute phase reactant, and pregnancy.

Haptoglobin is the third major component of the α_2 band. It is a protein that binds free hemoglobin; hence, it is found to be markedly decreased or absent in acute intravascular hemolysis. Since only tiny amounts of free hemoglobin are necessary to deplete the serum of haptoglobin, it is a very sensitive marker of hemolysis. It does not, however, bind myoglobin so that the serum haptoglobin is a useful analyte in discerning the cause of a positive urine dipstick for hemoglobin. There are several haptoglobin allotypes, relating to two main haptoglobin

alleles: type 1 and type 2. Based upon these alleles, three haptoglobin phenotypes are possible: 1-1, 1-2, and 2-2. The 2-2 phenotype appears to be an independent risk factor for cardiovascular disease in diabetics. Haptoglobin is an acute phase reactant.

Transferrin is the major β globulin. Its function is to transport ferric (Fe^{3+}) iron, with which it is normally about 30% saturated. There is a marked increase in serum transferrin in iron deficiency, a phenomenon that can produce an abnormal band masquerading as an M-protein. Transferrin is also increased in pregnancy and estrogen therapy. Like gamma globulins, transferrin decreases in the acute phase, but later increases if the inflammatory state persists. The blood-brain barrier transports transferrin into the CSF, but not before modifying a percentage of it to make asialated transferrin (so-called Tau protein), while the rest is unmodified. Thus, a second hallmark of CSF protein electrophoresis is a double transferrin peak. A form of transferrin in serum—carbohydrate-deficient transferrin—may be superior to GGT as a marker for alcohol use.

Fibrinogen is also considered a β globulin with a couple of caveats. Firstly, in the normal course of events there is no fibrinogen in serum, most of it having been consumed in the clot. However, if the specimen clots incompletely (eg, a heparinized patient), then fibrinogen may be seen. Secondly, fibrinogen can straddle the β-γ interface. All of these features may combine to form a pseudo-paraprotein on SPEP. Fibrinogen, when present in serum specimens, may be misinterpreted as an M protein. Fibrinogen may be present in the serum of patients with dysfibrinogenemia, APL syndrome, liver disease, vitamin K deficiency, or heparin. Fibrinogen is visible in the β-γ interface. Absolute ethanol can be used *in vitro* to selectively precipitate fibrinogen and obviate this interference.

C-reactive protein (CRP) is found in the γ region, with the immunoglobulins.

- CRP is produced in the liver. Its name derives from its reaction with Streptococcal capsular (C) polysaccharide. Formerly, assays for CRP had an analytical sensitivity of about 5 mg/L. This was appropriate, as the CRP test was used to support such diagnoses as bacterial endocarditis, appendicitis, active collagen vascular disease, and the like, in which CRP values tended to be well over 10 mg/L.

- However, attention has recently been turned to the apparent predictive value of low-level CRP elevations (> 2-3 mg/L) for cardiac events, and as a result high-sensitivity CRP (hsCRP) assays have become available which have analytical sensitivity of <0.5 mg/L. An exact cut-off for CRP, in the context of cardiovascular risk, is difficult to determine. About half the population have CRP > 2 mg/L, and about a third have CRP > 3 mg/L. Interestingly, a population distribution of CRP levels is not an evenly-distributed Gaussian curve; instead, it is a curve significantly skewed, with a dense cluster in the very lowest CRP levels and a long tail extending into the >10 range.

- Thus, there are 3 categories based upon CRP levels. Normal CRP levels are those less than 3 mg/L. High-level CRP elevations are those over 10 mg/L, usually indicative of active inflammation. Low-level CRP elevations are those between 3 and 10, indicative of cellular stress.

- Low-level CRP elevation may indicate a wide array of minor disease states, genetic factors, demographic variables, and behavioral patterns. CRP levels are mildly elevated in a fraction of unselected normal individuals, and an individual's set-point appears to be inherited.

- Low-level CRP elevation is known to predict poor outcome following cardiovascular events, but it has also been shown to correlate with mortality in non-cardiac diseases as well as in apparently healthy individuals. Several reports indicate that CRP is elevated in individuals who soon thereafter sustain coronary and cerebrovascular events. In the Physician's Health Study, men with CRP >2.11 mg/L had 3 times the risk of suffering an acute myocardial infarction as compared with men having CRP <0.55 mg/L.

Patterns in Serum Protein Electrophoresis (F1.7)

Normal serum has a nearly invisible pre-albumin band and a very large albumin band. This is followed by a small peaked α_1 band, an α_2 band, a bimodal β, and broad γ.

Bisalbuminemia is seen in heterozygotes for albumin allotypes. The SPEP shows double albumin spike. This is of no clinical consequence.

α_1-antitrypsin (AAT) deficiency can be diagnosed with SPEP, since AAT is the major component of the α_1 band. Genotypic PiZZ individuals have a visibly and quantitatively decreased band.

Nephrotic syndrome results in massive loss of small serum proteins, particularly albumin. In nephrotic syndrome due to minimal change disease, there is an especially selective loss of albumin (selective proteinuria). In other forms of nephrotic syndrome, nearly all proteins are lost, including gamma globulins. However, in all types of nephrotic syndrome, larger protein molecules are retained. The result is dimming of all the electrophoretic bands, most prominently the albumin band, with the conspicuous exception of the α_2 band which contains the large protein α_2-macroglobulin.

In ***acute inflammation***, the acute phase reactants account for an increase in the α_1 and α_2 bands. Albumin is slightly decreased. Initially, the gamma globulins are unchanged, but with prolonged inflammation, these are polyclonally increased.

β-γ bridging is the hallmark of cirrhosis. Additional features include hypoalbuminemia and blunted α_1 and α_2 bands. β-γ bridging is mainly attributed to increased serum IgA.

Serum Proteins>Patterns in Serum Protein Electrophoresis

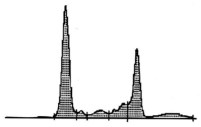
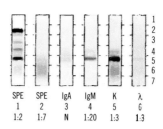

F1.7A IgM κ M-protein. Note that IgM paraproteins tend to migrate near the β-γ interface

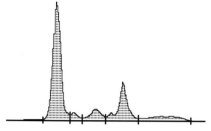
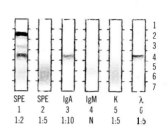

F1.7B IgM λ M-protein. Note that IgA paraproteins tend to migrate into the β region

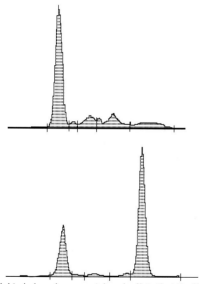
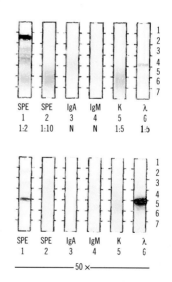

F1.7C λ light chain-only paraproteinemia. Note that the M-protein is essentially undetectable on the SPEP (upper left). It is quite prominent in the UPEP (lower left). It is confirmed in the serum IFE (upper right) and urine IFE (lower right)

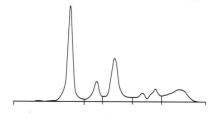

| | | | A/G Ratio: 0.62 | | |
| | | | TP: 6.5 | | |
Fractions	%	Ref %	g/dL	Ref g/dL	
Albumin	38.1	52.9-66.9	2.5 L	3.7-4.9
Alpha 1	9.9	3.9-5.8	0.6 H	0.2-0.4
Alpha 2	25.4	7.5-13.4	1.7 H	0.5-0.9
Beta	11.6	8.5-13.7	0.8	0.6-1.0
Gamma	15.0	8.8-19.2	1.0	0.6-1.4

F1.7C λ Acute inflammation pattern

Monoclonal gammopathy

- The SPEP shows a prominent, discrete, dark band (M-spike) usually within the gamma region but sometimes in β or α_2. A monoclonal gammopathy (paraproteinemia) is a condition in which there is an immunochemically homogeneous immunoglobulin (M protein) in the serum. This may be the result of several types of neoplastic proliferations in addition to multiple myeloma, including solitary plasmacytoma, MGUS, Waldenströms macroglobulinemia (lymphoplasmacytic lymphoma), and CLL/SLL.

- Biclonal gammopathy (two M-proteins) occurs in 3-4% of cases. When what appears to be a biclonal gammopathy turns out to be composed of IgA spikes having a single light chain, this is most likely due to the appearance of both monomers and dimers in the SPEP and should be considered monoclonal rather than biclonal.

- About 10% of patients with myeloma have an SPEP showing only hypogammaglobulinemia. Hypogammaglobulinemia, when not due to myeloma, may be due to congenital hypogammaglobulinemias, lymphoma, nephrotic syndrome, and corticosteroid treatment. Patients with myeloma whose SPEP shows only hypogammaglobulinemia are likely to have free light chains (Bence-Jones protein) in their urine.

- Immunofixation or immunosubtraction is indicated to characterize the M-protein. Even when an M-spike is not evident on SPEP, an immunofixation may be indicated if (a) there is a strong clinical suspicion of myeloma, (b) there is systemic AL amyloidosis, or (c) there is hypogammaglobulinemia. In patients with negative serum screens in whom the clinical suspicion is high, the urine should be screened by electrophoresis and immunofixation.

- An M protein is usually an intact immunoglobulin, composed of 2 heavy and 2 light chains. Sometimes it is composed of a light chain only and (rarely) a heavy chain only.

- Systemic AL amyloidosis is a condition that may result from a monoclonal gammopathy, when the M protein produced has unusual (amyloidogenic) properties.

- After making the diagnosis, the protein electrophoresis is used to follow disease progression and the efficacy of treatment. Three quantitative immunochemical results are important in disease monitoring. The M-protein quantity, routinely carried out by nephelometry (or turbidimetry), is important to classify the disease (see criteria for multiple myeloma) and to follow the disease. Secondly, it is important to quantify the other major immunoglobulin classes—IgG, IgA, and IgM—to determine the degree to which they are suppressed. Lastly, the quantity of serum free light chains is important in monitoring the disease. The serum free light chain assay can be used especially to follow those with light chain-only myelomas; furthermore, the free light chain assay finds abnormalities in the κ:λ ratio in the majority of patients previously classified as non-secretory. The free light chain assay is extremely sensitive to myeloma recurrence after treatment.

- Serum viscosity is normally in the range of 1.5 to 1.8 centipoise (cp). Hyperviscosity syndrome may develop when serum viscosity exceeds 3 cp. Hyperviscosity syndrome may present with nasal bleeding, blurred vision, retinal veins dilation (with flame-shaped retinal hemorrhages) and neurologic symptoms (headache, vertigo, nystagmus, tinnitus, hearing loss, ataxia, and diplopia). Serum viscosity should be measured when an IgM M-protein exceeds 4 g/dL or an IgA or IgG exceeds 6 g/dL.

- Cryoglobulins should be looked for in patients with M-proteins.

CSF Protein Electrophoresis (F1.8)

Electrophoresis of normal CSF appears distinctly different from serum. The CSF normally contains essentially all the proteins present in serum, although in smaller quantities. The most characteristic features of the normal CSF electrophoresis are: a prominent pre-albumin band and a double beta (transferrin) band; additional subtler features are a dim albumin and α_2 band.

The main purpose of CSF electrophoresis is to support a diagnosis of multiple sclerosis by finding oligoclonal bands—several distinct bands in the gamma region reflective of several clonal immunoglobulins. These bands should be absent from the patient's serum, run concurrently, to be specific.

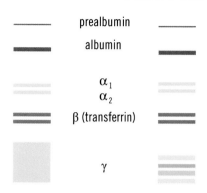

prealbumin

albumin

α_1
α_2

β (transferrin)

γ

F1.8 CSF protein electrophoresis. Left shows a normal pattern. Right shows oligoclonal bands

	1	2a	2b	2c
albumin				
α_1				
α_2				
β (transferrin)				
γ				

F1.9 Urine protein electrophoresis. 1 normal, 2a glomerular protein-uria, 2b tubular proteinuria, 2c overflow proteinuria

Urine Protein Electrophoresis (UPEP; F1.9)

The urine of a normal person contains little protein.

In **proteinuria**, the UPEP can be used to determine the source of the protein. In tubular proteinuria, tubuloint-erstitial nephritis or acute tubular necrosis is implied, while in glomerular proteinuria glomerulonephritis is usually responsible. In overflow proteinuria, a serum protein that is present in excess overwhelms the kidneys and overflows into the urine.

- **Glomerular proteinuria pattern.** The urine contains strong albumin, α_1 and β bands. Very large proteins, due to the persistence of some filtering function, and very small proteins due to tubular reabsorption, do not make their way into the urine. This leaves the proteins in between these, most notably albumin, AAT, and transferrin.

- **Tubular proteinuria pattern.** The urine contains a weak albumin band, and strong α_1 and β bands. This pattern results form the impaired tubular reabsorption of low molecular weight proteins normally filtered freely by the glomerulus such as α_2-macroglobulin, β_2-microglobulin, and light chains.

- **Overflow proteinuria pattern.** Most commonly this is a monoclonal light chain (Bence Jones proteinuria). Other possibilities include myoglobin & hemoglobin.

Cryoglobulinemia

Cryoglobulins are immunoglobulins that precipitate reversibly at low temperatures.

To detect cryoglobulins, blood is drawn and kept at 37° C until clotted, then centrifuged at 37° C. The remaining serum is stored at 4° C for at least 3 days, then centrifuged at 4° C. Any precipitate that forms is a cryoprecipitate. This can be subjected to electrophoresis for characterization.

Three types of cryoglobulins are recognized: type I and the mixed types, II & III.

- Type I: monoclonal immunoglobulins associated with multiple myeloma or Waldenström macroglobulinemia.

- Type II: a mixture of a monoclonal IgM and a polyclonal IgG. The IgM has rheumatoid factor activity (anti-IgG). This is the most common type of cryoglobulin.

- Type III: a mixture of two polyclonal immunoglobulins.

23

Mixed cryoglobulinemia (types II & III)

- **Etiology.** Mixed cryoglobulins can be found in the serum of individuals with a variety of clinical conditions, including lymphoproliferative disorders, chronic infections, chronic liver diseases, and autoimmune diseases (especially SLE). It is most common in women in the 4th and 5th decades. In the past, about 30-50% of cases, were associated with no underlying disorder (essential mixed cryoglobulinemia). With the advent of testing for hepatitis C virus, it was found that most of these had underlying hepatitis C virus infection. Currently, HCV is the most common cause of mixed cryoglobulinemia.

- **Clinical manifestations.** Cryoglobulinemia is a systemic immune complex disease characterized by a distinctive clinical syndrome of palpable purpura (leukocytoclastic vasculitis), arthralgias, hepatosplenomegaly, lymphadenopathy, anemia, sensorineural deficits, and glomerulonephritis. Purpura is a constant feature, usually distributed over the lower extremities. Most patients are variably hypocomplementemic, reflecting the immune complex nature of the disease. Renal involvement trails by 4-5 years, manifests as either nephrotic or nephritic syndrome, and is associated with severe hypocomplementemia. In renal biopsies, the most common finding is membranoproliferative glomerulonephritis (MPGN) type II. In some cases, usually when acute, the deposits produce the appearance of thrombotic microangiopathy. In all tissues, as in the kidney, the basic pathologic lesion is vasculitis. Electron microscopy demonstrates large subendothelial immune complex deposits with a fibrillary or tubular structure in a finger-print like pattern.

- **Treatment.** The treatment for mixed cryoglobulinemia consists of attempts at immune-modulation using corticosteroids, plasmapheresis, and α-interferon (in patients with HCV). Remissions are achieved in around 75% of patients, but 50% relapse.

Acid-Base & Electrolytes

Sodium

Hyponatremia

- Hyponatremia is defined as serum sodium <135 mmol/L. Hyponatremia is considered severe when <120 mmol/L.

- One caveat with regard to the differential diagnosis: a misdiagnosis of SIADH may be made in the presence of recent diuretic use when there is a brief reflex water retention. The diagnosis of SIADH should be made only when hyponatremia exists prima facie, with a urine sodium >20 mmol/L, euvolemia, normal renal function, no recent use of diuretics, and normal adrenal function.

- Too rapid correction can induce central pontine myelinolysis (CPM), while too slow correction can lead to cerebral edema.

- Differential diagnosis

  □ Pseudohyponatremia (serum osmolarity >280) may result from hyperglycemia, hyperlipidemia, hyperproteinemia

  □ True hyponatremia

    • Patient is hypovolemic

      ○ Renal losses (U_{na}>30 mmol/L): diuretics, medullary renal disease, Addison, RTA type I

      ○ Extrarenal loss (U_{na}<30): GI losses, third spacing

    • Patient is euvolemic: SIADH, psychogenic polydipsia, drugs with ADH-like (vasopressin-like) effect, including desmopressin, SSRIs, and tricyclic antidepressants. The recreational drug ecstasy is also thought to produce hyponatremia by this mechanism

    • Patient is hypervolemic: congestive heart failure, cirrhosis, nephrotic syndrome

Hypernatremia

- Hypernatremia is most commonly seen in an individual with dehydration (due to diarrhea or insensible water losses) and inability to respond to their thirst response: infants, ICU patients, and extremely debilitated adults.

- Differential diagnosis:

  □ Iatrogenic sodium administration: I.V. fluids, sodium bicarbonate, high-dose sodium-bearing antibiotics

  □ Water loss: diabetes insipidus, diabetes mellitus, diarrhea, osmotic diuretics, sweating

Potassium

Hypokalemia

- Differential diagnosis.

  □ GI losses (U_K<30mEq/day): vomiting, nasogastric tube, diarrhea, villous adenoma.

  □ Renal losses (U_K>30mEq/day): diuretics, hypomagnesemia, antibiotics (carbenicillin, amphotericin-B), mineralocorticoid excess, renal tubular acidosis (RTA) types I & II, Cushing syndrome, congenital adrenal hyperplasia, hyperreninism.

  □ Transcellular shifts: alkalosis, correction of diabetic ketoacidosis.

- Notes on hypokalemia: note that in diabetic ketoacidosis, the ketoacidosis is associated with hyperkalemia (like most acidotic states), but correction of DKA results in a profound hypokalemia unless supplemental potassium is given.

Hyperkalemia

- Pseudohyperkalemia is characterized by elevated serum potassium levels in the absence of clinical evidence of hyperkalemia (it is usually a good idea to confirm potassium status with an ECG). In this scenario, no therapy is required, and in fact treatment may be harmful. After blood is collected, potassium may be released from the cellular components of blood. When potassium is released from red cells as a result of *in vitro* hemolysis, the simultaneous release of hemoglobin serves as a visible warning that this has occurred. However, other not-so-visible mechanisms may cause a spurious elevation in potassium. Potassium is released as a result of *in vitro* clot formation, and this effect is more pronounced in patients with thrombocytosis. Passive transmembrane potassium leak from leukocytes may be pronounced, particularly when there is a leukocytosis. A passive transmembrane leak of potassium from red cells, without concomitant hemolysis, has

been associated with an autosomal dominant abnormal gene on chromosome 16 (familial pseudohyperkalemia).

- Differential diagnosis Acidosis, renal failure, potassium-sparing diuretics (spironolactone, triamterine, amiloride), adrenal insufficiency, iatrogenic, rhabdomyolysis.

- Nearly all cases of acidosis are associated with hyperkalemia. The main exception is renal tubular acidosis types I & II in which potassium is low.

Calcium

Hypercalcemia

- Differential diagnosis T1.8

  □ Primary hyperparathyroidism

    • **Primary hyperparathyroidism** is characterized by increased calcium, decreased phosphate, increased chloride, increased nephrogenous cAMP. This is in stark contrast to many other forms of hypercalcemia in which the phosphate is high (leading to an increased calcium × phosphate product). This is because PTH has the dual effect, on renal tubules, of increasing calcium reabsorption while increasing phosphate excretion.

T1.8
Differential Diagnosis of Hypercalcemia

Etiology	Notes
Primary hyperparathroidism	Parathyroid adenoma (most common), 4-gland hyperplasia, parathyroid carcinoma
Tertiary hyperparathyroidism	Post-renal transplant
Malignancy	Squamous cell carcinoma, multiple myeloma, breat carcinoma, islet cell tumors, paraganglioma, renal cell carcinoma, hepatocellular carcinoma, T-acute lymphoblastic lymphoma, small cell carcinoma of ovary (hypercalcemic type)
Familial hypocalciuric hypercalcemia	*CASR* gene on 3q
Drugs	Thiazides calcium-containing antacids or calcium supplements (milk-alkali syndrome), hypervitaminosis
Endocrine	Hyperthyrodism, Addison, acromegaly
Granulomatous disease	Sarcoidosis, mainly
Paget disease	Only if the patient is immobilized

- Primary hyperparathyroidism is due in 90% of cases to solitary parathyroid adenoma, 9% 4-gland hyperplasia, 1% carcinoma.

- Primary hyperparathyroidism may be inherited as part of multiple endocrine neoplasia syndrome, including MEN 1 (parathyroid adenoma, pituitary adenoma, pancreatic islet cell tumors) and MEN 2A (parathyroid adenoma, pheochromocytoma, medullary thyroid carcinoma). The locus on chromosome 11 that, in germline form, leads to MEN 1 has been found to contain somatic mutation in about 25% of sporadic parathyroid adenomas.

  □ **Secondary hyperparathyroidism** is due to peripheral resistance to the action of PTH (see below) and is associated with hypocalcemia

  □ **Tertiary hyperparathyroidism** is hyperparathyroidism that persists in patients post-renal transplant; ie, the parathyroids become autonomous—essentially primary hyperparathyroidism.

  □ **Malignancy** may produce hypercalcemia either in association with bone metastases or in the absence of bone metastases (humoral hypercalcemia of malignancy). The latter situation may be seen in association with renal cell carcinoma, hepatocellular carcinoma, squamous cell carcinoma, islet cell tumors, paragangliomas, and a variety of hematolymphoid neoplasms. The most common mediator of this syndrome is PTHrP. An increased nephrogenous cAMP in the presence of normal PTH is highly suggestive of humoral hypercalcemia of malignancy.

  □ **Hypervitaminosis D** results from long-term ingestion of vitamin supplements (recall that A, D, E, and K are lipophilic vitamins that, when taken in excess, are not readily excreted). Vitamin D, unlike PTH, enhances reabsorption of both calcium and phosphate by the kidneys, potentially leading to calciphylaxis.

  □ The histiocytes of sarcoidal granulomas appear to have the capacity to activate vitamin D to the active forme (1,25 di-hydroxy vitamin D). This phenomenon is rarely seen in other types of granulomatous disease.

  □ **Milk-alkali syndrome**, which for a time appeared to be disappearing, seems to be making a resurgence, thanks to compulsive calcium supplementation for the prevention of osteoporosis.

- Clinical presentation

  □ Hypercalcemia may present with nephrolithiasis, lethargy, hypo-reflexia, slowed mentation, nausea, vomiting, constipation, pression, and high peaked T waves on ECG. Hypercalcemia increases the risk of both pancreatitis and peptic ulcer disease.

  □ When long-term hypercalcemia is associated with concomitant hyperphasphatemia (increased calcium × phosphate product), there may be so-called metastatic calcification of vessel walls and soft tissue (calciphylaxis). This may be seen in skin and GI biopsies and often presents with pruritus.

- Laboratory evaluation

  □ In practical terms, the vast majority (80%-90%) of cases of hypercalcemia are due to hyperparathyroidism and malignancy. Distinguishing these two is easiest with clinical correlation; however, modern assays allow distinction of PTH (associated with hyperparathyroidism) and PTHrP (associated with some malignancies).

  □ Assays for parathyroid hormone (PTH), which are immunoassays, are sensitive to particular portions of the PTH molecule. PTH is initially synthesized as an 84 amino acid protein (intact or nascent PTH) which is subsequently broken down, both within the parathyroid and in the blood, into smaller fragments—an amino terminal fragment, a mid fragment, and a carboxy terminal fragment—while some persists as intact PTH **T1.9**. N-terminal and intact PTH have biological activity and, like other biologically active hormones, there are mechanisms in place to rapidly clear them from the blood.

Acid-Base & Electrolytes>Calcium

T1.9
Forms of Parathyroid Hormone (PTH)

	Biologic Activity	Half-Life
Intact PTH	+	Short
N-terminal PTH	+	Short
Mid-region PTH	−	Long
C-terminal PTH	−	Long

□ Early assays were somewhat indiscriminate and tended to include C-terminal and mid-fragments in their measurements. This is problematic, because the body makes no special effort to quickly clear these fragment from the blood; furthermore, these are cleared mainly by the kidneys, producing false elevations in renal insufficiency. Measuring mid-region and C-terminal PTH suffers from an additional problem: they can be elevated in hypercalcemia of other causes, since hypercalcemia suppresses PTH secretion but not PTH production, and intra-glandular destruction of PTH leads to normal/high levels in some patients.

□ Current, so-called 2nd generation, assays are capable of a high degree of specificity for the N-terminal or intact hormone. This specificity, combined with the rapid in vivo degradation of these peptides, has permitted the use of the PTH assay to assess intra-operatively the adequacy of parathyroid resection.

□ About 50% of serum calcium is bound to protein, mainly albumin. The free fraction is biologically active and is a more accurate reflection of the clinical calcium status. The effect of protein binding is relevant, for example, in patients with significant hyperproteinemia due to multiple myeloma or hypoproteinemia due to malnutrition. Conditions such as these may be associated with a markedly abnormal total calcium despite a normal ionized calcium.

● Acidosis increases the proportion of free calcium by competing for binding sites on albumin. Likewise, alkalosis decreases free calcium.

● The sample for ionized calcium measurement must be obtained from an artery; it must not be exposed to air (metabolism will change pH); it must not be drawn in calcium-chelating anticoagulants (EDTA, citrate); fist clenching and prolonged tourniquet application, capable of altering the local pH, are to be avoided; it must be kept cool and delivered to the laboratory rapidly.

● The measurement is usually performed on the blood gas analyzer. A rule-of-thumb correction for low protein is 0.8 mg/dL Ca per 1 g/dL protein lost. While this formula often provides a good estimate of the ionized calcium, its use should be avoided in patients with acid-base disturbances, renal insufficiency, liver disease, and neonates.

□ Old (biologic assay) techniques could not separate PTH from PTH-related protein. PTH-related protein (PTHrP) is secreted by some normal epithelia (squamous epithelium and lactating breast epithelium) and certain tumors (squamous cell carcinomas of lung, head & neck, skin, cervix, and esophagus, breast carcinoma, T-cell lymphomas). It is responsible for many cases of so-called humoral hypercalcemia of malignancy. PTHrP is encoded by a gene on chromosome 12 and has homology with the amino-terminal, biologically active component of PTH. Current immunologic assays do not suffer tremendously from cross-reactivity, and PTHrP can be specifically assayed.

■ Differential diagnosis **T1.10**

◻ Hypoparathyroidism is most often acquired. It is characterized by a low PTH, low calcium, and increased phosphate. $1,25(OH)_2D$ levels are also low, due to the dependence upon PTH for production.

◻ Hereditary hypoparathyroidism can occur as an isolated anomaly or in association with the DiGeorge syndrome.

◻ Secondary hyperparathyroidism (a.k.a. pseudohypoparathyroidism) is due to peripheral resistance to the action of PTH. This form of hyperparathyroidism is most commonly seen in chronic renal failure but may also be seen in vitamin D deficiency (osteomalacia, rickets). The calcium is low, while the PTH is normal to high. Phosphate is retained by the kidneys in this setting, creating the potential for tissue deposition of calcium salts. This persistent hyperparathyroid state produces marked activation of osteoclasts in bone, leading to so-called brown tumors of bone (renal osteodystrophy).

◻ Hypomagnesemia is capable of suppressing PTH secretion by the parathyroid gland. In fact, mild transient decreases in serum magnesium actually cause increased PTH secretion, an attempt on the part of the parathyroids to maintain the balance of divalent cations. However, persistent or marked hypomagnesemia somehow inhibits PTH secretion, leading to hypoparathyroidism.

■ Clinical presentation

◻ Hypocalcemia causes neurologic exciteability, presenting with muscle spasms, hyper-reflexia, paresthesias, lengthening of the QT interval, low-voltage T waves, and dysrhythmias.

◻ Severe hypocalcemia may cause laryngeal spasm, tetany, and respiratory arrest.

Acid-Base Disorders (T1.11)

Definitions

■ Acidemia refers to an arterial pH <7.40.

■ Alkalemia refers to an arterial pH >7.44.

■ Acidosis refers to a condition tending to lower the pH (the pH may not actually be lowered, due to compensation).

■ Alkalosis refers to a condition tending to raise the pH (the pH may not actually be raised, due to compensation).

■ Respiratory acidosis is due to too little elimination of CO_2 by the lungs (hypoventilation). The primary change is in CO_2.

T1.10
Differential Diagnosis of Hypocalcemia

Etiology	Notes
Vitamin D deficiency	
Chronic renal failure	
Drugs	Heparin, glucagons, osmotic diuretics, loop diuretics (Lasix), aminoglycosides, mithramycin
Hypoparathyroidism	Post-surgical, hypomagnesemia, DiGeorge syndrome, autoimmune
Medullary thyroid carcinoma	Rarely affects serum calcium
Hypoproteinemia	Often associated with a normal ionized calcium
Hyperphosphatemia	Calcium chelation
Pancreatitis	Extensive calcium deposition
Massive transfusion	Citrate

T1.11
Normal Values

Analyte	Normal Adult Range
pH	7.40-7.44
pCO_2	40-44 mm Hg
Bicarbonate	24-28 mEq/L
Anion gap	3-10
Albumin	3.5-5.0 gm/dL
PaO_2	90-100 mm Hg
O_2 saturation	95%-98%

Acid-Base & Electrolytes>Acid-Base Disorders

- Respiratory alkalosis is due to too much elimination of CO_2 by the lungs (hyperventilation). The primary change is in CO_2.

- Metabolic disorders are due to excessive intake, excessive production, or too little renal elimination of an acid or a base. The primary change is in (HCO_3^-).

- Compensation in primary respiratory disorders involves buffers and alterations in renal handling of bicarbonate (HCO_3^-).

- Compensation in primary metabolic disorders involves buffers and alterations in pulmonary handling of CO_2.

- A simple disorder is present when there is only a primary acid-base disturbance and associated compensation.

- A complex disorder is present when there are more than one primary acid-base disturbances.

Acid base homeostasis is somewhat understandable in light of the **Henderson-Hasselbach equation**

$$pH = pK + \log(base/acid)$$

- In normal individuals,

  □ pH = 7.4

  □ pK = 6.1,

  □ base = [bicarb] = 24

  □ acid = dissolved $PaCO_2$ = 0.03 × $PaCO_2$ = 0.03 × 40 = 1.2

- Substituting these into the equation, $7.4 = 6.1 + \log(24/1.2) = 6.1 + 1.3 = 7.4$

- Furthermore, the hydrogen ion concentration, $[H^+] = 24 \times (pCO_2/[HCO_3^-])$

- The body makes every attempt to maintain the validity of this equation. Since it must maintain a pH of 7.4, and the pK is a constant, it can only alter [bicarb] and $PaCO_2$. Note also that in order to maintain the validity of the formula, the ratio of these must remain 20:1. So whenever one goes up so must the other.

- Methods

  □ ABG (arterial blood gas) analyzers use a pH electrode, a $PaCO_2$ electrode, and PaO_2 electrode to measure these variables directly. They usually also derive a percent saturation of oxygen through a calculation that assumes a normal hemoglobin oxygen affinity.

  □ The pulse oximeter measures hemoglobin oxygen saturation directly, by measuring the absorbance of transdermally transmitted light. It emits two wavelengths of light, one that deoxyhemoglobin absorbs, and one that oxyhemoglobin absorbs.

  □ The co-oximeter is a spectrophotometric device that measures absorbance of multiple wavelengths of light. It is thus able to measure (not calculate) the proportions of oxyhemoglobin, deoxyhemoglobin, methemoglobin, and carboxyhemoglobin. Oxygen saturation is then the ratio of oxyhemoglobin to the total. Co-oximetry has great utility in critical care settings, where pulse-oximeters may fail for numerous reasons (not the least of which is poor peripheral perfusion where the device is attached). Furthermore, when the patient has undergone red cell transfusion and levels of 2,3-DPG are low in the transfused cells, ABG calculations of oxygen saturation can be very misleading. Whenever oxygen variants (methemoglobinemia, etc) are present, co-oximetry is superior to other modalities (often does not, however, detect sulfhemoglobin). Co-oximetry is the method of choice for detecting carbon monoxide poisoning.

Classifying an acid-base disorder

- Calculate:

  $$anion\ gap = [Na] - ([Cl] + [HCO_3])$$

  □ normal <12

  □ hypoalbuminemia can mask the anion gap.

  □ correction formula

  $$corrected\ anion\ gap = [Na] - ([Cl] + [HCO_3]) + 2.5(4-albumin)$$

  □ low anion gap (regardless of acid-base status) can be caused by paraproteinemia, hypoalbuminemia, hypermagnesemia, hypercalcemia, lithium therapy, and hypophosphatemia.

  □ Δ bicarb = normal bicarb − patient's bicarb

  □ Δ CO_2

□ Osmolal gap

osmolal gap $= osm_{measured} - (2[Na] + [Glu]/18 + BUN/2.8)$

□ normal < 10

□ the delta-delta is a comparison of the Δ bicarb and the Δ anion gap. These changes should be essentially 1:1 (within $\pm$ 2) in simple acid-base disorders. A delta-delta greater than that is indicative of a complex disorder.

■ Determine what is the primary abnormality

□ Acidosis:

- Metabolic acidosis: pH and $[HCO_3]$ go same direction (bicarb usually < 25 mEq/L)

- Respiratory acidosis: pH and $[HCO_3]$ go opposite direction (pCO_2 usually > 44 mm Hg)

□ Alkalosis:

- Metabolic alkalosis: pH and $[HCO_3]$ go same direction (bicarb usually > 25 mEq/L)

- Respiratory alkalosis: pH and $[HCO_3]$ go opposite direction (pCO_2 usually < 40 mm Hg)

■ Determine if the compensation is appropriate

□ Metabolic acidosis: for each 1.3 mEq fall in $[HCO_3]$, the pCO_2 decreases by 1.0 mm Hg.

□ Metabolic alkalosis: for each 0.6 mEq rise in $[HCO_3]$, the pCO_2 increases by 1.0 mm Hg.

□ Respiratory alkalosis or acidosis:

- Acute: for each 1 mmHg change in pCO_2, the $[HCO_3]$ changes by 0.1 in the same direction

- Chronic: for each 1 mmHg change in pCO_2, the $[HCO_3]$ changes by 0.4 in the same direction

Differential diagnosis of metabolic acidosis

■ Disorders are categorized by presence or absence of anion gap T1.12 and osmolal gap T1.13.

□ In non-anion gap acidosis, the chloride level is often elevated (hyperchloremic metabolic acidosis).

□ Remember to correct for hypoalbuminemia if present. For every 1.0 g/dL drop in albumin, there is a 2.5 mEq change in the anion gap; thus corrected anion gap = anion gap + 2.5 (4.0 – actual serum albumin)

Differential diagnosis of metabolic alkalosis

■ Disorders are categorized by chloride responsiveness or resistance T1.14.

T1.12
Metabolic Acidosis

Increased Anion Gap (>12)	Normal Anion Gap (<12)
methanol	diarrhea
uremia	recovery phase DKA
ketoacidosis (diabetic, EtOH, starvation)	ureterosigmoidostomy
paraldehyde	NH_4Cl
lactic acidosis	carbonic anhydrase inhibitors
ethylene glycol	TPN
salicylate	RTA

T1.13
Increased Osmolal Gap

With metabolic acidosis	methanol propylene glycol diethylene glycol paraldehyde ethanol (sometimes)
Without metabolic acidosis	isopropyl alcohol glycerol sorbitol mannitol acetone ethanol (sometimes)

T1.14
Metabolic Alkalosis

Chloride responsive (U_{cl}<10)	Chloride resistant (U_{cl}>10)
Didiuretic therapy Vomiting NGT suction Villous adenoma Carbenicillin Contraction alkalosis	Hyperaldosteronism Cushing syndrome Exogenous steroids Licorice (glycrrhizic acid) Bartter syndrome Milk-alkali syndrome

Renal Function

Renal Function Tests

Blood urea nitrogen (BUN)

- There are several nonprotein nitrogenous compounds in the blood, collectively termed nonprotein nitrogen (NPN), including urea, individual amino acids, urate, creatinine, and ammonia. These are principally derived from the breakdown of protein and nucleic acids.

- Urea, the end-product of the urea cycle, is the largest component of NPN. Urea nitrogen is measured by first splitting ammonium ion from urea through the use of the enzyme urease, then quantifying ammonium ion by any one of a number of methods. The urea concentration is calculated from the measurement of urea nitrogen. Methods to directly measure urea are also available.

- Urea is freely filtered and partially reabsorbed by the nephron; this reabsorption has the consequence that BUN always slightly underestimates GFR.

- Reabsorption increases with hypovolemia; thus BUN underestimates GFR even more in hypovolemic states.

- An increase in BUN is called azotemia, and a condition associated with very high BUN and its toxic effects is called uremia.

Creatinine and GFR calculations

- The creatinine concentration was classically determined, and is still often determined, by the Jaffe reaction—alkaline picrate (which may detonate) forms a colored complex with creatinine. Alternative enzymatic (using creatinase) and colorimetric assays are available.

- The serum creatinine varies inversely with the GFR. Creatinine is an endogenously produced substance that passes freely through the glomerulus. A small amount is secreted by the tubules, and the quantity of tubular secretion increases with increasing serum creatinine concentration. Thus, at all serum concentrations, creatinine slightly overestimates GFR. The simplest way to calculate GFR is based upon the creatinine clearance:

$$Cl_{Cr} = U_{Cr} \times V_{Ur} / P_{Cr}$$

U_{Cr} is urine creatinine (mg/dL)
V_{Ur} is volume of urine (mL/24 hours)
P_{Cr} is plasma creatinine (mg/dL)

- However, this formula turns out to be overly simplistic. While it is true that by far the greatest influence on serum creatinine is the GFR, and serum creatinine within an individual patient varies little from day to day, two phenomena conspire to weaken the suitability of the clearance formula for clinical use:

  □ Nonlinearity: the inverse relationship between GFR and creatinine is nonlinear. That is, mild to moderate degrees of GFR impairment do not cause appreciable increases in the creatinine concentration. At a certain point, however, when GFR is about half normal, creatinine rises precipitously and begins to linearly reflect changes in GFR.

  □ Nonglomerular influences upon creatinine: the serum creatinine concentration is increased by muscle mass, muscle activity, muscle injury (trauma, surgery), and protein intake. It tends to decrease with age, and it is influenced by race, sex, and numerous medications.

- This has led to the development of formulas to calculate estimated GFR (eGFR) from plasma creatinine, taking into account such factors as age and body weight. The Modification of Diet in Renal Disease (MDRD) Study equation is the most widely recommended formula.

  □ The MDRD equation has been studied and validated in adult Caucasian and African American populations with impaired kidney function (GFR < 60) between the ages of 18 and 70 years. It has not been validated for use in pregnant women, children, the elderly, the very sick hospitalized patient, or those with essentially normal GFR.

  □ The MDRD equation requires knowledge of the serum creatinine (S_{cr}), patient age (in years), sex, and race (African American or not African American). To make matters slightly more complicated, labs may produce a S_{cr} result in terms of either mg/dL (conventional units) or μmol/L (SI units), and a different equation exists for each. To make things even more complicated, the originally published MDRD equation is recommended for labs using a creatinine assay that has not been calibrated to be traceable to an isotope dilution mass spectrometry (IDMS) reference method. A different formula is recommended for labs with creatinine assays that have been calibrated to be traceable to IDMS (check package insert or contact manufacturer). Below are the many formulas:

Original (non-traceable), S_{Cr} in mg/dL

$$eGFR = 186 \times (S_{Cr})^{-1.154} \times age^{-0.203}$$

Original (non-traceable), S_{Cr} in μmol/L:

$$eGFR = 186 - (S_{Cr}/88.4)^{-1.154} - age^{-0.203}$$

Traceable, S_{cr} in mg/dL:

$$eGFR = 175 \times (S_{Cr})^{-1.154} \times age^{-0.203}$$

Traceable, S_{cr} in μmol/L:

$$eGFR = 175 \times (S_{Cr}/88.4)^{-1.154} \times age^{-0.203}$$

The result is multiplied by 0.742 if the patient is female, and by 1.210 if African American. The units for eGFR are given as mL/min/1.73 m²

□ The National Kidney Foundation recommends that eGFRs >60 mL/min/1.73 m² be reported simply as ">60 mL/min/1.73 m²" rather than with a specific number

BUN/creatinine ratio

Due to the ways that renal handling of BUN and creatinine differ, useful information can be obtained by comparing these two analytes.

- The normal BUN/creatinine ratio is about 10:1. When BUN and creatinine are elevated and this ratio is maintained it is suggestive of intra-renal disease—glomerulonephritis and tubulointerstitial nephritis. This is often referred to as *renal azotemia.*

- When the BUN/creatinine ratio is elevated, this suggests either prerenal azotemia or postrenal azotemia. *Prerenal azotemia* exists whenever there is poor renal perfusion—hypovolemia, hypotension, et cetera—and results from the effect described above in which BUN reabsorption is increased. *Postrenal azotemia* results from renal obstruction.

- A decreased BUN/Creatinine ratio is rare and may result from dietary protein insufficiency or severe liver disease.

Cystatin C is a cysteine protease inhibitor produced by nearly all cells in the body that is freely filtered by the glomerulus and metabolized by the proximal tubular epithelium. It has demonstrated superiority over creatinine for estimating the GFR and appears to be independent of age, sex, or muscle mass. It has been known for some time that chronic kidney disease, as estimated by the creatinine, is a risk factor for death from cardiovascular causes. Due possibly to all the factors that affect creatinine, cystatin C has been found to be a stronger predictor of mortality in this setting. Cystatin C concentrations appear to be strongly and independently associated with future cardiovascular events, independent of the serum creatinine.

Urine protein and urine albumin

- Normal proteinuria does not exceed 150 mg/day. This consists mainly of Tamm-Harsfall protein and minute amounts of albumin. The normal glomerulus filters protein based on size and charge. Some proteins are small enough to be freely filtered by the glomerulus, but most of these proteins are reabsorbed in the proximal tubules. Normally albumin does not freely cross the glomerular membrane.

- Significant proteinuria is usually defined as exceeding 300mg/day, and the definitive measurement has traditionally been based upon a 24-hour urine collection.

- The urine protein assay is sensitive to all kinds of protein (albumin, globulins, Bence-Jones), and its lower limit of detection is about 3 mg/dL. While the urine protein concentration of a random urine sample ('spot urine') can be misleading for innumerable reasons, the urine protein:creatinine ratio is an excellent test for significant proteinuria and appears to be as good (if not better considering a host of practical problems with a 24 hour urine collection) as the 24 hour urine for excluding significant proteinuria.

■ The urine dipstick result (1+ to 3+) has excellent cor-relation with the spot urine protein concentration; however, the urine dipstick test is most sensitive to albumin. It is not sufficiently sensitive to albumin to detect microalbuminuria, is not sensitive to globulins, andis not sensitive to even very high levels of Bence-Jones protein. The lower limit of detection of the urine dipstick test for albumin is about 18 mg/dL.

■ The microalbumin assay is capable of detecting as little as 0.3 mg/dL of albumin. Significant microalbuminuria is currently defined in terms of the albumin:creatinine ratio of a spot urine rather than a 24-hour timed urine collection. The albumin:creatinine ratio is reported in units of mg/g (protein:creatinine ratio is reported as mg/mg, a possible source of confusion). Since the microalbumin assay is a homogeneous immunometric one, *it is subject to the Hook effect*. In fact, the differen-tial diagnosis of a high urine protein concentration with negative microalbumin assay includes Bence-Jones protein and Hook effect. The Hook effect can be checked by running a urine protein on all specimens or performing a urine dipstick on all specimens.

■ The β_2-microglobulin & lysozyme assays can be used to detect tubular dysfunction. These proteins are freely fil-tered by the glomerulus then completely reabsorbed by the normally functioning proximal convoluted tubule. Their presence in urine suggests **tubular dysfunction.**

Laboratory Screening for Chronic Kidney Disease

■ The current recommendation of the national kidney foundation is annual testing for those at high risk for chronic kidney disease. High-risk individuals are those who have: diabetes mellitus, hypertension, or a family history of renal disease.

■ Recommended screening for high risk groups includes an eGFR and a microalbuminuria screen (urine albumin:creatinine ratio), where albumin is measured by a microalbumin assay.

■ Chronic kidney disease is defined by either

(1) GFR <60 mL per minute per 1.73 m² of body surface area, or

(2) albuminuria for 3 or more consecutive months

■ The degree (or stage) of chronic kidney disease: stage 1 equates to kidney damage (albuminuria) without decreased GFR, stage 2 is kidney damage with a mild decrease in GFR, stage 3 is a moderate decrease in GFR, stage 4 is a severe decrease in GFR, and stage 5 is renal failure (GFR <15 mL per minute per 1.73 m² or dialysis-dependence).

Laboratory Evaluation in Acute Renal Failure

■ There is no broadly accepted definition of ARF, but the term implies a rapid and sustained decrement in renal function.

■ The causes of ARF are categorized as prerenal, renal, or postrenal **T1.15, T1.16.**

□ Prerenal ARF is the result of decreased renal perfusion, leading to a physiologic reduction in glomerular filtration rate (GFR). A sustained benefit by expansion of intravascular volume with colloid is characteristic; fluid replacement ('fluid challenge') is therefore both a therapeutic and a diagnostic maneuver in this setting.

T1.15
Prerenal vs Renal

Parameter	Prerenal ARF	Renal ARF
BUN/creatinine ratio	>20:1	<20:1
Urine specific gravity	High (>1.020)	Low (<1.010)
Urine osmolarity	High (>500 mmol/kg)	Low (300-500)
FENa	<1%	>2%
FE urea	<35%	>35%

T1.16
Causes of Acute Renal Failure

Prerenal	Renal	Postrenal
Hypovolemia Congestive heart failure Cirrhosis NSAIDs ACE Inhibitors Vasopressors	Acute tubular necrosis (contrast media, aminoglycosides, amphotericin, tumor lysis syndrome, rhabdomyolysis); Acute glomerular injury (penicillamine, cyclosporine, acute glomerulonephritis, thrombotic microangiopathy, malignant hypertension); Acute tublointerstitial nephritis (NSAIDs) Vasculitis	Bladder outlet obstruction (prostatism); Bilateral ureteral obstruction (tumor, retroperitoneal fibrosis)

1: Clinical Chemistry

Renal Function>Laboratory Evaluation in Acute Renal Failure; Hepatorenal Syndrome (HRS) I
Laboratory Tests in Pregnancy>Amniotic Fluid Bilirubin

□ Postrenal ARF is caused by an obstruction of the renal collecting system.

□ Renal causes of ARF produce injury to the nephron (glomeruli, tubules, vessels, or interstitium). The most common cause of renal ARF is acute tubular necrosis (ATN), and the most common causes of ATN are ischemia and nephrotoxins. Acute glomerulonephritis (AGN) may also cause renal ARF.

■ A patient with new-onset ARF must have a battery of laboratory tests and a renal ultrasound (the latter to exclude hydronephrosis indicative of postrenal ARF).

□ Initial and serial serum BUN and creatinine. In addition, there must be serial monitoring of variables that may require the initiation of dialysis. Indications for dialysis include refractory volume overload, hyperkalemia, metabolic acidosis, end-organ damage due to uremia (eg, pericarditis), or BUN >100 gm/dL.

□ Urine volume monitoring. Most cases of renal failure are oliguric. Non-oliguric renal failure may occur in renal or postrenal ARF, but rarely in prerenal ARF.

□ BUN/Cr ratio, urine osmolarity, urine specific gravity, and fractional excretion of sodium (FENA) are helpful for distinguishing renal from prerenal causes. The FENA is almost always low (<1%) in prerenal ARF (the exception being when the patient has been given diuretics or has glycosuria, in whom fractional excretion of urea can be a useful alternative).

□ Urinalysis provides important information in renal failure. A lack of findings or isolated hyaline casts suggest prerenal ARF. Dysmorphic red blood cells and red blood cell casts suggest glomerulonephritis. Pigmented casts suggest acute tubular necrosis. Leukocytes (in the absence of infection—sterile pyuria), white blood cell casts, and/or eosinophils suggest tubulointerstitial nephritis.

Hepatorenal Syndrome (HRS)

■ Hepatorenal syndrome is the development of progressive renal impairment in patients with severe end-stage liver disease in the absence of another identifiable cause of renal disease (shock, bacterial sepsis, nephrotoxin exposure, etc).

■ HRS has an incidence of about 5% per admission for decompensated cirrhosis, and about 50% over the course of cirrhosis.

■ Spontaneous bacterial peritonitis (SBP) is the most common cause of renal failure in the cirrhotic patient, and this must be excluded. Also common in hospital admissions for cirrhosis are the use of nephrotoxic agents (aminoglycosides, NSAIDs, radiocontrast dyes). The renal biopsy is essentially normal in HRS, but an abnormal biopsy must be interpreted cautiously—many patients with cirrhosis due to hepatitis viruses have an associated glomerulonephritis, and cirrhosis can by itself lead to an IgA-like nephropathy.

■ HRS in most instances is not present at admission but arises following profound fluid shifts such as occur in the treatment of ascites. It is felt to be due to dysregulation of renal blood flow.

Laboratory Tests in Pregnancy

Amniotic Fluid Bilirubin

Method

The concentration of bilirubin is proportional to absorbance. The maximal absorbance of bilirubin is at 450 nm. After amniotic fluid is obtained, preferably with minimal blood contamination, the specimen should be protected from light (a brown plastic tube is usually provided in the amniocentesis tray). Light significantly diminishes the absorbance peak for the specimen. A scanning spectrophotometer is used to measure absorbances at intervals from 340 to 560 nm.

Determination of the amniotic fluid bilirubin is part of the clinical evaluation of the pregnancy complicated by alloimmunization. The amniotic fluid bilirubin reflects the degree of fetal hemolysis.

Interpretation

- On semilog paper, the absorbances are plotted against wavelength. A straight line from the point at 350 nm to the point at 550 nm. This line reflects the theoretical plot if there were no pigments in the fluid. The difference between the line and the actual absorbance at 450 nm is the 'ΔOD 450' which reflects the bilirubin concentration.

- The ΔOD 450 is then plotted against the estimated gestational age (EGA) on a Liley chart.

- Unless a result falls into zone III on the Liley chart, serial measurements are usually indicated. If results are in zone III or rising in zone II, then immediate delivery for EGA > 36 wks, determination of FLM for EGA 35-36 weeks, or intrauterine transfusion may be considered.

Maternal Serum Human Chorionic Gonadotropin (hCG)

Method

hCG is a glycoprotein heterodimer composed of an α and a β chain. The α subunit is identical to that found in TSH, FSH, and LH. The predominant methodologies involve immunoassay directed against the β subunit. The concentration of hCG is expressed in mIU/mL and ng/mL (100 mIU = 8 ng). Both qualitative and quantitative assays are available.

- False negative hCG can occur with the urine testing, especially if the urine is dilute. When there is a high suspicion of pregnancy, or when certainty is required, a negative urine hCG should be confirmed with a serum hCG test. In the presence of a negative serum test, pregnancy is exceedingly unlikely.

- False positive hCG may be encountered, due to heterophile antibody interference. When suspected, it can be helpful to repeat the measurement on a different analyzer, pretreat with heterophile binding reagent, or to run serial dilutions.

- True positive, low-level, 'phantom' hCG, not associated with pregnancy or overt gestational trophoblastic disease, is an increasingly recognized clinical problem. Some of the patients in this group have been diagnosed as having so-called quiescent gestational trophoblastic disease; that is, despite having had an identified hydatidiform mole or other gestational trophoblastic disease that was appropriately treated with evacuation and/or chemotherapy, they are found to have persistent low levels of hCG for long periods of time. No demonstrable persistent lesion is found, and multiple rounds of chemotherapy and/or surgery do nothing to alter the hCG. Other patients in this group have no history of trophoblastic disease, have a positive hCG as part of a routine pre-procedure or pre-medication check, and this hCG persists for many months or years. Rarely, a clinically inapparent pituitary tumor is identified. Certain investigations may be warranted: imaging of the uterus and ovaries, lungs, mediastinum, and retroperitoneum, and the pituitary fossa. The published accounts appear to support watchful waiting if no anatomic lesion is identified.

hCG in normal gestation

- hCG becomes detectable about 6-8 days following conception (about the time of implantation), when levels are around 10-50 mIU/mL.

- The hCG level doubles every two days until the concentration of 1200 mIU/mL at about 10 weeks.

- It then doubles every three days between 1200 and 6000.

- It doubles every four days above 6000 until it peaks near the end of the first trimester at around 100,000.

- By early second trimester, it plateaus at around 10,000 (800 ng/mL).

- Causes of elevated levels, aside from those discussed below, include multiple gestations, polyhydramnios, eclampsia, and erythroblastosis fetalis.

- After delivery, hCG normally remains detectable for 2 weeks. The disappearance of hCG after term pregnancy is best viewed as triphasic, with rapid, medium, and slow half-lives of 3.6 hours, 18 hours, and 53 hours.

hCG in ectopic pregnancy

- Ectopic pregnancy is the most common cause of maternal death in the 1st trimester and an easy diagnosis to miss. It usually presents with abdominal pain or mild vaginal bleeding (spotting) in a woman of child-bearing age who may or may not know she's pregnant.

- Ectopic pregnancy is defined as one implanted outside the uterine cavity. The vast majority (>95%) occur in the fallopian tube, the remainder in the ovary, abdomen, or cornu. Heterotopic pregnancy, in which there is simultaneous intrauterine and ectopic implantation, was once exceedingly rare; however, in those treated with fertility-enhancing agents the incidence is 1%.

- The clinician uses the β-hCG to first diagnose the pregnancy and then to assist with distinguishing a normal from ectopic pregnancy. The quantity (and rate of rise) of hCG tells the clinician how reliable an ultrasound test is. However, there is no hCG level below which rupture of an ectopic is impossible; levels below 100 mIU/mL have been associated with rupture.

- If the normal hCG dynamic is not seen, this suggests an abnormal pregnancy. Specifically, if serum hCG does not rise at least 66% in 48 hours, or if the hCG falls during this time, this suggests a abnormal pregnancy (either ectopic pregnancy or nonviable intrauterine pregnancy). However, a normal rate of rise can be seen in 15% of ectopics, and an abnormal rate of rise can be seen in 15% of normal intrauterine pregnancies (IUP).

- Further elucidation relies on ultrasonic demonstration of an intrauterine gestational sac. With transabdominal ultrasound, a gestational sac should be detectable when the hCG exceeds 6000 mIU/mL. When the hCG is greater than 1400 mIU/mL, the absence of an IUP detectable by transvaginal ultrasound is 90% specific for an ectopic. The detection of an IUP virtually excludes an ectopic, except in the case of heterotopic pregnancy which may be a consideration in the setting of fertility enhancement. The absence of an IUP beyond these thresholds is highly specific for an ectopic pregnancy.

- A useful adjunct is the serum progesterone level. A serum progesterone greater than 25 ng/mL virtually assures an IUP. Levels below 5 ng/mL are strongly (approaching 100%) predictive of an abnormal pregnancy. The bad news is that most patients fall somewhere between these thresholds.

- In summary, the combined clinical and laboratory approach is as follows:

  □ If a woman of child-bearing age presents with abdominal pain, vaginal bleeding, or hemodynamic instability, a pregnancy test should be performed.

  □ The unstable patient may need rapid surgical intervention following a positive hCG and negative ultrasound for IUP. In this case, Rh status should be determined to guide Rhogam therapy.

  □ The stable patient with a positive hCG should then have a quantitative hCG initiated while ultrasonography is performed. If an IUP is identified, then a threatened abortion is likely (though not assured). If ultrasound evidence of an ectopic is found, then ablation with either surgical intervention or methotrexate is indicated. When neither definite IUP nor definite ectopic is found, what happens next depends upon the quantitative hCG. If above the threshold where IUP should be visible, then the patient should be considered at high risk for ectopic pregnancy with the differential diagnosis including a completed spontaneous abortion. A progesterone level may help if very low or very high. In the patient with a progesterone level less than 5 ng/mL, the absence of chorionic villi in material from a D&C indicates a high likelihood of ectopic pregnancy. Above 5 ng/mL, the risk of evacuating a normal IUP is sufficiently high to dissuade most practicioners from performing this procedure. In these patient and in patients whose initial quantitative hCG was not above the threshold value, comparison with a 48-hour interval quantitative hCG is required. A normal rise in βhCG (> 66%) is consistent with a normal, intrauterine, pregnancy. However, a significant minority—about 20%— ectopic pregnancies will also have a normal rise, so these patients require further monitoring until the hCG reaches the threshold and ultrasound confirms an IUP. Furthermore, an abnormal rise in hCG is not diagnostic of ectopic; it is seen in about 20% of normal IUPs and in pregnancies abnormal for other reasons.

- After removal of an ectopic pregnancy, hCG normally remains detectable for 4 weeks. Levels have to be monitored to exclude persistent trophoblastic tissue.

1: Clinical Chemistry

Laboratory Tests in Pregnancy>Maternal Serum Human Chorionic Gonadotropin;
Prenatal Screening for Trisomy and Neural Tube Defects

hCG in spontaneous abortion Serial quantitative hCGs demonstrate an abnormal rate of change as in ectopic pregnancy. At this point, either an IUP is visible by transvaginal ultrasound, or spontaneous passage of tissue has occurred. After spontaneous abortion, hCG remains detectable for 4-6 weeks.

hCG in gestational trophoblastic disease

- Women with GTD usually produce a greater amount of hCG than normal gestations. Furthermore, average hCG levels are higher in complete moles than partial moles.

- In actual practice, most partial moles are diagnosed based upon the histological features of uterine contents. In contrast, most complete moles are diagnosed clinically. Complete moles have a characteristic clinical presentation, including uterine enlargement out of proportion for the gestational age, vaginal bleeding, hypertension, absence of fetal heart tones, and a characteristic ultrasound. Both types of molar pregnancy must be monitored for (1) persistence and (2) the development of malignant trophoblastic disease. The risk of malignancy is <5% for partial moles and about 20% for complete moles.

- After evacuation of a molar pregnancy, hCG levels must be monitored weekly until undetectable for 3 consecutive weeks. HCG is then measured monthly for 1 year. After evacuation of an uncomplicated molar pregnancy, hCG remains detectable for up to 10 weeks.

- So long as hCG is falling, there is no need for intervention. If the hCG plateaus or rises, then persistent GTD is suspected. Most often this is an indication for chemotherapy following a metastatic workup.

- Uterine choriocarcinomas may not be preceded by a molar pregnancy. Half of all cases follow a normal term pregnancy, and about 25% follow a histologically normal spontaneous abortion. The remaining 25% derive from molar pregnancy.

Prenatal Screening for Trisomy and Neural Tube Defects

Available approaches to screening

- The "triple screen" is the traditional panel of hCG, AFP, & unconjugated estriol (uE) performed on maternal serum drawn during the 2nd trimester, ideally around 18 weeks. The sensitivity of this panel for Down syndrome is 70%.

- The 'Quad test,' combining the above three analytes with the dimeric inhibin A (DIA), has become the standard screening method. Unlike the analytes of the triple screen, the concentration of DIA is fairly stable throughout the 2nd trimester. The improved performance of the Quad test comes mainly from amelioration of the effects of inaccurate gestational age which plague the triple screen. The sensitivity of this panel for Down syndrome is about 80%.

- The 'integrated screen' combines 1st and 2nd trimester serum testing. PAPP-A and hCG are measured in the 1st trimester, ideally between weeks 10-13; later, a 2nd trimester measurement of AFP, uE, and DIA is made, and the data combined. The sensitivity for Down syndrome is about 85%. If combined with a sonographic measurement of nuchal fold thickness, the sensitivity can be improved to >90%.

Clinical considerations

- In diabetic mothers, both the uE and hCG are decreased mildly.

- In mothers who smoke, MSAFP is increased, while uE and hCG are decreased.

- Twin gestations remain a challenge. Down syndrome occurs more frequently in twin than singleton pregnancies—both twinning and DS increase with maternal age. However, the sensitivity of routine screening in twin pregnancies is just under between 50%-70% (better for monozygotic twins, both of which would have DS, than dizygotic, in which usually only one has DS).

- Trisomy 18 (Edward syndrome) usually shows a characteristic pattern: ↓AFP, ↓hCG, ↓uE. About 80% of cases are detected with screening, and about 10% of cases identified with this pattern turn out to be affected.

- **Neural tube defect** shows a pattern of ↑AFP, normal hCG, ↓uE. About 2%-3% of MSAFPs will be elevated, and of these, about 10% are due to an actual NTD. If a MSAFP is borderline elevated (2.5-3.0 MOM) and was obtained somewhat early (<18 weeks), there is value in repeating it. Otherwise, an ultrasound is required to confirm gestational age, exclude multiple gestations, look for overt anatomic abnormalities, and exclude fetal demise. Having excluded these possibilities, an amniocentesis is performed to obtain amniotic fluid for AFP and acetylcholinesterase (AChE). The sensitivity of MSAFP screening is about 90 percent. The sensitivity is worse (about 30%) for multiple gestations.

- **Trisomy 21 (Down) syndrome** has a characteristic pattern: ↓AFP, ↑hCG, ↓uE. Dimeric inhibin A is increased in Down syndrome. Follow-up should include high-resolution ultrasound and amniocentesis for confirmatory cytogenetics.

Analytes

- **Maternal age** was the first analyte by which risk of Down syndrome was assessed. It is a powerful marker of DS risk, and maternal age remains a critical variable in the calculation of risk. Based on 2007 ACOG recommendations, all women, regardless of age, should be offered noninvasive screening. Prior to 2007, the recommendation was to perform invasive testing on women over 35; noninvasive screening was limited to those under 35. Women under 35 years of age were be offered serum screening to determine *if their risk is that of a 35 year old woman,* and therefore if they should be offered invasive testing.

- **AFP.** α-fetoprotein is the principle plasma protein in the fetus. Maternal serum AFP (MSAFP) rises progressively during the first and second trimesters. Adjustments to the MSAFP interpretation are routinely made for maternal weight, race, number of fetuses, and maternal diabetes. Increased maternal weight can have a dilutional effect on the AFP, providing a falsely low value. Levels tend to be much higher in multiple gestations, and levels are much lower in maternal diabetes.

  - □ MSAFP is > 2.5 multiples of the median (MOM) in > 80% of neural tube defect (NTD). Values > 2.0 MOM are considered abnormal in maternal diabetes. In twin gestations, MSAFP is considered abnormal only above 4.5 MOM.

- □ Conditions associated with increased MSAFP

  - neural tube defects
  - omphalocele and gastroschisis
  - renal anomalies
  - sacrococcygeal teratoma
  - cystic hygroma
  - hydrops fetalis
  - Turner syndrome
  - bowel obstruction
  - twins
  - wrong gestational age
  - fetal demise
  - fetal-maternal hemorrhage

- **hCG.** Maternal serum HCG is roughly 2 times higher in fetal Down syndrome. Adjustments are typically made for maternal weight, multiple gestation, maternal diabetes, and race.

- **uE.** Fetal Down syndrome is associated with decreased maternal serum unconjugated estriol. uE is a somewhat weakly sensitive to Down syndrome pregnancies but is a very good indicator of trisomy 18 (Edward syndrome), Smith-Lemli-Optiz syndrome (SLOS), and inherited (fetal) deficiencies of steroid sulfatase.

- **DIA** is a glycoprotein produced by the placenta. In a Down syndrome fetus, DIA is increased to an average of 1.9 multiples of the median (MOM). What makes DIA such an splendid addition to the panel is that, unlike the other analytes in the triple screen, levels of DIA are relatively constant throughout the second trimester testing period, which minimizes the effect of erroneous gestational age estimates. Maternal serum DIA is elevated in Down syndrome.

Assessing the Risk of Preterm Birth

Preterm labor is defined as regular contractions, with associated cervical change, prior to 37 weeks. Prematurity is the single most important cause of perinatal morbidity and mortality. A test that serves as a predictor of preterm labor would permit appropriate hospitalization and treatment of affected women. Markers which have demonstrated limited utility in this regard include serum estradiol and salivary estriol (both increase before the onset of preterm labor), screening for bacterial vaginosis (independently associated with preterm labor), and others.

Fetal fibronectin is a protein found normally at placental fetomaternal interface. Cervicovaginal fluid contains fetal fibronectin protein briefly during early gestation, after which time it is absent until just before labor. Specimens for fetal fibronectin should be collected ideally greater than 24 hours after the last cervical examination or intercourse. Several trials have demonstrated that the absence of fetal fibronectin protein has very high negative predictive value and can exclude impending preterm birth. A positive result suggests the onset of preterm labor, but the overall positive predictive value is low. The only other test that shows similar performance is transvaginal cervical ultrasound to assess cervical length.

Determination of Fetal Lung Maturity

- Mature type II pneumocytes produce a mixture of phospholipids composed predominantly of lecithin. The vast majority of lecithin is disaturated phosphatidylcholine (DSPC). Lesser amounts of phosphatidylglycerol (PG), phosphatidylinositol (PI), phosphatidylethanolamine (PE), and sphingomyelin also comprise lecithin.

- *Fetal lung maturity (FLM)* is necessary to avoid respiratory distress syndrome (RDS). Assessment of fetal lung maturity is really an issue for gestations between 34-37 weeks' gestation. Prior to this time, fetal lung maturity is unlikely, and the risk of RDS is very high. After 37 weeks the risk of RDS is exceedingly low, and FLM testing is generally not indicated, except in the presence of poorly controlled maternal diabetes.

- *Specimen.* Uncontaminated amniotic fluid obtained by amniocentesis is the optimal specimen for determination of FLM. Vaginal pool specimens from women with premature rupture of membranes (PROM) should be avoided as should specimens with blood or meconium contamination. Sometimes these things are unavoidable, and, in general, the best results from suboptimal specimens are obtained with a phosphatidyl glycerol (PG) determination.

- *Testing strategy.* Most tests for FLM are better at predicting maturity than immaturity. Therefore, a mature result by almost any method is fairly reliable. If an initial result is below the maturity cut-off, then a second test, with another technique, is often warranted to clarify.

Lecithin/sphingomyelin (L/S) ratio

- Lecithin increases with gestational age, while sphingomyelin remains at a relatively constant 2% of total surfactant phospholipid. Until about 26 weeks, the ratio is around 1:1.

- After that, the L:S ratio increases until the ratio of 2:1 is reached around 35 weeks. The ratio of 2:1 is generally taken to indicate fetal lung maturity. Above 2:1, around 2% of premature infants will develop RDS. Below 2:1, nearly 60% will.

- Problems in interpretation of L/S ratio

  □ In diabetes mellitus, a ratio of 2:1 does not ensure fetal lung maturity. The phosphatidylglycerol concentration is more reliable in this scenario.

  □ The presence of meconium falsely decreases the L:S ratio.

  □ The presence of blood normalizes the L:S ratio to around 1.5.

  □ The CV of the L:S ratio is high.

Phosphatidylglycerol (PG) concentration. Phosphatidylglycerol is first detected around 36 weeks. Its presence is indicative of fetal lung maturity. Neither blood nor meconium interfere with PG determinations, making it the test of choice when the only available specimen is a contaminated one. PG can be measured by TLC, with its attendant logistical limitations, or by agglutination, which is felt to be equally reliable.

Foam stability. When pulmonary surfactant is present in amniotic fluid in sufficient concentration, the fluid is able to form a highly stable film that can support the structure of a foam. The amniotic fluid is serially diluted with ethanol, and the highest concentration of ethanol at which a complete ring of bubbles is seen is the foam stability index (FSI). An FSI greater than 0.47 is considered indicative of fetal lung maturity.

Lamellar body number density (LBND). Surfactant lamellar bodies (LBs) are approximately the size of platelets, and the platelet channel of a cell counter (Coulter) can be used to quantify them. An LBND greater than 50,000/mL is predictive of maturity.

Disaturated phosphatidylcholine (DSPC) concentration: an alternative to the L:S ratio is to determine the DSPC, the major component of lecithin, directly. Since it doesn't rely on a ratio with sphingomyelin, it is unaffected by meconium and blood contamination.

Fluorescence polarization assay: now the most commonly used method, this test is rapid and at least as predictive of fetal lung maturity as the L/S, with considerably lower CV. A fluorescence polarization value less than 260 is considered mature. Values greater than 290 are considered immature. If there is less than 0.5% blood, results are unaffected. Greater amounts tend to lower high values and raise low values. Even in the presence of blood, values <230 are considered mature.

Laboratory Evaluation of Diseases in Pregnancy

Physiologic changes and altered reference ranges in pregnancy

- Expected chemical changes T1.17

T1.17
Common Laboratory Values in Pregnancy

Analyte	Change in Pregnancy
Albumin	↓1 gm/dL
Calcium (total)	↓10%
Creatinine	↓0.3 mg/dL
Fibrinogen	↑1-2 g/L
Albumin	↓0.5-1 g/dL
BUN	↓50%
Urine protein	↑approximately double
Amylase	↑50%-100%
Hct	↓4%-7%
Hgb	↓1.5-2 g/dL

- Increased circulating fatty acids. Serum triglycerides are increased by about 40%, and a low-level ketosis is often seen.

- Decreased albumin and total protein result from hemodilution.

- Increased transport proteins such as thyroid-binding globulin (TBG) result from increased estrogen.

- Increased GFR. This is felt to be due to the increased blood volume, and it is reflected in decreased BUN, Creatinine, and urate.

- Increased insulin resistance. Until the mid-2nd trimester, glucose tolerance actually improves. After that, however, relative insulin resistance emerges, reflected in prolonged elevations in serum glucose after meals. Perhaps the most important cause of this change is human placental lactogen (hPL) which has anti-insulin effects similar to growth hormone (GH). Note that in infants of poorly controlled diabetic mothers, potentially life-threatening neonatal hypoglycemia is a risk.

- Sodium and potassium remain relatively constant throughout pregnancy. Calcium falls slightly throughout pregnancy.

Medical conditions of particular importance in pregnancy

- Thromboembolism: the incidence of deep venous thrombosis (DVT) is 1/2000 antepartum and 1/700 postpartum. The incidence of PE is about 1/2500

- Diabetes mellitus

- Autoimmune diseases

  - Though extremely common among women of childbearing age, most women with autoimmune diseases do no worse than women without them. In fact, pregnancy seems to have a palliative effect on some, notably rheumatoid arthritis and Graves disease. However, systemic lupus erythematosis (SLE) is often exacerbated by pregnancy, and both Graves disease and myasthenia gravis are notorious for postpartum exacerbations. In idiopathic thrombocytopenic purpura (ITP) antibodies can cross the placenta and lead to neonatal thrombocytopenia. It is important to distinguish this from neonatal alloimmune thrombocytopenia (NATP). Life-threatening neonatal intracranial hemorrhages are a common complication.

Laboratory Tests in Pregnancy>Laboratory Evaluation of Diseases in Pregnancy

□ Systemic lupus erythematosis (SLE) activity is affected by pregnancy, and both pregnancy and the neonate can be affected by SLE.

- Although the subject of ongoing research and debate, it appears that pregnancy increases the likelihood of an SLE flare. The risk is highest early in pregnancy and during puerperium, with relative quiescence in the latter half of pregnancy. Renal deterioration that occurs in lupus during pregnancy is often irreversible. A lupus flare may be difficult to distinguish from pregnancy-induced hypertension, as the features of hypertension, edema, and proteinuria are shared. This distinction may be aided by complement levels (low in SLE flare, normal in PIH).

- Mortality is increased in pregnant women with SLE, with most deaths occurring as a result of pulmonary hemorrhage due to lupus pneumonitis and other complications (transverse myelitis, stroke, corticosteroid complications). Pregnant women with SLE have an increased incidence of pregnancy-induced hypertension (PIH). While it is often difficult to distinguish PIH from a flare of SLE, the treatments are very different (delivery for PIH, corticosteroids for SLE). Lastly, SLE is a cause of recurrent miscarriage, abortion, and preterm labor. The lupus anticoagulant is thought to mediate these pregnancy loss effects, and these may occur without SLE; furthermore, SLE may occur without lupus anticoagulant. In this regard, the appropriate treatment is anticoagulation, not corticosteroids.

- In addition to an increased incidence of IUGR and preterm labor, neonates born to mothers with SLE have a risk of congenital heart block Antibodies to SS-A and SS-B (Ro and La) are thought to mediate this complication.

■ Genitourinary diseases

□ Chronic renal disease may be first detected during pregnancy (since proteinuria is routinely tested during pregnancy) or exacerbated by pregnancy. Pregnancy normally has the effect of increasing the creatinine clearance. In addition, a slight increase in normal urinary protein excretion is expected, up to 300 mg/day. This increase in GFR is somewhat protective early in pregnancy, with most profound exacerbations of underlying renal disease occurring late in pregnancy, during the third trimester. The greatest risk posed to the pregnant woman with chronic renal disease is significant hypertension.

□ Pregnant women are at increased risk for urinary tract infection, the consequences of which may be grave. Asymptomatic bacteriuria, therefore, is dealt with more aggressively in pregnant women. Asymptomatic bacteriuria is diagnosed based upon a clean-catch voided urine specimen containing >100,000 colonies/mL. Asymptomatic bacteriuria is present in 10%-20% of women and an equivalent proportion of pregnant women; however, while largely inconsequential in most women, it is associated with the development of urinary tract infection, with an attendant high risk of pyelonephritis, in 40% of pregnant women. *Escherichia coli* is responsible for most cases.

■ Endocrine

□ Hypopituitarism. Sheehan syndrome (postpartum pituitary apoplexy) is due to the conspiring effects of pregnancy-associated pituitary enlargement and severe blood loss during delivery. It is considered to be the most common cause of hypopituitarism in women of childbearing age. In fact, about 90% of affected women have a history of severe puerperal bleeding. They then experience the inability to lactate, amenorrhea, lethargy, weakness, and weight loss.

□ Thyroid disorders. In the normal pregnancy, there is increased demand placed upon the thyroid gland, due to an increase in an estrogen-driven increase in thyroid-binding globulin (TBG) and the TSH-like stimulatory effect of hCG. Patients with borderline thyroid function or those with borderline availability of iodine will be unable to meet these demands. As a consequence, hypothyroidism is a more common problem in pregnancy than hyperthyroidism. The serum TSH is the single best test of thyroid status.

□ Hyperthyroidism must be distinguished from the syndrome of transient hyperthyroidism of hyperemesis gravidarum. Transient hyperthyroidism of hyperemesis gravidarum, due to high levels of hCG, is thought to be the most common cause of hyperthyroidism in pregnancy.

- Hepatic

  - Acute fatty liver of pregnancy is a rare but serious condition—a medical emergency usually complicated by disseminated intravascular coagulation (DIC). It affects about 1 in 10,000 pregnancies but has a case fatality rate as high as 30%. Acute fatty liver usually presents in the third trimester, with nausea, vomiting, and right upper quadrant tenderness. This is followed by jaundice and altered mental status. Several metabolic defects contribute to morbidity, including metabolic acidosis, renal failure, hypoglycemia, and a prolonged protime with or without DIC. Histologic examination of the liver shows widespread microvesicular steatosis, accentuated paracentrally (zone 3), with a paucity of inflammatory activity or hepatocellular necrosis. An oil-red-O stain (on frozen tissue) highlights the microvesicles. Immediate delivery is the treatment of choice.

  - Intrahepatic cholestasis presents with jaundice and pruritus, usually in the third trimester. While the jaundice is usually mild, the pruritus is distressing. Serum alkaline phosphatase levels are increased 5- to 10-fold (recall that alkaline phosphatase is normally increased in pregnancy due to the placental isoenzyme), with parallel increases in GGT and 5'-nucleotidase. Bilirubin is elevated, but usually remains below 5 mg/dL, and is composed largely of the direct (conjugated) form. Transaminase levels are usually normal or very mildly elevated. Serum bile acids (chenodeoxycholic acid, deoxycholic acid, and cholic acid) are increased, often to levels 10 times the upper limit of normal, are this is considered the most characteristic laboratory finding. Histologically, the change is in the pericentral (zone 3) region, which shows dilated canaliculi containing bile plugs.

Recurrent Pregnancy Loss

- Investigation is often undertaken following two or more spontaneous abortions.

- Laboratory evaluation usually involves:

  - Parental karyotyping. Karyotyping of an abortus is often indicated as well.

  - Endometrial biopsies may be obtained to exclude luteal phase defect (endometrial histology that is 2 or more days discrepant with dates). Endometrial culture may be ordered to exclude subclinical infection with *Ureaplasma urealyticum* or *Chlamydia trachomatis*.

  - Thyroid function tests

  - Tests for lupus anticoagulants

Toxicology

Toxicology can be thought of as consisting of three clinical applications: drugs of abuse screening (forensic toxicology), management of overdose, and therapeutic drug monitoring. There is of course some overlap between these categories.

Half-life

- The half-life ($T\frac{1}{2}$) is the time it takes for the concentration of drug to reach $\frac{1}{2}$ of the starting amount. Generally speaking, a drug is dosed according to its $T\frac{1}{2}$; that is, if a drug's half-life is 12 hours, then doses are given every 12 hours.

- Drugs are eliminated by a limited number of mechanisms: renal clearance, metabolism (usually in the liver), or both.

- Elimination of most agents follows so-called first-order (1°) kinetics, meaning that the rate of loss is exponential, with a graph that is asymptotic.

- A concept important in therapeutic drug monitoring is the steady state, which exists when the amount of drug leaving the body equals the amount entering. With many drugs, this point is reached after 5 half-lives (ie, after 5 doses given at intervals of 1 half-life each). When in the steady state, concentration of drug is lowest (trough) right before a dose, and highest shortly after (peak).

Free vs bound. Like many small molecules, a variable fraction of circulating drug is bound, usually to protein (such as albumin), and the remaining drug is free. The free drug is the therapeutically (and toxicologically) active component. When total protein is decreased, more free drug is available for a given dose; conversely, when total protein is increased, less free drug is available for a given dose. Furthermore, small molecules compete for binding spots, and a second drug may displace the first, leading to increased free drug concentrations.

Volume of distribution (V_d) The properties of a drug, in particular its size and solubility, influence how widely the drug is distributed in the body. Some drugs—that are extremely hydrophilic (lipophobic)—remain confined within the vascular space. Others are capable of distributing within the vascular and extravascular aqueous (interstitial) spaces, and others (very hydrophobic) distribute within the vascular, extravascular aqueous, and adipose tissue. The more of these spaces a drug can distribute into, the greater its V_d. A drug's V_d is usually expressed in liters and can be calculated, based upon the quantity of an administered dose (D) and resulting measured plasma concentration (C):

$$V_d = D \div C$$

Drugs of Abuse Screening (Forensic Toxicology) T1.18

- These drugs are often screened in the workplace, as part of a drug treatment program, in emergency care, and in legal settings. In emergency settings, a drug screen may be ordered to support the evaluation of patients with altered mental status, psychiatric presentations, certain metabolic disturbances, chest pain, and hypertension. Sometimes urine opiate screens are utilized to ensure that a prescribed opiate is being taken and not sold.

- Urine is the usual specimen for drug screening. In most cases, the urine is subjected to a panel of screening tests (a 'drugs of abuse screen'). These tests are designed for high sensitivity, and their specificity is fairly low. Screening drug tests are usually based upon an immunoassay. Several substances can cause cross-reacting false positives for any given assay in the panel, and every positive needs confirmation.

- If the screen is positive for a substance or if the history strongly implicates a particular substance, a confirmatory test can be ordered. These assays are designed for high specificity, and gas chromatography/mass spectrometry is the typical method.

T1.18
Selected Drugs of Abuse

Drug	$T_{1/2}$	$T_{detectable}$	Key Metabolite
Cocaine	1 hour	24-72 hours	benzoyl ecgonine methyl ester
Morphine	3 minutes	72 hours	N-acetyl morphine
Amphetamines	30 minutes	72 hours	norepinephrine & phenylacetone
PCP	30 minutes	72 hours	hydroxylated & glucuronated
Cannabis	8 hours	weeks	Δ-9-THC-COOH

■ In some settings, a witnessed collection is required to ensure that the urine sample has not been altered. In some settings, eg, federal workplaces, the specimen must be divided into two aliquots so that retesting can be performed if a positive result is obtained.

■ Chain of custody precautions are a requirement for any test that may have implications in criminal proceedings; eg, the specimens of a sexual assault kit or some instances of urine drug testing. This simply requires that the specimen is always in the custody of someone and that all times from the point of collection until the time of testing are accounted for. A document accompanies the specimen that is first endorsed by both the person contributing the specimen and the person collecting, labeling, and sealing the specimen and subsequently signed with a note of time and date by both parties each time the specimen changes hands. The specimen cannot be left unattended unless in locked storage.

■ **Adulterant detection.** Numerous substances have been added to urine for the purposes of producing a false-negative result. Several products are commercially available for this purpose. To detect these substances, it is routine to check the specimen color (eg, for the blue tinge of toilet water), odor (eg, for bleach), temperature (suspicious if cool), pH (suspicious if less than 4.5 or greater than 8.0), specific gravity (suspicious for dilution if <1.005), creatinine (suspicious if <5 mg/dL) and/or nitrite (suspicious if >500µg/mL).

Cocaine

■ The usual routes of administration are sniffing (the drug is absorbed across the nasal mucosa into the blood), injection, and smoking (crack, free-basing). Prolonged cocaine sniffing can lead to ulceration of the nasal mucosa and necrosis and collapse of the nasal septum. Laboratory testing for cocaine is primarily applied to detecting abuse, but testing may support the evaluation of patients in the emergency setting who present with chest pain or acute intoxication.

■ Chest pain

 □ Cocaine-induced chest pain has its basis in coronary vasoconstriction. This effect is compounded by an increase in heart rate and arterial blood pressure, which, over time, leads to left ventricular hypertrophy. There appears to be an atherogenic effect of prolonged cocaine use. While vasospasm can produce chest pain without myocardial infarction, in many patients a full myocardial infarction occurs.

 □ Cocaine must be considered in the differential diagnosis of chest pain, particularly in young patients with no risk factors for coronary artery disease. Chest pain usually arises within minutes of cocaine use, but may present many hours later. Patients are often not forthcoming with the history of cocaine use. Knowing that cocaine is involved influences both the immediate treatment and follow-up for chest pain, so a drug screen and confirmation has considerable clinical significance.

 □ Even when cocaine is known to be a factor, however, the differential diagnosis of cocaine-associated chest pain is lengthy. Considerations include pneumothorax (due to inhalational barotraumas), aortic dissection (due to hypertension), pulmonary embolus (due to clotting activation), and endocarditis (due to injection of cocaine).

 □ Due to skeletal muscle effects, the specificity of both myoglobin and CK-MB is lower in cocaine-induced acute myocardial infarction. The specificity of troponin I is equally good, however.

■ **Acute intoxication.** Cocaine induces the sympathetic nervous system, leading to tachycardia, hypertension, diaphoresis, mydriasis, and agitation. Severe intoxication may present with altered mental status or seizures. Patients often have raised temperature, and on hot days may present with hyperthermia. Hypertension may be quite severe and lead to a hypertensive emergency (defined as hypertension with end-organ damage). Lastly, a life-threatening arrhythmia may be induced.

Opiates

■ There are several abused opiates, including heroin, morphine, hydromorphone (dilaudid), oxycodone (oxycontin), and fentanyl (duragesic).

■ **Acute intoxication.** Opiates produce sedation, pinpoint pupils, constipation, bradycardia, and hypotension. Severe intoxication can present with altered mental status and respiratory arrest. Naloxone (narcan) and nalmefene are synthetic opioid antagonists that can be administered to treat opiate intoxication. Their use can be diagnostic as well as therapeutic, since failure to respond to an adequate dose essentially excludes opiate intoxication.

■ Symptoms of opiate withdrawal include increased lacrimation, rhinorrhea, diaphoresis, dilated pupils, tachycardia, irritability and restlessness. The symptoms can be lightened by the use of clonidine or methadone (dolophine) in tapering doses. Methadone is a long-acting, orally administered, opioid agonist with fewer central nervous system effects which is less addictive. However, methadone has itself become a substance of abuse. Clonidine does not interact with opioid receptors at all; rather, it antagonizes many of the sympathetic symptoms of opioid withdrawal.

■ Propoxyphene is an opioid which, in addition to producing the usual opioid-related toxicities, can cause unusual toxicities, such as cardiac conduction abnormalities and seizures. This is because both propoxyphene and its major metabolite (norpropoxyphene) cause a quinidine-like interference with sodium channels.

Barbiturates

■ Barbiturates are CNS depressants which can be life-threatening in both intoxication and withdrawal. They act through stimulating the release of γ-aminobutyric acid (GABA), an inhibitor in the central nervous system.

■ A large number of barbiturates are available, varying in onset and duration of pharmacologic effect. These include brevital (methohexital), pentothal (thiopental), nembutal (pentobarbital), seconal (secobarbital), and others.

■ Intoxication results in suppression of consciousness and respiratory suppression through direct action on the medulla. In addition, barbiturates impair myocardial function. Severe intoxication presents with altered mental status, hypotension, hypothermia, pulmonary edema, or respiratory arrest.

Amphetamines

■ Amphetamine and methamphetamine have stimulant properties mediated predominantly by the release of dopamine in the central nervous system.

■ An unfortunate consequence of long-term use is destruction of the dopamine-secreting cells upon which amphetamines exert their effect, resulting in an irreversible Parkinsonian syndrome.

■ Acute intoxication manifests with hyperpnea, hyperthermia, tachycardia, hypertension, anxiety and irritability. Severe intoxication may present with altered mental status, cerebral bleeds, or seizure.

Phencyclidine (PCP)

■ PCP may be ingested, injected, or smoked (by "dusting" tobacco or marijuana). It exerts its effects through blocking catecholamine re-uptake.

■ The psychiatric effects of PCP (aggressive or paranoid) are the usual cause of an emergency room visit. The effects of intoxication include hyperpnea, hypertension, and tachycardia. Horizontal nystagmus is often present and provides a clue to PCP use. The behavioral manifestations are characteristically fluctuating, thought to be a reflection of the marked lipid solubility of PCP, resulting in fluctuating blood levels. The behavioral effects include periods of remarkable calm and sedation interrupted by marked agitation, aggression, and incoordination. Many PCP-related emergencies, in fact, are trauma-related.

■ Severe intoxication, however, may present instead with hypoglycemia, hypotension, bradycardia, hypopnea, altered mental status, seizures, and/or life-threatening hyperthermia. Rhabdomyolysis may be induced by PCP.

■ In addition to toxicology testing, patients with PCP intoxication require immediate and serial glucose monitoring, CK, and BUN. Leukocytosis is a frequent nonspecific finding.

Ethanol T1.19

■ Ethanol is tested both as a drug of abuse and as a potential poisoning.

T1.19
Clinical Effects of Blood Alcohol

Blood Alcohol Concentration (%)	Clinical Effects
<0.05	Sobriety
0.05-0.1	Euphoria
0.1-0.2	Excitement
0.2-0.3	Confusion
0.3-0.4	Stupor
>0.4	Coma and death

- Ethanol is metabolized by hepatic alcohol dehydrogenase to acetaldehyde which is converted by aldehyde dehydrogenase to acetic acid.

- **Measurement.** The type of specimen depends on the clinical situation. Alcohol testing in an overdose evaluation is usually based upon serum or plasma. In forensic testing, either breath alcohol or whole blood alcohol is measured. Whole blood should be submitted in sodium fluoride and potassium oxalate to prevent both increases (due to fermentation) and decreases in ethanol concentration. Use of alcohol swabs on the venipuncture site should be avoided.

  - **Blood alcohol.** Using serum, plasma, or whole blood, an enzymatic procedure utilizing alcohol dehydrogenase is most often employed. This method is fairly specific for ethanol and doesn't measure other alcohols such as methanol.

  - **Breath alcohol.** This test is based on the principle that blood alcohol diffuses across alveolar septa and is excreted in expired air. The ratio of blood:breath alcohol is 2100:1. Thus, many statutes define the legal limit according to either the blood alcohol per dL or the breath alcohol per 210 L.

  - **Urine alcohol.** The urine alcohol can be correlated roughly with blood levels and clinical effects, it is mainly useful as a qualitative test of alcohol consumption.

- Most states define the legal limit for operation of a motor vehicle as 80-100 mg/dL (0.08-0.1 g/dL, 0.08%-0.1%, 0.8-1.0 g/L) in whole blood. Whole blood ethanol tends to run lower than serum or plasma ethanol concentration, and legal definitions are usually in terms of whole blood. One should not attempt to use a conversion formula, as conversion varies with hematocrit (**T1.19**).

- Gamma glutamyl transferase (GGT) is increased in heavy consumers of alcohol (more than 4 drinks per day for more than 4 weeks). Four or more weeks of abstinence are usually required for normalization of GGT.

- Carbohydrate-deficient transferrin (CDT) has been widely investigated as a biological marker of heavy alcohol consumption.

  - In general, CDT is at least as sensitive and probably more specific than gamma-glutamyl transferase (GGT). CDT levels require only about 1-2 weeks of heavy consumption before levels are raised. Because the two analytes are not highly correlated, their use in parallel enhances the sensitivity of detection of heavy alcohol consumption, especially in clinical populations.

  - Women produce more CDT under natural conditions and may produce less CDT in response to heavy drinking. In addition, there are some conditions such as severe liver disease in which higher than normal levels of CDT are produced, thereby reducing the specificity of this marker for detecting heavy drinking under certain conditions.

  - In the monitoring of alcoholics during treatment, changes in CDT individual baseline values seem to be more sensitive to lower level relapse drinking than is the use of raw cut-off values.

- The mean corpuscular volume (MCV) in increased in heavy alcohol consumption. Its sensitivity and specificity are modest, and at least 4-8 weeks of consumption are required to produce a measurable effect.

Overdose

- Laboratory evaluation of the apparent overdose may be guided by multiple considerations, including a history, when present, of exposure to a specific agent or the finding of a particular toxidrome. Toxidromes are constellations of findings that suggest a particular agent or group of agents (**T1.20**).

- Laboratory evaluation may include:

  - **Toxicology screening**

  - **Calculation of the anion gap.** An increase in the anion gap to >20 mEq/L is significant. It is important to note that some common conditions may lower the anion gap or mask a mildly increased anion gap. Chief among these is hypoalbuminemia; for every 1 gram decrease in albumin, there is a 2.5 mEq decrease in the anion gap. The differential diagnosis for an altered anion gap was given previously. Specific toxins that cause an increased anion gap metabolic acidosis include: acetaminophen, salicylates, ascorbate, hydrogen sulfide, ethylene glycol, methanol, ethanol, formaldehyde, carbon monoxide, nitroprusside, epinephrine, and paraldehyde.

Toxicology>Drugs of Abuse Screening; Overdose

T1.20
Common Toxidromes

Class	Signs	Agents
Anticholinergic	Hyperthermia, dry skin, flushing, altered mental status, psychosis ("hot as a hare, dry as a bone, red as a beet, mad as a hatter"), mydriasis, constipation	Atropine, Antihistamines, Tricyclics, Scopolamine
Cholinergic	Salivation, lacrimation, urination, diarrhea, GI cramps, emesis ("SLUDGE"); diaphoresis, miosis, and wheezing	Organophosphates, Pilocarpine, Carbamate
Adrenergic	Hypertension, tachycardia, mydriasis, anxiety, hyperthermia	Amphetamines, Cocaine, Pseudoephedrine Ephedrine, PCP
Sedative	Altered mental status, slurred speech, hypopnea/apnea	Barbiturates Alcohols Opiates
Narcotic	Altered mental status, hypopnea/apnea	Opiates
Hallucinogenic	Hallucinations, anxiety, hyperthermia	LSD PCP Amphetamines Cocaine

☐ **Calculation of the osmolal gap.** Sodium, glucose, and BUN normally account for all but about 5-10mOsm of the serum osmolarity (normal 285-295 mOsm/L). Some agents **T1.21** are capable of significantly altering serum osmolarity, and when they are present, the sum of the contributions of sodium, glucose, and BUN will not approximate serum osmolarity as well. Serum osmolarity is generally measured by freezing point depression osmometry, and this method will measure most alcohols (including ethanol, methanol, ethylene glycol, etc). However, the less commonly used vapor pressure method does not detect ethanol and methanol; thus, these two agents will not give an osmolal gap if vapor pressure osmometry is used. The difference between the measured serum osmolarity and the osmolarity calculated from sodium, glucose, and BUN is the osmolal gap. The osmolarity is calculated as: $2Na + BUN/2.8 + glucose/18$.

T1.21
Agents that Increase the Osmolal Gap

Ethanol
Ethylene glycol
Methanol
Isopropyl alcohol
Propylene glycol
Glycerol
Acetone
Mannitol
Radiocontrast media
Hypermagnesemia

☐ **Measurement of blood gases**

● Calculation of the oxygen saturation gap is the difference between the saturation given by co-oximetry and the saturation given by the ABG analyzer. Normally, the difference between these two determinations should be <5. An arterial blood gas (ABG) analyzer measures the oxygen tension (pO_2) and pH of blood and, assuming a standard hemoglobin oxygen affinity, calculates the percent oxygen saturation (percent oxyhemoglobin). A co-oximeter measures the light absorption of blood at numerous wavelengths and is capable of determining the proportion of oxyhemoglobin and deoxyhemoglobin (in addition to carboxyhemoglobin and methemoglobin, if present) directly. Thus, if there is a species of hemoglobin that cannot bind oxygen (eg, carboxyhemoglobin, methemoglobin), the ABG analyzer is likely to give a falsely normal (falsely high) reading. Furthermore, in these circumstances there will be a difference between percent oxyhemoglobin given by the ABG analyzer and that given by the co-oximeter. This difference is often called the oxygen saturation gap. Causes of an increased oxygen saturation gap include: carbon monoxide poisoning (carboxyhemoglobin), methemoglobin, hydrogen sulfide poisoning (sulfmethemoglobin), and cyanide poisoning.

T1.22
Toxic Alcohol Poisoning

Alcohol	Source	Anion Gap Acidosis	Osmolal Gap	Increased Ketones	Metabolite
Ethanol		–/+	+	–/+	
Ethylene glycol (1,2-ethanediol)	antifreeze	+	+	–	oxalate & glycolate
Isopropyl alcohol (isopropanol)	rubbing alcohol	–	+	–	acetone
Methanol (wood alcohol)	windshield washer fluid	+	+	–	formate & formaldehyde

- Confusingly, the term oxygen saturation gap is sometimes also used to refer to the difference between the percent oxyhemoglobin given by the ABG analyzer and that given by the pulse oximeter. The pulse oximeter measures transdermally by measuring absorption at two wavelengths. It measures oxyhemoglobin and deoxyhemoglobin directly, and does not differentiate carboxyhemoglobin and methemoglobin. When these abnormal hemoglobins are present, they will absorb light and give a falsely high reading to either the oxyhemoglobin or the deoxyhemoglobin, often in difficult to predict ways. For example, in the setting of methemoglobinemia: oxygen saturation by pulse-oximetry may be falsely high in severe methemoglobinemia and falsely low in mild methemoglobinemia. Carboxyhemoglobin has a maximal absorption similar to oxyhemoglobin, leading to a falsely high oxyhemoglobin by pulse-oximetry.

- Lastly, the difference between arterial and venous oxygen tension can be informative. An abnormally high venous oxygen content (arteriolization of venous blood) is seen in cyanide and hydrogen sulfide poisoning.

  □ Measurement or urinary pH may be required to monitor the efficacy of pH manipulation. Treating physicians commonly employ manipulation of the urinary pH to enhance drug excretion. Generally, the limits of urinary pH manipulation are 4.5 to 7.5 under conditions of enhanced acidification and alkalinization. Agents whose pKa are well outside this range pKa<3 or >8) tend to be unaffected by these maneuvers.

Toxic alcohol (ethylene glycol, methanol, and isopropyl alcohol) poisoning (T1.22)

- A toxic alcohol ingestion is suspected if the osmolal gap exceeds 10, suspected strongly if it exceeds 20. Direct laboratory tests for methanol and ethylene glycol are not available in most places, so the osmolal gap is used as a surrogate marker.

- Ethanol is often present in conjunction with toxic alcohol ingestion, and ethanol can by itself widen the osmolal gap. Thus, it may be useful to calculate this effect, based upon the measured ethanol concentration, so that the toxic alcohol level can be more accurately estimated:

$$2[Na] + [BUN]/2.8 + [glucose]/18 + [ethanol]/4.6$$

Toxicology>Overdose

■ Ingestion of ethylene glycol or methanol is in the differential diagnosis of metabolic acidosis with an increased anion gap and increased osmolal gap. Isopropyl alcohol (like ethanol) does not cause acidosis but does create an osmolal gap.

■ Ethylene glycol (found in antifreeze), methanol (windshield washer fluid, paint removers, wood alcohol) or isopropyl alcohol (rubbing alcohol) may be ingested accidentally, as readily available and cheap intoxicants, or in suicide attempts.

■ Ethylene glycol is metabolized to glycolic acid and then to oxalate by the action of alcohol dehydrogenase. Oxalate binds calcium to produce calcium oxalate, which is deposited in tissues. Glycolic acid is responsible for the CNS manifestations and for the anion gap acidosis. Calcium oxalate crystals can be found in the urine, where they appear envelope-shaped, translucent, and birefringent. In renal biopsies, they are found within renal tubules.

■ Methanol is metabolized to formaldehyde and then formic acid by alcohol dehydrogenase. These metabolites result in ocular toxicity, anion gap acidosis, and an osmolal gap.

■ Isopropyl alcohol (isopropanol) is metabolized to acetone. Isopropyl alcohol ingestion is strongly suspected when there is an increased osmolal gap, ketonemia/ketonuria, and neither acidosis nor increased anion gap.

■ Treatment consists of inhibiting the activity of alcohol dehydrogenase, since it is the metabolites that create the toxicity in the case of ethylene glycol and methanol. Traditionally, this was accomplished with the administration of ethanol. Ethanol competitively inhibits the formation of glycolic acid, oxalate, formaldehyde, and formic acid. A clinically significant consequence of this is that, in methanol or polyethylene glycol poisoning, concurrent ethanol use *delays the development of increased anion gap metabolic acidosis.* In such instances, the elevated osmolal gap may be the only clue to the correct diagnosis. Newer approaches include the administration of fomepizole and, if needed, dialysis.

Lead poisoning (plumbism)

■ Sources

□ **Household.** Lead paint, lead pipes

□ **Environmental.** Lead gasoline

□ **Industrial.** Manufacture of lead batteries, lead smelters, refurbishing lead-painted buildings

■ Mechanism

□ Lead enters the body through inhalation and ingestion. About 95% of ingested lead is distributed in erythrocytes and bone. Some also goes to the kidney where it is toxic to renal tubular cells. Lead is toxic to cells in 2 ways: it nonspecifically binds to and inhibits enzymes bearing sulfhydryl groups, and it is directly toxic to mitochondria.

□ Among the enzymes inhibited are many of the key enzymes involved in heme synthesis, particularly Δ-ALA-dehydratase and ferrochelatase. This leads to an accumulation of the immediate precursor of heme, protoporphyrin (free erythrocyte protoporphyrin or FEP). FEP binds non-enzymatically to available zinc, yielding zinc protoporphyrin (ZPP). Both FEP and ZPP are also raised in iron deficiency.

□ Lead inhibits sodium channel ATPases, leading to increased osmotic fragility and shortened red cell survival.

□ Basophilic stippling results from the inhibition of 5'-nucleotidase, an enzyme whose function is to breakdown RNA.

■ Iron deficiency and lead toxicity frequently coexist. The effect of iron deficiency is to enhance the toxic effects of lead in two ways:

□ The final step in biosynthesis of heme, in which iron is incorporated into protoporphyrin, is further inhibited by a deficiency of iron.

□ In an attempt to upregulate intestinal absorption of iron, there is the unintended effect of increased absorption of lead.

- Manifestations

  □ **Hematologic manifestations** include a microcytic, hypochromic anemia with basophilic stippling.

  □ **Neurologic manifestations** range from mild cognitive impairment to encephalopathy. Severity correlates somewhat with the rate of lead toxicity and absolute lead level.

  □ **Renal manifestations** occur following long-term lead toxicity. Mitochondrial toxicity leads to reduced ATP available to drive the numerous ATP-dependent channels involved in tubular epithelial function. The end-result is aminoaciduria, glycosuria, and phosphaturia (similar to Fanconi renal syndrome). Lead inclusions are detectable ultrastructurally as highly electron-dense rounded intracellular bodies.

  □ **Peripheral neuropathy** results in a classic (though rarely observed) bilateral wrist drop. It is also thought that the common presentation of abdominal pain in lead toxicity is due at least in part to sensory neuropathy.

- Testing

  □ Nonspecific laboratory findings in lead poisoning

    - anemia, microcytic and hypochromic, with basophilic stippling

    - elevated FEP and ZPP

    - proteinuria & glycosuria

  □ **Laboratory methods.** The CDC recommendation, made in 1978 and still upheld today, is that a blood lead level ≥10 g/dL should be considered elevated. Thus, screening requires an assay capable of detecting lead levels this low.

    - In the past, FEP or ZPP were used to screen for lead exposure. However, these tests are insensitive at levels of lead below 35 mg/dL. Furthermore, they may be elevated in other conditions, most notably iron deficiency. Their advantage is that they can be performed on capillary blood samples and they easily detect moderate to severe lead toxicity. One further advantage is that blood lead levels tend to misleadingly 'rebound' during treatment, so that the FEP and ZPP can be used to distinguish this phenomenon from a true increase in lead toxicity.

- A blood lead level, determined by atomic absorption spectrophotometry, is the preferred method screen for lead toxicity. It is capable of detecting lead levels below the 10 μg/dL threshold . A venous sample is necessary for this determination, as capillary blood obtained from heel- or finger-sticks can give erroneous results. Furthermore, a repeat for confirmation of any abnormal screening test is advised.

- The calcium disodium ethylenediaminic acid (CaNa-EDTA) test is designed to assess the degree to which lead will be mobilized by chelation therapy. An intravenous dose of CaNa-EDTA is given followed by an 8-hour urine collection. The amount of lead excreted in the urine is determined. This test is sometimes administered prior to initiation of chelation therapy.

- **Treatment.** At low levels (10-20 μg/dL), environmental interventions may be all that is indicated. Beyond that, both environmental interventions and chelation therapy are indicated. A level >70 μg/dL is considered an indication for inpatient monitoring and treatment. Chelators include dimercaprol (also known as British antilewisite or BAL), CaNa-EDTA, D-penicillamine, and succimer.

Carbon monoxide (CO) poisoning T1.23

- CO binds tightly (with 200 times the affinity of oxygen) to hemoglobin forming carboxyhemoglobin (Hb-CO), thus reducing the available binding sites for oxygen. CO has even greater avidity for fetal hemoglobin, placing infants (and fetuses) at great risk. Furthermore, CO is directly toxic to intracellular oxidative mechanisms and appears to enhance production of nitric oxide (NO).

T1.23
Clinical Effects of Carbon Monoxide Poisoning

Level of CO	Clinical Findings
0.4%-2%	Normal nonsmoker
2%-6%	Normal smoker
10%-20%	Mild symptoms: dyspnea on exertion
20%-50%	Severe symptoms: intoxication, with headache, lethargy, loss of consciousness
>50%	Coma and death

- CO is produced in the environment when there is partial combustion of carbon-containing fossil fuels (complete oxidation leads to CO_2 production). It is produced endogenously from only one source: the breakdown heme. Endogenous production usually results in Hb-CO levels ≤ 1%. Carbon monoxide is also generated in the hepatic metabolism of dichloromethane (methylene chloride), found in paint and varnish removers.

- Accidental poisoning results most often from house fires, engine exhaust, indoor heaters, and stoves. In fact, unventilated burning of charcoal or gas is a common source of poisoning during power outages in the winter. Intentional poisoning is a common means of suicide.

- Hb-CO can be measured by the co-oximeter, and venous blood is as good as arterial for this determination. Hb-CO levels correlate well with clinical effects **T1.23**; however, there is some variability in the clinical effects of the 20%-60% range. Remember that blood gas analyzers, in contrast to co-oximeters, do not measure hemoglobin variants and determine oxyhemoglobin by calculation. Pulse oximetry may give a falsely reassuring oxygen saturation. The oxygen gap (difference between pulse oximetry and co-oximetry) reflects the level of Hb-CO.

- Additional laboratory testing in support of the patient with CO poisoning may include measurement of lactate, calculation of the anion gap, myocardial markers, and cyanide levels (smoke inhalation also poses a risk of cyanide inhalation, depending upon the materials present in the fire).

- CO is eliminated by slowly being replaced by oxygen on hemoglobin molecules. The half-life of CO depends on the oxygen tension. The $T_{1/2}$ on room air is about 6 hours, while the $T_{1/2}$ on 100% O_2 is 1 hour.

Acetaminophen (Tylenol®) poisoning

- The clinical course of acute acetaminophen overdose is polyphasic. Initially (phase I), there may be mild nausea and abdominal discomfort, which is self-limited and abates over a matter of hours. Later, often days later (usually >24 hours), there is progressive liver injury (phase II). This leads to fulminant hepatic failure (phase III), after which there is resolution (phase IV) in the form of complete recovery, liver transplant, or death.

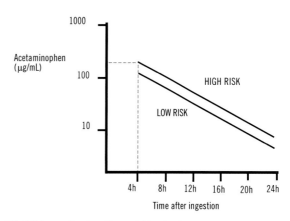

F1.10 Acetaminophen (Rumack-Matthew) nomogram

- The great danger is hepatic failure, but the majority of acetaminophen poisonings do not result in significant hepatic necrosis. For patients who present in the first phase, practitioners may utilize the Rumack-Matthew nomogram **F1.10** to predict which patients are at risk. If the approximate time of ingestion is known, the initial blood samples should be drawn no earlier than 4 hours following ingestion (this is the time it takes for full absorption). The serum acetaminophen concentration and time since ingestion can predict hepatic necrosis and whether ICU admission and N-acetyl cysteine treatment are indicated. The nomogram stratifies patients into: probable hepatic toxicity, possible hepatic toxicity, and no hepatic toxicity. N-acetylcysteine is indicated for patients falling into the first two categories. ICU admission is indicated for those falling into the first category. The Rumack-Mathew nomogram should be used only in the setting of a single acute ingestion.

- In cases presenting late, samples drawn greater than 2-3 hours apart can be used to estimate the elimination half-life of acetaminophen in the patient. If the half-life is >4 hours, then hepatic necrosis is likely. Furthermore, any single acetaminophen level >5 μg/mL places the patient at high risk.

- In healthy individuals, the potentially toxic dose is any over about 150 mg/kg.

- False positive acetaminophen levels have been reported in hyperbilirubinemic patients. Because of its broad spectrophotometric absorbance, bilirubin can interfere with numerous assays based upon this format, but bilirubin's interference with acetaminophen assays appears to be more complex than this and nonlinear.

- The liver handles acetaminophen in two main pathways. Most of it is conjugated with glucuronide or sulfate to form *nontoxic* metabolites. A small amount is metabolized by the P_{450} system into the *toxic* metabolite N-acetyl-p-benzoquinoneimine (NAPQI). NAPQI is normally detoxified by glutathione, but glutathione reserves are quickly overwhelmed in toxic ingestions. Furthermore, any agent that induces the P_{450} system increases the proportion of acetaminophen processed to NAPQI, enhancing toxicity. Chronic ethanol use, for example, has this effect.

- NAPQI is the primary cause of hepatotoxicity. This toxic metabolite induces centrilobular (zone 3) hepatic necrosis with periportal sparing. Its formation within hepatocytes makes the liver the primary target, but other organs may be affected.

- *N*-acetylcysteine (mucomyst) is the mainstay of treatment. Mucomyst promotes metabolism via the conjugation pathways, thereby decreasing the formation of the toxic metabolite NAPQI.

Cyanide poisoning

- Cyanide poisoning may be due to inhalation of smoke from a fire (present in insulation), industrial exposure (present in pesticides and other industrial materials), or suicide/homicide attempt.

- Cyanide binds to and inhibits cytochrome a3, thus uncoupling the electron transport system. This results in diminished oxygen-dependent metabolism and severe anion-gap metabolic (lactic) acidosis. Oxygen accumulates in the blood, giving rise to the typical bright cherry-red skin color.

- Patients exposed to very high concentrations develop hyperpnea and loss of consciousness, followed within several minutes by apnea. Those exposed to smaller quantities may follow a slower course, complaining initially of headache, weakness, dyspnea, and altered mental status, but obtundation and death will usually occur even with small exposures. Due to the presence of HCN gas, an exposed patient's breath often has a bitter almond odor; however, only about 50% of the population is capable of detecting this odor.

- Cyanide levels can be measured, but cyanide is rapidly metabolized to thiocyanate. Thiocyanate persists for a long period of time and is more reliable for the diagnosis of cyanide exposure. Neither test is commonly available acutely, however, so that a clinical suspicion in conjunction with surrogate markers are important in making the diagnosis.

- While not specific, all patients exposed to cyanide should have an elevated serum lactate and an anion gap metabolic acidosis. Furthermore, the plasma lactate concentration correlates linearly with the cyanide concentration, and a normal lactate essentially excludes the diagnosis.

- Cyanide-poisoned patients usually have an elevated serum glucose (due to decreased utilization).

- Blood gases, performed by co-oximetry, can be extremely informative. First, if compared to venous blood, a decrease in the arterial-venous oxygen gap (due to decreased utilization) is consistent with cyanide toxicity. Second, the co-oximeter can specifically measure carboxyhemoglobin and methemoglobin, removing them from the differential diagnosis.

- Treatment Administration of sodium nitrite and amyl nitrite leads to formation of methemoglobin, which binds available cyanide. Sodium thiosulfate, which reacts with cyanomethemoglobin to form thiocyanate, a harmless compound that can be cleared by the kidneys, is administered next.

Salicylate (Aspirin)

- Aspirin exerts conflicting effects upon acid-base balance. First, it directly stimulates the respiratory center within the medulla oblongata, promoting respiratory alkalosis. Second, it uncouples oxidative phosphorylation and inhibits Krebs cycle, shunting energy production towards anaerobic pathways with the development of a metabolic acidosis.

- The earliest manifestations of salicylate toxicity include tinnitus and dizziness.

- The acid-base disorder caused by salicylate is triphasic:

  □ Initially, direct stimulation of the respiratory center leads to hyperventilation and respiratory alkalosis. This effect is maximally exerted between 3-8 hours following ingestion.

  □ The physiologic response creates is a compensatory metabolic acidosis. It is in this stage, between 12-24 hours, that patients usually present.

  □ Alterations in metabolic pathways, in addition to a progressive loss in buffering capacity, finally conspire to cause an **increased anion gap metabolic acidosis**. At this stage, CNS depression may contribute to hypoventilation and a compounding respiratory acidosis.

- Mortality is best correlated with the 6-hour plasma salicylate concentration, with values of >130 mg/dL having a high fatality rate.

- Chronic salicylate intoxication manifests as a chronic metabolic acidosis, hypoglycemia, and possible hearing loss.

Arsenic

- Though technically a metalloid, arsenic appears in the toxicology literature within the category of heavy metal toxicity (in addition to lead, mercury, and others).

- Arsenic is a traditional agent in attempted homicide. It usually acquired accidentally, however, through exposure to various pesticides, wood preservatives, and leather tanning. It occasionally contaminates water supplies. It is found in gaseous form (arsine gas) in certain industries, particularly the production of metal alloys and semiconductor manufacture. Arsine gas is the most toxic form of arsenic, capable of producing acute renal failure, hemolysis, and death within 24-48 hours.

- Ingested arsenic is largely excreted in urine, with most of the remainder distributed into skin, nails, and hair.

- Through a variety of mechanisms, arsenic inhibits oxidative production of ATP. Thus, initial toxicity is manifested in dividing tissue such as GI mucosa, with nausea, vomiting, bloody diarrhea, and abdominal pain. The marrow is affected, causing cytopenias (with erythrocyte basophilic stippling similar to that seen in lead toxicity). Chronic toxicity results in peripheral neuropathy, nephropathy, skin hyperpigmentation and hyperkeratosis (particularly palms and soles), and transverse Mees lines in the nails.

- Samples for the diagnosis of chronic intoxication may include fingernails, hair, or urine. The most reliable test is a quantitative 24-hour urinary arsenic excretion; however, this result may be misleadingly elevated due to recent seafood ingestion. A blood arsenic level is highly unreliable, as the substance is rapidly cleared from circulation. Arsenic detection in hair and nails may reflect prolonged exposure.

Tricyclic antidepressants (TCAs)

- TCAs exert their beneficial effect by blocking reuptake of dopamine and epinephrine from the synaptic space.

- There are also anticholinergic effects, more or less profound depending upon the particular agent (strongest for amitriptyline). Many of the adverse reactions within the therapeutic range (dry mouth, constipation, urinary retention), and some of the adverse effects in toxic ranges (papillary dilation, hyperthermia, lethargy, confusion) relate to this effect.

■ The major adverse consequences of tricyclic overdose take place within the central nervous and cardiac conduction systems. TCAs cause widening of the QRS complex (QRS prolongation) that can lead to ventricular arrhythmias. A QRS interval longer than 0.16 seconds is strongly associated with arrhythmia. Furthermore, the duration of the QRS is predictive of the likelihood of seizures, with a QRS interval longer than 0.1 seconds associated with a high risk of seizure.

Organophosphates and Carbamates

■ Organophosphates and carbamates are found in insecticides used in agriculture.

■ These chemicals inhibit acetylcholinesterase, the enzyme involved in breakdown of the neurotransmitter acetylcholine at synaptic and neuromuscular junctions. This results in over stimulation of cholinergic processes.

■ The classic presentation is a farmer who presents with miosis (pinpoint pupils), diaphoresis, excess salivation, lacrimation, gastrointestinal hypermotility, bradycardia and bronchospasm. This constellation of symptoms is often referred to as the muscarinic toxidrome.

■ The laboratory's role is to test the level of erythrocyte cholinesterase activity. Alternatively, metabolites can be detected in the urine up to 1 week after exposure.

Mercury

■ Mercury is an occupational hazard, most notorious for intoxication of hat makers ("mad hatter's disease"). Elemental mercury is a liquid at room temperature, and toxic exposure to mercury usually occurs through inhalation of the vapor. Ingestion of elemental mercury is largely inconsequential, as GI absorption does not occur to any significant degree. Recently, however, intoxication with organic mercury has been increasingly recognized, resulting from the ingestion of fish. Organic mercury is readily absorbed in the GI tract.

■ While acute elemental mercury toxicity manifests as respiratory distress and renal failure, chronic mercury toxicity takes the form of either one of two characteristic syndromes: acrodynia or erethism.

□ Acrodynia (Feer syndrome) manifests with autonomic manifestations (sweating, hemodynamic instability) and a desquamative erythematous rash on the palms and soles. Feer syndrome is associated with increased urinary catecholamines and can in many ways mimic pheochromocytoma.

□ Erethism is a central nervous system disorder manifesting as personality changes, irritability, and fine motor disturbances.

■ Organic mercury toxicity manifests as visual field constriction, peripheral neuropathy, tremor, and hearing loss. Importantly, inorganic mercury readily crosses the placenta, resulting in infants with severe neurologic impairment.

■ A 24-hour urine collection is essential for diagnosis or elemental mercury poisoning. Organic mercury, however, is not significantly excreted in urine. Whole blood or hair analysis is needed for the diagnosis of organic mercury toxicity.

Therapeutic Drug Monitoring (TDM)

Digoxin

■ Routine measurement of digoxin concentrations in patients who are stable on therapy is not widely recommended. Monitoring may be indicated, however, when there is a change in dose, a change in the patient's renal function, or a change in concomitantly administered medications. Digoxin is primarily excreted by the kidneys and has a long half-life, around 36 hours. Samples for digoxin levels should be drawn approximately 8-12 hours after the last dose, ideally about 8-10 days after a dose change.

■ While serum samples are important, both the efficacy and the toxicity of digoxin may best measured by clinical parameters (heart rate, etc).

■ Renal function tests should be performed initially do guide initial dosing.

■ Factors that increase digoxin toxicity: hypokalemia, hypercalcemia, hypomagnesemia, hypoxia, hypothyroidism, quinidine, and calcium channel blockers.

■ Quinidine, in addition to enhancing end-organ effects of digoxin, frees digoxin from protein binding sites and impairs digoxin clearance. For all these reasons, digoxin levels and the risk of digoxin toxicity are markedly enhanced by concomitant administration of quinidine.

■ Digoxin-like Immunoreactive Substances (DLIS) or Endogenous Digoxin-Like Substances (EDLS). Digoxin cross-reactivity is found in the blood of some individuals who are not taking digoxin. This finding is particularly common in neonates, pregnant women, liver failure and renal failure.

Procainamide

- Procainamide is cleared predominantly by the liver. Hepatic impairment leads to slower excretion.

- Procainamide is metabolized to N-acetylprocainamide (NAPA), which has pharmacologic activity of its own. The rate of conversion to NAPA is determined by the concentration of hepatic acetyltransferase, which is genetically determined. So-called fast acetylators, who have genetically high levels of acetyltransferase, will have higher levels of NAPA. Furthermore, NAPA clearance is predominantly renal clearance. Thus, high levels of NAPA are found in renal insufficiency and in fast acetylators.

- Both procainamide and NAPA have biologic activity, and the levels of both should be measured. Usually the sum of procainamide and NAPA are considered for making dosing decisions.

- Procainamide is a cause of drug-induced lupus that is not dose-dependent.

Aminoglycosides (eg, gentamicin)

- Aminoglycosides are mainly cleared by the kidneys. Patients with renal impairment require lower doses, less frequent doses, or both.

- Ideally, the gentamicin trough specimen is drawn immediately before a dose, and the peak is drawn 30 minutes after the completion of a dose.

Quinidine

- The class IA antiarrhythmic agents include quinidine, disopyramide, and procainamide, which function by blocking sodium and potassium channels in cardiac conduction fibers.

- The typical manifestations of quinidine toxicity include altered mental status, cinchonism (tinnitus, vertigo, blurred vision), a widening of the QRS complex, a prolonged QT interval, and hypotension (without compensatory tachycardia). Conditions associated with a prolonged QT interval raise the likelihood of ventricular arrhythmias, particularly a polymorphic ventricular tachycardia called Torsades de pointes. This sort of presentation, particularly the prolonged QT interval, CNS changes, and hypotension, can result from numerous conditions, including tricyclic antidepressants, phenothiazines, and electrolyte abnormalities.

- Quinidine is cleared by the liver. Quinidine levels are not routinely used to predict toxicity, and the ECG is more reliable in this regard. It is important to check and correct electrolyte levels.

Phenytoin

- Early manifestations of phenytoin toxicity include ocular dysmotility (particularly horizontal gaze nystagmus), ataxia, and incoordination. More severe toxicity is associated with altered mental status and cardiac conduction disturbances. Interestingly, oral phenytoin overdose has not been associated with significant cardiac conduction abnormalities; whereas, intravenous overdose often produces a prolonged PR interval (AV block), hypotension, and a risk of arrhythmia. It appears that this discrepancy and the arrhythmogenic effects of IV intoxication are due to the propylene glycol diluent instead of quinidine.

- Phenytoin toxicity may result from overdosage as concomitant use of agents that decrease clearance (inhibition of the cytochrome P_{450} system) or increase free drug concentrations (hypoproteinemia, drugs that compete for albumin binding sites).

- Fetal hydantoin syndrome is the result of intrauterine exposure. It is characterized by intrauterine growth retardation, microcephaly, mental retardation, midfacial hypoplasia, hypertelorism, a flattened philtrum, and shortened nose.

Lithium

- The margin between therapeutic effect and toxicity is a narrow one for lithium. The therapeutic range varies from 0.4–1.2 mmol/L. And while some toxicity can be seen in the upper reaches of this range, 1.5 mmol/L is the level at which the risk of adverse effects becomes extremely high.

- Several guidelines have been proposed for the routine monitoring of lithium therapy (patients who are stable on therapy) with a range of recommended monitoring intervals of 1-3 months. For routine monitoring, a sample should be taken at 12 hours following the last dose.

- Following initiation of lithium and following a change in dose, since the half-life for lithium varies from 8-40 hours (depending largely upon age and renal function) steady state conditions would be expected between 2 and 8 days. Checking levels after a period of 3 days to 1 week is recommended.

Amiodarone

- Amiodarone levels should not necessarily be routinely monitored in the stable patient. In this situation, many advocate the use of other monitors such as the function of organs known to be affected by amiodarone toxicity or the monitoring of desethylamiodarone (an amiodarone metabolite) or the amiodarone to desethylamiodarone ratio.

- The major risks due to amiodarone include pulmonary toxicity (incidence of 1% annually), thyroid toxicity (hypothyroidism 5%-15%, hyperthyroidism 1%-2%), hepatotoxicity (0.6%), and peripheral neuropathy (0.3%). Thus, at baseline and every 6 months it is recommended that there be thyroid function testing and liver function testing, in addition to annual chest X-ray and ECG.

- Amiodarone reduces the clearance of warfarin, and can thereby prolong the INR. This effect is usually fully manifest by 7 weeks of co-treatment with amiodarone and coumadin, so that close INR monitoring needs only be carried out for that period of time.

- Amiodarone increases digoxin concentrations, and doses of digoxin must be reduced while closely monitoring digoxin concentrations.

Lipids and Carbohydrates

Lipids

Brief review of lipids

- The major lipids found in plasma are cholesterol, triglyceride (TG), and phospholipid.

  □ TG is composed of 3 fatty acids extending from a glycerol group. Fatty acids are linear hydrocarbons that come in several lengths: short chain (4-6 carbons), medium chain (8-12 carbons), and long chain (>12 carbons). In addition, some fatty acids have only single bonds between carbons and thus

have the maximum number of attached hydrogen ions (saturated fatty acids), some have one double bond somewhere along their length and thus have 1 fewer hydrogen (monounsaturated), and some have several double bonds (polyunsaturated). In general, unsaturated fatty acids provide more fluidity than saturated fatty acids.

  □ Phospholipid is composed of two fatty acids extending from a glycerol group, with the third spot on glycerol occupied by a phosphatidyl group (such as phosphatidylcholine).

  □ Cholesterol is composed of 4 rings, a hydrocarbon side chain, and a hydroxyl group.

- Lipids are insoluble in aqueous media such as plasma and therefore must be packaged into lipoprotein particles that have a hydrophilic exterior by virtue of a phospholipid coat. Embedded in the external phospholipid layer are the various apolipoproteins. In the center of the lipoprotein particle are cholesterol and TG. Every lipoprotein contains cholesterol, TG, phospholipids, and apolipoproteins. However, 5 different lipoprotein classes are identified based on the various proportions of these 4 constituents and the particular apolipoproteins they possess **T1.24**.

- Ingested lipids are internalized by small bowel enterocytes and packaged into the first class of lipoproteins, called chylomicrons. These have low density due to a large TG component and, among others, contain the apolipoprotein B-48. The chylomicron is the lipoprotein that transports lipid from enterocytes to other somatic cells, particularly hepatocytes, into which they are endocytosed via apolipoprotein E.

- In the liver, cholesterol and TG undergo additional metabolism before being packaged, for secretion into the blood, into another class of lipoproteins called very low density lipoprotein (VLDL). VLDL has low density due to a large TG component and bears the apolipoproteins B-100, C, and E. VLDL is the vehicle for transport of TG to somatic cells.

T1.24
Lipoprotein Classes

Lipoprotein	Electrophoretic Mobility	Average Density (g/mL)	Major lipid	Protein (%)	Apolipoproteins
Chylomicrons	origin	0.95	TG	1	B-48, A-1, C, E
VLDL	pre-β	1.0	TG	8	B-100, C, E
IDL	pre-β/β	1.02	Cholesterol	15	B-100, E
LDL	β	1.04	Cholesterol	20	B-100
HDL	α	1.10	Cholesterol	50	A-1, C, E

- In the blood, the TG in VLDL undergoes progressive hydrolysis by the endothelium-based enzyme, lipoprotein lipase (LPL). Over time, enough TG is removed from VLDL to increase its density to that of intermediate density lipoprotein (IDL) and, eventually, low density lipoprotein (LDL). The typical LDL particle has lost most of its TG and a good bit of its apolipoproteins C and E, leaving predominantly phospholipid, cholesterol and apolipoprotein B-100. LDL is the main vehicle for transporting cholesterol to somatic cells where LDL particles undergo endocytosis mediated by the LDL receptor and apolipoprotein B-100.

- The liver also produces a class of lipoproteins called high density lipoprotein (HDL) that contains a small amount of lipid, mainly phospholipid and cholesterol, the enzyme lecithin cholesterol acyl transferase (LCAT), and apolipoproteins, especially apolipoprotein A-1. The function of HDL appears to be the scavenging of cholesterol from the periphery and returning it to the liver.

Methods

- **Quantification of lipids.** Since lipid levels are affected by diet, alcohol consumption, physical stress such as exercise, smoking, and posture, standard conditions, including a 12-hour fast, should surround the blood collection. Initially, the total cholesterol, HDL, and TG are determined, and LDL is usually calculated.

  - Total cholesterol is usually measured enzymatically. A series of enzymatic reactions is used to produce a color change in a dye, measured by a spectrophotometer. The spectrophotometric reading is calibrated to be proportional to a quantity of cholesterol.

- G measurement, like total cholesterol measurement, is usually carried out by a sequence of enzymatic reactions, a dye product of which is measured spectrophotometrically. VLDL cholesterol is often estimated as TG ÷ 5 (when expressed in mg/dL) or TG ÷ 2.2 (when expressed in mmol/L). This estimation is valid in most circumstances but fails when TG is greater than 400 mg/dL, chylomicrons are present, or there is β-VLDL characteristic of the very rare type III dyslipidemia.

- HDL cholesterol is usually measured by an enzymatic sequence similar or identical to that for total cholesterol, after removal of non-HDL lipoproteins. This initial removal step may take the form of selective precipitation by manual chemical pretreatment, followed by a cholesterol determination performed on the supernatant. This method may also require ultracentrifugation to remove VLDL and chylomicrons when they are increased. Alternatively, in what are called homogenous assays, a polymer, detergent, or enzyme is used to inactivate non-HDL cholesterol, followed by a cholesterol determination. The *homogenous* assays are amenable to automation, without a manual step.

- Separation of LDL from other lipoproteins, in order to directly measure LDL cholesterol, is extremely difficult. Consequently, LDL is usually calculated, using the Friedewald equation.

- The Friedewald equation: LDL cholesterol = total cholesterol—HDL cholesterol—TG/5

- The Friedewald calculation is not considered valid for TG>400, if chylomicrons are present, or in type III dyslipidemia.

● Direct methods for measuring the LDL choles-terol include ultracentrifugation, electrophoresis, and homogeneous assays. Ultracentrifugation is a tedious and technically difficult technique not well-suited for routine use. Ultracentrifugation remains the gold standard for method compari-son, however. In a way similar to SPEP, lipopro-teins can be subjected to electrophoresis on agarose gel then scanned densitometrically to give quantitative results. Current electrophoretic techniques yield fairly reliable quantitation; fur-thermore, they provide a display that can be ana-lyzed visually to help classify lipid disorders. Still, the electrophoretic technique, due to the labor and expertise required, is not suitable for routine use in all labs. Most recently, so-called homoge-neous assays were introduced that can be auto-mated. These assays employ detergents to block or dissolve all but LDL, permitting direct enzy-matic measurement of LDL-cholesterol.

■ **Quantifying lipoproteins**

☐ The individual lipoproteins differ in density from one another, so that by ultracentrifugation, they can be separated into the various types and quantified. It is uncommon to have access to ultracentrifugation in routine laboratory practice; however, its use remains integral in reference methods for lipopro-tein measurement.

☐ Lipoprotein electrophoresis is performed on a gel in a manner similar to protein electrophoresis, and stained with a fat stain such as Oil Red O or Sudan Black B. Chylomicrons do not move from the point of application. LDL migrates in the β region, VLDL in the pre-β region, and HDL in the α **T1.25**. For these reasons, LDL is often referred to as β-lipopro-tein and HDL is called α-lipoprotein. This method is employed as a basis for qualitative analysis of lipoprotein classes but is not suitable for quantita-tive analysis.

☐ Overnight refrigeration produces characteristic pat-terns in plasma, depending upon the lipoprotein profile. The presence of a creamy layer atop the plas-ma indicates the presence of excess chylomicrons. Turbidity or opacity of the plasma below this indi-cates abundant VLDL. LDL and HDL, even when present in excess, do not visibly alter the plasma.

T1.25

Classification of Lipid Disorders by Lipoprotein Electrophoresis

Phenotype	Lipoprotein Electrophoresis	Lipoproteins Increased
Normal	origin β pre-β α	None
I	Chylomicrons (origin) increased	Chylomicrons
IIa	β increased	LDL
IIb	pre-β & β increased	LDL & VLDL
III	β increased and very *broad* β	IDL
IV	pre-β increased	VLDL
V	Chylomicrons & pre-β increased	VLDL & Chylomicrons

Lipids and Carbohydrates>Lipids

- **Quantifying specific apolipoproteins.** The apoproteins currently thought to be clinically relevant are: Apo B, Apo A1, and Lp(a). Immunoassays are available for the measurement of each.

  □ Apo B is the major apolipoprotein of LDL and VLDL.

  □ Apo A1 is the major apolipoprotein of HDL.

  □ Lp(a).

Lipid disorders

- **Classification.** A confusing aspect of lipid disorders is that there are two major ways of conceptually classifying them. In the first, one looks at the lipoprotein profile, while the second is concerned more specifically with the serum concentrations of cholesterol and TG. If one recalls that VLDL and chylomicrons contain predominantly TG, while LDL contains predominantly cholesterol, the two concepts correlate fairly well.

- **Clinical manifestations T1.26.** Premature atherosclerosis is the most notorious consequence of hyperlipidemia. This complication is seen whenever there is abnormally high LDL or IDL; that is, whenever the cholesterol is too high. It is not a prominent feature when only the TG is elevated. Eruptive xanthomas, presenting as crops of yellow, pruritic, papulonodules, are seen with elevated TG (chylomicrons or VLDL). Tendinous (tuberous) xanthomas are seen near the knees or elbows and appear when there are simultaneous elevations in TG and cholesterol (elevated IDL). Xanthelasma are yellow periorbital papules that are associated with high cholesterol (LDL). Acute pancreatitis is associated with elevated TG (chylomicrons or VLDL), particularly when > 5-10 mmol/L.

- **Predominant hypercholesterolemia.** Generally considered to exist when the plasma total cholesterol exceeds 200 mg/dL, hypercholesterolemia is usually related to elevated LDL. In lipoprotein electrophoresis, it may fall into patterns II or III. Secondary causes of hypercholesterolemia are hypothyroidism, diabetes mellitus, nephrotic syndrome, cholestasis, cyclosporine, thiazide diuretics, or loop diuretics. The most common primary cause of hypercholesterolemia is familial hypercholesterolemia, an autosomal dominant deficiency in LDL receptors.

T1.26

Classification of Lipid Disorders by Predominant Lipids

Disorder	Phenotype	Cholesterol	TG	Clinical features
Familial LPL deficiency	I	↑	↑↑↑	Eruptive xanthomas, pancreatitis
Familial apo C-II deficiency	I or V	↑	↑↑↑	Pancreatitis
Familial hypercholesterolemia	IIa	↑↑↑	→↑	Tendinous xanthomas, premature atherosclerosis
Apolipoprotein E deficiency	IIb	↑↑↑	↑↑↑	Eruptive xanthomas, premature atherosclerosis
Familial dysbetalipoproteinemia	III	↑↑↑	↑↑↑	
Familial combined hyperlipidemia	II or IV	↑	↑	Premature atherosclerosis
Familial hypertiglyceridemias	IV or V	↑	↑↑↑	Eruptive xanthomas, pancreatitis

- **Predominant hypertriglyceridemia.** This is related to elevated chylomicrons or VLDL. Hypertriglyceridemia is not an independent risk factor for coronary artery disease when considered together with the LDL and HDL. A very common secondary cause of this is heavy alcohol consumption. It may also be secondary to: obesity, diabetes mellitus, hepatitis, pregnancy, renal failure, b-blockers, isotretinoin, corticosteroids, nephrotic syndrome, and gout. Primary causes include familial combined hyperlipidemia, familial LPL deficiency, familial apo C-II deficiency, and familial hypertriglyceridemia.

- **Mixed hypertriglyceridemia and hypercholesterolemia.** This finding is most common in severe examples of diabetes mellitus, hypothyroidism, or nephrotic syndrome. It may also be seen with type III hyperlipidemia, thiazides, loop diuretics, and b-blockers. Primary causes include familial combined hyperlipidemia.

- **Low levels of HDL cholesterol.** This, defined as HDL <35 mg/dL, is an independent risk factor for premature atherosclerosis. A high HDL, greater than 70 mg/dL, is protective. Tangier disease is an autosomal recessive disorder of lipid metabolism characterized by low cholesterol, normal to increased TG, absent HDL, and absence of APO-A1. Cholesterol esters deposit in the tonsils, lymph nodes, vasculature, and spleen, and corneal opacities develop. HDL cholesterol may also be reduced by smoking, obesity, sedentary lifestyle, and anabolic steroids.

Lipids in the assessment of coronary artery disease (CAD) risk

- **The National Cholesterol Education Program** (NCEP) has been providing guidelines for cholesterol testing and treatment since 1988. Their most recent guidelines, the 3rd Adult Treatment Panel report (ATP III) reaffirms the traditional major risk factors for coronary artery disease: smoking, hypertension, low HDL, family history of premature CAD, and age (>45 years for men and >55 years for women). ATP III is also the first iteration to recognize the potential significance of the metabolic syndrome (syndrome X).

T1.27
ATP III Cholesterol Classification

Total Cholesterol (mg/dL)	Desirable <200 Borderline 200-239 High >240
LDL (mg/dL)	Optimal < 100 Near optimal 100-129 Borderline 130-159 High 160-189 Very high >190
HDL (mg/dL)	Low <40 High >60

- Whereas ATP II recommended a screening measurement of TC and HDL-C (fasting not required) and a fasting lipoprotein profile only in those at increased risk, ATP III recommends a fasting lipoprotein profile (including total cholesterol (TC), LDL cholesterol, HDL cholesterol, and triglyceride) in all. In a non-fasting patient, the TGs and calculated LDL-C are not considered valid.

- ATP III further recommends specific cholesterol and LDL targets (**T1.27, T1.28**)

Carbohydrates

- Insulin leads to an increase in cellular uptake of glucose from the blood and leads to an increase in overall intracellular anabolic activity: conversion of glucose to glycogen (glycogenesis), increased conversion of carbohydrates to fatty acids (lipogenesis), etc. This is noted in the peripheral blood as a decrease in blood glucose.

- Several agents act counter to the effects of insulin, including glucagon, epinephrine, glucocorticoids, growth hormone, thyroxine, and somatostatin. In pregnancy, human placental lactogen (HPL), also called somatomammotropin, has anti-insulin and is responsible for the relative glucose intolerance of pregnancy.

T1.28
ATP III Recommended LDL Targets

Risk Group	Notes	Target LDL
Presence of coronary heart disease (CHD) or CHD-equivalents	CHD equivalents include: diabetes, noncoronary atherosclerotic vascular disease, Framingham risk of MI within 10 years of >20% (a complex formula determines this risk)	<100 mg/dL
2 or more major risk factors	Major risk factors include: smoking, hypertension (>140/90), HDL <40, Family history of premature CHD (male 1st degree relative <55 or female 1st degree relative <65), age (men >45, women >55).	<130 mg/dL
<2 major risk factors		<160 mg/dL

■ Methods

  □ Immunometric assays are available for the measurement of insulin and C peptide. Insulin is synthesized as proinsulin, a single amino acid chain 51 amino acids long. Though it is a single polypeptide chain, by convention the first (amino terminus) several amino acids are called the B-chain, the next several amino acids are called the C-peptide, and the carboxy-terminal amino acids are called the A-chain. Disulfide bonds form between the A and B chains, and the C-peptide is proteolytically cleaved post-translationally to make insulin. When the b cells are induced to secrete, they secrete disulfide-linked A-B chains (insulin) and C-peptides simultaneously. Although C-peptide and insulin are produced in equimolar quantities, the ratio of C-peptide:insulin is about 5-15:1. This is because insulin is rapidly metabolized compared to C-peptide.

  □ Glucose measurement in the laboratory is an enzymatic assay, using glucose oxidase or hexokinase coupled with glucose-6-phosphate dehydrogenase, and measuring a reaction product. The latter method is considered most specific for glucose. The test is usually performed on plasma. Note that when blood is left in an un-separated test tube, glycolysis will reduce the glucose by about 5-10 mg/dL/hour depending on the temperature and white cell count. Fluoride added to the tube will arrest this process for 24 hours.

  □ Glucose is a frequent point-of-care analyte, and in this setting is usually performed on whole blood.

Most are calibrated to give results that correlate with plasma, but un-calibrated whole blood glucose usually runs 10%-15% lower than plasma glucose (depending upon the hematocrit). These measurements are inappropriate for the initial diagnosis of diabetes.

  □ Interstitial glucose monitoring, using an electro-chemical method, is a recent development with which continuous monitoring is possible. Changes in interstitial glucose lag changes in blood glucose by up to 30 minutes.

  □ Glycosylated hemoglobin is formed when hemoglobin undergoes nonenzymatic reaction with glucose. The resulting glycosylation product is known as glycosylated hemoglobin, and one type of glycosylated hemoglobin—HgbA$_{1c}$—can be easily measured.

   ● The concentration of HgbA1c depends on the concentration of serum glucose and, since glycosylation increases over time, the lifespan of the patient's red cells. Shortened red cell survival leads to decreased HgbA1c.

   ● In patients with normal red cell survival, the concentration of HgbA1c is an indicator of glucose concentrations over the preceding 3 months (the average red cell lifespan is 120 days; the average red cell in your body is about 60 days old). In actual fact, it's not this linear. Younger red cells are disproportionately represented, and most (a little over 50%) A1c reflects glucose control in the past 1 month.

Lipids and Carbohydrates>Carbohydrates

T1.29
ATP III Cholesterol Classification

Insulinoma
Nesidioblastosis
ILGF-like hormone secreting tumors (sarcomas, HCCa)
Advanced malignancy
Anti-insulin receptor antibodies
Autoimmune insulin syndrome
Post-gastric surgery
Alcohol consumption
Drug induced (exogenous insulin, sulfonylureas, salicylates, quinine, haloperidol, β-blockers)
Hepatic failure
Inborn errors of metabolism (glycogen storage disease, hereditary fructose intolerance, galactosemia, carnitine deficiency)
Starvation

- There are several ways to measure HgbA1c, including affinity chromatography, immunoassays, high-pressure liquid chromatography (HPLC), and ion-exchange chromatography. Normal HgbA1c is under 6%. Diabetics with excellent control have around 7%-9%.

Hypoglycemia T1.29

- Symptoms of hypoglycemia are referable to one of two phenomena

  □ The brain relies heavily on glucose for metabolism, and hypoglycemia directly leads to altered mental status. These symptoms predominate in so-called 'fasting' hypoglycemia in which the drop in serum glucose is moderate and gradual.

  □ Hormonal responses to hypoglycemia include excess adrenergic activity leading to sweating, palpitations, tachycardia, and nervousness. These symptoms predominate in 'reactive' hypoglycemia that tends to be more profound and rapid in onset.

- Drug-induced hypoglycemia is caused by insulin, sulfonylureas (oral hypoglycemic agents), alcohol, and quinine.

- Fasting hypoglycemia is the abnormal gradual-onset of hypoglycemia occurring following a prolonged fast or prolonged exercise. Causes include: proliferations of islet β cells (nesidioblastosis or insulinoma), several inherited metabolic defects, certain large sarcomas, and end-stage liver disease. Insulinomas are tumors of the endocrine pancreas, consisting of neoplastic proliferations of islet β cells, resulting in high insulin levels. They present with the classic Whipple triad of: hypoglycemic symptoms, plasma glucose <45 mg/dL, and relief of symptoms with glucose administration. In patients with insulinomas, the absolute insulin concentration may be normal, but it is inappropriately high for the degree of hypoglycemia. Thus, the diagnosis depends on the insulin:glucose ratio, which is often >180 with insulinoma.

- Reactive hypoglycemia is the abnormal rapid-onset of hypoglycemia following a meal. Its causes include: hereditary fructose intolerance, galactosemia, post-vagotomy states (dumping syndrome), and (sometimes) early type 2 DM.

- The diagnostic approach involves (1) documenting hypoglycemia, then (2) identifying a cause.

  □ Documenting hypoglycemia requires that a blood sample be obtained during a symptomatic period. This may require provocative testing such as: fasting with or without exercise (when fasting hypoglycemia is suspected); or a carbohydrate-rich meal (when reactive hypoglycemia is suspected).

  □ C peptide and insulin are secreted together by pancreatic islet cells in equimolar amounts; however, insulin is metabolized much faster than C peptide, resulting in a concentration of C peptide that is several times higher than insulin. Its major clinical use is in the detection of exogenous insulin administration. In interpreting this, recall that C peptide is cleared by the kidneys, and is therefore raised in renal impairment.

  □ Proinsulin, which normally represents less than 10% of circulating insulin, is useful in the diagnosis of insulinoma.

  □ Anti-insulin antibodies can be raised in response to exogenous insulin, but this is rare in the era of human insulin administration. Anti-insulin auto antibodies may rarely occur in patients never exposed to exogenous insulin, and may cause reactive hypoglycemia (autoimmune insulin syndrome (AIS)). However, anti-insulin antibodies may be found rarely in patients with insulinoma.

Lipids and Carbohydrates>Carbohydrates

T1.30
Lipoprotein Classes

Diagnosis	Fasting Plasma Glucose	Random Non-Fasting Plasma Glucose	Plasma Glucose 2 Hours After 75 g OGTT
Diabetes mellitus	>125 mg/dL	>199 mg/dL	>199 mg/dL
Impaired fasting glucose (pre-diabetes)	>99 mg/dL (< 126 mg/dL)	—	—
Impaired glucose tolerance (pre-diabetes)	—	—	>139 mg/dL (< 200 mg/dL)

□ Anti-insulin receptor antibodies (AIRAs) may cause either hyperglycemia or, more rarely, hypoglycemia.

□ An important concept is the distinction of hyperinsulinemic from hypoinsulinemic hypoglycemia: hyperinsulinemic hypoglycemia is (when not exogenous) most commonly due to insulinoma; while hypoinsulinemic hypoglycemia typifies most other causes. Hypoinsulinemic hypoglycemia is divided into ketotic (high beta-hydroxy butyrate) and non-ketotic (low beta-hydroxy butyrate) types. Non-ketotic hypoglycemia suggests the presence of insulin-like activity and may be seen in autoimmune hypoglycemia, liver failure, or starvation. All other causes of hypoglycemia are associated with ketosis.

□ Note that serum calcium should be measured in patients diagnosed with insulinoma, because insulinomas may be a feature of type 1 MEN.

□ Hypoglycemia is virtually impossible to diagnose after death. However, insulin, C peptide, and proinsulin may remain detectable for several days after death.

Diabetes mellitus

■ Types

□ Type 1 diabetes results from autoimmune islet β-cell destruction, causing a deficiency of insulin.

● Type 1 represents about 10% of all diabetics. It most commonly presents in childhood.

● Autoantibodies can frequently be detected. In particular, at least one of anti-GAD65, anti-ICA512, or anti-IAA is present in nearly all cases.

T1.31
Diagnostic Criteria for Gestational Diabetes, Based Upon 100 gram Oral Glucose Tolerance Test

Time of Collection	Plasma Glucose
Fasting	>95 mg/dL
1 hour	>180 mg/dL
2 hours	>155 mg/dL
3 hours	>140 mg/dL

□ Type 2 diabetes results from progressive insulin resistance, compounded by a progressive defect in insulin secretion.

□ Gestational diabetes mellitus (GDM).

□ Miscellaneous forms of diabetes result from an assortment of genetic defects, cystic fibrosis, medications, and toxins.

■ Diagnosis **T1.30, T1.31**

□ The fasting plasma glucose (FPG) is the recommended test to diagnose diabetes in nonpregnant persons (both children and adults). A FPG of 126 mg/dL (7.0 mmol/L) or higher is considered diagnostic.

□ Alternatively, in persons with classic symptoms of diabetes, a random (non-fasting) plasma glucose (casual plasma glucose) of 200 mg/dL (11.1 mmol/L) is diagnostic.

□ An oral glucose tolerance test (OGTT) can be administered by giving a 75 g glucose load. A 2-hour plasma glucose of 200 mg/dL (11.1 mmol/L) or higher is diagnostic.

□ In pregnancy, early screening at the first prenatal visit should be offered to high-risk women. Risk factors for GDM include obesity, GDM during a previous pregnancy, glycosuria, and family history of diabetes. An FPG of 126 mg/dL or random plasma glucose of 200 mg/dL is diagnostic of GDM in these women. Subsequently

(1) those high-risk women who have normal tests at the initial visit and

(2) average-risk women should undergo oral glucose tolerance testing (OGTT) with a 100-gram glucose load at 24-28 weeks.

□ Criteria for a positive 100-gram OGTT in pregnancy are any two of

● >95 mg/dL fasting plasma glucose

● >180 mg/dL 1-hour plasma glucose

● >155 mg/dL 2-hour plasma glucose

● >140 mg/dL 3-hour plasma glucose

□ In many instances, the need for a 100-g test is determined by first performing a 50-g OGTT. A plasma glucose measurement at 1 hr that exceeds 140 mg/dL indicates the need for a 100 g oral glucose tolerance test. Some women, considered to be at very low risk, can avoid OGTT altogether: age <25, normal pre-pregnancy weight, low-risk ethnic group, no family history of diabetes, *and* no prior obstetric complications.

□ Women who have been diagnosed with GDM should be tested for (nongestational) diabetes at 6-12 weeks postpartum.

□ The hemoglobin A1C should not be used to diagnose diabetes.

■ Conditions considered 'pre-diabetic' include impaired glucose tolerance (IGT) and increased fasting glucose (IFG). IGT is diagnosed when an oral glucose tolerance test is abnormal but does not meet criteria for diabetes; that is, a 2-hour plasma glucose of 140 mg/dL (7.8 mmol/L) to 199 mg/dL (11.0 mmol/L). Increased fasting glucose (IFG) is diagnosed when a fasting glucose is abnormal but does not meet the criteria for diabetes; that is, a FPG of 100 mg/dL (5.6 mmol/L) to 125 mg/dL (6.9 mmol/L).

■ Initial and repetitive laboratory testing in diabetes

□ The hemoglobin A1C testing is used to monitor glycemic control. The frequency of testing is often individualized. The American Diabetes Association (ADA) currently recommends GHb testing at least twice a year in stable patients and more frequently in others. The ADA-recommended goal of therapy is a GHb concentration of <7%.

□ Adult patients with diabetes should be screened annually for lipid disorders.

□ An annual test for microalbuminuria should be performed.

□ The serum creatinine should be measured annually for calculation of the estimated glomerular filtration rate (eGFR).

□ Hypomagnesemia is a common problem in diabetics. Furthermore, hypomagnesemia appears to complicate glycemic control. Magnesium levels should be checked periodically.

Diabetic ketoacidosis (DKA)

■ DKA occurs in insulin-dependent diabetics. Type 1 DM is more prone to DKA than type 2. Generally, DKA follows some sort of provocation such as infection, trauma, or failure to take insulin. In early DKA, the patient experiences polyuria, polydipsia, nausea, and abdominal pain. Later there is the altered breathing pattern referred to as Kussmaul respiration, the onset of altered mental status progressing to coma and, if untreated, death.

■ Diagnosis

□ Hyperglycemia, ketosis, and metabolic acidosis are the usual requirements for the diagnosis of DKA. Occasionally the diagnosis is made solely on the basis of the typical clinical presentation coupled with urine dipstick findings of glycosuria and ketonuria.

□ More specifically, the glucose should be at least 200 mg/dL, and the venous pH <7.30 (or bicarbonate < 15 mmol/L). Normoglycemic DKA is rare.

□ Additional common, though nonspecific, findings include left-shifted neutrophilia, hyperamylasemia, and hyperlipasemia. The mechanism for these is unclear. Neutrophilia appears to directly result from DKA and does not necessarily imply underlying infection.

■ Monitoring

◻ Serum ketones

- The major serum ketones are acetone, acetoacetic acid, and β-hydroxybutyrate. These are in a dynamic balance with one another and undergo continual interconversion.

- Ketones are measured by the nitroprusside technique, a semi-quantitative method that is sensitive to acetone and acetoacetic acid but not β-hydroxybutyrate. In normal circumstances, these are present in roughly equimolar concentrations. Due an altered metabolic milieu, acetone and acetoacetic acid account for only around 20% of serum ketones in DKA, and the remaining 80% are β-hydroxy butyrate.

- Thus, it is important to understand that when you measure 'ketones' you are only measuring a small fraction of serum ketones. In the treatment of DKA an initial apparent increase in 'ketones' is seen, which is due to β-hydroxybutyrate being converted to the other two forms as total serum ketones decrease.

◻ **Glucose** is initially >200 mg/dL in typical DKA.

◻ **pH and bicarbonate** are initially decreased and there is an anion gap.

◻ **Sodium** is initially decreased due to urinary losses.

◻ **Potassium** is tricky in DKA. The initial serum potassium is nearly always elevated, but due to transcellular shifts with loss of intracellular potassium and additional urinary losses of potassium, total body potassium is usually severely diminished in DKA. Furthermore, insulin treatment of DKA leads to transcellular shifts of both glucose and hydrogen ions, taking potassium with them. This can result in rapid and profound hypokalemia in the treated DKA patient. Thus, the administration of potassium during the treatment of DKA is crucial.

◻ **BUN** is initially increased due to severe volume depletion resulting in prerenal azotemia.

Hyperglycemic hyperosmolar nonketotic coma (HHNC)

■ Patients with type 2 (non-insulin dependent) diabetes, especially the elderly, are particularly prone to this complication. It is not seen much in insulin-dependent DM. HHNC is about one tenth as common as DKA but has a mortality rate 10 times that of DKA.

■ It presents with altered mental status, profound hyperglycemia, hyperosmolarity, dehydration, and essentially normal pH. Seizures and 'localizing' neurologic deficits such as hemiplegia are common features, and the mortality rate varies from 15%-50%.

■ **Diagnosis.** Relies on the typical clinical presentation in addition to extreme hyperglycemia (at least 600 mg/dL, usually >1000 mg/dL), hyperosmolarity (>330 mOsm/L), and essentially normal bicarbonate and ketones. Sodium and potassium tend to be elevated at presentation, and there is a deep total body potassium deficit as seen in DKA. The BUN is often markedly elevated, with an increased BUN:Cr ratio, reflective of profound dehydration.

The metabolic syndrome

■ Also known as syndrome X, the insulin resistance syndrome, and the deadly quartet, this refers to a cluster of findings that appear to occur together in an individual more often than might be expected by chance and that are risk factors for cardiovascular disease.

■ It consists of a constellation of metabolic abnormalities, including impaired glucose tolerance, insulin resistance, central obesity, dyslipidemia (increased VLDL, increased TG, increased small dense LDL particles, decreased HDL), increased PAI-1, increased CRP, and hypertension.

■ These individuals manifest accelerated atherosclerosis.

Tumor Markers

Screening for cancer through the use of tumor markers is generally not cost-effective. The reason for this is the dependence of a test's positive predictive value (PPV) on the disease prevalence in the population. PPV is directly proportional to prevalence. Hence, the cost of evaluation of false positives can negate any cost-savings from early detection of true positives when no selection criteria are applied to the population.

If, however, screening is applied to a selected population, then tumor marker screening may be cost-effective. A few examples exist, including the use of alpha-feto-protein (AFP) to screen for hepatocellular carcinoma in China, the use of serum prostate-specific antigen (PSA) to screen for prostate cancer in older American men, and the use of calcitonin to screen for medullary thyroid carcinoma in multiple endocrine neoplasia (MEN) kindreds.

Detection of tumor recurrence can be thought of as an example of this application. The pre-test probability of a positive result is high in this select group, and it is in this arena that serum tumor markers have enjoyed their greatest success.

Assays for tumor markers must have very low analytic sensitivity (defined as the lowest analyte concentration that will yield a result other than zero). Furthermore, they must have high between-run precision, since the time interval between measurements is often several months or a year. One strategy for dealing with this is to freeze samples, and thaw them to run parallel with later samples; thus, direct comparisons can be made.

The Hook effect can be a problem in certain immunoassay formats, and immunoassays are heavily applied in tumor marker testing. In this scenario, very high concentrations of an analyte give a falsely low result. If the sample is sufficiently diluted, the assay will give an appropriate result. In some patients with widely metastatic disease, serum tumor concentrations can be so high that they exceed the binding capacity of both the binding capture antibodies and the signal-bearing antibodies, preventing their association. This phenomenon, known as the high-dose Hook effect, mostly affects one-step immunometric assays. It is for this reason that it is common practice to analyze samples at several different dilutions.

Heterophile antibodies can cause significant interference in any immunoassay. These are antibodies that may be present in the patient which manifest broad reactivity with antibodies of other animal species (which are often the source of the assay antibodies). So-called 'sandwich' immunoassays are particularly susceptible to this interference. Heterophile antibodies may give false positives (by bridging the capture and signal antibody) or false negatives (by blocking one or the other). Both detecting and deterring this interference is not easy. One option is to repeat the test using a different assay. Various heterophile blocking reagents, steps to remove immunoglobulins, and serial dilutions may correct the problem.

PSA

Prostate cancer screening

- PSA has proven to be the prototype tumor marker, with high specificity, high sensitivity, and relatively low cost. Currently, an annual PSA, in addition to digital rectal examination (DRE), is recommended for men over age 50. The tests are sometimes performed at a younger age for men at high risk.

- However, while PSA is organ-specific, it is not cancer-specific, and it may be elevated in benign prostatic hyperplasia (BPH), prostatitis, prostatic infarct, and following prostate needle biopsy. PSA > 10 ng/mL is rarely associated with benign disease. Small elevations following DRE are not large enough to be clinically relevant, but elevations following prostate needle biopsy (PNB) may be. PSA undergoes significant physiologic variation within an individual, with great enough magnitude to be clinically significant, and serial measurements are recommended to support clinical decisions. Finasteride lowers the PSA, and PSA varies with race, with levels being significantly higher in blacks.

- Only about 30-40% of men with elevated PSA (>4.0 ng/mL) will be found to have prostate cancer, particularly when the PSA falls within the 4-10 ng/mL 'gray zone.'

- Many men with prostate cancer, especially organ-confined prostate cancer, have PSA values less than 4.0 ng/mL. In order to achieve a survival advantage, it is these men that we seek to identify.

- In an effort to improve the performance of PSA, numerous derivative formulations have been studied, including age-specific PSA, PSA density, and PSA velocity.

  □ PSA increases normally with age. Age-specific cut-offs increase sensitivity of PSA for younger men, while increasing specificity at older ages. However, it appears that the latter effect is obtained at the expense of sensitivity in older men.

  □ PSA density is defined as the PSA divided by the estimated prostatic volume. It was hoped that this might improve specificity by mitigating the effect of BPH. A PSA density of >0.15 is considered abnormal. However, due possibly to the difficulty in assessing prostatic volume or of knowing the gland to stroma ratio in any given prostate, this calculation does not perform significantly better than PSA.

  □ PSA velocity refers to the rate of change in successive PSA determinations. A PSA velocity of >0.75 ng/mL/year is considered abnormal. While this appears to improve the sensitivity and specificity, the magnitude of improvement is limited by biologic variation in PSA from non-malignant causes.

- In addition, different molecular forms of PSA have been studied, including free PSA, pro-PSA, benign PSA, intact PSA, and complexed PSA.

  □ Free PSA

    • PSA is a protease (whose function appears to be to minimize the viscosity of the ejaculate); thus, the small quantity of PSA that is released into circulation is quickly bound to protease inhibitors. In fact, most PSA (75%-90%) circulates bound, mostly to α_1-antichymotrypsin (ACT), but also to α_2-macroglobulin (A2M) and α_1-protein inhibitor (API). Methods exist that measure strictly free PSA.

    • A lowered free PSA fraction (or elevated bound PSA fraction) correlates with the presence of prostate cancer. The likelihood of cancer is quite low in men with free PSA (ratio of free PSA to total PSA) >25%, while it is very high with free PSA <10%.

    • The percent free PSA has proven to be more sensitive and specific than total PSA and has greatly aided decision-making in men with PSA<10.

  • Prostatic manipulation and instrumentation have been shown to affect the in ratio free to total PSA. While the total serum PSA is only minimally affected by urethral instrumentation and digital rectal examination, the % free PSA is markedly affected. It has been recommended that these measurements be taken either before or several weeks after such manipulation.

  • The advantage of % free PSA is only seen when prostatic volume is <60 cc.

  • Specimen handling is of utmost importance in % PSA determinations. Free PSA is less stable than bound PSA, and specimens should be processed rapidly to prevent this effect. Specimens that cannot be processed within 2 hours should be separated and frozen.

  □ PSA isoforms

    • PSA is released from glandular cells as pro-PSA (pPSA). A 7 amino acid leader peptide is clipped from pro-PSA to make mature PSA. Anomalous clipping gives rise to several additional (truncated) forms of pro-PSA having 2, 4, or 5 amino acids of the original leader sequence. In prostate cancer, there is an increase in both pro-PSA and these truncated forms. Detection of these has significantly improved diagnosis in men whose total PSA is in the 2.5 to 4.0 range.

    • Benign PSA (bPSA) refers to a form of PSA that was first isolated in the transition zone of benign prostatic hyperplasia (BPH). It appears to discriminate BPH from non-BPH prostatic enlargement, and it is being studied for a possible role in cancer detection. Intact PSA (a form of PSA identified in some forms of carcinoma that appears intact, proteolytically inactive, and does not complex with serum anti-proteinases) and complexed PSA (the sum of bound PSA) are also undergoing evaluation.

Prostate cancer prognosis and recurrence detection

- Preoperatively, the serum PSA quantity roughly reflects tumor volume and stage.

- Following radical prostatectomy, serum PSA should drop to undetectable levels and can be used to screen for tumor recurrence or metastases.

- The correlation between PSA and tumor recurrence is somewhat weak in the first 5 years following treatment but improves thereafter.

- While post-treatment PSA nadir appears to correlate with the likelihood of cancer cure, no specific value has been established which conclusively establishes disease eradication or treatment failure, particularly within the first 5 years. Various authors have placed the cut-off somewhere between 0.2 and 0.4 ng/mL. Guidelines put forth by the American Society for Therapeutic Radiology and Oncology (ASTRO) are as follows: PSA recurrence was defined as three consecutive increases in PSA, or a single rise so great as to trigger the initiation of hormone therapy, and the date of failure is the midpoint between the post-radiation nadir PSA and the first of the three consecutive increases.

- Furthermore, a rising post-treatment PSA (so-called biochemical failure) does not distinguish locoregional failure (local recurrence) from distant failure (metastases).

- While it appears that biochemical failure precedes clinical failure by approximately 6-18 months, it is not entirely clear that this lead time provides a survival benefit.

- PSA doubling time may address some of these limitations; for example, several studies suggest that doubling time kinetics may be associated with local *versus* systemic recurrence, and doubling time may be a better indicator of impending treatment failure.

Carcinoembryonic Antigen (CEA)

In patients with colorectal carcinoma, the degree of CEA elevation is known to be affected by tumor stage, tumor grade, tumor ploidy, tumor site, obstruction, liver function, and smoking.

- CEA varies inversely with grade, with well-differentiated tumors producing more CEA than poorly differentiated tumors.

- CEA is elevated in only 25% of tumors confined to the colon, 50% with positive nodes, and 75% with distant metastases.

- Left-sided tumors generally have a higher CEA than right-sided tumors, and bowel obstruction produces a higher CEA.

- Aneuploid tumors produce higher concentrations of CEA than diploid tumors.

- Since the liver is the primary site for its metabolism, liver dysfunction can increase the CEA.

- The median CEA values for smokers is higher than that for nonsmokers.

- Patients with high preoperative CEA concentrations can be predicted to have a worse outcome than those with low concentrations.

- For post-treatment surveillance, serial CEA measurements can detect recurrence with a sensitivity of 80% and specificity of 70%. CEA is most sensitive to the presence of liver metastases (94% sensitivity) and overall poorly sensitive to locoregional recurrences (about 60%).

CEA elevations also occur with other malignancies, including gastric adenocarcinoma (particularly well-differentiated intestinal type), breast cancer, lung cancer, pancreatic adenocarcinoma, medullary thyroid carcinoma, cervical adenocarcinoma, and urothelial carcinoma.

Nonneoplastic conditions associated with elevated CEA include smoking, peptic ulcer disease, inflammatory bowel disease, pancreatitis, hypothyroidism, biliary obstruction, and cirrhosis. Levels exceeding 10 ng/mL are rarely due to benign disease.

Thyroglobulin

The mainstay for detection of tumor recurrence in so-called differentiated (follicular and papillary) thyroid carcinomas is the serum thyroglobulin. Thyroglobulin is not elaborated by medullary or anaplastic thyroid carcinoma. Circulating thyroglobulin has a half-life of about 65 hours, and it takes nearly a month before thyroglobulin becomes undetectable following total thyroidectomy. In normal circumstances, thyroglobulin is cleared from the circulation by the catabolism in the liver and recycling in the thyroid.

Anti-thyroglobulin antibodies are present in 10% of normal individuals and >20% of those with thyroid carcinoma and pose a major problem in thyroglobulin testing. These usually result in underestimation but sometimes cause overestimation (in a macro-thyroglobulin sort of mechanism) of the serum thyroglobulin. Assays are available to detect thyroglobulin antibodies, making identification of the problem (once suspected) fairly straightforward. What to do about it is not so simple. On the bright side, serial quantitative serum anti-thyroglobulin antibody measurements may be able to serve as a surrogate tumor marker. Antibodies are expected to progressively diminish after thyroid ablation. Any increase is indicative of antigenic stimulation, suggesting recurrence.

A thyroglobulin assay is only sufficiently specific if all functional thyroid tissue has been ablated (total thyroidectomy followed by radioactive iodine). To enhance sensitivity either TSH (thyrotropin) can be administered to the patient or thyroxine replacement therapy (generating an endogenous TSH response) can be withheld prior to testing.

Tumor-Associated Trypsin Inhibitor (TATI)

TATI has been used as a marker for mucinous ovarian carcinoma, urothelial carcinoma, and renal cell carcinoma. It was first discovered in the urine of patients with ovarian carcinoma.

TATI is cleared by the kidneys, and it is elevated in renal failure. Pancreatitis invariably causes increased TATI; in fact, the degree of elevation correlates with severity, and TATI over 70 µg/L are associated with a poor prognosis.

About 50% of stage I mucinous ovarian carcinomas are associated with increased TATI, and nearly 100% of stage IV tumors. It is complementary to CA-125 which shows greatest sensitivity for non-mucinous epithelial tumors.

About 85-95% of pancreatic adenocarcinomas are associated with increased TATI; however, the common finding of increased TATI in pancreatitis limits specificity.

TATI is elevated in about 60% of gastric carcinomas, particularly diffuse (infiltrative, signet-ring) types. In this setting, it complements CEA which tends to be elevated only in intestinal type adenocarcinoma.

In urothelial carcinoma, TATI expression varies with stage: from about 20% of low-stage tumors to 80% of high-stage tumors.

TATI has about 70% sensitivity for renal cell carcinoma. Again, however, increased TATI is most likely in advanced-stage disease.

In nearly all tumor types studied, TATI expression is an adverse prognostic factor.

Cancer Antigen (CA) 125

CA 125 is elevated in non-mucinous epithelial ovarian neoplasms and has a major role in the monitoring of these patients.

CA 125 has not proven useful in screening for ovarian neoplasms. This marker is elevated in only about 50% of patients with stage I disease, and CA 125 has a poor positive predictive value in unselected women.

CA 125 may be elevated in a number of nonneoplastic abdominopelvic disorders (pregnancy, fibroids, benign ovarian cysts, pelvic inflammation, ascites, and endometriosis), and in some non-ovarian neoplasms (endometrium, fallopian tube, pancreas, breast, and colon).

CA 125 <35 U/mL is considered normal. In post-menopausal women, it tends to decrease. Normal values are lower for African American and Asian women. The value also increases slightly during the follicular (prolif-erative) phase of the menstrual cycle. Values above 35 may be found in up to 2% of normal women.

CA 125 has utility in differentiating pelvic masses. In post-menopausal women with palpable adnexal masses, CA 125 levels > 65 U/mL have a positive predictive value of >95% for ovarian malignancy.

It is in patients with known ovarian malignancy that CA 125 finds its greatest utility:

- A fall in CA 125 during initial treatment suggests treat-ment efficacy, and the duration of disease-free survival seems to correlate best with the rate of fall. Conversely, an increase in CA 125 during treatment is indicative of treatment failure, and following treatment is a predic-tor of disease recurrence.

- A persistent elevation of CA 125 (>35 U/mL) predicts residual disease at the time of a second-look laparotomy with a specificity of > 95%.

- Rising CA 125 suggests relapse. In fact, the rise often precedes clinical evidence of disease by a median inter-val of 3-6 months.

- Prognosis relates to both the initial and post-treatment CA 125 value. A preoperative CA 125 > 65 U/mL portends an unfavorable prognosis and is associated with a many-fold increased risk of death from tumor. Persistent elevations following chemotherapy indicate a poor prognosis. Furthermore, the half-life of CA 125 after chemotherapy correlates with prognosis, with those patients demonstrating a CA 125 half-life <20 days having improved survival. Lastly, the time to normalization of CA 125 impacts prognosis, with those patients whose levels normalized within 3 cycles of chemotherapy having improved survival.

Cancer Antigens (CA) 27.29 and 15-3

CA 27.29 (also called BR 27.29) and CA 15-3 measure different epitopes of a single antigen—the protein product of the breast cancer-associated MUC1 gene. They are elevated in many cases of breast cancer. Due to enhanced sensitivity and specificity, CA27.29 has supplanted CA 15-3 as the preferred serum marker for breast cancer. It is elevated in about 30% of low-stage disease and 60%-70% of advanced-stage disease.

Both CA 27.29 and CA 15-3 may also be elevated in patients with benign ovarian cysts, benign breast disease, and benign liver disease. CA 15-3 can be elevated in cirrhosis, sarcoidosis, and lupus. CA 27.29 levels over 100 units/mL and CA15-3 levels over 25 U/mL are rare in benign conditions.

CA 27.29 may be elevated in non-breast malignancies, including colon, stomach, pancreas, prostate, and lung.

Presently the best markers of prognosis in breast cancer are tissue-based: estrogen receptor (ER), progesterone receptor (PR), and Her-2 (c-erbB-2).

- ER and PR assays are now performed almost exclusively by immunohistochemistry and graded according to the proportion of cells expressing intense nuclear staining. Grading systems vary, but one approach is to grade results as 0 (<1% of cells staining), 1+ (1%-10% of cells staining), and 2+ (>10% of cells staining). While 1% appears quite low, it seems that a good proportion of tumors in the 1%-10% range will respond to hormonal therapy. While biochemical (ligand-binding) assays are no longer widely used, it is important to note that a great quantity of the literature supporting the role of ER and PR is based upon this methodology.

Immunohistochemical determination of ER and PR, however, appears to correlate well with, and perhaps even to be superior to, biochemical assays. Care must be taken to ensure appropriate tissue fixation (particularly the avoidance of extended formalin fixation), appropriately reacting controls, and the assessment of only nuclear staining. When results appear to be in conflict with the observed histology (eg, lack of ER staining in a very well-differentiated tumor), repeat testing should be undertaken.

- Her-2 may be determined by immunohistochemistry, FISH, or a combination of both. The purpose of Her-2 staining is to determine suitability for treatment with trantuzumab. As with immunohistochemical staining for ER/PR, rigorous attention to detail is essential: proper fixation, appropriate controls, assessment of only the invasive component, and assessment of only membrane staining. Tumor immunohistochemical expression is graded 0-3+. Furthermore, it is important to appreciate the limitations of immunohistochemical staining; in particular, all tumors grade 2+ should be submitted to FISH testing.

Cancer Antigen (CA) 19-9

CA 19-9 is thus far the best marker for pancreaticobiliary adenocarcinoma. In fact, in one study of patients with pancreatic lesions, a combination of weight loss >20 lb, bilirubin >3 mg/dL, and CA 19-9 >37 U/L had a positive predictive value approaching 100% for predicting pancreatic adenocarcinoma. With any 2 of these, the positive predictive value decreases to around 90%.

CA 19-9 is sometimes elevated in association with malignancies of the esophagus and intestines. It may also be elevated in benign conditions such as pancreatitis, cholestasis, cholangitis, and cirrhosis. Only about 3% of those with CA 19-9 >100 U/L have benign disease, however, and virtually nobody with CA 19-9 >1000 U/L has benign disease.

At the moment, CA 19-9 is most useful in assessing the response to treatment.

CA 19-9 is identical to the Lewis blood group antigen. It is not produced by Lewis-negative people.

Alpha Fetoprotein (AFP)

AFP is a major component of fetal serum, having physiologic effects similar to albumin. It is synthesized in the yolk sac, fetal liver, and fetal gastrointestinal tract. After birth, it rapidly recedes to undetectable levels. Normal adults have AFP under 5.4 ng/mL. While elevations may be seen in a number of benign conditions, values above 500 ng/mL are not seen in benign disease.

AFP is elevated in normal pregnancy (usually not more than 100 ng/mL), cirrhosis, and hepatitis.

AFP has utility in detection of hepatocellular carcinoma and yolk sac tumors. It may also be elevated sporadically in other tumors, notably hepatoid variants of gastric carcinoma.

- In yolk sac tumors, the magnitude of AFP correlates with prognosis (AFP >10,000 ng/mL associated with poor prognosis).

- In hepatocellular carcinoma, the reported rate of AFP elevation is 80%; however, this may not be the case in the Western world. It appears that this number may reflect old literature, when tumors were quite large at the time of diagnosis, and a high proportion of AFP elevation may be seen in certain populations (eg, Southeast Asia), where in fact AFP has been used successfully for screening. Furthermore, the magnitude of AFP elevation is in a range (500-1000 ng/mL) that overlaps with many benign diseases.

Human Chorionic Gonadotropin (HCG)

HCG is elevated in pregnancy, trophoblastic disease, and choriocarcinoma.

Marijuana use has been associated with low-level elevation of HCG.

In the initial evaluation of germ cell tumors, the magnitude of elevation correlates with prognosis (HCG>50,000 mIU/mL associated with a poor prognosis).

HCG may is elevated in about 15% of pure seminomas and in rare examples of tumors from numerous sites (GI tract, GU tract). By itself, this finding does not imply a choriocarcinoma.

β2-Microglobulin (β2M)

β2M is expressed on the surface of most nucleated cells. It is a small molecule linked non-covalently to class I MHC molecules, and when cells die β2M is released into the extracellular fluid. Thus, β2M can be expected to be elevated whenever there is increased cell turnover, and in fact it proves to be a good though nonspecific marker for several types of tumor.

It has been studied as a marker of solid tumors and hematolymphoid neoplasms. It is an independent prognostic factor in multiple myeloma. β2M can be used to monitor transplant rejection. It is cleared by the kidneys and may be nonspecifically elevated in renal insufficiency. Its level is raised in a number of inflammatory states (rheumatoid arthritis, lupus, inflammatory bowel disease).

Lipid-Associated Sialic Acid in Plasma (LASA-P)

Like β2M, LASA-P is a highly nonspecific marker. Elevated LASA-P has been demonstrated in hematolymphoid neoplasms and tumors of the breast, GI tract, lung, and ovary.

LASA-P may be useful in monitoring the response to therapy and detecting disease recurrence in certain patients.

Alkaline Phosphatase

Alkaline phosphatase must be considered a highly non-specific tumor marker, but it has a place in certain settings.

A raised alkaline phosphatase may be an indication of osteoblastic activity; thus, it may be elevated in osteogenic sarcoma or bone metastases. It is also markedly elevated in active Paget disease of bone.

Alkaline phosphatase is the most sensitive liver function test to the presence of hepatic metastases. In some settings, such as primary intra-abdominal carcinoids, the concentration of alkaline phosphatase correlates with prognosis.

Some tumors, particularly when advanced, are associated with elevated alkaline phosphatase due to the Regan isoenzyme.

Markers of Neuroendocrine Tumors

Neuroendocrine tumors include, among others, carcinoids, islet cell tumors, medullary thyroid carcinomas, pheochromocytomas, and neuroendocrine carcinoma (small and large cell types).

Carcinoid tumors

- Carcinoids are neoplasms of enterochromaffin cells, which are capable of producing serotonin (5-hydroxytryptamine, 5-HT). In the biosynthesis of serotonin, the rate-limiting step is conversion of tryptophan to 5-hydroxytryptophane (5-HTP) by tryptophan hydroxylase. 5-HTP is converted to 5-HT by the action of dopa-decarboxylase. 5-HT is either stored (in the neurosecretory granules) or secreted. Most of the secreted 5-HT is taken up by platelets and stored in their secretory (dense) granules. Some makes it into the renal tubules, where it is converted into 5-hydroxyindoleacetic acid (5-HIAA) by renal tubular monoamine oxidase and aldehyde dehydrogenase.

- Carcinoids arising in the foregut (stomach, proximal duodenum, lung) often produce, in addition to modest quantities of 5-HT, histamine, catecholamines, and 5-hydroxytryptophane (5-HTP). Midgut carcinoids (distal duodenum, jejunum, ileum, appendix, right colon) usually produce only serotonin; however, they tend to produce it in great quantity. The serotonin they produce is dumped largely into the portal circulation and cleared by the liver. However, if there are metastases to or beyond the liver, a carcinoid syndrome may be seen, characterized by diarrhea, flushing, wheezing, etc. Hindgut carcinoids are most often non-secretory for indoles, but they may produce HCG.

- Both 5-HIAA (a serotonin metabolite) and serotonin can be assayed in a urine sample. Urinary 5-HIAA and serotonin may be within normal limits in 20-30% of patients with a carcinoid tumor, particularly foregut and hindgut tumors. Furthermore, these analytes may be falsely elevated in patients with a tryptophan-rich diet. Platelets take up serotonin from the serum at a constant rate that is unaffected by serotonin in diet. Platelet serotonin appears to be the most accurate marker for the detection of a carcinoid tumor.

- Other peptides that may be produced in excess include synaptophysin, neuropeptide K, pancreatic polypeptide (PP), and chromogranin A (CGA). The plasma CGA has been used as a measure of tumor burden and treatment response. Elevated serum levels of chromogranin A have been found in pheochromocytoma, carcinoid tumors, islet cell tumors, and small cell neuroendocrine carcinoma.

Markers of medullary thyroid carcinoma

- Plasma calcitonin is useful to detect medullary carcinoma and its recurrences.

- Mature, biologically active calcitonin is a 32 amino acid polypeptide that results from from post-translational modification of a larger 141 amino acid precursor called preprocalcitonin. Currently used assays are specific for the mature 32 amino acid form of calcitonin.

- Normal individuals have calcitonin values <10 ng/L.

- Some affected individuals have calcitonin values this low. Provocative testing, using pentagastrin, omeprazole, or calcium infusions, is a more sensitive test that may be employed in MEN II families.

- Note that calcitonin may also be increased in Hashimoto thyroiditis, C-cell hyperplasia, small cell lung carcinoma and breast carcinoma. It may be secondarily increased in chronic renal failure and Zollinger-Ellison syndrome.

- CEA is also very commonly elevated in medullary carcinoma. Higher CEA values correlate with greater dedifferentiation in the tumor and suggest a worse prognosis.

- Thyroglobulin is not elevated in medullary carcinoma.

Markers of paraganglioma and pheochromocytoma

- These are tumors of chromaffin cells, which are capable of secreting catecholamines. Conventionally, those arising in the adrenal medulla are called pheochromocytomas, and those arising extra-adrenally are called paragangliomas. Chromaffin cells are nearly always capable of producing norepinephrine. Norepinephrine can be converted to epinephrine by the action of the enzyme PNMT (phenolethanolamine-N-methyltransferase); however, significant quantities of norepinephrine are converted to epinephrine predominantly in tumors of the adrenal medulla. Thus, adrenal tumors usually secrete both epinephrine and norepinephrine, while extra-adrenal tumors tend to secrete mainly norepinephrine. Norepinephrine is metabolized to normetanephrine. Most normetanephrine is conjugated with sulfate and excreted in urine, and some is metabolized to vanillymandelic acid (VMA). Epinephrine is metabolized to metanephrine. Most metanephrine is conjugated with sulfate and excreted in urine, and some is metabolized to vanillymandelic acid (VMA).

- Therefore, fractionation of catecholamines (separate quantification of norepinephrine and epinephrine) or of metanephrines (separate quantification of normetanephrine and metanephrine) can be useful in suggesting the site of a pheochromocytoma.

- Available laboratory tests are urinary vanillymandelic acid (VMA), urinary metanephrines, urinary catecholamines, plasma metanephrines or plasma catecholamines. Certain antihypertensive drugs can interfere with these assays: imipramine, reserpine, guanethidine, nitroglycerin, MAO inhibitors.

- Among all these tests, the free (unconjugated) plasma metanephrine is considered the most accurate for initial screening. The urine metanephrine and catecholamine tests perform only slightly worse. Due to the episodic nature of release, plasma catecholamines have poor sensitivity (plasma metanephrines better reflect long-term catecholamine secretion).

- The clonidine suppression test can be used to clarify equivocal serum and urine tests.

Neuroblastoma

- Urine vanillymandelic acid (VMA) and homovanillic acid (HVA) are elevated in most cases. HVA is the final metabolic product of DOPA and dopamine, while VMA is the product of norepinephrine and epinephrine.

- Interestingly, the more poorly differentiated tumors make more HVA than VMA. A low VMA:HVA ratio portends a worse prognosis.

- Most neuroblastomas do not secrete large amounts of epinephrine or normetanephrine.

- Neuron-specific enolase (NSE), lactic dehydrogenase (LDH), and ferritin are nonspecific markers often used to follow disease activity.

Urine Markers for Urothelial Carcinoma

The NMP 22 (nuclear matrix protein 22) test detects a nuclear matrix protein, called NuMA (nuclear mitotic apparatus), that is released from the nuclei of tumor cells when they die. Elevated urinary levels of NMP 22 have been demonstrated in subjects with urothelial carcinoma. At the moment, this test is mainly applied to the monitoring of patients with a known history of bladder cancer. In this setting, it has proven quite sensitive but fairly nonspecific. When performed shortly (1-6 weeks) after tumor resection, >70% of patients with elevated NMP 22 have recurrent disease. >80% of patients with normal results have no evidence of disease. Other causes of rapid cell turnover (inflammation) may produce a positive test, and, in fact, leukocytes may be the source of these false positives.

The bladder tumor antigen (BTA) test detects complement factor H and complement factor H-related proteins (CFH-rp) in the urine. It demonstrates about 60%

1: Clinical Chemistry

Tumor Markers>Urine Markers for Urothelial Carcinoma; Urine PCA3/DD3 for Prostatic Carcinoma I
Endocrine>Thyroid Chemistry

sensitivity and 70% specificity. False positives appear to be related to stone disease, inflammation, and benign prostatic hyperplasia.

In direct comparisons, both the NMP22 and BTA tests have compared favorably with urine cytology in regard to sensitivity to low-grade neoplasms. There is not a significant advantage in sensitivity for high-grade tumors, nor is there a specificity advantage.

Multi-target fluorescence *in situ* hybridization (FISH) exploits the high incidence of aneuploidy in urothelial carcinoma. Centromere probes for specific to chromosomes (eg, 3, 7, 17 and 9) are applied, and the signals are counted.

Urine PCA3/DD3 for Prostatic Carcinoma

A problem with serum PSA testing is that a significant number of cancers occur in men with PSA <4 ng/dL, leading to a search for more sensitive assays. The prostate cancer 3 gene (PCA3) appears to be expressed only in prostatic glandular epithelium, and only to be strongly expressed in malignant prostatic glandular epithelium (prostatic adenocarcinoma). PCA3 encodes a non-translated mRNA known as differential display code 3 (DD3), which is over expressed in 95% of prostatic adenocarcinomas, up-regulated more than 60-fold as compared to adjacent benign epithelium.

In contrast, the *KLK3* gene, that encodes PSA, is not up-regulated in prostatic adenocarcinoma (its increased concentration in serum seems to be related to an increase in leakage into the extracellular matrix rather than increased production). Thus, the KLK3 (PSA) mRNA can be used to control for varying numbers of prostatic cells obtained in the urine sample.

A molecular assay for DD3, performed on urine, is now commercially available. Urine samples are obtained following prostatic massage. RNA is extracted from the urine sediment and subjected to quantitative real-time PCR to determine the number of DD3 RNA transcripts.

A specific cut-off has not been established. In one study, a cut-off point of 200×10^{-3} DD3 transcripts per PSA transcript gave a sensitivity of 67% and specificity of 83%.

Endocrine

Thyroid Chemistry

Thyroid function tests (TFTs) T1.32

- **Total T3 & T4** (thyroxine) will be elevated in most hyperthyroid individuals and decreased in hypothyroidism. Usually only T4 is measured, but T3 can be useful to diagnose the <5% of hyperthyroid individuals who have so-called T3 toxicosis. Since T3 and T4 are highly protein-bound, mainly to prealbumin (transthyretin) and thyroid binding globulin (TBG), total T3 and T4 are affected by levels of these serum proteins. Thus, a patient can be clinically euthyroid but have abnormal total T4 and/or T3. TBG is increased by pregnancy, oral contraceptives, estrogen therapy, cirrhosis, and hypothyroidism. TBG is decreased by hypoproteinemic states, androgen therapy, and cortisol.

- **T3 resin uptake (T3RU).** A conceptually confusing test whose purpose is to circumvent the limitations of total T4 or T3 measurements. In this test, an excess of ^{125}I-labeled T3 is added to the patient's serum. This ^{125}I-T3 binds to available unoccupied sites on TBG. Then a resin is added to the serum, which binds any unbound ^{125}I-T3. The amount of ^{125}I-T3 on the resin is measured. This amount is inversely proportional to the number of available binding sites on TBG and directly proportional to the amount of T3 present. Thus, in hypothyroidism, fewer sites are occupied on TBG, more ^{125}I-T3 binds to TBG and less is left over to bind to resin (low T3 resin uptake). In hyperthyroidism, the opposite occurs (high T3 resin uptake). The free thyroxine index (FTI) is obtained by multiplying the T3RU by the total thyroxine.

- **Free T4** (FT4) and **free T3** (FT3) measurement has always been theoretically advantageous, and recently developed direct immunoassay has made this practical. Measuring the FT4 can get around the intricacies of protein binding and correlates well with the patient's clinical thyroid status. Measurement of FT3 is usually unnecessary but may diagnose cases of so-called 'T3 thyrotoxicosis.'

- **rT3.** When T4 is metabolized in the peripheral blood, most of it is metabolized to T3. A smaller amount is metabolized to rT3. The amount of serum T3 and rT3 varies reciprocally. rT3 assays have little clinical utility other than to confirm the suspicion of the so-called euthyroid sick syndrome, in which rT3 is elevated.

- **Radioactive iodine uptake (RAIU).** The patient is given a dose of radioactive iodine then scanned for thyroid radioactivity. The expectation is that a hyperthyroid patient will have increased thyroid uptake. The hyperthyroid patient with normal or decreased RAIU may have struma ovarii or exogenous thyroid administration.

- **Thyroid stimulating hormone (TSH, thyrotropin)** has become widely accepted as the best first-line test for diagnosing hypo- and hyperthyroidism.

- **Thyroid releasing hormone (TRH)** stimulation test is used in the evaluation of hypothyroidism. In primary hypothyroidism (hypothyroidism due to intrinsic thyroid hypofunction), there is exaggerated secretion of TSH in response to TRH. It is useful to remember that TRH stimulates not only TSH but also GH and prolactin.

- **Testing strategy.** In most patients, particularly otherwise well ambulatory patients, the TSH assay alone will diagnose all cases of hypo- or hyperthyroidism. Some advocate corroborating TSH results with a free T4 measurement. In pregnancy, neonates, and inpatients with significant comorbidities, there is a chance that TSH-only testing strategies may miss a small number of cases. In these populations, a broader panel including at least free T4 is advised. Most of the other tests listed above are rarely indicated.

Hyperthyroidism

- The most common cause is Graves disease. Other causes are toxic multinodular goiter, toxic adenoma (Plummer syndrome), transient hyperthyroidism in various kinds of thyroiditis, exogenous thyroxine, and (very rarely) pituitary adenoma & thyroid carcinoma.

- Graves disease is further characterized by the typical ocular manifestations of retro-orbital infiltration leading to exophthalmos and pretibial myxedema. Patients are highly likely (>95%) to have thyroid-stimulating immunoglobulins (TSI), also called long-acting thyroid stimulating (LATS) antibodies which are capable of acting upon TSH receptors as agonists. In addition, it is important to know that a proportion have either anti-microsomal (60%) or anti-thyroglobulin (30%) antibodies and that these antibodies are not restricted to Hashimoto thyroiditis.

- Hyperthyroidism is a generalized hypermetabolic state in which the patient experiences anxiety, tachycardia, palpitations, weight loss (without anorexia), diarrhea, and heat intolerance. Due to the 5:1 female:male ratio in Graves disease, most patients are women.

- T3 thyrotoxicosis is an uncommon form of hyperthyroidism, affecting less than 5% of hyperthyroid patients, in which there are normal free T4 levels but elevated T3 levels.

T 1.32
Thyroid Function Tests

	TSH	T3	T4 (total)	rT3	T3RU	Serum Cholesterol	Creatine Kinase
Hyperthyroidism	↓	↑	↑	→↑	↑	↓	→↑
Hypothyroidism	↑	↓	↓	→↓	↓	↑	→↑
Euthyroid sick syndrome	→	↓	→↓	↑	→	→	→↑
Excess TBG	→	↑	↑	→	↓	→	→

- Hyperthyroidism is diagnosed when there is suppressed TSH and high serum FT4. When FT4 is normal despite a low TSH, free T3 should be measured to look for T3 thyrotoxicosis. When both FT4 and FT3 are normal, mild or subclinical hyperthyroidism is usually diagnosed. However, medication effect should be excluded in this latter setting.

Hypothyroidism

- The most common cause is Hashimoto thyroiditis. Others include thyroidectomy, lymphocytic and granulomatous (de Quervain) thyroiditis, 131I therapy, radiation, & drugs (iodine, lithium, IL-2, and a-IFN). A rare cause of hypothyroidism, Refetoff syndrome, is due to peripheral resistance.

- Hashimoto thyroiditis is characterized by anti-microsomal (>90%) and anti-thyroglobulin (>90%) antibodies. LATS and TSI are not identified in Hashimoto thyroiditis.

- Secondary hypothyroidism is quite uncommon. It is due to pituitary hypofunction with decreased TSH secretion or to hypothalamic dysfunction with decreased TRH secretion.

- Hypothyroidism manifests as a generalized hypometabolic state, with symptoms of fatigue, cold intolerance, slowed mentation reflexes and speech, and periorbital edema.

- Hypothyroidism is usually diagnosed with an elevated TSH and low free T4. Some patients have a normal free T4 in spite of a raised TSH, and these should be considered to have 'subclinical' or 'mild' hypothyroidism.

- When a low free T4 is found in the face of a normal or low TSH, this may indicate anterior pituitary pathology. In such cases, TSH is rarely the only deficient anterior pituitary product, and a complete evaluation of the pituitary gland is warranted.

Neonatal hypothyroidism

- The cause of neonatal hypothyroidism is most often the abnormal development of the thyroid gland (thyroid dysgenesis). Most cases are sporadic, and some familial (inherited mutations in PAX8 or TTF genes). There may be complete (agenesis) or partial (dysgenesis) absence of thyroid tissue; both manifest with elevated serum TSH, with either absence or deficiency of serum T4 and thyroglobulin.

- Other causes include familial thyroid dyshormonogenesis, peripheral hormone resistance (autosomal dominant Refetoff syndrome), hypopituitarism, and maternal factors (maternal autoantibodies, maternal medications) that usually produce transient neonatal hypothyroidism.

- Hypothyroidism in neonates manifests as dry skin, a hoarse cry, macroglossia, hypothermia, edema, neonatal jaundice, and inactivity. Many cases, however, are subclinical. If untreated, there is a great risk of mental retardation and growth retardation.

- Most commonly, the TSH assay alone is used to screen for this condition, with samples taken between 48-72 hours of age.

- Early initiation of thyroid hormone replacement prevents sequelae.

- In the normal neonate, the TSH peaks at about 1 hour after delivery (at around 60-80 mU/L) then drops to approximately 20 mU/L by 24 hours and to 10 mU/L by 1 week. The initial TSH peak stimulates a rise in serum T4, free T4, and T3, with their peak occurring at about 24-36 hours, falling gradually thereafter. Several conditions can alter this pattern; for example, preterm and sick neonates have smaller peaks but usually follow a similar pattern, and some sick neonates have a delayed TSH response to hypothyroidism.

- These confounding factors have led to the proposal of numerous disparate approaches to the detection of neonatal hypothyroidism, and some have advocated a second screening specimen at approximately 2 to 6 weeks of life. Approaches include primary T4 with follow-up TSH, simultaneous T4 and TSH, and primary TSH-only screening methods. All of these detect congenital hypothyroidism cases at essentially similar rates but all suffer from false negatives. The TSH-only approach will miss cases of delayed TSH rise and central hypothyroidism. All methods are likely to miss mild hypothyroidism. Presently, evidence supports a second discretionary screening test in very low birth weight infants, infants with significant perinatal complications, and same-sex twins.

Euthyroid sick syndrome

- A 'syndrome' consisting entirely of abnormal thyroid function tests in a euthyroid individual who is suffering from a non-thyroidal illness. The typical case involves a critically ill, elderly, hospitalized individual.

- Thyroid function tests in the euthyroid sick syndrome are typically: decreased T3, increased rT3, and normal TSH. The TSH is actually decreased in 5-9% of cases.

Exogenous estrogens

A common problem in TFT interpretation involves the patient taking exogenous estrogen, usually in the form of oral contraceptives. Such agents increase circulating thyroid-binding globulin (TBG), thus elevating total thyroxine (T3 & T4). The free thyroxine is still normal. Excess TBG is associated with the euthyroid state with a normal TSH.

Amiodarone

Due to a combination of its direct thyroid toxicity and its large quantity of iodine, amiodarone exerts effects on thyroid function. The effect is largely unpredictable, but a general rule-of-thumb is that in developed (iodine-rich) parts of the world, amiodarone causes hypothyroidism, and in underdeveloped (iodine-poor) places, amiodarone causes hyperthyroidism.

Adrenal Cortex

Tests

- **Serum cortisol.** It is essential to recall that cortisol secretion normally undergoes diurnal variation. It is secreted at low levels with, intermittent small surges, throughout the day with a relative trough around midnight and a significant peak around 8 am. Thus, interpretation of a single random serum cortisol is difficult. Furthermore, the quantity of serum cortisol depends upon highly variable levels of cortisol binding globulin. Patients with Cushing syndrome demonstrate elevated serum cortisol with loss of diurnal variation. A single elevated midnight serum cortisol, when levels should be relatively low, is highly suggestive of Cushing syndrome.

- **Urine free cortisol.** This test is more accurate than serum cortisol but requires a 24-hour urine collection. It is free (unbound) cortisol that passes into the urine, so this test reflects the amount of free cortisol. Furthermore, since measured in a 24-hour specimen, this test is independent of time-of-day considerations. An elevated urine free cortisol is highly suggestive of Cushing syndrome; however, like the serum test, false positive results may be seen in stress, depression, and chronic alcoholism. A negative test is incapable of excluding Cushing syndrome, and should be repeated. The test is invalid if there is renal insufficiency.

- **Dexamethasone suppression test (DST).** Dexamethasone is an agent capable of suppressing ACTH without cross-reacting with assays for cortisol. In patients with normal endocrine function, a dose of dexamethasone will suppress CRF, ACTH, and cortisol.

  □ **Rapid DST and low-dose DST.** Both of these tests are aimed at answering the question: does the patient have Cushing syndrome (hypercortisolism)? In the rapid test, 1 mg of dexamethasone is administered at 11 pm, and the plasma cortisol is measured at 8 am. In the low-dose DST, 0.5 mg are given every 6 hours for 48 hours. Normal individuals experience suppression of plasma cortisol in this test. Impaired suppression of plasma cortisol levels by these tests confirms the diagnosis of Cushing syndrome; however, abnormal suppression can also be seen in severe stress, alcohol abuse, and major depression.

  □ **High-dose DST.** This test is used to answer the question: is the patient's Cushing syndrome (hypercortisolism) due to a pituitary adenoma (Cushing disease)? 2 mg dexamethasone every 6 hours for 48 hours should suppress pituitary adenoma-related hypercortisolism (Cushing disease). Non-suppression points to either ectopic ACTH production by tumor or primary adrenal hypercortisolism. The latter two can be distinguished by serum ACTH measurement.

- **Cortisol-Releasing Hormone (CRH) stimulation test.** Like the high-dose DST, this test is aimed at determining the cause of Cushing syndrome. After IV administration of CRH, an exaggerated elevation in ACTH and cortisol suggests Cushing disease (pituitary adenoma). With adrenal tumors or ectopic ACTH, no response is seen.

- **Metyrapone stimulation test.** The metyrapone stimulation tests is used to determine whether the pituitary is to blame when a patient is deficient in cortisol (Addisonian). Metyrapone blocks the conversion of 11-deoxycortisol to cortisol. The decreased cortisol leads to increased ACTH production by the pituitary. In normal subjects, this increased ACTH can sufficiently increase the 11-deoxycortisol to overcome the metyrapone-induced block, thus increasing serum cortisol. Patients who cannot overcome this block have impaired pituitary function.

■ The late-night (11:00 pm) salivary cortisol is perhaps the best screening test for Cushing syndrome. It has a reported 100% specificity and 91%-93% sensitivity for Cushing syndrome. It appears that salivary cortisol correlates well with serum cortisol, independent of salivary flow rates. Furthermore, it is free cortisol that crosses into the saliva; thus this assay reflects free serum cortisol and therefore does not have the problem of variation with changes in cortisol binding globulin that significantly hampers the interpretation of serum cortisol levels. Cortisol is stable in saliva for up to 1 week, so patients may collect the sample at home.

Cushing syndrome (hypercortisolism)

■ Causes of Cushing syndrome include adrenal hypercortisolism (about 20%), pituitary hypersecretion of ACTH (Cushing disease—about 70%), and ectopic ACTH production by tumor. Iatrogenic Cushing syndrome—administration of corticosteroids for the treatment of inflammatory disease—is very common as well, perhaps more common than all of the above.

   □ In Cushing disease, the cause is usually a pituitary microadenoma of basophilic cells. There is bilateral adrenal hyperplasia, and ACTH levels are elevated along with cortisol levels.

   □ Ectopic ACTH is most commonly associated with a pulmonary neoplasm, usually small cell (oat cell) carcinoma.

   □ Primary adrenal hypercortisolism may be due to bilateral adrenal hyperplasia, adenoma, or carcinoma. In adults, adenomas and carcinomas have roughly equal incidence. In children, carcinomas actually outnumber adenomas. Carcinomas are associated with higher mean levels of serum cortisol than adenomas.

■ In all these, there is elevated serum cortisol, elevated urinary free cortisol, elevated salivary cortisol, loss of the normal diurnal variation, and abnormal suppression by dexamethasone.

■ The biochemical results of hypercortisolism include hyperglycemia, hypokalemia, hypernatremia, protein catabolism, and osteoporosis.

Addison syndrome (hypocortisolism)

■ Addison syndrome may be due to Addison disease (primary adrenal insufficiency) or pituitary hypofunction (secondary adrenal insufficiency). Most cases are related to the administration of exogenous cortisol that can lead to irreversible (or very slowly reversible) suppression of endogenous ACTH production by the pituitary. The most common cause in the past related to primary destruction of the adrenal gland by autoimmunity or granulomatous infection such as tuberculosis. Addison disease may also be due to metastatic tumor, amyloidosis, bilateral adrenal hemorrhage (Waterhouse-Friderichsen syndrome), or administration of drugs such as ketoconazole. Adrenal failure is frequent in severe sepsis, with a reported incidence as high as 61%. Liver failure is well recognized to cause renal (hepatorenal syndrome) and pulmonary (hepatopulmonary syndrome) disease; it has recently been recognized that patients with liver failure and patients undergoing liver transplantation have a very high rate (>70%) of adrenal failure (hepatoadrenal syndrome).

■ In the typical case, a patient presents with altered mental status, weakness, hypotension, and the typical biochemical abnormalities including hypoglycemia, hyponatremia and hyperkalemia with a metabolic acidosis. In patients with primary adrenal causes of Addison syndrome, co-hypersecretion of melanocyte stimulating hormone (MSH) results in diffuse hyperpigmentation of the skin.

T1.33
Congenital Adrenal Hyperplasia (CAH)

Enzyme Deficiency	Adrenal Hyperplasia	Virilization	Salt Wasting	Hypertension
21-hydroxylase	+	+	+	−
11-hydroxylase	+	+	−	+

- Diagnosis depends fairly straightforwardly on the demonstration of low serum cortisol. If the cortisol is not low, then additional testing with a cortosyn stimulation test and/or plasma ACTH levels are necessary. Cortosyn (cosyntropin) is an ACTH analog whose administration should result in a measurable bump in serum cortisol. Absence of this response confirms primary adrenal insufficiency. A good response with low serum ACTH suggests secondary adrenal insufficiency.

Conn syndrome (hyperaldosteronism)

- This is usually due to an adrenal adenoma. Secondary hyperaldosteronism is seen in hyper-reninemic states such as renal artery stenosis or the rare renin-producing juxtaglomerular cell tumor of the kidney.

- In primary hyperaldosteronism, serum renin is low. The aldosterone/renin ratio is useful for screening; however, interpretation of the result requires an appreciation that many factors (diet, posture, time of day, day-to-day variation, presence of hypokalemia, medications, age, and renal function) can affect the results. Control of these factors and repeated testing on separate days is necessary before a decision to pursue primary hyperaldosteronism is made. Renin is measured by the plasma renin activity (PRA) assay, which measures the rate of conversion of angiotensin I to angiotensin II.

- The consequences of hyperaldosteronism include hypertension with hypervolemia, hypernatremia, hypokalemia, and metabolic alkalosis. Conn syndrome is a surgically treatable form of hypertension that may account for up to 3% of new hypertensives.

Congenital adrenal hyperplasia T1.33

- At least 8 different inherited enzyme deficiencies of the adrenal cortex are known, all of which are autosomal recessively inherited. 21-hydroxylase deficiency is the most common, followed by 11-hydroxylase deficiency, and the others are vanishingly rare.

- The incidence varies geographically, and the U.S., the disease is particularly common in Native Americans and Yupic Eskimos (incidence of 1/280). Among American Caucasians, the incidence is about 1/15000. A high rate of the disease is found on the island of La Réunion (1/2100), Brazil (1/7500), and the Philippines (1/7000).

- The gene for 21-hydroxylase is found on 6p21.3, within the HLA complex. 21-hydroxylase deficiency results from a fairly unique sort of mutation. The gene consists of two highly homologous near-copies in series—an active gene (CYP21A), and an inactive pseudogene (CYP21P). Mutant alleles result from recombination between the pseudo and active genes in a process called gene conversion.

- The severity of disease varies (depending upon the nature of the mutation). In general, a compensatory increase in ACTH by the pituitary leads to increased production of steroid hormone precursors in the adrenal cortex. The resulting adrenal hyperplasia and altered hormonal milieu results in some degree of salt wasting, hypertension, and virilization. Affected individuals have increased 17-hydroxy progesterone, decreased cortisol, increased ACTH, increased androgens, increased 17-ketosteroids, and decreased aldosterone. The effect on serum electrolytes is an increase in potassium and decrease in sodium T1.27.

- Female infants with classic CAH have ambiguous genitalia because of exposure to high concentrations of androgens in utero, and CAH due to 21-hydroxylase deficiency is the most common cause of ambiguous genitalia in 46XX infants. Less severely affected girls can present with early pubarche, or as young women with polycystic ovarian syndrome (hirsutism, oligomenorrhea polycystic ovaries, and acne).

- Boys with classic CAH have no signs of CAH at birth, except subtle hyperpigmentation and possible penile enlargement. Thus, the age at diagnosis in boys varies according to the severity of aldosterone deficiency. Boys with the non-salt-losing form present with early virilization at age 2–4 years.

- A very high concentration of 17-hydroxyprogesterone (more than 242 nmol/L; normal less than 3 nmol/L at 3 days in full-term infant) in a randomly timed blood sample is diagnostic of classic 21-hydroxylase deficiency. Typically, salt-losing patients have higher 17-hydroxyprogesterone concentrations than non-salt losers. False-positive results from neonatal screening are common with premature infants, and many screening programs have established reference ranges that are based on weight and gestational age. A corticotrophin stimulation test can be used in borderline cases. Genetic analysis can be helpful to confirm the diagnosis. Treatment involves replacement of glucocorticoids and mineralocorticoids.

Pituitary

- Physiologic control of anterior pituitary hormone secretion comes from feedback acting directly on the anterior pituitary as well as hypothalamic hormones.

- The anterior pituitary (adenohypophysis) houses a heterogeneous population of cells, some of which are acidophilic with acridine orange while others are basophilic with this stain.

  □ The acidophils consist of two cell types: growth hormone-secreting cells and prolactin-secreting cells.

  □ The **b**asophils include four cell types that secrete: **f**ollicle-stimulating hormone (FSH), **l**uteinizing hormone (LH), **a**drenocorticotrophic hormone (ACTH), and **t**hyroid stimulating hormone (TSH). An easy way to remember this is the mnemonic **B-FLAT.**

- The posterior pituitary (neurohypophysis) contains the axon-termini of neurons that originate in the supraoptic and paraventricular nuclei in the hypothalamus and produce oxytocin and anti-diuretic hormone (ADH; vasopressin).

- Hypersecretion of any of the anterior pituitary hormones is nearly always the result of a pituitary adenoma. Prolactinomas are the most common secretory tumors of the pituitary. Most prolactinomas are so-called microadenomas (measuring <1 cm).

- **Panhypopituitarism (hypofunction of the pituitary)** Pituitary hypofunction rarely involves a single hormone. Usually there is global hyposecretion. Causes include tumors impinging on the pituitary (nonsecretory pituitary adenomas, craniopharyngiomas), infarction (Sheehan syndrome, sickle cell anemia), sarcoidosis, histiocytosis X, hemochromatosis, irradiation, and autoimmune destruction. Hypothalamic disorders and interruption of the pituitary stalk may produce depression of all anterior pituitary hormones except prolactin. This pattern prolactin-sparing hypopituitarism is called 'stalk effect.'

Growth hormone (GH)

- GH is secreted by acidophils (called somatotrophs) in the anterior pituitary. GH release is stimulated by growth hormone releasing hormone (GHRH) from the hypothalamus. It is inhibited by somatostatin (SS) from the pancreas. Stimulants of GHRH and GH release are: stress, hypoglycemia, and increased amino acid levels, particularly arginine.

- GH may be undetectable in normal adult individuals. Increases in GH levels occur in association with a number of events: it is highest during sleep—particularly the first two hours, a small increase is seen with exercise, and it rises with hypoglycemia and stress.

- **GH hyposecretion.** In children, GH deficiency causes dwarfism. In adults, it is relatively asymptomatic. Undetectable fasting GH levels occur frequently in healthy subjects and are not diagnostic of hyposecretion. Thus, provocative testing is required, performed by measuring GH in the fasting state, during sleep, following exercise, or following insulin or arginine administration. An insulin tolerance test is performed by injecting insulin then serially measuring GH every 15 minutes. The hypoglycemia that results should cause a GH rise of greater than 20 ng/mL. Similar provocative tests can be carried out with exercise, arginine injection, or oral clonidine.

- **GH hypersecretion.** GH hypersecretion causes acromegaly in children and gigantism in adults. GH hypersecretion cannot be excluded with a single normal GH level. A good test for GH excess is IGF-1. As it does not undergo diurnal variation and is consistently elevated in GH hypersecretion, a single normal IGF-1 determination is reliable for excluding GH excess. GH hypersecretion can also be diagnosed by

  □ a markedly elevated GH from a random blood sample

  □ a relatively normal level that fails to suppress with glucose administration.

Endocrine>Pituitary

Follicle stimulating hormone (FSH) and luteinizing hormone (LH)

- Secretion of FSH and LH is stimulated by hypothalamic gonadotropin releasing hormone (GnRH), also called luteinizing hormone releasing hormone (LHRH).

- A unique property of GnRH activity is that when GnRH receptors are continuously stimulated, GnRH soon becomes inhibitory. This is the principle exploited by therapeutic GnRH agonists.

- FSH assays can be useful in younger women (eg, < 45 years) presenting with possible early menopause. The finding, on two separate determinations taken >4 weeks apart, of FSH >40 IU/L suggests ovarian failure.

Prolactin

- Prolactin is unique among the anterior pituitary hormones in that it does not have a dedicated stimulator for its release; instead, the hypothalamus produces a potent inhibitor, dopamine. If connections between the hypothalamus and pituitary are severed, all anterior pituitary hormones decrease (due to lack of stimulation) except prolactin which markedly increases (due to lack of inhibition). In fact, this constellation of endocrine findings is often referred to as "stalk effect", referring to its frequent relation to some kind of impingement upon the pituitary stalk.

- In women, hyperprolactinemia produces the so-called amenorrhea-galactorrhea syndrome. In men, testicular atrophy, impotence, and gynecomastia are the result.

- Hypoprolactinemia is rare. Hyperprolactinemia is usually due to a prolactin-secreting pituitary adenoma. Other causes include pregnancy, lactation, stalk compression, macroprolactinemia, & phenothiazine therapy.

Adrenocorticotropic hormone (ACTH)

- Corticotrophin-releasing hormone (CRH) stimulates secretion of ACTH. ACTH is the product of post-translational cleavage of a large precursor molecule called pro-opio melanocortin (POMC). POMC is cleaved into ACTH, melanocyte-stimulating hormone (MSH), and b-endorphin.

Anti-diuretic hormone (ADH)

- Is secreted from the posterior pituitary in response to increased serum osmotic pressure and volume depletion.

- Diabetes insipidus (DI), the condition that results from inadequate ADH activity, is characterized by polyuria and polydipsia. Patients produce a large quantity of very dilute urine. Either ADH secretion is inadequate (central DI) or renal tubules are unresponsive to ADH (nephrogenic DI). Causes of central DI include head trauma, mass lesions involving the pituitary, and an X-linked recessive familial form. Nephrogenic DI may be due to hypercalcemia, hypokalemia, a very low-protein diet, demeclocycline therapy, lithium therapy, relief of longstanding obstruction, and familial causes. Normal aging may by itself be associated with a partial nephrogenic DI. The diagnosis is suspected in any hypernatremic individual who has low urine osmolarity. It is confirmed by an overnight water deprivation test followed by administration of ADH (vasopressin). In healthy individuals, urine osmolarity progressively increases during water deprivation. Administration of exogenous ADH has no additional effect on urine concentration. In central DI, there is failure to appropriately concentrate the urine in response to dehydration and a rise in urine osmolarity in response to administered ADH. In nephrogenic DI, urine cannot be concentrated in either case.

- The syndrome of inappropriate ADH (SIADH) is suspected in the hyponatremic individual who is relatively normovolemic and has high urinary sodium (>20 mmol/L) and high urine osmolarity (>100 mOsm/Kg). It may be caused by: tumors (especially small cell carcinoma of the lung, pancreatic adenocarcinoma, and intracranial tumors), interstitial lung disease, cerebral trauma, and the drug chlorpropamide.

Postmortem Chemistries

Samples

There are significant differences in glucose, insulin, pH, oxygen tension, LDH, alkaline phosphatase, and many drugs between specimens taken from the left and right sides of the heart and between central (cardiac) and peripheral blood. The exact source of blood submitted is therefore important to know, and blind cardiac puncture is to be avoided.

Up to 3 mL of vitreous can be obtained from the typical adult. It is important to obtain as much vitreous as can be extracted, as there is variation in the concentrations of many solutes between vitreous next to the retina and central vitreous.

DNA testing works quite well in postmortem tissue.

Glucose

Serum glucose tends to increase after death, due to postmortem hepatic glycogenolysis. Samples from the right heart or inferior vena cava (IVC) will usually have extremely high glucose, but even peripheral vessels cannot be relied upon to give useful measurements. The postmortem diagnosis of diabetes mellitus should not be made on the basis of postmortem blood glucose alone. Adjunctive tests include the $HgbA_{1c}$, glycosuria, ketonuria, and serum acetone.

Vitreous glucose falls after death, due to glycolysis. Vitreous is preferred for the postmortem diagnosis of diabetic ketoacidosis (DKA) which is diagnosed in the presence of high vitreous glucose and ketones.

Hypoglycemia cannot be reliably diagnosed in the postmortem state.

Blood Urea Nitrogen (BUN) and Creatinine

Both BUN and creatinine are remarkably stable after death.

In addition to its value in diagnosing renal insufficiency, mild nitrogen retention in conjunction with hypernatremia is useful to diagnose dehydration.

Sodium and Chloride

Sodium and chloride levels begin to decrease immediately after death, both at a rate of approximately 0.9 mEq/L/hour. Individual variation precludes their use in determining the postmortem interval.

Vitreous sodium and chloride are very stable. Both reflect antemortem electrolyte status, and can be used in conjunction with BUN and K^+ to categorize the patient into one of several patterns T1.34.

Potassium

Serum and CSF potassium rise quite abruptly after death.

Vitreous potassium rises more linearly after death and is probably the most reliable chemical test for postmortem interval.

Normal vitreous K^+ is anything under 15 mEq/L.

T1.34
Postmortem Chemistry Patterns

Pattern	Sodium	Chloride	Potassium	BUN	Creatinine
Dehydration	↑	↑	→	↑	↑
Uremic	→	→	→	↑	↑
Low-salt	↓	↓	↓	→	→
Decomposition	↓	↓	↑	→	→

Digoxin

Digoxin is a lipotrophic drug in vivo. After death, digoxin is released from tissues and reenters the serum.

Thus, postmortem digoxin levels rise progressively, and the postmortem diagnosis of digoxin toxicity should not be made on this basis alone.

Another source of error is the presence of endogenous digoxin-like substances (EDLS). EDLS are found in patients with volume overload, hepatorenal failure, pregnancy, hypertension, and in normal infants.

Tryptase and the Postmortem Diagnosis of Anaphylaxis

The postmortem anatomic findings reported in anaphylaxis are numerous and somewhat nonspecific, including pulmonary and laryngeal edema. The postmortem serum tryptase has been advocated as a means to establish a diagnosis of anaphylaxis. Tryptase appears to be stable in serum for several days after death.

An elevated serum tryptase is not an entirely specific finding, and has been reported in non-anaphylactic deaths. However, a normal postmortem serum tryptase has a high negative predictive value. The overall sensitivity of postmortem serum tryptase is about 85-90%. Specific IgE assays may be of some use if a particular stimulus is suspected.

Body Fluids

Urine

Urine chemistry

- **Glucose.** The two methods widely employed for detecting glucose in urine are

    □ the dipstick

    □ the copper sulfate method (eg, Clinitest)

    Glucose begins to spill over into urine when the 'renal threshold' for serum glucose is reached, at around 180 mg/dL. The dipstick method relies on the enzymes glucose oxidase and peroxidase to

convert glucose to gluconate with the resulting hydrogen peroxide by-product reacting with a chromogen. This method is sensitive mainly to glucose, and other 'reducing substances' do not tend to give a positive reaction. In contrast, the copper sulfate method (Benedict reaction) reacts with a wide range of 'reducing substances'.

- **Protein.** Only albumin is detected by the dipstick reagent. Although semi quantitative, trace positive reactions correspond to around 15-30 mg/dL and 4+ positives correspond to around 2.0 g/dL. Normal urine protein amounts to about 150 mg/day of predominantly Tamm-Harsfall (tubular) protein. Greater amounts of protein may be seen following vigorous exercise, dehydration, and fever. Benign types of proteinuria include postural and intermittent proteinuria, which together occur in up to 5% of the population. Precipitation techniques, such as sulfosalicylic acid (SSA) or trichloroacetic acid (TCA), can establish the presence of other proteins. To detect Bence-Jones proteins, a unique solubility property of light chain proteins can be exploited: when heated, Bence-Jones proteins precipitate at 40°C then re-dissolve at 100°C. When cooled, the proteins precipitate at 60°C the re-dissolve at 40°C. A urine protein electrophoresis (UPEP) may also be helpful.

- **Ketones.** The dipstick test for ketones is sensitive only to acetoacetic acid, but not β-hydroxybutyrate or acetone.

- **Hemoglobin.** Hemoglobinuria must be distinguished from hematuria, the latter referring to the finding of red blood cells in the urine and can only be confirmed by urine microscopy. Most cases of hemoglobinuria are due to hematuria, but uncommonly hemoglobin may be present alone in the urine, indicating intravascular hemolysis. Myoglobinuria, resulting usually from rhabdomyolysis, also results in a positive dipstick test for hemoglobin. The best way to distinguish myoglobinuria from hemoglobinuria is by history and additional lab tests. Specifically, myoglobinuria is accompanied by a history of severe muscle tenderness following strenuous exercise and additional laboratory findings of elevated serum CK, elevated serum aldolase, and normal haptoglobin. Immunochemical methods can also be used to separate the two. In the past, various poorly reproducible precipitation methods were employed, including ammonium sulfate (NH_4SO_4) in which Mgb is soluble while Hgb precipitates.

■ **Bilirubin and urobilinogen.** Since unconjugated bilirubin does not pass through the glomerulus, urinary bilirubin is indicative of conjugated hyperbilirubinemia. Urobilinogen, on the other hand, is more complicated. Urobilinogen is the product of hydrolysis of bilirubin by intestinal bacteria. In the usual course of events, a certain amount of the bilirubin that is dumped into the intestine through the bile duct is converted into urobilinogen by the bacterial flora. A fraction of this urobilinogen is absorbed by the enterocytes and passed into the portal circulation where most of it goes to the liver to be re-excreted, and a small amount makes it to the kidneys to be excreted in urine. Whenever there is (1) liver disease preventing the re-excretion step or (2) increased bilirubin excretion leading to increased urobilinogen formation thus exceeding the capacity of the re-excretion step, one sees increased urobilinogen in the urine. In the jaundiced patient, the interpretation of urinary bilirubin and urobilinogen is shown in **T1.35**.

■ **Nitrite.** Most agents that cause urinary tract infections (UTI) are nitrite + organisms such as *E. coli*. Thus, this test will be positive in the presence of most urinary tract infections. Urine must have been standing in the bladder for 4 hours to give a positive test. Nitrite negative organisms that may cause UTI include enterococci, *N. gonorrhea,* and *M. tuberculosis.*

■ **Leukocyte esterase.** Also useful to screen for UTI, this test is a reflection of the number of urinary neutrophils. Trichomonads and eosinophils are possible sources of esterases giving false-positive results.

■ **Specific gravity.** The normal adult specific gravity ranges from 1.003-1.029. It is increased in dehydration, diabetes mellitus, proteinuria, congestive heart failure, Addison disease, and the syndrome of inappropriate anti-diuretic hormone (SIADH). It is decreased in polydipsia, diuretic therapy, and diabetes insipidus (DI). It is fixed at around 1.010 in isosthenuria, in which tubular damage results in the urine specific gravity equaling that of the glomerular filtrate. Isosthenuria results from renal medullary dysfunction and is a common finding in sickle cell disease.

■ **pH.** Normal urinary pH varies between 4.6 and 8.0. In renal tubular acidosis (RTA) the urine is inappropriately alkaline relative to the blood pH, and the kidneys cannot acidify the urine beyond pH 6.5.

■ **Ascorbic acid.** Ascorbate inhibits several dipstick tests, including glucose, hemoglobin, bilirubin, nitrite, and leukocyte esterase.

Nephrolithiasis (kidney stones)

■ The majority (70%) of kidney stones are composed of calcium oxalate. In decreasing order of incidence, the remaining stones are composed of: calcium phosphate, struvite (also know as magnesium ammonium phosphate stones, triple phosphate stones, or staghorn calculi), urate, and cystine.

■ Stone formation requires a nidus; thus, not all patients with a predisposing metabolic state will form a stone. One regularly sees crystals in the urine of people without a history of stones **T1.36**

■ Nonetheless, knowing the chemical composition of a stone helps to illuminate treatable underlying metabolic conditions. The chemical composition of stones is most often carried out by x-ray crystallography or infrared spectroscopy.

T1.35
Urine Bilirubin Interpretation

Test	Normal	Unconjugated Hyperbilirubinemia	Conjugated Hyperbilirubinemia	Hepatitis
Urine bilirubin	–	–	+	+
Urine urobilinogen	+/–	–	+++	+++

- The most common stone, calcium oxalate, is promoted by low urine volumes (a factor common to all types of stone), low urinary citrate, hypercalciuria, and oxaluria. Oxaluria is increased in patients who have Crohn disease, who have undergone small bowel resection or small bowel bypass, or who ingest excessive amounts of oxalate (rhubarbs, spinach, and nuts). Urinary pH has little effect on calcium oxalate crystallization. Primary hyperoxaluria is a rare autosomal recessive condition which results in a very high oxalate excretion with stone formation that begins in childhood. Tubulointerstitial nephritis develops, ultimately leading to renal failure.

- Calcium phosphate stones are promoted by low urinary volumes, hypercalciuria, and elevated (alkalotic) pH. Many types of stones are promoted by systemic hypercalcemia, and this should be diagnosed and treated. X linked nephrolithiasis (Dent disease) is a very rare condition caused by a mutation in the voltage-gated chloride channel 5 (CLCN5) gene, leading to a renal calcium leak, hypercalciuria, and stone formation. Formers of calcium-containing stones who demonstrate hypercalciuria may benefit from thiazide diuretics (which increase calcium reabsorption). Citrate functions as a stone inhibitor because it binds calcium.

T1.36
Urine Crystals

Crystal	Comments
Calcium oxalate	'Envelopes' May also form 'dumbbells' Most common component of kidney stones
Uric acid	Pleomorphic crystals, most often diamond, square, or rod-shaped, which polarize in a variety of colors
Hippurate	
Triple phosphate (magnesium ammonium phosphate; struvite)	'Coffin lids' Form in alkaline pH, related to *P. mirabilis* Cause 'staghorn calculi'
Ammonium biurate	'Thorn apples'
Cysteine	Hexagonal crystals Related to cystinuria
Tyrosine	'Silky' or 'sheaves of wheat' crystals
Cholesterol	'Broken panes of glass'
Sulfa	'Fans'
Bilirubin	Yellow-brown needles

- Struvite stones are promoted by urinary infection by urea-splitting organisms (*Proteus mirabilis*) which contribute to markedly elevated (alkalotic) urine pH.

- Urate stones are promoted by acidotic pH and hyperuricosuria. While patients with chronic ulcerative colitis and Crohn disease tend to develop hyperoxaluria and oxalate stones, up to 30% of stones identified in these patients are urate stones. Urate stones are particularly common in patients after colectomy. Hyperuricosuria can be treated with allopurinol (xanthine oxidase inhibitor) that reduces the endogenous formation of urate. Urine alkalinization is also helpful.

- Cystine stones are seen in the setting of the inherited disease cystinuria (not cystinosis), an autosomal recessive disease characterized by defective renal and intestinal dibasic amino acid transport, affecting cystine, ornithine, lysine, and arginine (COLA). Of these, cystine is the least soluble and the most likely to precipitate as a stone. Cystine stone formation can be inhibited by urine alkalinization and dietary protein restriction.

- 2,8-Dihydroxyadenine stones are extremely rare, representing about 1 in 1000 stones, and are due to an autosomal recessive deficiency of adenine phosphoribosyl transferase, which is necessary for purine metabolism. In its absence, 2,8-dihydroxyadenine appears in urine resulting in stone formation. Treatment is with allopurinol.

Urine microscopy

- **Red blood cells (hematuria).** Some insight into the source of urinary red blood cells can be gained by observing the red cell morphology. In glomerular pattern bleeding, the red cells are polymorphous, with various shapes and hemoglobin concentrations. Furthermore, there are often red blood cell casts and erythrophagocytosis. In non-glomerular pattern bleeding, the red cell morphology is relatively uniform, red cell casts are absent, and no erythrophagocytosis is seen.

T1.37
Urine Microscopy in Acute Renal Failure

Finding	ATN	RPGN	AIN
Red blood cells	Normal numbers or slightly increased with nonglomerular pattern	Increased with glomerular pattern	Normal numbers or slightly increased with nonglomerular pattern
Casts	Granular & waxy; tubular casts	Granular & waxy; red cell casts	Granular & waxy; tubular casts
Erythrophagocytosis	–	+	–
Granulocytes	Scant	Scant	Numerous, including neutrophils and eosinophils

- Casts

    - **Hyaline casts.** These are clear, colorless casts that are difficult to see and are relatively nonspecific. Though they may be seen in renal disease, they may also be the consequence of dehydration or vigorous exercise.

    - **Red cell casts.** Relatively specific for glomerulonephritis, these casts have lumpy edges and are composed of anucleate, slightly reddish, pale discs.

    - **White cell casts.** This finding is typical of tubulointerstitial nephritis, particularly pyelonephritis. The casts are composed of nucleated cells with the typical lobated nuclei of neutrophils.

    - **Tubular casts.** These are composed of renal tubular cells characterized by their mononuclear, cuboidal, cells and generally indicate acute tubular necrosis.

    - **Granular casts.** These casts are somewhat nonspecific but are typically present when there is significant renal disease. They are casts that are acellular and characterized by a rough, granular, surface. The granules may be fine or coarse.

    - **Waxy casts.** Also indicative of some kind of renal disease, these casts are acellular and characterized by blunt ends, a pale yellow color, and cracks along their length.

    - **Broad casts.** These can be any of the above that are unusually broad and indicate end-stage renal disease. They correspond to the widely dilated collecting ducts seen in advanced atrophy.

    - **Fatty casts.** These are indicative of nephrotic syndrome, in which lipiduria is a common feature. They consist of cellular casts in which lipid droplets are absorbed. With polarized light, the absorbed lipid has a Maltese-cross appearance.

- **Urine microscopy in the patient with acute renal failure.** For practical purposes, the differential diagnosis of acute renal failure includes: acute tubular necrosis (ATN), rapidly progressive (crescentic) glomerulonephritis (RPGN), and acute interstitial nephritis (AIN) **T1.37**.

Cerebrospinal Fluid (CSF)

CSF chemistry

- **Xanthochromia** is defined as pink or yellow-tinged fluid following centrifugation. Pink xanthochromia is due to free hemoglobin and is detected following subarachnoid hemorrhage. Yellow xanthochromia is due to bilirubin from hemoglobin metabolism and begins around 12 hours, peaking at 72 hours, and disappearing in 2-4 weeks. Artifactual xanthochromia may be due to: hyperbilirubinemia, CSF protein >150 mg/dL, carotinoids, melanin, rifampin, or delay of >1 hour prior to examination.

- **Distinguishing truly bloody from traumatic taps.** If the fluid becomes progressively clearer from tube 1 to tube 4, then it is likely traumatic. If xanthochromia is present, then it is probably truly bloody. Erythrophagocytosis, hemosiderin-laden macrophages, and a positive latex for D-dimer all indicate a true bleed and are negative in traumatic taps.

- CSF protein is normally 15-45 mg/dL. CSF protein is so scant that it must be precipitated with trichloroacetic acid (TCA) or sulosalicylic acid (SSA) before quantitation. Increased CSF protein is seen in inflammatory states such as meningitis, hemorrhage, and CSF obstruction.

- Assessment of the integrity of the blood-brain barrier can be made with the CSF/serum albumin ratio (should be <1:230).

- CSF leak, such as when a patient has post-traumatic rhinorrhea or otorrhea, may be diagnosed by

  □ **glucose measurement**, which is very nonspecific, looking for the typical glucose content of CSF

  □ **protein electrophoresis**, looking for the typical twin transfusion peak and pre-albumin bands of CSF

  □ measurement of **asialated transferrin**, whose presence is suggestive of CSF

- Supporting the diagnosis of multiple sclerosis (MS)

  □ Two cerebrospinal fluid findings support the diagnosis of MS: intrathecal IgG synthesis and oligoclonal bands.

  □ The ratio of CSF:serum IgG is elevated whenever there is intrathecal immunoglobulin production or increased blood-brain barrier permeability. One can exclude the effect of increased permeability by using the albumin CSF:serum ratio as a control; thus, the IgG index is obtained by dividing the CSF IgG/serum IgG ratio by the ratio of CSF albumin/serum albumin (all determined by nephelometry). Intrathecal IgG synthesis (CSF IgG index) has a sensitivity of about 90% for MS.

  □ Oligoclonal bands (several distinct bands in the gamma region) by agarose gel electrophoresis has a sensitivity of 50-75% and a specificity of 95-97% for MS. Isoelectric focusing (IEF) appears to be more sensitive for the detection of oligoclonal bands, with a reported sensitivity of 90% and specificity of 95%. Recall that in simple electrophoresis, after voltage has been applied to the sample for a period of time, the gel is fixed and stained; whereas, in IEF anti-IgG antibody is added prior to staining. This step ampli-

fies any bands that may be present. In simple electrophoresis, 2 or more bands are typically considered positive; whereas, in IEF, 4 or more bands are considered positive.

- Immunoglobulin isotypes in cerebrospinal fluid: increased intrathecal production of IgA is the most sensitive marker for cerebral adrenoleukodystrophy.

- CSF glucose levels are normally 60% of serum levels (ie, somewhere around 60 mg/dL), varying from 40-80%. Hypoglycorrhachia (<30%) is seen in bacterial meningitis.

- CSF glutamine is elevated in hepatic encephalopathy.

- Latex agglutination has around 90% sensitivity for *H. influenzae*, 60% for *S. pneumoniae* and *N. meningitidis*, and 90% for Group B Streptococci. For neurosyphilis, the FTA-ABS is essentially 100% sensitive and 95% specific. The CSF VDRL is around 60% sensitive but nearly 100% specific. Thus, counter to what is true for serum, the CSF FTA-ABS is used for screening, and the CSF VDRL is confirmatory. The RPR is inappropriate for CSF.

CSF microscopy

- The normal cell count is 0-5 per mL for adults and 0-30 per mL for neonates. In a traumatic tap, some WBCs may be from peripheral blood, as may some protein. For normal individuals, about 1 WBC can be expected for every 700 red cells, and about 8 mg/dL protein for each 10,000 RBC/mL.

- Normal CSF differentials **T1.38**

T1.38
Normal Cerebrospinal Fluid Differential Counts

Cell Type	Adults	Neonates
Lymphocytes	30%-90%	10%-40%
Monocytes	10%-50%	50%-90%
Neutrophils	0-6%	0-10%
Ependymal	rare	rare
Eosinophils	rare	rare

T1.39
Cerebrospinal Fluid Differential Counts in Meningitis

Type of Infection	Leukocyte Count	Protein	Leukocyte Differential	Glucose	Comment
Bacterial	1000-10,000	>100	Polys predominate	<40	Partially treated infections may be lymphocyte-predominant
Viral	50-500	20-100	Polys early, lymphs late	Normal	Decreased glucose is characteristic of HSV encephalitis
Fungal and mycobacterial	50-500	20-100	Lymphs predominate	<50	

- CSF differentials in infection **T1.39**

Pleural Fluid

Pleural fluid chemistry

- **Light criteria** help to classify effusions as exudative or transudative. Generally speaking, most transudates are due to congestive heart failure (CHF), cirrhosis, or nephrotic syndrome (the latter two relating to decreased serum osmotic pressure). Nearly all other causes of pleural effusions cause exudative effusions. Causes of exudative pleural effusions include, but are not limited to, bacterial pneumonia (parapneumonic pleural effusion), malignancy (usually bloody), tuberculosis (noted for lymphocyte predominance and paucity of mesothelial cells), pulmonary embolus (may be transudative), collagen vascular diseases (especially rheumatoid arthritis), pancreatitis (classically left-sided), esophageal perforation, chylothorax, asbestos exposure, post-myocardial infarction (Dressler syndrome), uremia, and ovarian fibromas (Meig syndrome). According to Light criteria, the presence of any of the following indicates an exudative effusion

  □ Pleural fluid:serum protein ratio >0.5

  □ Pleural fluid:serum LDH ratio >0.6

  □ Pleural fluid LDH >200 (later modified to two thirds the laboratory's upper limit of normal for serum LDH to reflect interlaboratory differences in LDH)

- Other features that have been demonstrated to correlate with the presence of an exudate:

  □ Specific gravity >1.016

  □ Pleural fluid protein >3 g/dL

  □ Pleural fluic cholesterol > 45 mg/dL

  □ Pleural fluid bilirubin:serum bilirubin ratio >0.6

- **Congestive heart failure (CHF)** is the most common cause of transudative pleural effusions. In treated congestive heart failure, a transudate may be 'converted' into an exudate when progressive reabsorption of effusion fluid leads to increasing specific gravity and increasingly concentrated solutes such as protein and LDH. Effusions due to CHF tend to be larger on the right or, when unilateral, are usually right-sided.

- **Parapneumonic pleural effusions.** Whenever there is bacterial pneumonia, an exudative pleural effusion may develop. Generally these effusions are sterile or contain few bacteria and are associated with low numbers of neutrophils. If a frank bacterial infection arises as a complication of bacterial pneumonia, this is called an empyema. Empyema is diagnosed when the pleural fluid contains: >100,000 neutrophils/mL, pH <7.2, and bacteria on gram stain.

- **Pulmonary embolism (PE).** Up to 50% of patients with PE have an associated, usually small, pleural effusion. About 1/3 of these are transudates, and the remaining 2/3 are exudates.

T1.40
Chylous vs Pseudochylous Effusions

	Chylous	Pseudochylous
Gross appearance	milky	milky
Microscopic appearance	lymphocytes	mixed leukocytes, cholesterol crystals
Triglycerides	>110 mg/dL	<50 mg/dL
Chylomicrons (by electrophoresis)	+	−

- **Collagen vascular diseases.** Nearly any systemic collagen vascular disease may cause a pleuritis and exudative pleural effusion. The one most likely one to do so is rheumatoid arthritis. The pleural fluid chemistries are distinctive: pH <7.2, LDH >700, and glucose <30. In addition, rheumatoid factor (RF) is often elevated.

- **Chylous vs pseudochylous effusions.** True chylous effusion (chylothorax) is caused by lymphatic (thoracic duct) obstruction. In older studies, over half of cases were due to malignancy. Lymphoma was the most common malignancy, followed by bronchogenic carcinoma. In more recent series, trauma and surgery are the most common causes. Other cases are due to lymphangioleiomyomatosis (LAM) of the lung, sarcoidosis, and infection. A creamy top layer of chylomicrons may form if the fluid is allowed to stand. Pseudochylous effusions result from the gradual accumulation of lipids from cellular breakdown in conditions such as tuberculosis, rheumatoid pleural effusion, and myxedema **T1.40**.

- Amylase is elevated in pleural effusions related to esophageal perforation, pancreatitis, and malignancy. Pleural effusions associated with pancreatitis are classically left-sided.

- The combination of low pH (<7.30) and low glucose (<60 mg/dL) indicates empyema, malignancy, or rheumatoid pleuritis. A low pH alone, often <6.0, is seen in esophageal perforation.

Pleural fluid microscopy

- Neutrophils, when numerous, suggest empyema.

- Lymphocytic pleural effusions, particularly when mesothelial cells are sparse, is strongly suggestive of tuberculous effusions.

- Eosinophils are most commonly seen following a prior tap and have little additional significance.

- Mesothelial cells are conspicuously decreased or absent in rheumatoid pleuritis, tuberculous pleuritis, and post-pleurodesis pleuritis.

Peritoneal Fluid (Ascites Fluid)

Peritoneal fluid chemistry

- In peritoneal fluid, using criteria similar to Light criteria is an unreliable guide to sorting out the cause of ascites. The serum-ascites albumin gradient is perhaps the most useful index and can distinguish portal hypertension (cirrhosis)-related ascites from others. The serum-ascites albumin gradient is simply the arithmetic difference between the albumin measured in serum and that measured in ascites fluid. In portal hypertension, the serum-ascites albumin gradient is >1.1 g/dL. In ascites from other causes, it is less than 1.1.

Peritoneal fluid microscopy

- The diagnostic peritoneal lavage (DPL) is an extremely useful test for the trauma surgeon interested in whether the trauma patient has an indication for exploratory laparotomy. Criteria for a positive DPL are

  □ >15 mL gross blood

  □ RBCs >100,000/mL

  □ WBCs >500/mL

  □ DPL fluid in the chest tube or Foley catheter

  □ Bacteria present on gram stain

Synovial Fluid

Synovial fluid chemistry

■ Mucin clot test This test is an antiquated approach to determining whether there is inflammation in a synovial fluid. In it, acetic acid is added to the fluid which normally should lead to congealing of the hyaluronic acid, forming a 'mucin clot.' In the presence of ongoing inflammation, the fluid's hyaluronic acid is largely degraded, leading to a poor mucin clot.

■ Lactate is elevated in septic arthritis, often above 250 mg/dL.

■ Complement is lowered in rheumatoid arthritis and lupus.

Synovial fluid microscopy

■ Cell count T1.41

■ Crystals

  □ Monosodium urate crystals are found in gout. These are seen as needle-shaped rods, varying from 2-20 microns in length, that manifest strong birefringence, rapid extinction, and negative birefringent. Rapid extinction refers to the fact that when the compensator is rotated just a few degrees from parallel or perpendicular to a crystal, the crystal rapidly fades back into the red background. Negative birefringence refers to a particle that appears yellow when parallel to the compensator and blue when perpendicular. An easy way to remember this is the mnemonic 'you lose money when U PAY PEB'. The 'losing money' part reminds you that it's negatively birefringent, the 'U' refers to urate, the 'PAY' to parallel yellow, and the 'PEB' to perpendicular blue.

  □ Calcium pyrophosphate crystals are found in pseudogout, also called calcium pyrophosphate deposition disease (CPPD). These are seen as rods or rhomboids, varying from 2-20 microns, that are weakly birefringent, show slow extinction, and positive birefringence.

  □ Hydroxyapatite crystals are small and non-birefringent. They are largely undetectable unless one does an Alizarin Red S stain.

  □ Corticosteroid crystals may be seen following therapeutic steroid injection and appear as blunt jagged-ended crystals with variable birefringence.

T1.41
Synovial Fluid

Condition	WBC Count	Neutrophils (%)	Glucose (Difference Between Serum and Synovial)	Other
Normal	0-150	<25	0-10	Clear-straw colored
Noninflammatory effusion	0-3000	<25	0-10	Clear-straw colored
Inflammatory effusion	3000-75,000	30-75	0-40	Turbid and opaque
Septic, urate and rheumatoid arthritis	>100,000	>90	30-100	Yellow and purulent

Enzymes

Alpert JS, Thysegen K, Antman E, Bassand JP, et al. Myocardial infarction redefined—a consensus document of the Joint European Society of Cardiology/American College of Cardiology. *J Am Coll Cardiol* 2000;36:959-969.

Apple FS, Wu AH. Myocardial infarction redefined: role of cardiac troponin testing. *Clin Chem* 2001; 47(3): 377-379.

Arndt T. Carbohydrate-deficient transferrin as a marker of chronic alcohol abuse: a critical review of preanalysis, analysis, and interpretation. *Clin Chem* 2001; 47: 13-27.

Balk EM. Accuracy of biomarkers to diagnose acute cardiac ischemia in the emergency department. *Ann Emerg Med* 2001; 37(5):478-494.

Banks PA. Practice guidelines in acute pancreatitis. *Am J Gastroenterol* 1997; 92(3): 377-386.

Bar-Or D, Winkler JV, VanBenthuysen K, Harris L, Lau E, Hetzel FW. Reduced albumin-cobalt binding with transient myocardial ischemia after elective percutaneous transluminal coronary angioplasty: a preliminary comparison to creatine kinase-MB, myoglobin, and troponin I. *Am Heart J* 2001; 141: 985-991.

Caragher TE, Fernandez BB, Barr LA. Long-term experience with an accelerated protocol for diagnosis of chest pain. *Arch Pathol Lab Med* 2000; 124: 1434-1439.

Dervenis C, Johnson CD, Bassi C. Diagnosis, objective assessment of severity, and management of acute pancreatitis. *Int J Pancreatol* 1999; 25:195-210.

Dufour DR, Lott JA, Nolte FS, Gretch DR, Koff RS, Seeff LB. Diagnosis and monitoring of hepatic injury: I. performance characteristics of laboratory tests. *Clin Chem* 2000; 46: 2027-2049.

Harris KR, Dighe AS. Laboratory testing for viral hepatitis. *Am J Clin Pathol* 2002; 118: S18-25.

Keffer JH. Myocardial markers of injury. *Am J Clin Pathol* 1996; 105: 305-319.

Kemppainen EA, Hedstrom J, Puolakkainen P. Rapid measurement of urinary trypsinogen-2 as a screening test for acute pancreatitis. *N Engl J Med* 1997; 336:1788-93.

Maisel A. B-type natriuretic peptide levels: a potential novel "white count" for congestive heart failure. *J Card Fail*. 2001; 7:183-193.

Matull WR, Pereira SP, O'Donohue JW. Biochemical markers of acute pancreatitis. *J Clin Pathol* 2006;59:340-344.

Morrison LK, Harrison A, Krishnaswamy P, Kazanegra R, Clopton P, Maisel A. Utility of a rapid B-natriuretic peptide assay in differentiating congestive heart failure from lung disease in patients presenting with dyspnea. *J Am Coll Cardiol* 2002; 39: 202-209.

Mueller C, Scholer A, Laule-Kilian K, Martina B, Schindler C, Buser P, Pfisterer M, Perruchoud AP. Use of b-type natriuretic peptide in the evaluation and management of acute dyspnea. *NEJM* 2002; 350:647-654.

Munoz SJ. Prothrombin time in fulminant hepatic failure. *Gastroenterology* 1991; 100: 1480-1481.

O'Grady JG, Alexander GJM, Hayllar KM, Williams R. Early indicators of prognosis in fulminant hepatic failure. *Gastroenterology* 1989; 97: 439-445.

Ottani F, Galvani M, Nicolini FA, Ferrini D, Pozzati A, Di Pasquale G, Jaffe AS. Elevated cardiac troponin levels predict the risk of adverse outcome in patients with acute coronary syndromes. *Am Heart J* 2000; 140(6): 917-927.

Papachristou GI, Whitcomb DC. Inflammatory markers of disease severity in acute pancreatitis. *Clin Lab Med* 2005; 25: 17-37.

Peacock F, Morris DL, Anwaruddin S, Christenson RH, Collinson RO, Goodacre SW, Januzzi JL, Jesse RL, Kaski JC, Kontos MC, Lefevre G, Mutrie D, Sinha MK, Uettwiller-Geiger D, Pollack CV. Meta-analysis of ischemia-modified albumin to rule out acute coronary syndromes in the emergency department. *Am Heart J* 2006;152: 253-262.

Petersen JR, Okorodudu AO, Mohammad A, Fernando A, Shattuck KE. Association of transcutaneous bilirubin testing in hospital with decreased readmission rate for hyperbilirubinemia. *Clin Chem* 2005;51: 540-544.

Pezzilli R, Billi P, Plate L, Barakat B, Bongiovanni F, Miglioli M. Human pancreatic secretory trypsin inhibitor in the assessment of the severity of acute pancreatitis. A comparison with C-reactive protein. *J Clin Gastroenterol* 1994;19:112-117.

Pincus MR, Schaffner JA. Assessment of liver function. *Clinical Diagnosis and Management by Laboratory Methods,* 19th ed. (Philadelphia: W.B. Saunders Company, 1996).

Pincus MR, Zimmerman HJ, Henry JB. Clinical enzymology. *Clinical Diagnosis and Management by Laboratory Methods,* 19th ed. (Philadelphia: W.B. Saunders Company, 1996).

Pratt DS, Kaplan MM. Evaluation of abnormal liver-enzyme results in asymptomatic patients. *NEJM* 2000; 342: 1266-1271.

Scouller K, Conigrave KM, Macaskill P, Irwig L, Whitfield JB. Should we use carbohydrate-deficient transferrin instead of γ-glutamyltransferase for detecting problem drinkers? a systematic review and metaanalysis. *Clin Chem* 2000; 46: 1894-1902.

Smotkin J, Tenner S. Pancreatic and biliary disease: laboratory diagnostic tests in acute pancreatitis. *J Clin Gastroenterol* 2002;34:459-462.

Wilson JW. Inherited elevation of alkaline phosphatase activity in the absence of disease. *N Engl J Med* 1979; 301:983.

Yadav D, Agarwal N, Pitchumoni CS. A critical evaluation of laboratory tests in acute pancreatitis. *The Am J Gastroenterol* 2002; 97: 1309-1318.

Zaninotto M. Strategies for the early diagnosis of acute myocardial infarction using biochemical markers. *Am J Clin Pathol* 1999; 111: 399-405.

Proteins

Baskin L, Jialal I. Detection of oligoclonal bands in cerebrospinal fluid by immunofixation electrophoresis. *Am J Clin Pathol* 1998; 109: 585-588.

Fortini AS, Sanders EL, Weinshenker BG, Katzmann JA. Cerebrospinal fluid oligoclonal bands in the diagnosis of multiple sclerosis: isoelectric focusing with IgG immunoblotting compared with high-resolution agarose gel electrophoresis and cerebrospinal fluid IgG index. *Am J Clin Pathol* 2003; 120: 672-675.

Gabay C, Kushner I. Acute-phase proteins and other systemic responses to inflammation. *NEJM* 1999; 340: 448-454.

Heeschen C, Hamm CW, Bruemmer J, Simoons ML. Predictive value of C-reactive protein and troponin t in patients with unstable angina: a comparative analysis. *J Am Coll Cardiol* 2000; 35(6): 1535-1542.

Kallemuchikkal U, Gorevic. PD Evaluation of cryoglobulins. *Arch Pathol ab Med* 1999; 123: 119-125.

Katzmann JA, Clark R, Sanders E, Landers JP, Kyle RA. Prospective Study of Serum Protein Capillary Zone Electrophoresis and Immunotyping of Monoclonal Proteins by Immunosubtraction. *Am J Clin Pathol* 1998; 110(4):503-509.

Keren DF, Alexanian R, Goeken JA, Gorevic PD, Kyle RA, Tomar RH. Guidelines for clinical and laboratory evaluation of patients with monoclonal gammopathies. *Arch Pathol Lab Med* 1999; 123: 106-107.

Keren DF. Procedures for the evaluation of monoclonal immunoglobulins. *Arch Pathol Lab Med* 1999; 123: 126-132.

Keren DF. *Protein Electrophoresis in Clinical Diagnosis* (London: Arnold, 2003).

Koenig W, Sund M, Fröhlich M, Fischer HG, Löwel H, Döring A, Hutchinson WL, Pepys MB. C-reactive protein, a sensitive marker of inflammation, predicts future risk of coronary heart disease in initially healthy middle-aged men. results from MONICA (Monitoring Trends And Determinants In Cardiovascular Disease) Augsburg Cohort Study, 1984 To 1992. *Circulation* 1999; 99(2): 237-242.

Kushner I, Rzewnicki D, Samols D. What does minor elevation of C-reactive protein signify? *Am J Med* 2006; 119: 166.e17-166.e28.

McPherson RA. Specific Proteins. *Clinical Diagnosis and Management by Laboratory Methods,* 19th ed. (Philadelphia: W.B. Saunders Company, 1996).

Pearson TA, Mensah GA, Alexander RW, Anderson JL, Cannon RO 3rd, Criqui M, Fadl YY, Fortmann SP, Hong Y, Myers GL, Rifai N, Smith SC Jr, Taubert K, Tracy RP, Vinicor F. Markers of inflammation and cardiovascular disease application to clinical and public health practice: a statement for healthcare professionals from the centers for disease control and prevention and the american heart association. *Circulation* 2003; 107(3): 499-511.

Qiu LL, Levinson SS, Keeling KL, Elin RJ. Convenient and effective method for removing fibrinogen from serum specimens before protein electrophoresis. *Clin Chem* 2003; 49(6): 868-872.

Rajmkumar SV, Kyle RA, Therneau TM, Melton LJ III, Bradwell AR, Clark RJ, Larson DR, Plevak MF, Dispenzieri A, Katzmann JA. Serum free light chain ratio is an independent risk factor for progression in monoclonal gammopathy of undetermined significance. *Blood* 2005; 106: 812-817.

Rifai N, Ridker PM. High-sensitivity C-reactive protein: a novel and promising marker of coronary heart disease. *Clin Chem* 2001; 47: 403-411.

Skowasch D, Jabs A, Andrié R, Lüderitz B. Bauriedel G. Progression of native coronary plaques and in-stent restenosis are associated and predicted by increased pre-procedural C-reactive protein. *Heart* 2005; 91:535-536.

Tate JR, Gill D, Cobcroft R, Hickman PE. Practical considerations for the measurement of free light chains in serum. *Clin Chem* 2003; 49(8): 1252-1257.

Acid-Base and Electrolytes

Carter AB, Howanitz PJ. Intraoperative testing for parathyroid hormone: a comprehensive review of the use of the assay and the relevant literature. *Arch Pathol Lab Med* 2003; 127: 1424-1442.

Gabow PA, Kaehny WD, Fennessey PV, Goodman SI, Gross PA, Schrier RW. Diagnostic importance of an increased serum anion gap. *N Engl J Med* 1980; 303:854-858.

Gao P, Scheibel S, D'Amour P, John MR, Rao SD, Schmidt-Gayk H, Cantor TL. Development of a novel immunoradiometric assay exclusively for biologically active whole parathyroid hormone 1-84: implications for improvement of accurate assessment of parathyroid function. *J Bone Miner Res* 2001; 16: 605-614.

John MR, Goodman WG, Gao P, Cantor TL, Salusky IB, Juppner H. A novel immunoradiometric assay detects full-length human pth but not amino-terminally truncated fragments: implications for pth measurements in renal failure. *J Clin Endocrinol Metab* 1999; 84: 4287-4290.

Saeed BO, Beaumont D, Handley GH, Weaver JU. Severe hyponatraemia: investigation and management in a district general hospital. *J Clin Pathol* 2002; 55: 893-896.

Seifter JL. Acid-base disorders. *Cecil Textbook of Medicine,* 22nd ed. (Philadelphia: W.B. Saunders Company, 2004).

Sevastos N, Theodossiades G, Efstathiou S, Papatheodoridis GV, Manesis E, Archimandritis AJ. Pseudohyperkalemia in serum: the phenomenon and its clinical magnitude. *J Lab Clin Med* 2006;147:139-144.

Yamashita H, Gao P, Cantor T, Noguchi S, Uchino S, Watanabe S, Ogawa T, Kawamoto H, Fukagawa M. Comparison of parathyroid hormone levels from the intact and whole parathyroid hormone assays after parathyroidectomy for primary and secondary hyperparathyroidism. *Surgery* 2004; 135: 149-156.

Renal Function Tests

Carvounis CP, Nisar S, Guro-Razuman S. Significance of the fractional excretion of urea in the differential diagnosis of acute renal failure. *Kidney Int* 2002; 62: 2223-2229.

Dagher L, Moore K. The hepatorenal syndrome. *Gut* 2001;49:729-737.

Dufour DR. Laboratory evaluation of renal function. *Professional Practice in Clin Chem, A Companion Text,* 1999 edition (Washington, DC: American Association for Clinical Chemistry, 1999).

Esson ML, Schrier RW. Diagnosis and treatment of acute tubular necrosis. *Ann Intern Med* 2002; 137: 744-752.

Kaplan AA, Kohn OF. Fractional excretion of urea as a guide to renal dysfunction. *Am J Nephrol* 1992; 12: 49-54.

Koenig W, Twardella D, Brenner H, Rothenbacher D. Plasma concentrations of cystatin c in patients with coronary heart disease and risk for secondary cardiovascular events: more than simply a marker of glomerular filtration rate *Clin Chem* 2005; 51: 321-327

Lameire N, Van Biesen W, Vanholder R. Acute renal failure *Lancet* 2005; 365: 417-30

Levey AS, Bosch JP, Lewis JB, Greene T, Rogers N, Roth D. A More accurate method to estimate glomerular filtration rate from serum creatinine: a new prediction equation. *Ann Intern Med* 1999;130:461-70.

Price CP, Newall RG, Boyd JC. Use of protein:creatinine ratio measurements on random urine samples for prediction of significant proteinuria: a systematic review. *Clin Chem*2005; 51: 1577-1586.

Rabb H. Evaluation of urinary markers in acute renal failure. *Curr Opin Nephrol Hypertens* 1998; 7: 681-685.

Sarnak MJ, Levey AS, Schoolwerth AC, Coresh J, Culleton B, Hamm LL, McCullough PA, Kasiske BL, Kelepouris E, Klag MJ, Parfrey P, Pfeffer M, Raij L, Spinosa DJ, Wilson PW. Kidney disease as a risk factor for development of cardiovascular disease. *Circulation* 2003;108:2154.

Shlipak MG, Sarnak MJ, Katz R, Fried LF, Seliger SL, Newman AB, Siscovick DS, Stehman-Breen C. Cystatin C and the risk of death and cardiovascular events among elderly persons. *N Engl J Med* 2005;352(20):2049-2060.

Stevens LA, Coresh J, Greene T, Levey AS. Assessing kidney function—measured and estimated glomerular filtration rate. *N Engl J Med* 2006; 354: 2473-2483.

Stevens LA, Levey AS. Chronic kidney disease in the elderly—how to assess risk *N Engl J Med* 2005; 352: 2122-2124.

Intrapartum Tests

ACOG Committee on Practice Bulletins and the SGO Education Committee. Diagnosis and treatment of gestational trophoblastic disease. *ACOG Practice Bulletin* 2004; 53.

Bender TM, Stone LR, Amenta JS. Diagnostic power of lecithin/sphingomyelin ratio and fluorescent polarization assays for respiratory distress syndrome compared by relative operating characteristic curves. *Clin Chem* 1994, 40: 541-545.

Benn PA, Fang M, Egan JF, Horne D, Collins R. Incorporation of inhibin-A in second trimester screening for Down syndrome. *Obset Gynecol* 2003; 101: 451-454.

Buyon JP, Cronstein BN, Morris M, Tanner M, Weissmann G. Serum complement values (c3 and c4) to differentiate between systemic lupus activity and preeclampsia. *Am J Med* 1986; 81(2):194-200.

Cole LA, Shahabi S, Butler SA, Mitchell H, Newlands ES, Behrman HR, Verrill HL. Utility of commonly used commercial human chorionic gonadotropin immunoassays in the diagnosis and management of trophoblastic diseases. *Clin Chem* 2001; 47: 308-315.

Derksen RH, Meilof JF. Anti-Ro/SS-A and anti La/SS-B auto-antibody levels in relation to systemic lupus erythematosus disease activity and congenital heart block. *Arthritis Rheum* 1992; 35(8): 953-959.

Dombrowski RA, Mackenna J, Brame RG. comparison of amniotic fliud lung maturity profiles in paired vaginal and amniocentesis specimens. *Am J Obstet Gynecol* 1981; 140: 461-464.

Dubin SB. Assessment of fetal lung maturity. *Am J Clin Pathol* 1998; 110:723-732.

Erickson JA, Ashwood ER, Gin CA. Evaluation of a dimeric inhibin A assay for assessing fetal Down syndrome. *Arch Pathol Lab Med* 2004; 128:415-420.

Flynn SD, Seifer DB. Clinical application of human chorionic gonadotropin. *Clinical Diagnosis and Management by Laboratory Methods,* 19th ed. (Philadelphia: W.B. Saunders Company, 1996).

Gimovsky ML, Montoro M, Paul RH. Pregnancy outcome in women with systemic lupus erythematosus. *Obstet Gynecol* 1984; 63(5): 686-692.

Grenspan JS, Rosen DJO, Roll K, et al. Evaluation of lamellar body number density as the initial assessment in a fetal lung maturity test cascade. *J Reprod Med* 1995; 40: 260-266.

Hadley AG. Laboratory assays for predicting the severity of haemolytic disease of the fetus and newborn. *Transpl Immunol* 2002; 10: 191-198.

Kjos SL, Walther FJ, Montero M, Paul RH, Diaz F, Stabler M. Prevalence and etiology of infants of diabetic mothers: predictive value of fetal lung maturation tests. *Am J Obstet Gynecol* 1990; 163: 898-903.

Klee GG. Human chorionic gonadotropin. *Mayo Clin Proc* 1994; 69: 391-392.

Korhonen J, Alfthan H, Ylöstalo P, Veldhuis J, Stenman UH. Disappearance of human chorionic gonadotropin and its α- and β-subunits after term pregnancy. *Clin Chem* 1997; 43: 2155-2163.

Kumpel BM. Quantification of anti-D and fetomaternal hemorrhage by flow cytometry. *Transfusion* 2000; 40: 6-9.

Kohorn EI. The new FIGO 2000 staging and risk factor scoring system for gestational trophoblastic disease: description and clinical assessment. *Int J Gynecol Cancer* 2001; 11: 73-77.

Livingston EG, Herbert WNP, Hage ML, Chapman JF, Stubbs TM. Use of the TDx-FLM assay in evaluating fetal lung maturity in an insulin-dependent diabetic population. *Obstet Gynecol* 1995;86:826-829.

Moniz CF, Nicolaides KH, Bamforth FJ Rodeck CH. Normal reference ranges for biochemical substances relating to renal, hepatic, and bone function in fetal and maternal plasma throughout pregnancy. *J Clin Pathol* 1985; 38: 468-472.

Ojomo EO, Coustan DR. Absence of evidence of pulmonary maturity at amniocentesis in term infants of diabetic mothers. *Am J Obstet Gynecol* 1990;163:954-957.

Piper JM, Langer O. Does maternal diabetes delay fetal pulmonary maturity? *Am J Obstet Gynecol* 1993; 168: 783-786.

Ramsey PS, Andrews WW. Biochemical predictors of preterm labor: fetal fibronectin and salivary estriol. *Clin Perinatol* 2003; 30(4): 701-733.

Reichlin M. Systemic lupus erythematosus and pregnancy. *J Reprod Med* 1998; 43(4): 355-360.

Repke JT. Hypertensive disorders of pregnancy: differentiating preeclampsia from active systemic lupus erythematosus. *J Reprod Med* 1998; 43(4): 350-354.

Usta IM, Barton JR, Amon EA, Gonzalez A, Sibai BM. Acute fatty liver of pregnancy: an experience in the diagnosis and management of fourteen cases. *Am J Obstet Gynecol* 1994; 171(5): 1342-1347.

Wald NJ, Watt HC, Hackshaw AK. Integrated screening for Down's syndrome based on tests performed during the first and second trimesters. *NEJM* 1999; 341: 461-467.

Wenk RE, Rosenbaum JM. Examination of amniotic fluid. *Clinical Diagnosis and Management by Laboratory Methods,* 19th ed. (Philadelphia: W.B. Saunders Company, 1996).

Yeast JD, Lu G. Biochemical markers for the prediction of preterm labor. *Obstet Gynecol Clin N Am* 2005; 32: 369-381.

Toxicology

Amiodarone Trials Meta-Analysis Investigators. Effect of prophylactic amiodarone on mortality after acute myocardial infarction and in congestive heart failure: meta-analysis of individual data from 6500 patients in randomised trials. *Lancet* 1997; 350: 1417-1424.

Ammar KA, Heckerling PS. ethylene glycol poisoning with a normal anion gap caused by concurrent ethanol ingestion: importance of the osmolal gap. *Am J Kidney Dis* 1996; 27:130-133.

Baud FJ, Borron SW, Megarbane B, et al. Value of lactic acidosis in the assessment of the severity of acute cyanide poisoning. *Crit Care Med* 2002; 30(9): 2044- 2050.

Begg EJ, Barclay ML, Kirkpatrick CJM. The therapeutic monitoring of antimicrobial agents. *Br J Clin Pharmacol* 1999; 47: 23-30.

Bertholf RL, Johannsen LM, Bazooband A, Mansouri V. False-positive acetaminophen results in a hyperbilirubinemic patient. *Clin Chem* 2003; 49(4): 695-698.

Centers for Disease Control. *Prevention of Lead Poisoning in Children* Atlanta: US Dept of Health; 1978.

Centers for Disease Control and Prevention. *Preventing Lead Poisoning in Young Children* Atlanta: US Dept of Health and Human Services; 2005.

Connolly SJ. Evidence-based analysis of amiodarone efficacy and safety. *Circulation* 1999; 100: 2025-2034.

Cook DS, Braithwaite RA, Hale KA. Estimating antemortem drug concentrations from postmortem blood samples: the influence of postmortem redistribution. *J Clin Pathol* 2000;53:282-285.

Bibliography and Additional Reading>Toxicology

Dawson AH, Whyte IM. Therapeutic drug monitoring in drug overdose. *Br J Clin Pharmacol* 1999; 48; 278-283.

Gabow PA. Disorders associated with an altered anion gap. *Kidney Int* 1985; 27: 472-483.

Jürgens G, Graudal NA, Kampmann JP. Therapeutic drug monitoring of antiarrhythmic drugs. *Clin Pharmacokinet* 2003; 42: 647-663.

Keifer MC. The clinical laboratory in the diagnosis of over-exposure to agrochemicals. *Lab Med* 1998; 29: 689-695.

Ibrahim D, Froberg B, Wolf A, Rusyniak DE. Heavy metal poisoning: clinical presentations and pathophysiology. *Clin Lab* Med 2006; 26: 67-97.

Jones JH, Weir WB. Cocaine-associated chest pain. *Med Clin N Am* 2005; 89: 1323-1342.

Larsen LC, Fuller SH. Management of acetaminophen toxicity. *American Family Physician* 1996; 53: 185-190.

Linder M, Keck PE. Standards of laboratory practice: antidepressant drug monitoring. national academy of clinical biochemistry. *Clin Chem* 1998; 44: 1073-1084.

Litovitz TL, Felberg L, White S, Klein-Schwartz W: 1995 annual report of the American Association of Poison Control Centers: toxic exposure surveillance system. *Am J Emerg Med* 1996; 14:487

Mitchell PB. Therapeutic drug monitoring of psychotropic medications. *Br J Clin Pharmacol* 2000; 49: 303-312.

Morocco AP. Cyanides. *Crit Care Clin* 2005; 21: 691-705.

Piomelli S. Childhood lead poisoning. *Pediatr Clin N Am* 2002; 49: 1285-1304.

Peddy SB, Rigby MR, Shaffner DH. Acute cyanide poisoning. *Pediatr Crit Care Med* 2006; 7(1): 79-82.

Piomelli S, Rosen JF, Chisolm Jr JJ, et al. Management of *Childhood Lead Poisoning. J Pediatr* 1984;105: 523-532.

Reid LD, Horner JR, McKenna DA. Therapeutic drug monitoring reduces toxic drug reactions: a meta-analysis. *Ther Drug Monit* 1990; 12: 72-78.

Rumack BH, Matthew H. Acetaminophen poisoning and toxicity. *Pediatrics* 1975; 55(6): 871-876.

Sanoski CA, Bauman JL. Clinical observations with the amiodarone/warfarin interaction: dosing relationships with longterm therapy. *Chest* 2002; 121: 19-23.

Shannon M. Ingestion of toxic substances by children. *N Engl J Med* 2000; 342:186-191.

Soldin SJ. Free drug measurements: when and why? an overview. *Arch Pathol Lab Med* 1999; 123: 822-823.

Valdes R Jr, Jortani SA, Gheorghiade M. Standards of laboratory practice: cardiac drug monitoring. *Clin Chem* 1998; 44: 1096-1109.

Williams RH, Leikin JB. Medicolegal issues and specimen collection for ethanol testing. *Lab Med* 1999; 30: 530-536.

Williams RH, Erickson T. Evaluating toxic alcohol poisoning in the emergency setting. *Lab Med* 1998; 29: 102-108.

Wu AHB, McKay C, Broussard LA, Hoffman RS, Kwong TC, Moyer TP, Otten EM, Welch SL, Wax P. Recommendations for the use of laboratory tests to support poisoned patients who present to the emergency department. *Clin Chem* 2003; 49: 357-379.

Wu SL, Li W, Wells A, Dasgupta A. Digoxin-like and digitoxin-like immunoreactive substances in elderly people. *Am J Clin Pathol* 2001; 115: 600-604.

Lipids and Carbohydrates

American College of Cardiology / American Heart Association Task Force on Practice Guidelines. ACC/AHA guidelines for the evaluation and management of chronic heart failure in the adult. *Circulation* 2001; 104: 2996 -3007.

American Diabetes Association. Diagnosis and classification of diabetes mellitus. *Diabetes Care* 2005; 28 (Supplement 1): S37-S42

American Diabetes Association: Report of the expert committee on the diagnosis and classification of diabetes mellitus. *Diabetes Care* 1997; 20: 1183-1197.

American Diabetes Association. *Standards Of Medical Care In Diabetes* 2006

Bachorik PS, Ross JW. National cholesterol education program recommendations for measurement of low-density lipoprotein cholesterol: executive summary. *Clin Chem* 1995; 41(10): 1414-1420.

The Diabetes Control and Complications Trial Research Group. The effect of intensive treatment of diabetes on the development and progression of long-term complications in insulin-dependent diabetes mellitus. *N Engl J Med* 1993; 329: 977-979.

Eckel RH, Grundy SM, Zimmet PZ. The metabolic syndrome. *Lancet* 2005; 365: 1415-1428

Emancipator K. Laboratory diagnosis and monitoring of diabetes mellitus. *Am J Clin Pathol* 1999; 112: 665-674.

Gama R, Teale JD, Marks V. Clinical and laboratory investigation of adult spontaneous hypoglycaemia. *J Clin Pathol* 2003; 56: 641-646.

Grundy SM and the Expert Panel on Detection, Evaluation, and Treatment of High Blood Cholesterol in Adults. Executive summary of the third report of the National Cholesterol Education Program (NCEP) expert panel on detection, evaluation, and treatment of high blood cholesterol in adults (adult treatment panel III). *JAMA* 2001; 285(19): 2486-2497.

Nauck M, Warnick R, Rifai N. Methods for measurement of LDL-cholesterol: a critical assessment of direct measurement by homogeneous assays versus calculation. *Clin Chem* 2002; 48(2): 236-254.

Ogedegbe HO, DW Brown. Lipids, lipoproteins, and apolipoproteins and their disease associations. *Lab Med* 2001; 7:384-388.

Tumor Markers

Balk SP, Ko Y-J, Bubley GJ. Biology of prostate- specific antigen. *J Clin Oncol* 2003; 21(2): 383-391.

Bhatnagar J, Tewari H, Bhatnagar M, Austin GE. Comparison of carcinoembryonic antigen in tissue and serum with grade and stage of colon cancer. *Anticancer Res* 1999; 19: 2181-2188.

Bidart J-M, Thuillier F, Augereau C, Chalas J, Daver A, Jacob N, Labrousse F, Voitot H. Kinetics of serum tumor marker concentrations and usefulness in clinical monitoring. *Clin Chem* 1999; 45(10): 1695-1707.

Canto EI, Slawin KM. Early management of prostate cancer: how to respond to an elevated PSA. *Annu Rev Med* 2002; 53: 355-368.

Catalona WJ, Hudson MA, Scardino PT, Richie JP, Ahmann FR, Flanigan RC, et al. Selection of optimal prostate specific antigen cutoffs for early detection of prostate cancer: receiver operating characteristic curves. *J Urol* 1994; 152(6): 2037-2042.

Compton CC, Fielding LP, Burgart LJ, Conley B, Cooper HS, Hamilton SR, Hammond MEH, Henson DE, Hutter RVP, Nagle RB, Nielsen ML, Sargent DJ, Taylor CR, Welton M, Willett C. Prognostic factors in colorectal cancer. *Arch Pathol Lab Med* 2000; 124: 979-994.

Duffy MJ. Carcinoembryonic antigen as a marker for colorectal cancer: is it clinically useful? *Clin Chem* 2001; 47: 624-630.

Duffy MJ. Predictive markers in breast and other cancers: a review. *Clin Chem* 2005; 51: 94-503.

Eustatia-Rutten CFA, Smit JWA, Romijn JA, van der Kleij-Corssmit EPM, Pereira AM, Stokkel MP, Kievit J. Diagnostic value of serum thyroglobulin measurements in the follow-up of differentiated thyroid carcinoma, a structured meta-analysis. *Clin Endocrinol* 2004; 61: 61-74.

Fleisher M. Criteria for tumor marker evaluation and utilization. *MLO* 2003; April: 16-18.

Freedland SJ, Partin AW. Detecting prostate cancer with molecular markers: uPM3. *Rev Urol* 2005; 7(4): 236-238.

Fritsche HA, Bast RC. CA125 In Ovarian cancer: advances and controversy. *Clin Chem* 1998;44:1379-1380.

Gadducci A, Cosio S, Fanucchi A, Negri S, Cristofani R, Genazzani AR. The predictive and prognostic value of serum CA125 half-life during paclitaxel/platinum-based chemotherapy in patients with advanced ovarian carcinoma. *Gynecol Oncol* 2004;93:131-136.

Groskopf J, Aubin SM, Deras IL, Blase A, Bodrug S, Clark C, Brentano S, Mathis J, Pham J, Meyer T, Cass M, Hodge P, Macairan ML, Marks LS, Rittenhouse H. APTIMA PCA3 molecular urine test: development of a method to aid in the diagnosis of prostate cancer. *Clin Chem* 2006; 52(6): 1089-1095.

Harrison LE, Guillem JG, Paty P, Cohen AM. Preoperative carcinoembryonic antigen predicts outcome in node negative colon cancer patients: a multivariate analysis of 572 patients. *J Am Coll Surg* 1997; 185: 55-59.

Hessels D, Klein-Gunnewiek JMT, van Oort I, Karthaus HFM, van Leenders GJL, van Balken B, Kiemeney LA, Witjes JA, Schalken JA. DD3[PCA3]-based molecular urine analysis for the diagnosis of prostate cancer. *Eur Urol* 2003; 44(1): 8-15.

Hjiyiannakis P, Mundy J, Harmer C. Thyroglobulin antibodies in differentiated thyroid cancer. *Clin Oncol* 1999; 11(4): 240-244.

Malkasian GD Jr, Knapp RC, Lavin PT, Zurawski VR Jr, Podratz KC, Stanhope CR, et al. Preoperative evaluation of serum CA 125 levels in premenopausal and postmenopausal patients with pelvic masses: discrimination of benign from malignant disease. *Am J Obstet Gynecol* 1988; 159: 341-346.

Meijer WG, Kema IP, Volmer M, Willemse PHB, de Vries EGE. Discriminating capacity of indole markers in the diagnosis of carcinoid tumors *Clin Chem* 2000; 46(10): 1588-1596.

Bibliography and Additional Reading>Tumor Markers

Miyanaga N, Akaza H, Tsukamoto S, et al. Usefulness of urinary NMP22 to detect tumor recurrence of superficial bladder cancer after transurethral resection. *Int J Clin Oncol* 2003;8:396-373.

Pajak TF, Clark GM, Sargent DJ, McShane LM, Hammond ME. Statistical issues in tumor marker studies. *Arch Pathol Lab Med* 2000; 124:1011-1015.

Pass HI, Lott D, Lonardo F, Harbut M, Liu Z, Tang N, Carbone M, Webb C, Wali A. Asbestos exposure, pleural mesothelioma, and serum osteopontin levels. *N Engl J Med* 2005; 353: 1564-1573.

Pateron D, Ganne N, Trinchet JC, Aurousseau MH, Mal F, Meicler C, et al. Prospective study of screening for hepatocellular carcinoma in caucasian patients with cirrhosis. *J Hepatol* 1994; 20: 65-71.

Pincus MR, Brandt-Rauf PW, Nostro D. Cell biology and early tumor detection. *Clinical Diagnosis and Management by Laboratory Methods,* 19th ed. (Philadelphia: W.B. Saunders Company, 1996), Chapter 15.

Seaman E, Whang M, Olsson CA, Katz A, Cooner WH, Benson MC. PSA density (PSAD). Role in patient evaluation and management. *Urol Clin North Am* 1993; 20(4): 653-663.

Sherman M, Peltekian KM, Lee C. Screening for hepatocellular carcinoma in chronic carriers of hepatitis b virus: incidence and prevalence of hepatocellular carcinoma in a north american urban population. *Hepatology* 1995; 22: 432-438.

Soloway MS, Briggman J, and Carpinito GA, et al. Use of a new tumor marker, urinary nmp-22 in the detection of occult or rapidly recurring transitional cell carcinoma of the urinary tract following surgical treatment. *J Urol* 1996;156:363-367.

Stenman U. Tumor-associated trypsin inhibitor. *Clin Chem* 2002; 48(8): 1206-1209.

Spencer CA, Takeuchi M, Kazarosyan M, Wang CC, Guttler RB, Singer PA, et al. Serum thyroglobulin autoantibodies: prevalence, influence on serum thyroglobulin measurement, and prognostic significance in patients with differentiated thyroid carcinoma. *J Clin Endocrinol Metab* 1998; 83(4):1121-1127.

Tessler DA, Catanzaro A, Velanovich V, Havstad S, Goel S. Predictors of cancer in patients with suspected pancreatic malignancy without a tissue diagnosis. *Am J Surg* 2006; 191: 191-197.

Van Der Cruijsen-Koeter IW, Wildhagen MF, DeKoning HJ, Schröder FH. The value of current diagnostic tests in prostate cancer screening. *BJU International* 2001; 88: 458-466.

Vicini FA, Vargas C, Abner A, Kestin L, Horwitz E, Martinez A. Limitations in the use of serum prostate specific antigen levels to monitor patients after treatment for prostate cancer. *J Urology* 2005; 173: 1456-1462.

Ward JF, Moul JW. Biochemical recurrence after definitive prostate cancer therapy. part I: defining and localizing biochemical recurrence of prostate cancer. *Curr Opin Urol* 2005; 15(3): 181-186.

Woodrum DL, Brawer MK, Partin AW, Catalona WJ, Southwick PC. Interpretation of free prostate specific antigen clinical research studies for the detection of prostate cancer. *J Urol* 1998; 159(1): 5-12.

Wu JT. Diagnosis and management of cancer using serologic tumor markers. *Clinical Diagnosis and Management by Laboratory Methods,* 19th ed (Philadelphia: W.B. Saunders Company, 1996), Chapter 45.

Endocrine

Basaria S, Cooper DS. Amiodarone and the thyroid. *Am J Medicine* 2005; 118: 706-714.

Dorin RI, Qualls CR, Crapo LM. Diagnosis of adrenal insufficiency. *Ann Int Med* 2003; 139:194-204.

Ganguly A. Primary aldosteronism. *NEJM* 1998; 339: 1828-1834.

Lim PO, Young WF, MacDonald TM. A review of the medical treatment of primary aldosteronism. *J Hypertens* 2001; 19: 353-361.

Løvås K, Husebye ES. Addison's disease. *Lancet* 2005; 365: 2058-61.

Madison LD, LaFranchi S. Screening for congenital hypothyroidism: current controversies. *Curr Opin Endocrinol Diabetes Obes* 2005, 12: 36-41.

Marik PE, Gayowski T, Starzl TE.The hepatoadrenal syndrome: a common yet unrecognized clinical condition. *Crit Care Med* 2005; 33(6): 1254-1259.

Marik PE, Zaloga GP. Adrenal insufficiency during septic shock. *Crit Care Med* 2003; 31(1):141-145.

Marx SJ. Hyperparathyroid and hypoparathyroid disorders. *NEJM* 2000; 343: 1863-1875.

Oelkers W. Adrenal insufficiency. *NEJM* 1996; 335: 1206-1212.

Merke DP, Bornstein SR. Congenital adrenal hyperplasia *Lancet* 2005; 365: 2125-2136.

Pearce EN, Farwell AP, Braverman LE. Thyroiditis. *NEJM* 2003; 349: 2646-2655.

Raff H, Findling JW. A physiologic approach to diagnosis of the Cushing syndrome. *Ann Int Med* 2003; 138: 980-991.

Sands JM, Bichet DG. Nephrogenic diabetes insipidus. *Ann Intern Med* 2006; 144: 186-194.

Speiser PW, White PC. Congenital adrenal hyperplasia. *NEJM* 2003; 349: 776-788.

Weetman AP. Graves' Disease. *NEJM* 2000; 343: 1236-1248.

Stowasser M, Gordon RD. The aldosterone-renin ratio in screening for primary aldosteronism. *Endocrinologist* 2004; 14: 267-276.

Postmortem Chemistries

Coe JI. Postmortem chemistry update: emphasis on forensic application. *Am J Forensic Med Pathol* 1993; 14(2): 91-117.

Cook DS, Braithwaite RA, Hale KA. Estimating antemortem drug concentrations from postmortem blood samples: the influence of postmortem redistribution. *J Clin Pathol* 2000;53:282-285.

Edston E, Gidlund E, Wickman M. Increased mast cell tryptase in sudden infant death syndrome: anaphylaxis, hypoxia, or artifact? *Clin Exp Allergy* 1999; 29: 1648-1654.

Edston E, van Hag-Hamsten M. Beta-tryptase measurements postmortem in anaphylactic deaths in controls. *Forensic Sci Int* 1998; 93: 135-142.

Rodman JS. Struvite stones. *Nephron* 1999; 81(suppl 1): 50-59.

Randall D, Butts J, Halsey J. Elevated postmortem tryptase in the absence of anaphylaxis. *J Forensic Sci* 1995; 40: 208-211.

Body Fluids

Doerr CH, Allen MS, Nichols FC III, Ryu JH. Etiology of chylothorax in 203 patients. *Mayo Clin Proc* 2005; 80(7): 867-870.

Görögh T, Rudolph P, Meyer JE, Werner JA, Lippert BM, Maune S. Separation of α2-transferrin by denaturing gel electrophoresis to detect cerebrospinal fluid in ear and nasal fluids. *Clin Chem* 2005; 51(9): 1704-1710.

Heffner JE. Discriminating between transudates and exudates. *Clin Chest Med* 2006; 27: 241-252.

Henry JB, Lauzon RB, Schumann GB. Basic examination of urine. *Clinical Diagnosis and Management by Laboratory Methods* (Philadelphia: W.B. Saunders Company, 1996), Chapter 18.

Marton KI, Gean AD. The spinal tap: a new look at an old test. *Ann Int Med* 1986; 104: 840-848.

Owen WE, Roberts WL. Performance characteristics of four immunonephelometric assays for the quantitative determination of IgA and IgM in cerebrospinal fluid. *Am J Clin Pathol* 2003; 119: 689-693.

Pumphrey RSH, Roberts ISD. Postmortem findings after fatal anaphylactic reactions. *J Clin Pathol* 2000; 53: 273-276.

Romero-Candeira S, Hernández L, Romero-Brufao S, Orts D, Fernández C, Martin C. Is it meaningful to use biochemical parameters to discriminate between transudative and exudative pleural effusions? *Chest* 2002; 122: 1524-1529.

Runyon BA, Montano AA, Akriviadis EA, Antillon MR, Irving MA, McHutchison JG. The serum-ascites albumin gradient is superior to the exudate-transudate concept in the differential diagnosis of ascites. *Ann Int Med* 1992; 117:215-220.

Sassoon CS, Light RW. Chylothorax and pseudochylothorax. *Clin Chest Med* 1985; 6: 163-171.

Schieneman SJ. X-linked hypercalciuric nephrolithiasis: clinical syndromes and chloride channel mutations. *Kidney Int* 1998; 53: 3-17.

Sellebjerg F, Christiansen M, Nielsen PM, Fredericksen JL. Cerebrospinal fluid measures of disease activity in patients with multiple sclerosis. *Mult Scler* 1998; 4: 475-479.

Valentine VG, Raffin TA. The management of chylothorax. *Chest* 1992; 102: 586-591.

Yilmaz A, Tunaboyu İK, Akkaya E, Bayramgürler B. A comparative analysis of the biochemical parameters used to distinguish between pleural exudates and transudates. *Respirology* 2000; 5: 363-367.

Chapter 2

Blood Banking & Transfusion

Daniel D Mais & Emily E Volk

Allogeneic Donor Testing

History & Physical Examination

Questions must be asked of the prospective donor with regard to age, date of last donation, medical illnesses, pregnancy, drug therapy, at-risk behavior, receipt of blood or other human tissues, immunizations, and infectious diseases. The prospective donor must be 16 years old or conform to applicable state law. Donors should be asked to report any illness developing within a few days after donation and, especially to report a new positive HIV or hepatitis result within 12 months of donation.

Physical. The prospective donor must be checked for general appearance, temperature, weight, blood pressure, pulse, hemoglobin or hematocrit, and venipuncture sites. Specific requirements are:

- Temperature: shall not exceed 37.5°C (99.5° F).

- Pulse: should be regular and between 50 and 100 beats per minute. A prospective donor with heart rate < 50 may be accepted if an otherwise healthy athlete.

- Blood pressure: should be no higher than 180 systolic and 100 diastolic.

- Hemoglobin and hematocrit: ≥12.5 g/dL/38% for allogeneic donors, (11g/dL/33% for autologous donors) as determined from a sample of blood taken at the time of donation.

- The skin at the site of venipuncture must be free of lesions. Both arms must be examined for evidence of repeated parenteral entry (IV drug use).

Blood Collection

Donors must give written informed consent.

Donors must be notified of any significantly abnormal test results. Donors must be informed up front if there is a circumstance in which certain routine tests may not be performed on the unit.

Blood must be collected in an aseptic manner and drawn into a *closed* sterile system; that is, a pre-attached group of bags and *integral* tubing that, following blood collection, can be manipulated without ever entering the system again. If at any point in the life of this closed sterile system it is penetrated ('spiked') the shelf-life is shortened. Sterile connection devices (docking devices) exist that allow entering the system without compromising sterility.

At the time of collection, a certain amount of blood is left in the integral tubing which is then pinched (by a heat sealer) in several places to create several sealed segments of blood-filled tubing. These can be separated (without entering the bag) at any time for lab testing.

Volume drawn. For years, the *AABB Standards* stated that 450 ± 45 mL whole blood was to be drawn. If 300-404 mL are collected, the donation may be used, but a label must be attached reading "Low-volume unit: __ mL." Furthermore, this unit may not be used to make other products such as platelets. If <300 mL are collected, then the anticoagulant in the bag must be proportionately reduced. The current edition stipulates a maximum of 10.5 mL/Kg, including samples.

After collection, the blood must be stored at

- 1-6°C if used only for red cells.

- 20-24°C if used to make components first. It must be stored at 1-6°C within 8 hours if used for red blood cells.

The whole blood can be used to make packed red cells and/or components such as platelets and plasma. This is discussed further under Blood Components.

Donor adverse reactions

- Vasovagal reactions are recognized by a *slow heart rate* in addition to hypotension, syncope, and nausea. To treat vasovagal reactions, begin by elevating the feet and applying cold compresses to the donor's head or back of neck while continuing to monitor the donor.

- Hypovolemia is recognized by a *fast heart rate* with hypotension and possible nausea and syncope. In this case, the donor must be given fluids, often intravenously.

- Hyperventilation is characterized by an altered, rapid and shallow, respiratory pattern that results in hypercapnea. The donor may also manifest facial

Allogeneic Donor Testing>Blood Collection

T2.1 Donor Deferrals

Reason for Deferral	Deferral
Viral hepatitis after 11th birthday	Indefinite
Pregnancy	Defer until 6 weeks postpartum (exceptions for transfusion to the infant with physician approval)
Stigmata of parenteral drug use	Indefinite
Family history of Creutzfeld-Jacob disease	Indefinite
History of syphilis or gonorrhea, treatment for syphilis or gonorrhea, or positive syphilis screening test	12 months (after completion of therapy)
Receipt of blood products, human tissue, or plasma-derived clotting factors	12 months
Receipt of dura mater or pituitary growth hormone of human origin	Indefinite
Aspirin (and other medications that irreversibly inhibit platelet function)	36 hours for aspirin (and other medications as defined by the medical director). Only precludes use of the collected blood as the sole source of platelets
Recent blood donation	8 weeks for whole blood donation; 16 weeks for 2 unit red cell pheresis; 72 hours for autologous whole blood; >48 hours for plasma-, platelet-, or leukopheresis
Toxoids, synthetic or killed vaccines: anthrax, cholera, diptheria, hepatitis A, hepatitis B, influenza, lyme, paratyphoid, pertussis, plague, pneumococcal polysaccharide, polio (Salk injection), rabies, rocky mountain spotted fever, tetanus, typhoid (injection)	None (if donor is afebrile and symptom-free)
Live attenuated viral and bacterial vaccines: german measles and chicken pox (varicella)	4 weeks
Live attenuated viral and bacterial vaccines; measles, polio (Sabin oral), mumps, typhoid (oral), and yellow fever	2 weeks
Smallpox vaccine (vaccinia)	In those with no complications of vaccine, 21 days or until scab falls off, whichever is longer. In those with severe complications, 14 days after resolution. Asymptomatic contacts of vaccinia recipients need not be deferred
Hepatitis B immune globulin administration	12 months
Confirmed positive test for HbsAg or repeatedly reactive test for anti-HBc	Indefinite
Laboratory evidence of HCV infection	Indefinite
Laboratory evidence of HTLV-1 infection	Indefinite
Have donated the only unit of blood to a patient who developed HIV or HTLV and had no other probable cause of infection	Indefinite
Application of tattoo	12 months
Mucous membrane exposure to blood	12 months
Nonsterile skin penetration	12 months
Residing with or having sexual contact with an individual with viral hepatitis	12 months
Being incarcerated for >72 consecutive hours	12 months
Malaria	3 years (after becoming asymptomatic)
Immigrants from malaria-endemic areas	3 years (after departure, if symptom free)
Travelers to malaria-endemic areas	12 months (after departure, if symptom free, regardless of prophylaxis)
Travelers to variant Creutzfeld-Jacob areas	Indefinite
Use of bovine insulin manufactured in UK	Indefinite
History of babesiosis of Chagas disease	Indefinite
West Nile virus	14 days after resolved or 28 days after onset, whichever is longer. Positive West Nile antibody test, without illness, is not grounds for deferral
Stigmata of alcohol intoxication or habituation	Exclude donor, no specific period of time stated
Finasteride (Proscar, Propecia)	1 month after last dose
Dutasteride (Avodart)	6 months after last dose
Isotretinoin (Accutane)	1 month after last dose
Acitretin (Soriatane)	3 years after last dose
Etretinate (Tegison)	Indefinite
Receiving money or drugs for sex	Indefinite
Paying for sex	12 months

2: Blood Banking and Transfusion

Allogeneic Donor Testing>Blood Collection; Laboratory Testing of Donor Blood I
Pretransfusion Laboratory Testing>Proper Paperwork & Properly Identified Blood Samples

twitching and seizures. The donor should be assisted with breathing into a paper bag.

■ Citrate effect is only seen in apheresis donors in whom citrate must be used as an anticoagulant. Sometimes the citrate returning to the donor's circulation results in hypocalcemia manifested by perioral tingling possibly progressing to arrhythmias and seizures. The initial treatment, for mild symptoms, is to simply slow the infusion rate. Oral calcium may also be given.

■ Hematoma may occur during or after phlebotomy. Remove the tourniquet and needle from the donor's arm and, with the use of sterile gauze, apply digital pressure. Ice may also be helpful.

Laboratory Testing of Donor Blood

ABO & Rh. Determinations of the ABO and Rh type must be made on donor blood. ABO testing must be done with anti-A and anti-B reagents (forward typing) and with A and B test cells for serum ABO antibodies (reverse typing). The Rh type is determined with anti-D. If the anti-D test is negative, then testing must be performed for weak D (described further below). Only when both of these are negative can a unit be labeled Rh-negative.

Antibody screen. Blood from donors with a history of transfusion or pregnancy must be screened for

unexpected antibodies to red cell antigens. Blood testing positive for alloantibodies may be discarded.

Infectious disease screening. Multiple tests are currently required on donor blood: HbsAg, anti-HBc, anti-HCV, HCV nucleic acid (HCV RNA), anti-HTLV-I, anti-HTLV-II, anti-HIV-1, anti-HIV-2, HIV nucleic acid (HIV RNA), serologic testing for syphilis (RPR), and West Nile virus (WNV). These tests can be bypassed in an emergency of critical blood shortage, but this omission must be indicated on the label, and testing must still be completed as soon as it is possible.

Pretransfusion Laboratory Testing

Proper Paperwork & Properly Identified Blood Samples

Appropriate patient identification must accompany the paperwork and blood samples, and the two must match up. A zero-tolerance policy for clerical errors is critical, as *clerical error is the most common cause of fatal transfusion reactions.* Blood samples for potential recipients must be labeled with at least two unique identifiers (eg, name and unique armband number [B-number]), date of collection, and a way of identifying the phlebotomist.

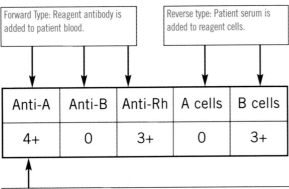

Forward Type: Reagent antibody is added to patient blood.

Reverse type: Patient serum is added to reagent cells.

Anti-A	Anti-B	Anti-Rh	A cells	B cells
4+	0	3+	0	3+

Strength of reaction is graded 0 to 4+ and mf+ (mixed field). The term mixed field reaction means some cells are reacting and others are not; it is best seen microscopically. It implies that two populations of red cells are present, as in recent transfusion or following stem cell/bone marrow transplant. In ABO typing, 3+ or 4+ reactions are expected. Weaker reactions (2+) may be seen, for example, if the cell type is a subgroup of A or there has been transfusion of type O cells.

F2.1 Initial blood typing. In this example, the patient types as A+, with the expected anti-B antibody.

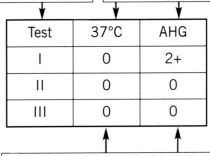

Test cells are selected so that all the important antigens are represented. The cells are type O. Some labs use only 2 cells.

Phase of reactivity. These tests are customarily performed LISS. In the antihuman globulin (AHG) phase, anti-IgG is added to the test tube.

Test	37°C	AHG
I	0	2+
II	0	0
III	0	0

All of these reactions should be negative (0) in order to proceed to crossmatch. In this case, the patient has reactivity against test cell I, of 2+ intensity, at AHG phase. This is an abnormal result that suggests an alloantibody and should lead to the performance of a complete panel.

F2.2 An antibody screen. This test is abnormal and should be followed by an alloantibody panel.

2: Blood Banking and Transfusion

Pretransfusion Laboratory Testing>Proper Paperwork & Properly Identified Blood Samples;
ABO & Rh Testing of Recipient Blood; Antibody Screen; Antibody Panel

If the intended recipient has been pregnant or transfused in the past 3 months, then the blood sample must be drawn within 3 days of transfusion.

Either serum or plasma is acceptable for traditional tube testing; plasma is preferred for newer platforms (gel testing). A hemolyzed sample may interfere with interpretation of tube testing.

The blood sample must be retained for 7 days after transfusion.

ABO & Rh Testing of Recipient Blood

ABO Testing F2.1, T2.2

- In *forward typing,* known antisera are added to the recipient's blood cells to determine which antigens are present on the red cell surfaces.

- In *reverse typing,* the recipient's serum is added to known test cells to determine which antibodies are present in the serum.

Rh testing is carried out with anti-D sera. Unlike donor blood, recipient blood need not be tested for weak D.

Antibody Screen (F2.2)

The antibody screen is a test for so-called unexpected antibodies. These are alloantibodies other than ABO that can cause hemolysis, (usually extravascular and of lesser severity than ABO), or hemolytic disease of the newborn.

These alloantibodies are nearly always acquired antibodies that result from prior transfusion or pregnancy.

Performance of the Antibody Screen

- The antibody screen is performed with 2 or 3 test cells, all type O negative, that are chosen so that, collectively, all the clinically significant antigens are represented.

- Only an indirect antiglobulin test (IAT) is required in the antibody screen. That is, to each test cell is added patient serum, followed by antihuman globulin (AHG).

- An autocontrol is run in parallel with the test cells, in which AHG is added to patient serum and patient blood.

T2.2
Results of Forward & Reverse Typing

Forward Typing		Reverse Typing		Blood Group
Anti-A	Anti-B	A cells	B cells	
0	0	4+	4+	0
4+	0	0	4+	A
0	4+	4+	0	B
4+	4+	0	0	AB

- If no reactions take place with any of the test cells, then the antibody screen is negative and one may proceed to crossmatch.

- If any of the cells react in the antibody screen, then the responsible antibody must be identified, usually with a panel. The antibody screen may be carried out at room temperature and 37°C, or at 37°C only. Room temperature incubation is omitted by many labs, since it mainly detects nuisance-type, clinically insignificant, alloantibodies such as anti-M, N, Lewis, I, and P.

Antibody Panel (F2.3)

A panel is like an expanded antibody screen. Usually 10 different test cells are used in the panel, all type O, which have known antigens on their surface. Panel interpretation is discussed more fully below, under section IV.

While many laboratories perform these studies in traditional test tubes, with macroscopic and microscopic inspection by a technologist, other methods exist. New methods such as testing in capillary tubes, microplates, solid-phase enzyme linked immuosorbent assays, and column agglutination (gel techniques) are being used more commonly. Several automated "walk away" testing platforms are now available. These systems perform all steps in the testing process from initial sample aliquoting, testing, to result reporting. These automated systems allow for multiple patient samples to be tested in parallel. Solid phase, gel-column, and microtiter technology may be employed in any one system. Ideally, these testing systems are interfaced with the blood bank information system. The use of barcode technology further enhances these systems by ensuring excellent efficiency without sacrificing accuracy.

Comparison with Prior Transfusion Records

Current results must be compared with prior pretransfusion testing results, if any. One looks for concurrence between current and previous ABO and Rh types and for previous alloantibodies that are currently undetectable. Certain alloantibodies, notoriously Kidd, become undetectable over time yet remain clinically significant.

Crossmatch

A crossmatch is the final check on issued blood, which is really aimed at detecting ABO incompatibility; although, other alloantibodies can be detected. The latter circumstance is most likely if the antibody screen is carried out at 37°C only, omitting the room temperature incubation.

Currently, either a serologic or computer crossmatch is allowed.

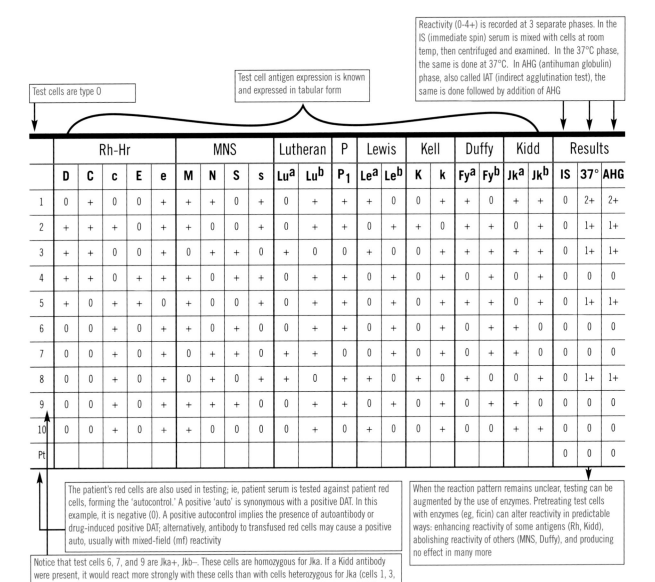

Reactivity (0-4+) is recorded at 3 separate phases. In the IS (immediate spin) serum is mixed with cells at room temp, then centrifuged and examined. In the 37°C phase, the same is done at 37°C. In AHG (antihuman globulin) phase, also called IAT (indirect agglutination test), the same is done followed by addition of AHG

Test cells are type O

Test cell antigen expression is known and expressed in tabular form

	Rh-Hr					MNS				Lutheran		P	Lewis		Kell		Duffy		Kidd		Results		
	D	C	c	E	e	M	N	S	s	Lu^a	Lu^b	P$_1$	Le^a	Le^b	K	k	Fy^a	Fy^b	Jk^a	Jk^b	IS	37°	AHG
1	0	+	0	0	+	+	+	0	+	0	+	+	+	0	0	+	+	0	+	+	0	2+	2+
2	+	+	+	0	+	+	0	0	+	0	+	+	0	+	+	0	+	+	0	+	0	1+	1+
3	+	+	0	0	+	0	+	+	0	+	0	0	+	0	0	+	+	+	+	+	0	1+	1+
4	+	+	0	+	+	+	0	+	+	0	+	+	0	+	0	+	0	+	0	+	0	0	0
5	+	0	+	+	0	+	0	0	+	0	+	+	0	+	0	+	+	+	0	+	0	1+	1+
6	0	0	+	0	+	+	0	+	0	0	+	+	0	+	0	+	0	+	+	0	0	0	0
7	0	0	+	0	+	0	+	+	0	+	+	0	0	+	0	+	0	+	+	0	0	0	0
8	0	0	+	0	+	0	+	0	+	+	0	+	+	0	+	0	+	0	0	+	0	1+	1+
9	0	0	+	0	+	+	+	+	0	0	+	+	0	+	0	+	0	+	+	0	0	0	0
10	0	0	+	0	+	+	0	0	0	0	+	0	+	0	0	+	0	0	+	+	0	0	0
Pt																					0	0	0

The patient's red cells are also used in testing; ie, patient serum is tested against patient red cells, forming the 'autocontrol.' A positive 'auto' is synonymous with a positive DAT. In this example, it is negative (0). A positive autocontrol implies the presence of autoantibody or drug-induced positive DAT; alternatively, antibody to transfused red cells may cause a positive auto, usually with mixed-field (mf) reactivity

When the reaction pattern remains unclear, testing can be augmented by the use of enzymes. Pretreating test cells with enzymes (eg, ficin) can alter reactivity in predictable ways: enhancing reactivity of some antigens (Rh, Kidd), abolishing reactivity of others (MNS, Duffy), and producing no effect in many more

Notice that test cells 6, 7, and 9 are Jka+, Jkb–. These cells are homozygous for Jka. If a Kidd antibody were present, it would react more strongly with these cells than with cells heterozygous for Jka (cells 1, 3, and 10). This is an example of dosage effect. Dosage effect is a feature of Kidd, Duffy, Rh, and MNS

F2.3 Antibody panel

2: Blood Banking and Transfusion

Pretransfusion Laboratory Testing>Crossmatch; Labeling and Visual Inspection of Blood Prior to Issue I
Blood Group Antigens>ABO

T2.3
Comparison of Carbohydrate and Protein Antigens

Carbohydrate Antigens	Protein Antigens
ABO, Le, I, M, N, P	All others, including Rh, Kidd, Kell, S, s, and Duffy
Naturally-occurring antibodies	Antibodies acquired only after exposure to products containing antigen
Antibodies usually IgM	Antibodies usually IgG
Antibodies usually reactive at room temperature	Antibodies usually reactive at 37°
"Agglutinating" antibodies	"Coating" antibodies
React at immediate spin (IS)	React at AHG phase

Serologic crossmatch. At room temperature, recipient serum is mixed with a sample of the donor blood obtained from one of the segments of integral tubing, followed by centrifugation. This is referred to as an immediate spin (IS) crossmatch and is the usual type of routine crossmatch performed.

- When a nuisance-type, cold-reacting, antibody is present, the crossmatch may be prewarmed to prevent interference by this clinically insignificant type of antibody.

- If clinically significant alloantibodies are known to be present, then the addition of a second, antiglobulin, step is required.

- A minor crossmatch (in which the donor's serum is tested against the recipient's red cells) is never required.

- Infant blood (up to 4 months old) need not be crossmatched if no clinically significant antibodies are detected. The serum of the neonate or the mother may be used to test for clinically significant antibodies.

Computer crossmatch. A computer crossmatch is permissible in patients with no detectable clinically significant alloantibodies. Certain conditions must be met for this to be an acceptable alternative to the serologic crossmatch, including, but not limited to, having a 'validated' computer system, and having had the recipient's ABO type determined at least twice.

Labeling and Visual Inspection of Blood Prior to Issue

The crossmatched units of blood must be labeled with the intended recipient's name and identification number. The units must also be visually inspected. Blood contamination should be suspected if units are discolored (purple), if there is a visible zone of hemolysis, or if clots can be seen. Also, visibly lipemic specimens should not be transfused.

Blood Group Antigens

ABO

ABO antigens are the single most important reason for most of what is done in blood banking. Without ABO compatibility, little else matters in pretransfusion testing.

- ABO antigens are carbohydrate antigens **T2.3**

- The genes for carbohydrate antigens often encode specific enzymes (glycosyltransferases) that transfer specific saccharides to a specific carbohydrate chain acceptor. Genes on chromosome 9 are responsible for A, B and O groups. The A and B alleles encode for enzymes that produce these antigens, which are formed by connecting specific saccharides on to the H antigen base. The O allele does not encode a functional enzyme, and, therefore, group O red cells contain lots of the H antigen that has not been converted into either an A or B antigen.

- H antigen is made from type 1 and type 2 precursor carbohydrate chains. In secretions (saliva, tears), type 1 chains are converted into H antigen by the enzymatic action (fucosylation) of the Se gene product. In blood, type 2 chains are converted to H antigen by the enzymatic action (fucosylation) of the H gene product. When no further modifications are made on the H antigen, the blood is type O. When the A gene product (N-acetyl-galactosaminyltransferase) acts enzymatically on the H antigen, resulting in the addition of N-acetyl galactosamine, the A antigen results. When the B gene product (galactosyltransferase) acts on the H antigen, D-galactose is added, and B antigen results.

- Bombay phenotype: When the h gene (an amorph) is inherited instead of H, no H substance can be produced in blood (although H can be produced in secretions if the Se gene is present), and the person has the Bombay phenotype. Such individuals, who are extremely rare, produce a dangerous anti-H.

T2.4
ABO Blood Types in the USA

ABO Type	Incidence (%)	
	Whites	Blacks
O	45	50
A	40	25
B	10	20
AB	5	5

■ The relative amount of H antigen in blood groups:
O >> A2 > B >A2B > A1 > A1B

O Blood Group

■ Results from inheritance of neither A nor B genes, resulting in an OO genotype.

■ Type O persons have naturally-occurring IgM anti-A and anti-B.

■ They also have IgG anti-A,B.

A Blood Group

■ Results from the AA or AO genotype T2.4.

■ Inheritance of A transferases of varying efficiencies results in subgroups of A that differ primarily in the quantity of A antigen on red cells. The two principal subgroups are A1 and A2. A1 cells express more A substance than A2 cells. 80% of blood group A individuals have the A1 phenotype, and most of the remaining 20% are A2.

■ A1 and A2 cells can be distinguished by the strength of their reactions with anti-A1 reagent prepared from the serum of blood group B individuals or with *Dolichos biflorus* lectin which has anti-A1 activity.

■ Clinically significant anti-A1 can be found in the serum of 5% of blood group A2 and 35% of group A2B individuals.

T2.5
Rh Nomenclature and Incidence

Weiner	Antigens	Whites (%)	Blacks (%)
R^1	CDe	40	15
R^2	cDE	10	10
R^0	cDE	5	45
R^Z	CDe	rare*	rare
r'	Cde	3	3
r''	cdE	2	rare
r	cde	40	30
r^y	Cde	rare	rare

* Found in 6% of Native Americans

B Blood Group

■ Results from the BB or BO genotype.

■ No important subgroups.

AB Blood Group

■ Results from the AB genotype.

■ Least frequent ABO phenotype.

Rh

Rh antigens are polypeptide antigens T2.5 encoded by closely linked gene loci C, D, and E. RHD and RHCE gene loci are found on chromosome 1. The *RHAG* gene which encodes the Rh associated glycoprotein (RhAG) is found on chromosome 6. The polypeptides produced from RHD and RHCE genes form a complex on the red blood cell membrane with the Rh associated glycoprotein on chromosome 6.

Gene frequencies. The most common genotype in Rh-negative individuals, both black and white, is r/r (cde/cde). The most common Rh-positive genotype is R1/R1 or R1/r in whites and R^0/R^0 or R^0/r in blacks. Note also that R^0 is the most common allele in blacks, while it is very uncommon in whites.

Blood Group Antigens>Rh

Weak D phenotype

- Formerly, weak D phenotype was mistakenly called D^u antigen .

- The term weak D refers to D+ red blood cells that do not react strongly with anti-D reagent. By definition, the reactions of weak D phenotype are as follows:

  □ negative at IS with anti-D reagent.

  □ negative after 37°C incubation with anti-D reagent

  □ positive at AHG phase with anti-D reagent

- The source of the weak D phenotype: quantitative weak D vs partial D

  □ Quantitative weak D is the most common basis for the weak D phenotype. It is caused by a gene alteration resulting in reduced D antigen expression on the red blood cell surface. Importantly, this altered D phenotype does not result in loss of D-antigen epitopes. This alteration is common in African Americans and often occurs as part of a Dce haplotype. Persons with the Dce/Ce genotype have weakened D expression due to the presence of the C allele situated *trans* (on the other homologous chromosome) to D (the Ceppelli effect).

  □ Partial D is the term used for persons whose red blood cells lack components (epitopes) of the D antigen. In the past, this was referred to as "D mosaic" or "D variant." Partial D phenotypes can be defined in terms of their D epitopes. Over 30 have been described. Partial D women are at risk for forming anti-D antibodies with D+ pregnancies.

- Transfusion of weak D cells into D– recipients does not elicit an immune response; however, transfusion of weak D cells into previously sensitized D– recipients can produce a hemolytic transfusion reaction.

- *AABB* Standards require that donor samples be tested for weak D and labeled D+ if found. The recipient need not be tested for weak D.

Rh null

- Rh null individuals have no Rh antigens (no Rh or RhAG).

- Due to lack of Rh antigens, Rh null cells lack LW and Fy5 and have weakened expression of S, s, and U antigens.

- Red cells lacking Rh/RhAG proteins have structural abnormalities, most commonly, stomatocytosis, which results in hemolytic anemia.

Rh Antibodies

- These are IgG antibodies that are acquired through exposure, unlike the naturally occurring ABO antibodies.

- D antigen is *the most immunogenic* of all the non-ABO antigens. 80% of D– individuals exposed to a single D+ unit will develop anti-D.

- All Rh antibodies *except* D display dosage. Recall that this refers to an antibody that reacts more strongly with red cells homozygous for an antigen (such as CC or EE) than with red cells heterozygous for the antigen (such as Cc or Ee).

- All Rh antigens are enhanced by enzymes. This means that the test red blood cells react more strongly with the patient's serum *in vitro* after treatment with enzymes such as ficin or papain.

- Rh antibodies may result in hemolytic transfusion reactions (HTR) with *extravascular* hemolysis and a severe form of hemolytic disease of the newborn (HDN).

- *If anti-E is detected in the serum, then the additional presence of anti-c should be suspected.* This is because most individuals who have anti-E have the R1R1 phenotype (CDe/CDe), and have been transfused with R2 blood, which has the phenotype cDE. Such individuals develop anti-E and too-weak-to-detect anti-c as well. Anti-c is a common cause of delayed hemolytic transfusion reactions (DHTR). It is common practice to select c-negative and E-negative blood for recipients with anti-E.

Kidd Blood Group System

Kidd antigens

- Kidd antigens are *enhanced* by enzymes.
- Kidd antigen frequencies **T2.6:**
    - □ Compatible blood: 23% of US population is Jka−, and 28% (60% of blacks) are Jkb−.

Kidd antibodies

- Kidd antibodies are warm-reacting IgG antibodies that are acquired only through exposure. They are notorious for being difficult to detect in the lab ("tricky Kidd") for many reasons elaborated below, not the least of which is that they tend to disappear over time. Kidd are potentially dangerous antibodies. Historical Kidd antibodies, despite the absence of currently detectable antibody, is reason enough to give Kidd antigen-negative blood.

- Kidd antibodies display dosage: red cells from homozygous [JkaJka or Jk(a+b−)] individuals express more antigen than heterozygous [JkaJkb or Jk(a+b+)] individuals. Since among the test cells in a panel some may be from homozygous individuals and some from heterozygous, this may give confusing panel results. In addition, it may be the cause of a false-negative crossmatch. Type all crossmatch compatible units with commercial antisera to make sure they are antigen negative.

- Kidd antibodies are often *weak:* anti-Jka and anti-Jkb fade quickly from the serum after sensitization. A strong antibody may be detected today that is undetectable in a few months. This is one of the main reasons to check blood bank records prior to transfusion. Furthermore, Kidd antibodies do not store well (eg, when serum is sent to a reference lab).

- Kidd antibodies most often *react only at the AHG phase.*

Clinical characteristics: despite the difficulties in detection of Kidd antibodies, they are very clinically significant ("Kidd kills").

- Kidd antibodies are a common cause of immediate hemolytic transfusion reactions (HTR). They are capable of binding complement and *can produce intravascular hemolysis* but most often produce acute extravascular hemolysis.

- Kidd antibodies are a notorious cause of delayed hemolytic transfusion reactions (DHTR).

T2.6
Kidd Phenotypes

Phenotype	Whites (%)	Blacks (%)
Jk(a+b−)	30	60
Jk(a+b+)	50	30
Jk(a−b+)	20	10
Jk(a−b−)	rare	rare

- Kidd antibodies *do not* usually cause hemolytic disease of the newborn (HDN) due to weak antigen expression by the fetus and neonate.

Lewis Blood Group System: the Tangled Web of Le, Se, H, and ABO

Lewis-related genes

- There are two precursor oligosaccharides: type 1 and type 2. Type 1 is found predominantly in secretions but also free in serum, while type 2 is found only on the red cell surface. There is no type 2 oligosaccharide on the red cell surface. Unbranched type 1 and 2 oligosaccharides represent *i antigen.* Branched type 1 and 2 oligosaccharides are *I antigens.* In the neonate, unbranched *(i antigen)* oligosaccharides predominate; thus, *cord blood* red cells are loaded with i antigen. Oligosaccharide branching is something that increases with age, and *adults* have mostly branched oligosaccharides, thus having little *i antigen* and mostly *I antigen.*

- As mentioned in the section on ABO genes, the H gene encodes a fucosyl transferase that adds fucose to type 2 precursor substances, on the surfaces of red cells, to make H antigen. The h gene is an amorph. When no further modifications are made on the H antigen, the person is type O. When the A gene product acts on the H antigen, resulting in the addition of N-acetyl galactosamine, the A antigen results. When the B gene product acts on the H antigen to add galactose, the B antigen results.

- The Le gene encodes a fucosyl transferase that adds fucose to type 1 precursors, both free in serum and in secretions, to make Lea antigen. The le gene is an amorph. Though Lewis antigens are synthesized on free type 1 precursor substance, *it becomes passively adsorbed onto red cell surfaces.*

Blood Group Antigens>Lewis Blood Group System

T2.7
Lewis Phenotypes

Phenotype	Whites (%)	Blacks (%)
Le(a−b+)	72	55
Le(a+b−)	22	22
Le(a−b−)	6	23
Le(a+b+)	0	0

- The Se gene has two functions:
  - It encodes a fucosyl transferase that adds fucose to type 1 precursor, *only if a fucose has already been added; ie, only if the Le gene product has acted on it,* resulting in Le^b antigen. There are two consequences of this: you can't make Le^b without a Le and Se gene, and Le^b is made at the expense of Le^a. Persons with both the Le and Se genes will have red cells bearing passively adsorbed Le^b with no Le^a. Persons with the Le but not Se genes will have red cells bearing passively adsorbed Le^a but not Le^b. Persons with no Le gene will have neither Le^a nor Le^b.
  - It produces the secretion equivalent of H substance from type 1 precursor and is thus responsible for the appearance of A, B, and H substances in secretions. Le substances are secreted independently of Se.

- Lewis antibodies: Are naturally occurring antibodies found almost exclusively in Le(a−b−) individuals who are commonly Black. Le(a−b+) persons do not make anti-Le^a antibodies. Lewis antibodies are nearly always IgM and insignificant. The rare significant Lewis antibody is always anti-Le^a. These antibodies are usually inconsequential because (a) transfused red cells shed their Lewis antigens and acquire the Lewis phenotype of the recipient and (b) Lewis antibodies are quickly adsorbed by free serum Lewis antigens.

- Lewis antigens in children: Lewis can't be reliably typed until the 2nd birthday. Those persons destined to be Le(a−b+) are as neonates Le(a−b−) then Le(a+b−) then Le(a+b+) and finally Le(a−b+).

- Lewis antigens are expressed weakly during pregnancy and the Le(a−b−) phenotype is not uncommonly seen during gestation.

- Lewis phenotype frequency **T2.7**

- Lewis quiz **T2.8**

T2.8
Lewis Quiz

	Lewis Genes	Hi Genes	Secretor Genes	ABO Genes	Red Cell Phenotype	Substances in Saliva
1	Le	H	Se	O	H, Le(a−b+)	H,↓Le^a, Le^b
2	le	H	Se	O	H, Le(a−b−)	H
3	Le	H	se	O	H, Le(a+b−)	Le^a
4	le	H	se	O	H, Le(a−b−)	none
5	Le	H	Se	A1	A1, Le(a−b+)	↓H, A,↓Le^a, Le^b
6	le	H	Se	A1	A1, Le(a−b−)	↓H, A,
7	Le	H	se	A1	A1, Le(a+b−)	Le^a
8	le	h	ee	A1	Bombay, Le(a−b−)	none
9	le	h	Se	A1	Bombay, Le(a−b−)	↓H, A, Le^a
10	Le	h	se	A1	Bombay, Le(a+b−)	Le^a
11	le	h	se	A1	Bombay, Le(a−b−)	none

Duffy

Duffy antigens

- Two antigens, Fya and Fyb, comprise the Duffy system.

- Fy(a+b–) is more common than Fy(a–b+).

- Fy(a–b–) is rare in Whites, but commonly found in Blacks (68%). This phenotype confers resistance to *P vivax* malaria.

- Duffy antigens are destroyed by enzymes.

Duffy antibodies

- Warm-reacting IgG antibodies acquired through exposure.

- Duffy antibodies show dosage effect.

- Can cause hemolytic transfusion reactions (HTR) with extravascular hemolysis and severe hemolytic disease of the newborn (HDN).

MNS System

- MNS antigens are found on red cell surface glycophorin A and glycophorin B molecules.

  □ The antigens included M and N (glycophorin A); S, s, and U (glycophorin B).

  □ M and N antigens are destroyed by enzymes:

- MNS antibodies

  □ MNS antibodies display dosage.

  □ Anti-M and anti-N antibodies are naturally occurring, cold-reacting, IgM antibodies that are usually clinically insignificant.

  □ Anti-S, anti-s, and anti-U antibodies are acquired following exposure and are warm-reacting IgG antibodies that are clinically significant.

Kell Blood Group

Kell antigens

- The k antigen is far more common (99.8%) than the K antigen (9%).

- Kell antigens are unaffected by enzymes (neither enhanced nor destroyed) but are destroyed by ZZAP and DTT.

- The McLeod phenotype refers to red cells with very weak expression of Kell antigens due to the lack of the Kx protein, a secondary supportive protein encoded on X chromosome (Kell encoded on chromosome 7), similar in function to the RhAG protein. Lack of this Kx protein, which is normally covalently linked to Kell protein, depresses the expression of Kell antigens and is associated with shortened red blood cell survival, reduced deformability and shortened survival. Hemolytic anemia and acanthocytosis result. This phenotype is associated with X-linked chronic granulomatous disease (CGD), acanthocytosis, and a late-onset type of muscular dystrophy.

Kell antibodies

- Most commonly these are anti-K and are acquired through exposure.

- They are warm-reacting IgG antibodies.

- They are associated with hemolytic transfusion reactions (HTR) with extravascular hemolysis and hemolytic disease of the newborn (HDN).

Lutheran

- Lutheran antigens: Lu^b is more common than Lu^a.

- Lutheran antigens are destroyed by enzymes.

- Lutheran antibodies: *usually clinically insignificant.*

P Blood Groups

- The P antigens are carbohydrate antigens that include P_1, P, and P^k.

- Note: the p antigen is not a part of the P system.

- Phenotypes: the phenotypes are defined by reactivity with the antibodies anti-P_1, anti-P, anti-P^k, and anti-PP_1P^k which reacts with the whole P complex of antigens.

  □ 80% of Whites and 95% of Blacks have the P_1 phenotype: anti-P_1+, P+, PP_1P^k+, and P^k−.

  □ 20% of Whites and 5% of Blacks have the P2 phenotype: anti-P_1−, P+, PP_1P^k+, and P^k−.

  □ The rare p phenotype refers to absence of P antigens (anti-P_1−, P−, PP_1P^k−and P^k−). p phenotype individuals make a potent anti-PP_1P^k. This antibody can be broken into its three component antibodies through adsorptions. Anti-PP_1P^k may be associated with delayed hemolytic transfusion reaction and hemolytic disease of the newborn. There is also an association between both anti-P_1 and anti-PP_1P^k antibodies and first trimester spontaneous abortion.

- Antibodies to P antigens are most commonly seen in P2 phenotype individuals. These are usually IgM anti-P_1 that are reactive at 4°C and are not clinically significant.

- The P antigens are the target of antibodies in paroxysmal cold hemoglobinuria (PCH). Auto-anti-P IgG antibodies act as a biphasic hemolysin. The cold-reacting IgG anti-P binds as blood passes through the cool (acral) portions of the body and activates complement, leading to hemolysis. This antibody is not usually detected in routine antibody screens, but can be detected with the Donath-Landsteiner test.

- The P antigen serves as the receptor for parvovirus B19 (fifth disease).

- The P antigens can be agglutinated by hydatid cyst fluid and pigeon eggs.

Human Leukocyte Antigens (HLA)

HLA is encoded on the major histocompatibility complex (MHC), a complex of several gene loci found on chromosome 6p. They are such closely linked loci that they are inherited en bloc from each parent, with no crossing over. Each locus has a multitude of possible alleles distributed through the population, making HLA genes the most polymorphic in the human genome.

The MHC is broadly divided into MHC class I, class II, and class III genes. Class III genes include complement proteins and are not relevant to blood banking. Also embedded in the MHC region are the genes for hemochromatosis, 21-hydroxylase, and tumor necrosis factor (TNF).

Class I genes encode HLA class I antigens that are found on the surfaces of *all nucleated cells and platelets.* Mature red cells have very little class I antigen. Class I genes are distributed among three loci, termed HLA-A, HLA-B, and HLA-C. For each locus there are several possible alleles, termed such things as HLA-A1, HLA-A2, etc. Class I genes encode a *single* polypeptide chain that has 3 domains very similar to the domains of an immunoglobulin heavy chain, in addition to a transmembrane domain. The class I molecules are embedded as a transmembrane protein in the cell membrane, and each is noncovalently associated with a single molecule of $\beta2$ microglobulin.

Class II genes encode HLA class II antigens that are found on 3 *cell types:* B cells, macrophages, and *activated* T cells. Class II genes are distributed among three loci, termed HLA-DR, HLA-DP, and HLA-DQ. For each locus, there are several possible alleles, termed, for example, HLA-DR3, HLA-Dw2, etc. The class II genes encode two polypeptide chains, termed α and β, each with two domains similar to the immunoglobulin light chains, in addition to a transmembrane domain.

HLA plays a small role in blood compatibility, but it is pivotal in platelet refractoriness, solid-organ compatibility, and some transfusion reactions (febrile nonhemolytic reactions, transfusion-related acute lung injury [TRALI], and transfusion-associated graft-vs-host disease [TAGVHD]). Red cells bear very small amounts of class I antigens, collectively referred to as Bg (Bennett-Goodspeed) antigens, which are rarely the cause of alloantibody-mediated hemolytic

2: Blood Banking and Transfusion

Blood Group Antigens>Kell Blood Group I
Investigating a Positive Antibody Screen or Unexpected Crossmatch Incompatibility>Panels

transfusion reactions. Platelets have generous amounts of class I antigens, particularly HLA-A and HLA-B antigens. Class II antigens are expressed on neither red cells nor platelets.

Since each MHC complex is closely linked and inherited en bloc, each parental chromosome can be thought of as a haplotype. Thus, *the chance that two siblings are HLA-identical is 25%.* The chance of having an HLA-identical sibling goes up with the number of siblings: with 1 sibling, the chance is 25%, with 2 it is around 45%, and with 3 it is nearly 60%.

See Chapter 7 for additional information.

Investigating a Positive Antibody Screen or Unexpected Crossmatch Incompatibility

Panels

When an antibody screen is positive, a red cell panel is used to determine the antibody responsible. The identity of the antibody is key to knowing (1) whether it is clinically significant and (2) the best strategy for finding antigen-negative blood.

A panel is essentially an expanded antibody screen. Recipient serum is tested against a panel of group O blood cells, usually 10 different cells, which have been selected so that it is possible to identify the antibody in question. Reagent cells licensed by the FDA must express the following antigens: D, C, E, c, e, M, N, S, s, P_1, Le^a, Le^b, K, k, Fy^a, Fy^b, Jk^a and Jk^b.

Usually panel reactions are carried out in some kind of enhancement media, designed to make antibody-antigen reactions more obvious. Enhancement media include such things as low ionic strength saline (LISS) and polyethylene glycol (PEG).

Panels typically involve both a 37°C incubation phase and an AHG phase using either polyspecific reagent or monospecific anti-IgG reagent. The particular phase during which reactivity is seen is important to note.

Panels usually are run in parallel with an autocontrol. This is to prevent confusing results due to a red cell autoantibody.

Types of reaction. As in the antibody screen, a positive test is indicated either by agglutination or hemolysis. Agglutination is characterized by red cell clumps seen either grossly or microscopically and is usually graded m+ (microscopic agglutination) to 4+. Hemolysis is identified by the presence of a pink supernatant.

Phases of testing. This refers to the conditions under which a test is run. For example, if serum is mixed with test cells and centrifuged at room temperature, this is said to be the *immediate spin (IS) phase.* Serum antibodies active at this phase are called 'cold-reacting.' If this is pre-heated before performance, then it is the *37° phase,* and active serum antibodies are called 'warm-reacting.' If serum and blood are mixed in the presence of antihuman globulin, then this is the *indirect antiglobulin test (IAT) or antihuman globulin (AHG) phase.* Warm-reacting antibodies are usually IgG antibodies and are considered at least potentially clinically significant. Cold-reacting antibodies are usually IgM and are likely to be clinically insignificant. *Notable exceptions* are ABO antibodies that are IgM but react over a broad thermal range and are, obviously, clinically significant, and the anti-P antibody of paroxysmal cold hemoglobinuria (PCH) that is a clinically significant, cold-reacting, IgG antibody. As a general rule-of-thumb, antibodies that are reactive at 37°C and/or reactive in

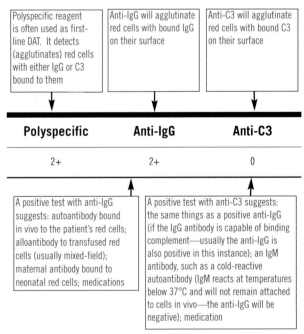

F2.4 DAT (direct antiglobulin test)

Investigating a Positive Antibody Screen or Unexpected Crossmatch Incompatibility>Panels

	Rh-Hr					MNS				Lutheran		P	Lewis		Kell		Duffy		Kidd		Results		
	D	C	c	E	e	M	N	S	s	Lu^a	Lu^b	P$_1$	Le^a	Le^b	K	k	Fy^a	Fy^b	Jk^a	Jk^b	IS	37°	AHG
1	0	+	0	0	+	+	+	0	+	0	+	+	+	0	0	+	+	0	+	+	0	0	2+
2	+	+	+	0	+	+	0	0	+	0	+	+	0	+	+	0	+	+	0	+	0	0	2+
3	+	+	0	0	+	0	+	+	0	+	0	0	+	0	0	+	+	+	+	+	0	0	2+
4	+	+	0	+	+	+	0	+	+	0	+	+	0	+	0	+	0	+	0	+	0	0	2+
5	+	0	+	+	0	+	0	0	0	0	+	+	0	+	0	+	+	+	0	+	0	0	0
6	0	0	+	0	+	+	0	+	0	0	+	+	0	+	0	+	0	+	+	0	0	0	0
7	0	0	+	0	+	0	+	+	0	+	+	0	0	+	0	+	0	+	+	0	0	0	0
8	0	0	+	0	+	0	+	0	+	+	0	+	+	0	+	0	+	0	0	+	0	0	0
9	0	0	+	0	+	+	+	+	0	0	+	+	0	+	0	+	0	+	+	0	0	0	0
10	0	0	+	0	+	+	0	0	0	0	+	0	0	0	0	+	0	0	+	+	0	0	0
Pt																					0	0	0

F2.5 Panel 1. The autocontrol is negative, suggesting that the reactions are due to alloantibody (not autoantibody). All the reactions are of similar strengths and at similar phases, suggesting that only one antibody is present. All antigens can be crossed out due to nonreactivity, except C. Even antigens known to show dosage (MNS, Kidd, C/c, E/e, & Duffy) can be excluded by nonreactivity with homozygous cells. The remaining specificity, C, fits perfectly with the observed reactions. Panel interpretation: anti-C

	Rh-Hr					MNS				Lutheran		P	Lewis		Kell		Duffy		Kidd		Results		
	D	C	c	E	e	M	N	S	s	Lu^a	Lu^b	P$_1$	Le^a	Le^b	K	k	Fy^a	Fy^b	Jk^a	Jk^b	IS	37°	AHG
1	0	+	0	0	+	+	+	0	+	0	+	+	+	0	0	+	+	0	+	+	0	2+	2+
2	+	+	+	0	+	+	0	0	+	0	+	+	0	+	+	0	+	+	0	+	0	1+	1+
3	+	+	0	0	+	0	+	+	0	+	0	0	+	0	0	+	+	+	+	+	0	1+	1+
4	+	+	0	+	+	+	0	+	+	0	+	+	0	+	0	+	0	+	0	+	0	0	0
5	+	0	+	+	0	+	0	0	0	0	+	+	0	+	0	+	+	+	0	+	0	1+	1+
6	0	0	+	0	+	+	0	+	0	0	+	+	0	+	0	+	0	+	+	0	0	0	0
7	0	0	+	0	+	0	+	+	0	+	+	0	0	+	0	+	0	+	+	0	0	0	0
8	0	0	+	0	+	0	+	0	+	+	0	+	+	0	+	0	+	0	0	+	0	1+	1+
9	0	0	+	0	+	+	+	+	0	0	+	+	0	+	0	+	0	+	+	0	0	0	0
10	0	0	+	0	+	+	0	0	0	0	+	0	+	0	0	+	0	0	+	+	0	0	0
Pt																					0	0	0

F2.6 Panel 2. The autocontrol is negative, suggesting that the positive reactions are due to alloantibody. The observation that there are different strengths of reactivity clues us in to the possibility that there may be more than one antibody or there is one manifesting dosage, or both. After the process of crossing-out, only K and Fy^a remain. In this case the reactions match both anti-Fy^a (showing dosage) and anti-K. Panel interpretation: anti-Fy^a & anti-K

the antiglobulin phase are more likely to be clinically significant.

The direct antiglobulin test (DAT) and indirect antiglobulin test (IAT). In the *direct* antiglobulin test **F2.4**, also known as the direct Coombs test, antihuman globulin (AHG) is added to blood. If the blood cells therein are coated with globulins, then there will be agglutination. In the *indirect* antiglobulin test, also called the indirect Coombs test, antibodies of known specificity are added to blood followed by the addition of antihuman globulin (AHG). If the blood cells contain the antigen of interest, then there will be agglutination. Thus, the DAT can be used to detect in vivo coating of red cells with antibody, while the IAT is used to detect in vitro coating of red cells with antibodies. In the addition of antihuman globulin, one may select either polyspecific (contains both anti-IgG and anti-C3d) or monospecific (contains either anti-IgG or anti-C3d) antihuman globulins.

Clinical significance of detected antibodies. An antibody has 'clinical significance' when it has the potential to cause hemolysis or hemolytic disease of the newborn. As a general *rule-of-thumb*, cold-reacting IgM antibodies are usually clinically insignificant, while warm-reacting or AHG-reacting IgG antibodies are considered significant.

Alloantibodies that are *nearly always insignificant* include: anti-M, N, Lewis, Lutheran, and I.

How to interpret the routine panel **F2.5, F2.6**.

- Look at the autocontrol. When panel cells are reactive with a negative autocontrol, then an alloantibody is present. When both the panel cells and autocontrol are positive, this may be due to autoantibody alone, but autoantibody with an alloantibody needs to be excluded. When only the autocontrol is positive, an autoantibody alone is likely (see section IV), although the possibility of alloantibody to recently transfused red cells (often giving an autocontrol with *mixed field* positivity) must be excluded.

- In the usual scenario where only a single antibody is present, one sees a few cells positive and some negative, but *all positive reactions are of the same strength and at the same phases*. For each cell with which the patient is nonreactive, cross out all the antigens for which that cell is positive. For example, if the recipient serum is

nonreactive with cell #1, which expresses the C antigen, then anti-C specificity can be tentatively excluded. Usually this simple process will leave one antigen that fits best with the reactivity seen. In actual practice, *reactivity with 3 positive cells and nonreactivity with 3 negative cells* are required to statistically establish a specific antibody.

- If the reactivity is still not clear-cut, then consider the possibility of more than one antibody, a single antibody showing dosage, antibodies to high-incidence antigens, antibodies to low-incidence antigens, antibodies to reagents, or polyagglutination (see p 120).

- In confusing cases, it may be helpful to phenotype the recipient blood cells. Antigens borne on recipient cells can be excluded as alloantibodies.

The Nonroutine Panel

Multiple antibodies are suspected when all or nearly all cells are positive but with differing strengths of reaction or at different phases. Various techniques can assist in clarifying the antibodies present, including the use of *enzymes, adsorption, and neutralization*.

Antibodies showing dosage

- An antibody showing dosage should be suspected when (1) there is weak reactivity with some cells, but the process of crossing-out has eliminated all specificities or (2) there is variable strength of reactivity.

- As mentioned previously, dosage means that an anti-body's strength of binding is influenced by the number of antigens on the red cell surface. Thus, antibodies with dosage effect react more strongly with cells from individuals homozygous for an antigen.

- Looking at the phenotype of the test cells, one notes that some of the cells are homozygous and some heterozygous; eg, cell #1 which is Fy^a positive, Fy^b negative is homozgyous for Fy^a, while cell #2 that is Fy^a positive, Fy^b positive is not. If anti-Fy^a were present, one might see weak reactivity with cell #1 and no reactivity with cell #2, even though both bear the antigen. Alternatively, one may see 3+ reactivity with cell #1 and 1+ or m+ with cell #2.

- The nice thing about dosage is that it is predictable. *Antigens that display dosage:* MNS, Kidd, C/c, E/e, Duffy.

- Dosage is a reason to routinely employ a slight alteration in the strategy for 'crossing out' antigens. Fully cross out, with an 'X', nonreactive antigens that do not manifest dosage, while only placing a single slash through nonreactive antigens that do display dosage. Place an 'X' through dosage-manifesting antigens *only if a homozygous cell is non reactive.* Only then can one confidently exclude MNSs, Kidd, C/c, E/e, and Duffy.

Antibodies to high incidence antigens or high-titer, low avidity (HTLA) antibodies.

- An HTLA antibody is suspected when there is weak reactivity in the AHG phase to all cells in the antibody panel. The antibody continues to react at dilutions >1:64.

- HTLA antibodies are a group of antibodies which

  □ Are directed against high incidence antigens (present in >99.9% of population)

  □ Usually show weak reactivity to all cells in an antibody panel at the AHG phase

  □ Continue to react at high dilutions (high titer, usually >1:64).

- The significance of HTLA antibodies is that they mask other alloantibodies.

- Some HTLA antibodies may be clinically significant themselves, and these include: Cartwright (Yt^a), Holley (Hy), and Gregory (Gy).

- HTLA antibodies that are *usually not clinically significant* include: Chido/Rogers (Ch/Rg), Sda, Bg, Csa, and York (Yka).

Antibodies to test reagents.

- This is suspected when the autocontrol is negative (because the reagents in question are in the diluent for the test cells) and there is across-the-board reactivity in the panel.

- The test cells can be washed to remove these antigens.

Antibodies to low-incidence antigens (Wr^a and Kp^a) may be suspected when only one test cell is reactive. Typically these antigens are not indicated on the panel, but the package insert for the test cells delineates a longer list of antigens for which the cell is positive.

Polyagglutination. Adult sera contain naturally-occurring IgM antibodies to T, Tn, Tk, and Cad. Some of these antigens (T, Tn, and Tk) exist only when normal red cell antigens are enzymatically altered by the action of bacterial neuraminidase, a process known as *T-activation.* This effect is transient and abates following the infection. Cad is a rare inherited antigen. The test for polyagglutination: polyagglutinable red cells are agglutinated by adult but not cord serum.

Other Special Techniques

Elutions. An antibody may be eluted from red cells. The eluate (that presumably contains antibody) can then be tested against a panel of red cells to determine its specificity.

Adsorption is a handy technique when there are allo- or auto-antibodies potentially masking other alloantibodies. The masking antibody can be adsorbed using red cells known to be positive for the antigen (in the case of an autoantibody, the patient's own (autologous) red cells are used). Adsorbed serum will contain any alloantibodies that were present.

Hemagglutination inhibition (neutralizing substances)

- Hemagglutination inhibition is a term that refers to the use of a substance **T2.9** that is known to contain or mimic a particular antigen. If a serum sample is thought to contain an antibody with specificity for this antigen, this suspicion can be confirmed by the abolition of (neutralization of) reactivity. Alternatively, neutralization of a particular antibody can assist in detecting additional antibodies that may be masked.

- Hemagglutination inhibition is also used to determine the secretor status (by detecting H substance in saliva).

Lectins **T2.9** are reagents derived from plants that will bind to specific antigens on red cells and agglutinate them (cause hemagglutination).

T2.9
Neutralizing Substances and Lectins

Neutralizing Substance	Antigenic Activity
Guinea pig urine	Sd$_a$
Hydatid cyst fluid	P$_1$
Saliva	H, Le^a
Breast milk	I
Pigeon eggs	P$_1$
Plasma	Chido, Rodgers

Lectin	Binds to
Dolichos biflorus	A1 (used to distinguish A1 phenotype from A subgroups).
Bandeiraea simplicifolia	B
Ulex europaeus	H (agglutinates group O erythrocytes). Useful in determination of secretor status
Lotus tetragonolobus	H
Arachis hypogaea	T
Vicea graminea	N

Proteolytic enzymes such as ficin, papain, and trypsin, when added to serologic tests, act to enhance the antigenicity of some antigens, while suppressing the antigenicity of others.

- Antigens *enhanced* by enzymes: Le, I/i, P, Rh, Kidd. Some Kidd antibodies can only be detected following enzyme enhancement.

- Antigens *destroyed* by enzymes: MNSs, Fy^a, Fy^b, Lutheran, Chido, Rodgers, and Yt^a.

- Antigens unaffected by enzymes: most remaining antigens, notably Kell.

Elution is used to remove antibody bound to red cells so that the antibody can be identified. The elution may be carried out in with the addition of heat, solvent, or acid.

The Positive Crossmatch

Causes of a positive crossmatch with positive antibody screen

- Alloantibodies.

- Autoantibodies.

- Antibodies to reagents.

Causes of positive crossmatch with negative antibody screen

- Anti-ABO antibodies.

- Antibodies to low incidence antigens.

Unusual findings in pretransfusion testing T2.10

Case 1 (T2.10) explanation: O-positive person with apparent anti-D antibody. This may be due to one of several causes:

- Autoantibody. The most common specificity in warm autoimmune hemolytic anemia (WAIHA) is anti-Rh.

- Anti-LW. The LW antigen is expressed more strongly on D+ cells than D−. If anti-LW antibodies are present, they may appear to be reacting with only D+ cells, thus simulating anti-D antibodies.

- D-variant. Such individuals may express antibodies to other D mosaics.

Case 2 (T2.10) explanation: B-negative individual manifesting the B(A) phenotype. Certain blood type B individuals have such high levels of glucosyltransferase that a small amount of A antigen is produced, and their red cells react weakly with anti-A reagent.

Case 3 (T2.10) explanation: A-negative individual with acquired B phenotype.

- In acquired B phenotype, the red cells of a blood type A individual acquire reactivity with anti-B reagent and thus type as AB, despite having serum anti-B antibodies.

Investigating a Positive Antibody Screen or Unexpected Crossmatch Incompatibility>Other Special Techniques

T2.10
Unusual Findings in Forward and Reverse Typing (see explanations p 121)

Case	Forward Typing			Reverse Typing			Antibody Screen
	Anti-a	**Anti-b**	**Anti-Rh**	**A Cells**	**B Cells**	**D+ Cells**	**All Cells**
1	–	–	4+	4+	4+	1-2+	Negative
2	1-2+	4+	–	4+	–	–	Negative
3	4+	1-2+	–	–	4+	–	Negative
4	4+	4+	–	1-2+	–	–	Negative
5	–	–	–	4+	4+	–	4+

- This occurs in subgroup A1 individuals when the A1 antigen is acted upon by bacterial deacetylases. Thus, the acquired B phenotype is associated with conditions that give rise to transient or persistent bacteremia such as colon cancer, colonic obstruction, and gram-negative sepsis.

- Due to the presence of anti-B in serum, this can also result in a positive DAT.

- To confirm this suspicion, several laboratory avenues are available. The altered A1 antigen with B antigenic activity can be re-acetylated in vitro with acetic anhydride. Further, the patient's own anti-B will agglutinate these red cells. Acidified human anti-B does not react with acquired B antigen. The patient's saliva will not contain the B antigen.

Case 4 (T2.10) explanation: AB-negative individual having anti-A1 antibodies. This is most likely due to the patient having the blood group A2B phenotype.

- Approximately 25% of A2B individuals have anti-A1 antibody.

- Anti-A1 is usually a clinically insignificant IgM, and compatible blood can be found with a pre-warmed crossmatch.

Case 5 (T2.10) explanation: Bombay phenotype.

Case 6 (T2.11) explanation: warm autoantibody. May also be positive at 37° phase. An autoadsorption may succeed in removing these antibodies, permitting further testing.

Case 7 (T2.11) explanation: high-titer, low avidity antibody to a frequently occurring antigen (eg, Chido, Rodgers). Can often neutralize with serum.

Case 8 (T2.11) explanation: cold autoantibody. If broad thermal amplitude, may also be positive in 37° phase. Since usually IgM, not reactive at AHG (IAT) phase. Can often work through with a prewarmed antibody screen and prewarmed crossmatch.

Case 9 (T2.11) explanation: antibody to reagents (LISS, PEG).

T2.11
Unusual Findings in Antibody Panel (see explanation pp 122-123)

Case	Finding
6	All cells (1-10 and autocontrol) positive at AHG only
7	All cells (1-10, except autocontrol) positive at AHG only, usually weak (1+ to 2+)
8	All cells (1-10 and autoconrol) positive at IS only
9	All cells (1-10 and autocontrol) positive at IS and 37°, not at AHG

2: Blood Banking and Transfusion

Investigating a Positive Antibody Screen or Unexpected Crossmatch Incompatibility>Other Special Techniques |
Autoantibodies>Warm-Reacting Antibodies

Other unusal findings

- Leukemia and Hodgkin lymphoma. In these individuals, there is often weakened expression of A or B antigens with mixed-field agglutination.

- Gastric carcinoma. Excess free serum A or B antigens may be present free in serum. This may have the effect in vitro of binding anti-A or anti-B reagents, hus giving the false impression that the patient has type O red cells.

Autoantibodies

Autoantibodies are suspected when there is a positive DAT or a positive autocontrol in the screening panel.

A positive DAT is very common, affecting up to 15% of hospitalized patients.

Whenever an autoantibody is suspected, several questions should be considered:

- Is the patient hemolyzing? If there is evidence of hemolysis, such as elevated LDH, depressed haptoglobin, elevated bilirubin, or anemia, then further workup may be indicated. Details of hemolytic anemia are presented in the hematopathology chapter. If there is no hemolysis, then the main significance of these antibodies has to do with their potential to disrupt pretransfusion testing.

- Is there an obvious explanation?

  □ Is there a history of recent transfusion? This may be the cause of the positive DAT or autocontrol. Typically this gives a mixed-field reaction. If the antibody responsible is not detectable in the serum, then an elution may be needed to characterize the antibody.

  □ What drugs is the patient taking? Drugs classically associated with a positive DAT (see below) are penicillin, cephalosporins, procainamide, and aldomet.

  □ Other uncommon causes of a positive DAT include post-bone marrow transplant patients (look for mixed field reactions) and patients receiving anti-lymphocyte globulin (ALG).

  □ If all these have been excluded, then a primary autoimmunity must be considered (see below).

Warm-Reacting Antibodies (see also Hematopathology Chapter 4)

The antibodies

- Warm-reacting antibodies react optimally at 37°C. Typically, they react with the patient's own red cells (produce a positive autocontrol/DAT) and react with all cells tested in the screen, panel, and crossmatch.

- Warm-reacting antibodies are usually IgG, uncommonly IgA or IgM.

- The AHG phase is positive with polyspecific antisera and anti-IgG antisera. In some cases (30%-50%), anti-C3 is also positive. It seems that the strength of reaction (m+ to 4+) correlates somewhat with the likelihood of hemolysis; it also appears that the presence and strength of C3 correlates with the likelihood of hemolysis.

- Most often the responsible antibody has *broad anti-Rh* specificity.

The significance of warm-reacting antibodies is two-fold. First, it may cause warm autoimmune hemolytic anemia (WAIHA), the most common type of autoimmune hemolytic anemia. However, not all warm-reacting antibodies cause hemolysis; in fact, most do not. Second, warm-reacting antibodies can interfere with pretransfusion testing for alloantibodies and crossmatching.

Transfusion. In a patient with a warm autoantibody, the best thing to do is avoid transfusions if possible, as there is a greater than usual risk of transfusion-related complications in these patients, and transfusion may exacerbate the underlying hemolytic anemia. When transfusion is required, the major challenge, if time permits, is to identify any underlying alloantibodies that may be present.

- This may require an autoadsorption procedure (to clear the autoantibody from the serum) followed by an antibody screen using the remaining (adsorbed) serum. Autoadsorption usually is performed using the patient's (autologous) red cells, after pretreatment with ZZAP, at 37°C (warm autoadsorption). Autoadsorption is ideally performed on a patient who has not been recently transfused (within the last 3 months).

- If the patient has been recently transfused, adsorption may be attempted using cells of the same Rh phenotype (if this is known) or using several different Rh phenotypes (if not known).

Cold-Reacting Autoantibodies

Benign cold autoagglutinins are the most commonly encountered autoantibodies

- Reactions: Nonpathologic cold *agglutinins react most strongly at 4°C,* but they have variably wide thermal amplitudes and may react up to 22°C. They usually do not interfere with routine tests, but they may do so when they react at or near room temperature, making such things as CBCs unreliable. *The only reliable CBC index in the presence of cold agglutinins is the hemoglobin.* The *titer* of benign cold agglutinins is *usually* <64 at 4°C. Most are IgM and can activate complement in vitro, thus reactions may be seen at the antiglobulin phase using polyspecific antisera. If monospecific reagents are used, the cells are agglutinated by anti-C3d but not anti-IgG.

- Antibody specificities: *most commonly anti-I.* The I antigen is strongly expressed on virtually all adult red cells but only weakly on cord red cells. Adult levels are reached around 2 years. The less common *anti-i* reacts with cord blood but not with adult blood. Anti-H reacts best with group O and A2 red cells because they have the most H substance. A_1 red cells have the least H substance and react weakly. It is important not to confuse this with the anti-H in O_h (Bombay) individuals that is a potent alloantibody reacting at 4-37°C and causing severe, life-threatening, hemolysis.

Pathologic cold autoagglutinins are less common than benign examples

- Reactions: reactive over a broad thermal range, up to 32-37°C and causes spontaneous autoagglutination in anticoagulated blood at room temperature. As with benign cold agglutinins, CBCs may be unreliable. The DAT is 2+ to 3+ with polyspecific reagent, positive with monospecific anti-C3d, but negative with monospecific anti-IgG. The titer is often >1000 when tested at 4°C.

- Clinical types
  - □ Idiopathic cold autoimmune hemolytic anemia (CAIHA) or cold agglutinin syndrome (CAS). A chronic idiopathic condition found predominantly in older individuals complaining of acrocyanosis and Reynaud phenomenon with a moderate hemolytic anemia. The responsible antibody is almost always an IgM with anti-I, anti-i, or rarely anti-Pr specificity, which is often monoclonal. The antibody causes agglutination in the extremities and fixing of complement, leading to eventual intravascular lysis.
  - □ Secondary CAIHA. A transient cold agglutinin, IgM anti-I, is seen in 50% of patients with *M. pneumonia* infection. This usually resolves within 2-3 weeks. A more persistent anti-I may be associated with lymphoproliferative disorders. Some of these are clinically significant. *Infectious mononucleosis less frequently causes the emergence of IgM anti-i.*

Mixed-type autoantibodies

- As the name implies, these patients have both cold-reacting IgM and warm-reacting IgG autoantibodies.

- Most often, they show reactions with both IgG and C3 at the antiglobulin phase.

- No particular antigen specificity has been consistently shown.

- Clinically, these patients present with an acute-onset hemolytic anemia, usually idiopathic or associated with lupus. It is markedly responsive to corticosteroid therapy, a fact that may help to avoid transfusion.

Paroxysmal cold hemoglobinuria (PCH)

- Clinical. The least common type of AIHA, responsible for about 1-2% of cases, most commonly affects *children with viral illnesses* such as measles, mumps, chickenpox, and infectious mono. It was originally described in *syphilis.* PCH presents with paroxysmal episodes of hemoglobinuria associated with cold exposure. These acute attacks are characterized by sudden fever, chills, abdominal and back pain, hemoglobinuria, and jaundice. The resultant anemia is usually severe (eg, Hgb<5 g/dL). Treatment consists of keeping the patient warm and transfusions as necessary.

T2.12

Example of a Positive Donath-Landsteiner Test

(blood sample 2 contains the Donath-Landsteiner antibody)

Procedure	Blood sample 1	Blood sample 2
30 minutes	37°C	4°C
30 minutes	37°C	37°C
Results	No hemolysis	Hemolysis

- **Lab.** The responsible antibody is an IgG biphasic hemolysin with *anti-P* specificity (Donath-Landsteiner antibody **T2.12**). It is called a biphasic hemolysin due to its capacity to produce hemolysis only when incubated at two different temperatures in vitro. Like CAIHA, the DAT is positive with polyspecific AHG, negative with anti-IgG, and positive with anti-C3. To confirm the diagnosis, the Donath-Landsteiner test is performed on 2 vials of blood at 2 different temperatures: 4°C and 37°C. A positive test is obtained if only incubation of the patient's red cells at 4° then 37° leads to hemolysis.

Blood banking considerations with a cold autoantibody

- The first objective is to determine whether the autoantibody is pathologic, based on its titer and thermal amplitude. Most pathologic examples have high titer and react over a broad temperature range, including temperatures greater than 30°C.

- The second is to find a way to carry out the search for alloantibodies in spite of the cold autoantibody. The first and most straightforward way to do this is to keep blood at 37°C and perform all tests at 37°C (prewarmed antibody screen and panel). Second, the use of monospecific anti-IgG AHG reagent will allow circumvention of the often C3-only positivity of the cold antibody. Lastly, the cold autoantibody can be adsorbed in the cold by autologous red cells.

Drug-Induced Positive DAT
(May Result From 1 of 4 Mechanisms):

Drug adsorption (hapten) mechanism

- Penicillin is the prototype.

- 3% of patients on penicillin develop a positive DAT.

- 5% of those with a positive DAT experience hemolysis.

- The effect is dose-dependent.

- Mechanism: the drug becomes adsorbed to the red cell membrane and the red cell subsequently becomes coated with anti-penicillin antibodies.

- Lab confirmation: the serum and eluate react with drug-treated red cells but not with untreated red cells.

Nonimmune protein adsorption

- Cephalothin is the prototype.

- Mechanism: the drug becomes adsorbed to the red cell membrane and the red cell subsequently becomes coated, nonspecifically, with all sorts of serum proteins, including antibodies.

- Lab confirmation: the red cells test positive with specific antisera for IgG, IgA, C3, etc, but the serum and eluate are nonreactive with red cells.

Immune complex

- Quinidine, phenacetin, and cephalosporins are prototypes.

- Mechanism: the drug elicits complement-fixing antibodies, leading to 'innocent bystander' lysis of red cells.

- Lab confirmation: the red cells test positive for C3d only.

True autoimmune hemolytic anemia

- This is seen with aldomet and procainamide in particular. These agents elicit a warm-reacting red cell autoantibody leading to a syndrome that resembles idiopathic types of warm autoimmune hemolytic anemias.

Neonatal and Intrauterine Transfusion

Blood for intrauterine transfusion should be fresh, washed, irradiated, type O, and negative for whatever (usually Rh) antigen is implicated.

Blood products for neonatal transfusion that contain *significant* plasma (eg, FFP, platelets) must be compatible with neonate's red cells.

Routine volume reduction for neonates is not warranted, because:

- very little volume is involved to begin with, and volume reduction only decreases it on average about 10%-20%.

- In the case of platelets, potential platelet loss and potential platelet functional defects.

- Potential bacterial contamination.

- Time delay.

CMV prophylaxis is routinely recommended for neonates under 1200 g who are CMV negative.

Maternal Immune Thrombocytopenic Purpura (ITP)

ITP is the immune-mediated destruction of platelets, usually on the basis of *auto*antibodies directed against platelet surface antigens such as PL^{A1}. In women with a history of ITP who become pregnant, or in women who have the onset of ITP during pregnancy, there is a risk of neonatal thrombocytopenia that is due to autoantibodies crossing the placenta.

Lab tests. There is no lab test that is a reliable predictor of neonatal thrombocytopenia. The risk of neonatal thrombocytopenia is highest with: previous maternal splenectomy for ITP, previous infant with ITP, & gestational (maternal) platelet count <100,000. It is recommended that serial neonatal platelet counts be monitored for a few days after delivery.

In infants of women with ITP, there is a low risk of severe thrombocytopenia (<50,000) and a low but definite risk of serious hemorrhage (intracranial hemorrhage in <1%, confined to neonates with platelets less than 20,000).

Treatment. Supportive platelet transfusions are sparingly given. The neonatal platelet count will begin to rise early, due to cessation of maternal autoantibody infusion. However, IV immunoglobulin (IVIG) may be necessary.

Neonatal Alloimmune Thrombocytopenia (NATP)

NATP is caused by maternal anti-platelet *allo*antibodies that cross the placenta and cause destruction of fetal platelets. Most commonly the maternal alloantibodies are directed against the platelet antigen PL^{A1}. In the general population, 2% of individuals are PL^{A1} negative, and can develop anti-PL^{A1} antibodies if exposed to the antigen such as through transfusion or pregnancy. In contrast to the analogous situation of hemolytic disease of the newborn (HDN), NATP can affect the *first* pregnancy.

Lab tests. Maternal and paternal platelet antigen phenotyping and screening of maternal serum for anti-platelet antibodies.

Neonatal platelet counts are commonly under 20,000. There is a 12% incidence of fatal intracranial hemorrhage, 20% incidence of intracranial hemorrhage overall, and 50% serious hemorrhage in utero.

Treatment. If known prior to delivery, intrauterine transfusion beginning at 18-20 weeks and C-section are recommended. Provide antigen-negative platelets, *preferably maternal platelets* that have been washed and irradiated. IV Ig and corticosteroids have limited utility. Platelet counts usually rise above 50,000 by 2-3 weeks.

Hemolytic Disease of the Newborn (HDN)

Hemolytic disease of the newborn results from maternal *allo*antibodies crossing the placenta, entering the fetal circulation, and causing hemolysis. This, depending on the severity, can lead to the appearance of bilirubin in the amniotic fluid, progressive fetal anemia, and eventual hydrops fetalis. To be significant, the maternal alloantibody must be of the IgG1, IgG3, or IgG4 class, since IgA, IgG2 and IgM do not cross the placenta.

Non-Rh HDN now is more common than Rh HDN, due to the success of prevention strategies.

■ HDN due to ABO is now the most common type of HDN. ABO incompatibility causes a mild form of HDN, and it is predominantly *seen in blood type O mothers bearing blood type A or B fetuses.* Hemolysis is caused by an IgG anti-A, B antibody. Since ABO antibodies are naturally occurring, this may be seen in the first pregnancy.

■ HDN due to Kell is now the most common cause of severe HDN. Anti-c is second.

Rh HDN

■ The classic form of HDN is so-called Rh HDN, which is caused by anti-D antibodies. Since anti-D antibodies are not naturally occurring, the woman must have had an exposure to D+ erythrocytes in order for HDN to occur. The most common sensitizing event is a prior pregnancy; thus, anti-D HDN *is usually not seen with the first pregnancy.* Sometimes, however, a woman may be sensitized by prior transfusion.

■ It is the first pregnancy that usually sensitizes the mom. In the course of a normal pregnancy, there is usually entry of fetal blood cells into the maternal circulation (fetomaternal hemorrhage), most often at the time of delivery. However, sensitization may occur as a result of other events **T2.13** and without the carriage of a pregnancy to term; at the very least, the second trimester must be reached, as this is when the fetus begins to circulate red cells.

■ Prior to the introduction of RhIg, the incidence of sensitization in an Rh-negative woman bearing an Rh-positive fetus was around 10%. The incidence is actually somewhat *lower* if the mom and fetus are also ABO *incompatible.*

■ Prevention of Rh HDN begins with checking every pregnant woman's D status.

  □ D– women should be checked for anti-D antibodies.

  □ D– women without antibodies: interventions in this scenario are aimed at preventing the development of anti-D antibodies. This is achieved through prophylactic doses of Rh immune globulin (RhIg), given at set intervals and whenever a fetal-maternal hemorrhage occurs. The idea is that the RhIg coats any

T2.13
Sources of Fetomaternal Hemorrhage and Rh(D) Sensitization

Normal pregnancy
Chorionic villus sampling
Amniocentesis
Cordocentesis
Abortion, threatened or completed (spontaneous or elective)
Abruption
Trauma

fetal red cells that enter the maternal circulation, thus preventing maternal immune sensitization.

  □ D– women with anti-D antibodies (previously sensitized): management is aimed at minimizing the effect on the fetus. A maternal antibody titer is first determined. Most often, if this titer is less than 1:16, then severe hemolysis is considered unlikely. However, once the titer exceeds 1:16, monitoring the degree of fetal hemolysis (discussed in Chapter 1) becomes the chief concern. If severe, then intrauterine transfusions and early delivery may be necessary to minimize the harm to the fetus.

■ Indications for and administration of Rh immune globulin (RhIg)

  □ In a D– woman bearing D+ or D-unknown fetus.

    ● 300 μg (1 full dose vial) at 28 weeks and at term. Without RhIg, the risk of developing anti-D is 8%; whereas, with RhIg at 28 weeks nd term, the risk is reduced to 0.1%.

    ● In the event of fetal-maternal hemorrhage of unknown quantity due to ectopic pregnancy, amniocentesis, chorionic villus sampling, spontaneous abortion, etc, then

      ○ within the first 12 weeks of gestation, a small vial (50 μg) dose is given

      ○ after 12 weeks, a full dose (300 μg) vial is given

2: Blood Banking and Transfusion

Autoantibodies>Hemolytic Disease of the Newborn |
Other Special Clinical Circumstances>Transfusion in Sickle Cell Disease

- ☐ RhIg is *not* indicated for D+ moms or D– moms who already have anti-D antibodies.

- ■ Calculating the dose of RhIg

Vials of RhIg =

$$\frac{\text{(maternal whole blood volume (mL))} \times \text{(\% fetal cells in mom's blood)}}{30}$$

- ☐ Maternal whole blood volume can usually be taken to be around 5000 mL. Otherwise, it is calculated as the mom's body weight (Kg) times 70 mL/Kg.

- ☐ The % fetal red cells is determined by a Kleihauer-Betke test (see below). If, for example, fetal cells comprise 3% of maternal blood, then substitute 0.03 into the formula.

- ☐ Divide by 30. Each full dose vial (300 μg) protects against 30 mL whole blood *or* 15 mL of red cells.

- ☐ The tricky part. You have to round up to the nearest integer if the number after the decimal is <5, and up two integers if >5. For example, if the result is 3.3, then give 4 vials, but if the result is 3.6, then give 5 vials.

- ■ Tests for fetal-maternal hemorrhage

- ☐ The rosette test uses D+ indicator cells to form rosettes around D+ fetal cells. It will detect as little as 10cc of fetal blood. The results are qualitative. If this test is positive, then a Kleihauer-Betke or ELAT is indicated.

- ☐ The Kleihauer-Betke (acid elution) test works on the principle that fetal hemoglobin (HbF) is resistant to acid elution, unlike adult hemoglobin. Thus when maternal blood is subjected to acid elution then Wright stained and examined under the microscope, any cells that take up stain (rather than appearing 'ghosted') represent red cells containing HbF. A cell count is performed to determine the percentage of fetal red cells.

- ☐ The enzyme-linked antiglobulin test (ELAT) is another quantitative assay for fetal-maternal hemorrhage.

- ☐ Flow cytometry is now commonly used to calculate the quantity of HbF.

Other Special Clinical Circumstances

Transfusion in Sickle Cell Disease

While in most respects transfusion in sickle cell disease does not differ from transfusion in other circumstances, there are some unique considerations. First, the high number of transfusions experienced in sickle cell disease lead to real concerns about iron overload and alloimmunization. Second, in both emergency and elective transfusion settings, patients with sickle cell disease should be considered for exchange transfusions rather than simple transfusion, because this lessens the risk of iron overload, hyperviscosity, and volume overload. Lastly, whereas transfusion is typically aimed at achieving a certain hemoglobin level, the end-point in sickle cell disease transfusion is a certain proportion of HbS.

Strong indications for emergency transfusion in sickle cell disease include stroke, retinal artery occlusion, splenic sequestration crisis, acute chest syndrome, and aplastic crisis. Some advocate emergency transfusion for priapism and severe acute pain crises.

Elective chronic transfusion is indicated for stroke prevention, for patients with progressive renal or cardiopulmonary disease, in preparation for some surgical procedures, and during some pregnancies. With regard to stroke prevention, the risk of stroke in children with sickle cell disease is about 10%, and transfusion is usually initiated in those considered to be at high risk, though the prediction of risk has been problematic. For practical purposes, this is often applied to those who have suffered a first stroke (risk of another is >70%) or those having adverse transcranial doppler examinations.

Some practitioners, however, liberally apply exchange transfusion to all sickle cell disease patients. The usual target HbS is <30% in children, and <50% in adults.

Alloimmunization eventually arises in 5-50% of multiply transfused sickle cell patients, with a rate of 3% per transfusion. The most common alloantibodies that develop are Kell, C, E, Jk^b. In large centers where it is possible to select blood typed for Cc, D, Ee, and Kell, the alloimmunization rate per transfusion can be reduced to 0.5%.

2: Blood Banking and Transfusion

Other Special Clinical Circumstances>Transfusion in Sickle Cell Disease; Emergency and Massive Transfusion |
Blood Components>Red Cell Components

Due to repeated exposures, the risk of transfusion-transmitted infection is high, and the risk of iron overload, ameliorated somewhat with exchange transfusion and chelation therapy, is high.

Emergency and Massive Transfusion

Emergency release of red cell products, implying that there is not time for completion of recipient blood testing, is sometimes required. There are differing levels of immediacy required, however, and in general routine practices should be followed when possible.

- When possible (ie, when clinical staff indicates that a 30-45 minute delay is acceptable), recipient blood should be typed and screened, with ABO/Rh-matched and crossmatch-compatible blood released.

- When greater urgency is needed, the ABO/Rh type can be determined and ABO/Rh-compatible blood released (without crossmatch).

- When no delay is acceptable (blood needed now), uncrossmatched O-negative blood can be released. Rh-positive blood can be released to males and older females.

Whenever emergency release is undertaken, the treating physician must sign a statement indicating that he/she is aware of the nature of the blood released. This need not be done prior to release.

In some cases, due to inventory considerations, the patient whose blood type is known must be given ABO-Rh-unmatched (but still compatible) blood. This switch requires medical director approval.

When Rh-positive blood must be given to an Rh-negative recipient, there is some benefit to giving RhIg, particularly in young women.

Massive transfusion definitions vary, including: transfusion of a quantity equal to the patient's whole blood volume within 24 hours and transfusion of >10 units within 24 hours. The point of making this distinction is that certain potential complications attend transfusion of a large volume of blood.

- Transfused blood does not immediately have the oxygen-carrying capacity of innate blood, due to depletion of 2,3-DPG and ATP. This results in a shift of the oxygen dissociation curve to the left (impaired release of oxygen from hemoglobin).

- Transfused blood may lower pH and raise potassium, lower the body temperature and raise the free hemoglobin.

- There is the potential for a 'dilutional coagulopathy.' Preparation of red cells involves the removal of most plasma and platelets, and whatever plasma is present in stored blood is rapidly depleted of multiple coagulation factors (especially the labile factors V and VIII).

Blood Components T2.14

Red Cell Components

How prepared and stored

- The first step in preparing nearly all of the blood components is blood collection from a donor. In most instances, red cells are administered to recipients in the form of packed red cells. This is obtained by separating most of the plasma and platelets from the original bag of whole blood (see below).

- Anticoagulant-preservative solutions. Blood is collected into bags containing a certain amount (usually around 60 mL) of anticoagulant-preservative solution T2.15. The different anticoagulant-preservative solutions vary in composition and in the duration over which red cells are considered acceptable for donation. These solutions are intended to maximize posttransfusion viability. All of them contain *dextrose,* a source of carbohydrate for the glycolytic production of ATP. Post-storage levels of ATP correlate with posttransfusion red cell viability. The solution known as CPDA has *adenine,* a substrate for the production of ATP. *Citrate* acts as an anticoagulant by chelating calcium. *Sodium phosphate* acts as a pH buffer. The additive solutions, known as AS-1 (Adsol), AS-3 (Nutricel), etc, contain additional dextrose, adenine, buffer, mannitol, and sodium chloride. Allowable storage time is the maximum time after which 75% of transfused red cells will be viable in the circulation 24 hours after transfusion.

Blood Components>Red Cell Components

T2.14
Summary of Blood Products

Blood Product	Composition	Volume	Contraindications	Storage Temp	Storage Time
Whole blood	Red cells (Hct 40%), plasma, WBC, platelets	500 cc	Relative: volume overload	1-6°C	Varies with preservative
Packed red blood cells	Red cells (Hct 60%-80%), reduced amount of plasma, WBC, platelets	250 cc	Relative: AIHA	1-6°C	Varies with preservative
Platelets (random donor)	Platelets ($>5 \times 10^{10}$), reduced amount of plasma, WBC, RBC	50 cc	Relative: ITP Absolute: TTP	22-24°C	5 days
Platelets (pheresis)	Platelets ($>3 \times 10^{11}$) reduced amount of plasma, WBC, RBC	300 cc	Relative: ITP Absolute: HIT & TTP	22-24°C	5 days
Fresh frozen plasma (FFP)	Plasma (all coag factors)	200 cc	–	−18°C	1 year
Cryoprecipitate	Cold-insoluble portions of plasma. Must contain at least *150 mg fibrinogen and 80 IU of factor VIII.* Also contains factors XIII, vWF.	15 cc	–	−18 °C	1 year
Granulocyte concentrate (pheresis)	Granulocytes ($>1 \times 10^{10}$)	200 cc	–	22-24°C	24 hours

T2.15
Additive Solutions

Solution	Contents	Allowable Storage	Comments
Heparin	Heparin	48 hours	Not used anymore
Citrate phosphate dextrose (CPD)	Citrate, dextrose, sodium phosphate	21 days	
Citrate phosphate dextrose adenine-1 (CPDA-1)	Citrate, dextrose, sodium phosphate & adenine	35 days	
Anticoagulant-preservative solution plus additive solution-1 (AS-1)	Dextrose, adenine, sodium phosphate, mannitol, sodium chloride	42 days	Must be added within 72 hours of collection

■ Storage 'lesion.' Stored red cells undergo progressive changes due to continued intracellular metabolism. 2,3-DPG (2,3-diphosphoglycerate) levels fall linearly. Red cell potassium falls (extracellular potassium increases), the pH decreases, and ATP levels fall. Decreased pH causes a shift in the hemoglobin saturation curve to the *right;* that is, *decreased pH enhances release of oxygen* from hemoglobin and inhibits oxygen binding. Decreased 2,3-DPG shifts it to the left. After transfusion, normal levels of 2,3-DPG, ATP, and pH are completely *restored within 24 hours.* There is always a slight degree of hemolysis in a bag of red cells, and some free hemoglobin is present in every unit. In the plasma contained in the unit, there is progressive diminution of clotting factors, particularly the *labile clotting factors V and VIII.* The platelets contained in the unit become rapidly dysfunctional and should *not* be considered therapeutic after the first few days.

Blood Components>Red Cell Components

- Transport and reissue

  □ Transport. Red cells must be transported in a monitored, refrigerated, device.

  □ Reissue. Units that have left the blood bank and have been returned unused may be reissued for transfusion if:

    • The unit has not been 'spiked' (entered).

    • The blood has been maintained continuously between 1-10°C in a monitored storage device and has not been outside a monitored storage device for more than 30 minutes.

    • At least one segment of sealed tubing remains.

- Red blood cell products **T2.16**

  □ Whole blood. This is what you get if you don't do anything to the unit of blood that you draw from the donor. It is not commonly found in blood banks anymore but is still considered by some to be ideal treatment for the patient with extreme blood loss. However, packed cells plus intravenous fluids has supplanted this in most cases. It contains approximately 450-525 mL of red cells, plasma (that contains clotting factors that diminish over time, particularly the labile factors V and VIII), and poorly functioning platelets.

  □ Red blood cells (packed cells). This is what's left over after removing most of the plasma and platelets via slow centrifugation of whole blood. *Standards* requires that the final hematocrit shall be <80%. *Red blood cells are stored at 1-6°C* within 8 hours of collection and for the duration of their storage. For transport, they must be kept between 1-10°C. *They expire in 21 days if stored in CPD, 35 days if stored in CPDA, and 42 days if AS.* If the system is opened ('spiked'), then the product expires in 24 hours.

  □ Red blood cells, leukocyte reduced (leukoreduced red cells). The typical unit of red cells contains around 5×10^9 white cells. To qualify as leukoreduced, *it must have <5×10^8 (a one-log reduction) if intended to prevent febrile reactions and <5×10^6 (a 3-log reduction) if intended to prevent HLA alloimmunization or CMV transmission.* The

T2.16
ABO Compatible Red Cell Components

Component	Recipient Type	Compatible Donor Type
Whole Blood	O, A, B, AB	ABO Identical
Red Blood Cells	O	O
	A	A or O
	B	B or O
	AB	AB, A, B, or O

leukoreduced unit must retain >80% of the original red cells. Normally, this is accomplished through bedside filtration, with a 3rd generation filter, at the time of transfusion; although, earlier filtration of blood products in the laboratory is perhaps even more effective. The normal blood filter (the 170-micron microaggregate filter) is inefficient at reducing white cells. Note that washed red cells and red cells that have been frozen, thawed, and deglycerolized (because extensive washing is involved) are considered leukoreduced. Note also that leukoreduction is not effective for the prevention of transfusion-associated graft-vs-host disease.

□ Washed red cells. Red cells may be washed and resuspended in normal saline for the purpose of removing the plasma contained in the product. Since washing requires an open system, the shelf-life a washed red cells is 24 hours. Washed red cells are used to prevent severe or recurrent allergic reactions, such as anaphylaxis in the IgA-deficient recipient.

□ Irradiated red blood cells, for the prevention of graft-vs-host disease, are good for 28 days post-irradiation, or the original outdate, whichever comes first.

□ Frozen red cells. Red cells, such as rare donor types or blood for autologous donation, may be frozen for prolonged storage. Freezing red cells can result in serious damage to the cells, unless so-called cryoprotective agents are used. Glycerol is a commonly used cryoprotective. After the slow addition of 40% glycerol, red cells can be placed in a −80°C freezer and kept at less than 65°C *for up to 10 years.* When thawed, the red cells must be immediately washed in a series of progressively more hypotonic solutions to remove the glycerol while preventing hemolysis. Once thawed, washed, and stored at 1-6 °C, the red cells must be transfused within 24 hours. Frozen and deglycerolized red cells are considered both leukoreduced and washed (free of IgA, for example).

What it contains. The total volume of a bag of red blood cells is around 250 mL. This is composed of about 200 mL of red cells, 50 mL plasma and anticoagulants. Note that each mL of red cells contains about 1 mg of iron; thus, a bag of packed cells contains about 200 mg iron.

Indications. Decreased oxygen-carrying capacity. Transfusion 'triggers' vary, but generally speaking healthy individuals can tolerate hematocrits down to around 20% without severe symptoms, while those with moderate cardiopulmonary insufficiency may need to be transfused at 30%. In the setting of trauma, it is generally held that the hypovolemic patient should be given a 'challenge' of 1-2 liters of intravenous crystalloids, and if this fails to stabilize the hemodynamic status, then blood may be indicated.

Contraindications. There are no absolute contraindications; although, crystalloids are a better choice for patients whose blood loss is less than 20% of blood volume (about a liter) or whose hematocrit is >30% in the absence of complicating factors. Additionally, some consider autoimmune hemolytic anemia a relative contraindication to blood transfusion, and at the very least other means of increasing oxygenation should be attempted first.

Dosing. The expected effect of a unit of red cells is a 1g/dL increase in hemoglobin and 3% increase in hematocrit. A pediatric dose of around 4 mL/Kg will achieve the same effect. All red cell products must be transfused through a filter, most commonly a 170-micron microaggregate filter. *The only fluid that may be transfused simultaneously through the infusion line is isotonic saline (0.9% saline).* No medications may be added to the infusion.

Platelets

How prepared and stored. When whole blood is slow-centrifuged, it separates into red blood cells and platelet-rich plasma. When the platelet-rich plasma is fast-centrifuged, it separates into platelet concentrate and plasma. The platelets are removed and *stored at 20-24°C with gentle agitation.* Platelets may also be collected by pheresis. They expire in 5 days unless the system is opened (such as for pooling), in which case they expire in 4 hours. As with red cells, one may prepare leukoreduced platelets & irradiated platelets.

What it contains. Each unit contains approximately 50 mL consisting of some plasma **T2.17**, a few white cells, approximately 80 mg fibrinogen, and a *minimum of 5.5×10^{10} platelets* (in at least 75% of units tested). Pheresis platelets contain about 100 mL, consisting of plasma, white cells, fibrinogen (about 150 mg), and a *minimum of 3.0×10^{11} platelets.*

Indications

■ The nonbleeding patient with thrombocytopenia. In these patients the idea is to prevent bleeding with prophylactic platelet transfusions whenever the patient falls below a certain threshold. Usually this transfusion 'trigger' is around 15,000 to 20,000 µL. The risk of spontaneous bleeding definitely increases below 10,000 µL.

T2.17

Compatibility of Components Containing Plasma (FFP, Platelets, or Plasma)

		Donor Blood Type			
		A	**B**	**AB**	**O**
Recipient Blood Type	**A**	compatible	incompatible	compatible	incompatible
	B	incompatible	compatible	compatible	incompatible
	AB	incompatible	incompatible	compatible	incompatible
	O	compatible	compatible	compatible	compatible

If group compatible platelets are not available, any type can be given to a patient >2 years of age.

No ABO criteria applied to cryoprecipitate.

D+ patients may receive either D+ or D−.
For D− patients, D− units preferred but not required.

- The bleeding patient with thrombocytopenia. In this case, platelets are often administered for platelet counts below 50,000 μL, although in some cases the threshold is moved all the way up to 100,000 μL.

- Functional platelet disorders. There is some role for platelets in patients with Glanzmann thrombasthenia, Bernard-Soulier syndrome, aspirin ingestion, and renal failure. In the latter, a trial of DDAVP or cryoprecipitate is first indicated.

Contraindications. Relative contraindications include immune thrombocytopenic purpura, in which platelet transfusion may actually enhance platelet destruction. *Absolute contraindications* include heparin-induced thrombocytopenia (HIT) and thrombotic thrombocy-topenic purpura (TTP), in which platelet transfusion may induce intravascular thromboses.

Dosing. Adults are given 4- or 6- packs of platelets at a time. Neonates are given 10-15 mL/Kg or 1 unit per 10 Kg. The expected result, in adults, of transfusing one unit (5.5×10^{10}) of platelets is an increase in the platelet count of about 5000/ μL. Hence, the average quad-pack will increase the platelet count around 20,000 μL, while the typical pheresis pack (which is roughly equivalent to a six-pack of platelets) will increase the platelet count around 30,000 μL. The average platelet life span is 9.5 days. Like red cells, platelets must always be transfused through at least a 170-micron microaggregate filter.

Prevention of platelet-transmitted infection. It is required by the AABB that a methods be employed to limit and detect platelet contamination by bacteria. See discussion under transfusion complications (p 135ff).

Granulocyte Concentrates

How prepared and stored. Granulocytes are often obtained by pheresis. They are stored at 20-24°C for up to 24 hours. The product should be administered *without* a filter.

What it contains. Each unit contains a certain amount of contaminating red cells, a large number of platelets, and around 10^{10} white cells.

Indications and contraindications. Granulocytes are usually employed for neutropenic sepsis.

Dosing. There is no agreed-upon dose, but several days of granulocyte therapy are generally required. As with all cellular blood products, a microaggregate filter is required, but a leukoreduction filter is obviously contraindicated.

Fresh Frozen Plasma (FFP)

How prepared and stored. When whole blood is slow-centrifuged, it separates into red blood cells and platelet-rich plasma. This latter product, when fast-centrifuged, can be separated into platelet concentrate and plasma. The plasma must be placed into an −18°C or colder freezer within 8 hours of blood collection to make FFP. It expires in 1 year. For administration, it must be thawed at 30-37°C. After thawing it expires in 24 hours.

What it contains. A unit of FFP contains about 200 mL and it usually contains approximately 1 IU per mL of all coagulation factors (by definition, an IU of coagulation factor is that amount contained in 1 mL normal plasma). The reason for freezing is to preserve the function of coagulation factors, particularly the so-called labile factors V and VIII.

Indications and contraindications. FFP is given for coagulopathies due to multiple factor deficiencies. In cases of single factor deficiencies (eg, factor VIII), recombinant factor or factor concentrates are preferred, and if that is not available, then cryoprecipitate is the second choice. Multiple factor deficiencies often arise in the setting of disseminated intravascular coagulation (DIC), warfarin therapy, or massive transfusion ('dilu-tional' coagulopathy occurs usually after the transfusion of 8-10 units of red blood cells in the absence of plasma or platelet transfusion). In DIC, both FFP and cryopre-cipitate are usually indicated, but this decision should be based on measurements of PT, PTT, and fibrinogen. In the setting of massive transfusion, it is best to give FFP based on measured coagulation parameters rather than prophylactically. FFP is also indicated as the replacement solution in plasmapheresis for thrombotic thrombocytopenic purpura (TTP) and for treatment of antithrombin III (ATIII) deficiency.

Dosing. Usually 2 units are given at a time for adult patients. 10-15 mL/Kg for neonates. Each unit is expected to increase factor activities by around 20%. FFP must be given through a standard 170-micron microaggregate filter. ABO compatibility is an issue, particularly for neonates. The plasma, which contains ABO antibodies, should be compatible with the recipient's red cell phenotype.

Cryoprecipitated Anti-Hemophilic Factor (aka Cryo or Cryoprecipitate)

How prepared and stored. When FFP is thawed to 1-6°C then centrifuged, a precipitate (the so-called cold-insoluble portion of plasma) forms. After removal of the thawed plasma, the precipitate must be replaced, within one hour, in a –18°C or colder freezer to make cryoprecipitate. It expires in 1 year. After thawing it expires in 24 hours.

What it contains. Each unit contains about 15 mL and *must* have a minimum of *150 mg fibrinogen and 80 IU of factor VIII* in all units tested. Units also contain factor XIII and von Willebrand factor (vWF). Cryo does *not* contain appreciable quantities of factor V. Note that each unit of cryo contains exactly the amount of factors present in each unit of FFP, but in a smaller volume.

Indications and contraindications

- Treatment for hemophilia A (factor VIII deficiency). Currently, the treatment of choice is factor VIII concentrate or recombinant factor VIII; however, for unusual situations (such as taking boards) it is still cryoprecipitate that is used for treatment.

$$\text{Bags of cryo} = \frac{\text{(Patient's plasma volume)} \times \text{(amount of factor VIII needed)}}{80}$$

□ The *patient's plasma volume* is calculated by:

(Patient's weight [Kg]) × (70 mL/Kg) × (1–hematocrit)

□ The *amount of factor VIII needed* is the desired factor VIII activity minus the current factor VIII activity. Recall that by definition an international unit (IU) of factor VIII is the amount of factor VIII contained in an mL of normal plasma.

A person with 100% factor VIII activity has 1 IU/mL. The usual hemophiliac has around 1-5% of factor VIII activity, or .01 to .05 IU/mL. Generally speaking, a factor VIII level of 50% is desirable to treat a spontaneous bleed, while a level of 100% is required for surgery. Thus in a hemophiliac with 3% activity who has a hemarthrosis, 47 is the number you would put into the equation.

- *Divide by 80.* This is because each bag of cryoprecipitate contains at least 80 IU of factor VIII. The formula above when not divided by 80 gives the number of units of factor VIII needed.

- You must know that the T ½ of factor VIII is 12 hours (T ½ of factor IX is 8 hours) and that this dose will need to be repeated in 12 hours. Alternatively, a continuous infusion to run over 12 hours may be administered.

- Treatment for von Willebrand disease. The initial treatment of choice is often DDAVP.

- Fibrinogen deficiency, most often seen in the setting of disseminated intravascular coagulation (DIC). Cryoprecipitate should not be used alone to treat DIC, as it lacks certain factors, notably factor V. FFP should be given as well.

- Others: bleeding in uremic patients, fibrin 'glue', factor XIII deficiency.

Dosing. The usual dose for adults is 10 bags. ABO compatibility is an issue as for FFP.

Recombinant factor VIIa. Recombinant f VIIa has demonstrated efficacy in hemophilia complicated by acquired inhibitors against f VIII or fIX. Furthermore, it has shown promise in trauma-associated bleeding and, of course, congenital f VII deficiency. It may also be useful in patients with excessive coumadinization, liver failure, and thrombocytopenia. The half-life of recombinant f VIIa is about 3.5 hours. In patients with f VIII or vIX inhibitors, the dose is 90µg/kg q 2-3 hours until hemostasis is obtained, after which doses are titrated for bleeding. Potential adverse effects include very rare thrombotic events.

Irradiated Products

How prepared and stored. Standards stipulates that 25 Gy (2500 cGy) are delivered to the midplane of the product. The minimum dose to any portion of the product shall be 15 Gy (1500 cGy). A method must be used to ensure that irradiation has occurred. For red cells, the storage time becomes *28 days or the original outdate, whichever is sooner.*

Indications. Irradiation is carried out solely for the purpose of preventing transfusion-associated graft-versus-host disease (GVHD), an often fatal complication of transfusion of cellular products to immunocompromised recipients. GVHD is mainly a risk in bone marrow transplant recipients, neonates, fetuses, recipients of blood from first-degree relatives, Hodgkin lymphoma, non-Hodgkin lymphoma, and patients with congenital T-cell defects (such as DiGeorge syndrome and severe combined immunodeficiency [SCID]) but not in B cell or macrophage defects. Irradiation is not effective in preventing CMV transmission.

Leukoreduced Products

How prepared and stored. Filtration is the usual method of leukoreduction. All cellular blood products are transfused through a microaggregate filter, but this filter is inefficient at reducing white cell numbers. The degree of leukoreduction depends on the goal. If meant to prevent febrile reactions, fewer than 5×10^8 white cells must be left in the unit. If meant to prevent alloimmunization or CMV transmission, then the unit must contain fewer than 5×10^6 white cells. Note that washed red cells and frozen, deglycerolized, red cells are considered leukoreduced. Blood banks differ on whether filtration is accomplished at the bedside during transfusion or at the time of collection.

Indications

- Preventing HLA alloimmunization. This is an issue in patients who are anticipated to require multiple transfusions, such as a leukemic patient. The acquisition of HLA alloimmunization is a cause of platelet refractoriness. Prevention of HLA alloimmunization requires less than 5×10^6 white cells per unit.

- Preventing febrile, nonhemolytic, transfusion reactions. This is a reaction felt to be largely due to white cells and their secreted cytokines. When a patient is experiencing refractory febrile reactions with every transfusion, filtering to reduce white cells is indicated. This requires a reduction only to 5×10^8 white cells to be effective.

- Preventing CMV transmission. It has been shown that leukoreduction is effective in preventing the transmission of CMV by CMV+ blood products given to CMV negative recipients. This, still somewhat controversial, indication requires a reduction to less than 5×10^6.

- Leukoreduction is *not* effective in preventing graft-vs-host disease.

Washed Red Cells

How prepared and stored. Red cells are washed to remove plasma proteins, a process that can delay transfusion by hours. Red cells that have been washed represent an open system and expire in 24 hours.

Indications

- Prevention of allergic reactions, particularly in IgA-deficient recipients who may suffer anaphylactic reactions to transfusion of IgA-containing products.

- Febrile nonhemolytic transfusion reactions. Since these are largely due to cytokines, washing can prevent them, though it may not be worth the time and expense.

- Transfusion to neonates from a parent or from ABO incompatible plasma.

Blood Substitutes

Suffice it to say that, at the moment, there is no substitute for blood. However, in some limited settings there may be a role for hemoglobin substitutes and volume-expanding fluids as adjuncts to blood transfusion.

Many putative hemoglobin substitutes have been studied and found to be limited mainly by their inability to persist in circulation and continue to carry oxygen for any length of time. Other major problems have included profound effects upon laboratory assays, renal toxicity, and vasoconstriction.

Resuscitation fluids for volume expansion do not carry oxygen, of course, but their role in maintaining blood volume and blood pressure assist in delivery of red cells to target tissue. The term crystalloid refers to aqueous solutions of inorganic ions and small organic molecules. These usually include NaCl and/or glucose and may be isotonic, hypotonic or hypertonic. On the other hand, colloids may be synthetic—gelatins, dextrans, and hydroxyethyl starch (HES)—or natural—fresh frozen plasma (FFP) and immunoglobulin solutions—and are presented dissolved in a crystalloid solution, most commonly normal saline. Gelatins are synthesized from hydrolyzed bovine collagen. Dextran is a high molecular weight D-glucose polymer. Hydroxyethyl starch (HES) is a D-glucose polymer with a branching structure.

The various fluids differ in the degree to which they expand intravascular volume and the duration of this expansion. For example, a 1 L infusion of normal saline will expand intravascular volume by approximately 250 mL (the other 750 mL contributing to tissue (and pulmonary) edema). The attractive feature of colloid solutions is that they persist in the intravascular space. The exact duration is a function of

(1) the rate of colloid molecule metabolism and

(2) the integrity of the endothelium, which may be compromised in sepsis and other conditions.

All colloid solutions have some capacity to impair hemostasis, at least through hemodilution, with many having direct effects upon clotting factors as well. Furthermore, all colloidal solutions have been associated with a small risk of anaphylactic or anaphylactoid reactions. Controversy over the best type of resuscitation fluid to use and in particular over the issue of colloid versus crystalloid permeates the medical literature. Crystalloids are favored for their relative safety—low risk of hemostatic anomalies, adverse drug reactions, and intravascular fluid overload. Colloids are favored for their enhanced intravascular persistence and lesser tendency to produce tissue edema. Controlled trials have not settled this question.

Transfusion Complications

The Workup of a
Suspected Transfusion Reaction

A transfusion reaction is suspected whenever the patient experiences unusual symptoms in proximity to a transfusion. The typical signs and symptoms of an acute intravascular hemolytic transfusion reaction are patient discomfort and apprehension, hemodynamic instability, back pain, fever, and chills.

When a transfusion reaction is suspected the very first thing to do is *stop the transfusion*. The intravenous line should be left open with a saline infusion.

Following this, supportive care is given to the patient, while the patient's physician evaluates the patient. If the reaction consists solely of a mild urticarial response or circulatory overload, then no further laboratory evaluation is necessary. If a transfusion reaction workup is initiated in the lab, then further transfusions should ideally await its completion.

The workup includes

- Paperwork and bag check to detect obvious clerical errors. The most common cause of hemolytic transfusion reactions is clerical error.

- Check blood for hemolysis (visually) and check urine for hemoglobin (dipstick).

  □ Serum or plasma is inspected visually for hemolysis (a pink or red discoloration). Blood drawn too late after the event (greater than 8 hours) may be negative visually despite significant hemolysis. In this event, a serum bilirubin will be elevated for up to 24-36 hours. Free serum myoglobin may give a false positive visual inspection. In this event there should be a clinical history of severe trauma.

  □ If a urine dipstick is positive, then examine the urine microscopically for hematuria. In a hemolytic transfusion reaction, there is free hemoglobin, usually without hematuria, in the urine. Myoglobinuria is another cause of a false-positive urine dipstick.

- Perform a direct antiglobulin test (DAT). Compare results to a pretransfusion sample. In a hemolytic transfusion reaction, the DAT is usually positive due to the presence of antibody on transfused red cells. If the hemolysis was quite severe, the DAT may be negative due to destruction of all the transfused cells.

2: Blood Banking and Transfusion

Transfusion Complications>Febrile, Nonhemolytic Transfusion Reactions; Acute Hemolytic Transfusion Reactions; Delayed Hemolytic Transfusion Reactions (DHTR)

■ If after all this the reaction is felt to be nonhemolytic, then additional transfusions can be administered with crossmatch-compatible blood. If, on the other hand, there is evidence of hemolysis, then additional workup, including repeat ABO and Rh typing and tests similar to the pretransfusion antibody panel must be carried out to identify the responsible antibody. Then antigen-negative, crossmatch-compatible blood can be given for transfusion.

Febrile, Nonhemolytic Transfusion Reactions

This is *the most common type of transfusion reaction,* with an incidence of around 1 in 200 transfusions, and is defined as an increase in temperature of *1°C or 2° F* with no other explanation (such as hemolytic transfusion reaction, bacterial contamination of the unit, or concurrent infection). Therefore, it is essentially a diagnosis of exclusion.

Etiology. This reaction is likely mediated by cytokines released by white blood cells in the stored unit of blood. This theory is supported by the observation that the incidence of febrile reactions can be reduced by early filtration of blood products at the time of collection or by washing of cellular blood products prior to transfusion. Though somewhat less efficiently, they can also be diminished by bedside filtration at the time of transfusion.

Treatment. As with any suspected transfusion reaction, the transfusion must be stopped and not restarted. The usual transfusion reaction workup is completed. In a patient with repeated febrile reactions, pre-treatment with antipyretics and/or any future transfusions to be done with leukocyte reduced products is recommended.

Acute Hemolytic Transfusion Reactions

This is the most feared transfusion reaction and may be fatal. Hemolytic transfusion reactions may be acute or delayed, intravascular or extravascular. It is the *acute intravascular* type that is very dangerous, and this is nearly always related to ABO incompatibility that most often results from clerical error. Rarely, non-ABO antibodies, most notoriously Kidd, may be responsible for acute intravascular hemolytic reactions. Most commonly, however, non-ABO alloantibodies are associated with either acute extravascular hemolysis or *delayed extravascular hemolysis.* These latter reactions

are also called delayed hemolytic transfusion reactions (DHTR). There are really no examples of delayed intravascular hemolysis. Importantly, not all hemolysis is immune-mediated. Nonimmune hemolysis may be due to prolonged storage, storage at inappropriate temperatures, the use of mechanical devices to infuse blood, blood warmers, needles of too small caliber, or the addition of anything other than normal saline to the infusion. In addition, bacterial contamination of the product, particularly with *Clostridia* spp, may cause hemolysis. Lastly, the donor may have an unrecognized intrinsic red cell defect causing hemolysis.

Etiology. ABO incompatibility (due to clerical error) is the most common cause of *acute* intravascular hemolysis. Acute extravascular hemolysis may be due to acquired alloantibodies of various specificities (Kell, Kidd, Duffy, etc).

Associated findings

■ **Clinical.** Intravascular hemolysis is accompanied by fever, chills, back pain, pain at infusion site, hypotension, disseminated intravascular coagulation (DIC). Extravascular hemolysis is often asymptomatic.

■ **Laboratory.** Positive DAT (both intra- and extravascular hemolysis), pink serum due to hemolysis (intravascular hemolysis), hyperbilirubinemia (extravascular hemolysis), hemoglobinuria (intravascular hemolysis), coagulation abnormalities (intravascular hemolysis), schistocytes (intravascular hemolysis), and/or spherocytes (extravascular hemolysis).

■ **Treatment.** Stop the transfusion, leaving the line open with a saline infusion. Support the patient hemodynamically. Perform transfusion workup. Also note that fatalities related to blood transfusion must be reported to the FDA within 24 hours by phone and in writing within 7 days.

Delayed Hemolytic Transfusion Reactions (DHTR)

This presents as progressive anemia, with or without fever and jaundice, occurring days to weeks after transfusion.

Etiology. Alloantibodies, most commonly directed against Kidd, Kell, and Duffy antigens.

Findings. Positive DAT (often with a mixed field reaction), icteric serum, anemia, spherocytes, usually no free hemoglobin (because it's extravascular hemolysis).

Treatment. Usually none is indicated except to identify the responsible antibody and avoid further exposure to it.

Bacterial Contamination

Transfusion-transmitted bacterial infection is now considered the most common cause of transfusion-related fatality in the United States. It is estimated that between 1:1000 to 1:4000 units are contaminated. Platelet products must now be screened for bacterial contamination, to prevent this serious complication.

Etiology. The bacteria are thought to originate either from the donor's blood (transient bacteremia) or skin. Bacterial proliferation *is most often a problem with platelets,* since they are stored at room temperature. Bacterial proliferation in cold-stored products (due to psychrophilic organisms) can also occur.

- Platelets are most likely to be associated with infection by gram-positive cocci. The estimated risk of bacterial infection per platelet unit transfused is between 1:2,000-1:4,000 on those units screened with gram stain, pH or glucose concentration methods.

- In red cell transfusion, the most commonly implicated organisms are *Yersinia enterocolitica, Serratia liquifaciens, Citrobacter* and *Pseudomonas* spp.

Findings. Bacterial contamination is suspected whenever the transfusion recipient experiences high fever and shock. Of course, a hemolytic reaction is also considered in this scenario and must be excluded. Bacterial contamination is equally grave, however, with 25% mortality. Upon inspection, the blood product may be visibly discolored, hemolyzed, or contain clots, all evidence of bacterial contamination. Generally, the patient's serum and urine will contain free hemoglobin, but the DAT is negative. A gram stain, though low yield, must be performed on the blood, and the blood product must be cultured at several temperatures.

Treatment. Stop the transfusion. Administer broad spectrum antibiotics and hemodynamic support.

Prevention. The AABB requires that the blood bank have methods to limit and detect bacterial contamination in platelet components.

- Methods to limit bacterial contamination include attention to donor history, scrupulous cleansing of the donor venipuncture site, and discarding the first (15-30 cc of) blood drawn. In addition, there is some evidence that preferential use of apheresis platelets may reduce the risk.

- Methods to detect bacterial contamination include visual inspection, culture (with rapid technology), grams staining, and nucleic acid tests.

Transfusion-Associated Graft-vs-Host Disease (TAGVHD)

TAGVHD may be caused by transfusion or solid-organ transplantation in which immunocompetent lymphocytes from the donor can engraft in the recipient. It is highly (>90%) fatal.

Etiology. An HLA reaction between donor white cells and recipient tissues. A peculiarity of this reaction is that in order for the donor cells to survive the recipient's defenses, the recipient must be immunocompromised or the donor white cells must be compatible with the recipient (while the recipient is not compatible with the donor). This latter circumstance arises in the case of *HLA-similar individuals.* As a very simplified example, if the donor is homozygous HLA-A1/HLA-A1 and the recipient is heterozygous HLA-A1/HLA-A2, then the recipient can't recognize the donor cells as foreign, while the donor does recognize the recipient tissues as foreign.

Findings. TAGVHD presents with the classic tetrad of dermatitis (periauricular, palmar and plantar erythroderma), enterocolitis (watery diarrhea), hepatitis (aminotransferase elevation), and bone marrow suppression (pancytopenia).

Treatment

- **Prevention.** *Irradiation* of blood products renders any contained white cells incapable of proliferation. All cellular blood products intended for transplant recipients, certain immunocompromised recipients, or for intrauterine transfusion must be irradiated. All cellular blood products transfused among first-degree relatives must be irradiated, even if the recipient is immunocompetent. The dose required by *Standards* is 2500 cGy to the center of the bag and a minimum of 1500 cGy to any part of the bag. Leukoreduction has *no role* in prevention of TAGVHD; and irradiation has *no role* in preventing CMV transmission.

- **Treatment.** There is no effective treatment, and most cases are fatal.

Transfusion-Associated Acute Lung Injury (TRALI)

TRALI is becoming a leading cause of transfusion-related death.

Etiology. Donor HLA antibodies are thought to react with recipient white cells to produce white cell microaggregates in the pulmonary circulation. While TRALI appears possible in any recipient, two groups seem to be at increased risk: those undergoing induction therapy for hematologic malignancies and those undergoing bypass surgery. Furthermore, it appears to be the case that both multiparous donors and prolonged blood storage raise the likelihood of TRALI. Plasma-containing blood components pose the greatest risk, with platelet concentrates and FFP being the most commonly implicated. The plasma fraction appears to contain the responsible agent for TRALI, thought to be anti-leukocyte HLA antibodies.

Findings. The presentation consists of tachypnea, cyanosis, dyspnea, fever (1°C or higher), hypoxemia, and diffuse, bilateral, fluffy infiltrates on CXR (resembling pulmonary edema). This presents within 8 hours of transfusion, but most cases present during or just after transfusion. The differential diagnosis in a patient with pulmonary insufficiency following transfusion includes volume overload (CHF), anaphylaxis, bacterial contamination and hemolytic transfusion reaction. Volume overload should present within minutes to hours of transfusion and respond just as rapidly to diuresis. Anaphylactic reactions are often characterized by wheezing, edema of the face and trunk, and urticaria, respond rapidly to epinephrine, and usually do not produce lung opacity. Transfusion-related sepsis manifests as pronounced fever and vascular collapse, with or without and usually out of proportion to respiratory distress. Lastly, evidence of hemolysis should accompany a hemolytic transfusion reaction. The histopathologic findings at autopsy resemble ARDS, with leukocyte infiltration, pulmonary edema, hyaline membranes, and destruction of the normal lung parenchyma.

Treatment. Supportive. Though there is up to a 25% mortality rate, most patients recover within 72 hours.

Allergic Transfusion Reactions

These range from mild reactions with urticaria (hives) and pruritus to severe, life-threatening, anaphylactic reactions.

Etiology. Plasma proteins to which the recipient is allergic. In the classic scenario with anaphylaxis, the recipient is IgA-deficient and has a reaction to IgA in the donor's plasma. IgA deficiency affects around 1/700 recipients, but only a minority of these will react adversely to IgA exposure.

Findings. Clinical findings depend on the severity and range from trivial reactions with pruritus to severe, life-threatening anaphylactic reactions with hemodynamic collapse. Usually there are no findings on the transfusion reaction workup.

Treatment. Stop the transfusion. For mild urticarial reactions, administer antihistamines and, if symptoms remit, then *the transfusion can be restarted.* The reaction is unlikely to be repeated with subsequent transfusions. For anaphylaxis, parenteral epinephrine is indicated, and subsequent transfusion must await determination of the causative protein. In the usual IgA-deficient scenario, either washed or IgA-deficient blood or platelets must be given. For FFP, only that obtained from IgA-deficient donors can be used.

Posttransfusion Purpura

This presents as profound thrombocytopenia 2-14 days following red cell or platelet transfusion. Affected recipients are almost always *multiparous women.*

Etiology. Platelet alloantibodies, most commonly anti-PL[A1], are responsible for destruction of donor and, mysteriously, native recipient platelets. About 98% of the population is PL[A1] positive. This reaction is a risk in the 2% of PL[A1] negative individuals when they receive PL[A1] positive platelets.

Findings. Thrombocytopenia, often less than 20,000.

Treatment. Steroids, plasma exchange, and intravenous gamma globulin have been tried.

Platelet Refractoriness

This presents as a progressive diminution in the quantity of platelet increase following platelet transfusion. It arises in patients who have required multiple transfusions in the course of their chemotherapeutic regimens.

- Platelet refractoriness has many causes, including systemic infection, splenomegaly, drugs such as amphotericin, and ongoing platelet consumption (eg, DIC).

- After all of these have been excluded, primary platelet refractoriness, due to alloimmunization, must be considered.

- In patients with AML, the incidence of platelet refractoriness (on any basis, including alloimmunization) arising during treatment is about 25%. Factors associated with refractoriness include a positive lymphocytotoxic antibody test, multiple (at least 2) pregnancies, male gender, heparin exposure, fever, bleeding, larger numbers of platelet transfusions, and a palpable spleen.

- In one large study looking at posttransfusion platelet increments (instead of formal refractoriness), the status of the spleen was the most important factor. Splenectomized patients had the largest posttransfusion increments, followed by patients with clinically normal spleens, followed by those with palpable spleens. Other factors that adversely affected increments included at least 2 pregnancies in a female, male sex, increasing weight and height (presumably reflecting greater volumes of distribution), amphotericin, heparin, fever, bleeding, and infection. Note that only a subset of these were associated with the development of true refractoriness. While DIC did not affect posttransfusion increments, it did decrease the time to next platelet transfusion.

Etiology. Primary platelet refractoriness is due to HLA-alloimmunization on the basis of HLA class I antigens (primarily HLA-A and HLA-B) present on platelet surfaces. It is the transfused white cells that elicit this response, however.

Findings. Definitions of refractoriness vary. Following transfusion of a single-donor unit of platelets, the expected increment is approximately 5000 per μL per unit transfused. Thus, a quad-pack would be expected to get an increment of approximately 20,000 per μL, and a pheresis pack or six-pack should get around 30,000. When these increments become progressively smaller, platelet refractoriness should be considered. Most patients with true refractoriness actually get no increment at all or even a slight decrement in their platelet count following transfusion. A more accurate assessment of response is the platelet count increment (CI), calculated as follows:

$$CI = \frac{(\text{posttransfusion plt count}) - (\text{pretransfusion plt count}) \times BSA}{(\text{platelets transfused} \times 10^{11})}$$

Treatment

- **Prevention.**

  - In patients undergoing chemotherapy or for any reason expected to require repeated platelet transfusions, prevention of HLA alloimmunization is essential, though not always possible.

  - The first step is to minimize transfusions, possibly through using a conservative transfusion trigger.

  - Second is to minimize donor exposures such as through using pheresis products instead of pooled platelets.

  - Third, leukoreduction filtration (to below 5×10^6 leukocytes per unit) can help prevent HLA alloimmunization.

  - In a large study of AML patients it was demonstrated that UV-B irradiation and leukoreduction were equally effective in preventing the development of lymphocytotoxic antibodies and platelet refractoriness due to alloimmunization.

- **Treatment.** Following alloimmunization, a PRA assay can help determine extent of immunization. Treatment may require HLA crossmatching, often with relatives or random pheresis donors.

Infections

Hepatitis B virus: The risk of acquiring HBV per unit transfused is around 1:100,000. All donors are screened by serology.

Hepatitis C virus: The risk of acquiring HCV per unit transfused is between 1: 800,000 and 1,700,000. All donors are screened by serology.

Hepatitis A virus: The risk of acquiring HAV per unit transfused is around 1: 1,000,000.

Human immunodeficiency virus (HIV) I/II: Currently, the risk of acquiring HIV infection per unit transfused is between 1:400,000 to 1:2,4,000,000. All donors are screened by serology and nucleic acid testing.

Blood Group Associations

Cytomegalovirus (CMV)

- CMV is transmitted by white blood cells in which it is carried intracellularly.

- Most individuals are already CMV positive, and those who are not will suffer no ill effects from its acquisition; however, it is particularly important to reduce the transmission of CMV in transplant candidates/recipients and low-birth-weight neonates.

- This is done by administering CMV-negative blood products, when available. If no CMV-negative blood is available, then leukoreduction (to $<5 \times 10^6$ WBCs) is generally considered an acceptable alternative.

Syphilis (Treponema pallidum)

- *Treponema pallidum* is transmitted by transfusion only very rarely, due to a very brief period of bacteremia.

- The RPR test that is required testing for all donated blood is not very useful to screen for syphilis, since RPR is usually *not* positive yet while individuals are experiencing the brief period of bacteremia. Furthermore, most positive RPRs are false positives.

- Thus, screening for syphilis is not the main reason to perform RPRs on donor blood. RPR is used as a *surrogate marker for* high-risk behavior for other transfusion-transmitted infections such as HIV.

Chagas disease (Trypanosoma cruzii)

- A disease prevalent in Latin America, this can be transmitted by transfusion.

- It is screened for mainly by history (living in thatched huts).

Malaria (Plasmodium spp)

- A disease prevalent throughout the world in discrete pockets.

- The risk of transfusion-transmitted malaria is 1 per 4 million transfusions.

- Screened for by history.

Babesiosis (Babesia microti)

- In areas endemic for babesiosis, the risk of transfusion-transmitted babesiosis is around 1 per 1000 transfusions.

- Screened for by history. Persons with a history of babesiosis are permanently deferred.

Creutzfeldt-Jacob disease (CJD)

- This prion-mediated disease has never been documented to be transmitted by transfusion. However, individuals at risk for CJD are excluded from donation by history.

Transfusion-Associated Metabolic Derangements

Circulatory Overload

Hypocalcemia (citrate toxicity). With large volumes of products, sufficient citrate can be infused to cause hypocalcemia.

Hypothermia. With large volumes of unwarmed products, the recipient's core body temperature can be reduced. Hypothermia exacerbates the effects of other metabolic derangements such as hypocalcemia and hyperkalemia. Prewarming is recommended for massive transfusion; however, *Standards* requires that the temperature not exceed 42°C.

Hyperkalemia. With every cellular blood product, there is a certain degree of unavoidable hemolysis, resulting in high extracellular potassium levels. The problem is proportional to the age of the product. Most patients can handle the extra potassium, but neonates and those who suffer from impaired renal function should be given the freshest units.

Hypokalemia. Some patients may experience hypokalemia due to transfusion of cells that are intracellularly potassium depleted, leading to transcellular shifts of serum potassium.

Iron overload. This is mainly a problem in chronically transfused patients. Each unit of red cells contains around 200 mg of iron. When the whole-body iron burden reaches about 500 mg/Kg, clinical iron overload can develop, affecting the heart and liver primarily. Iron chelation, such as with desferroxamine, can be helpful to prevent this complication.

Immunomodulation. Transfusion of cellular blood products appears to have a dampening effect on the immune system. This has been exploited for some time in renal transplantation recipients, in whom pre-transplant transfusion promotes graft survival. However, there is ongoing investigation into the question of whether there is an increased risk of infection or malignancy recurrence in transfused patients.

Assorted Blood Bank Take Home Points

Approximate risk of transfusion-associated complications (2004 data) **T2.18**

Naturally-occurring antibodies: I, i, ABO, Le, Lu, M, N, P.

Antigens that display dosage: MNS, Kidd, C/c, E/e, Duffy.

Antibodies that react at room temperature: Anti-M, N, P_1, Le^a, and Le^b.

The 4 most common antibodies implicated in immediate HTR: anti-A, anti-Kell, anti-Jk^a, and anti-Fy^a.

Antigens that are enhanced by enzymes: I/i, P, Le, Rh, Kidd.

T2.18
Approximate Risk of Transfusion Complications

Complication	Risk
HIV	1/1million-1/2 million
HTLV-1	1/1 million
HCV	1/1 million
HBV	1/100,000
EBV	1/200
CMV	7/100
ABO-Rh Incompatibility	1/5,000-1/20,000
TRALI	1/10,000
DHTR	1/3,000
GVHD	1/1,000
Allergic reaction	1/100
Febrile reaction	1/100

Assorted Blood Bank Take Home Points

Antigens that are destroyed by enzymes: MNSs, Fy^a, Fy^b, Lutheran, Chido.

Antigen frequency T2.19

The 4 most common antibodies implicated in delayed HTR: anti-Jk^a, anti-E, anti-D, anti-C.

Mixed field reactions are expected with: Lutheran, Sid, A$_3$, and post-bone marrow transplant.

Antibodies that commonly produce intravascular hemolysis: ABO, Kidd, P (paroxysmal cold hemoglobinuria).

The 4 most common antibodies implicated in HDN: anti-AB, anti-D, anti-Kell, anti-c.

Some hard-to-remember shelf lives (outdates):

- Red blood cells, saline washed or thawed and deglycerolized—24-hour shelflife

- Thawed fresh frozen plasma—24-hour shelflife (after 24 hours, re-labeled as plasma)

- Thawed plasma—5-day shelflife

- Pooled platelets—4-hour shelflife

- Thawed cryoprecipitated AHF, unpooled— 6-hour shelflife

- Thawed and pooled cryoprecipitated AHF— 4-hour shelflife

Antibodies that, when detected, are nearly always clinically insignificant: M, N, P, Lewis, Lutheran, and I.

Frequencies of common red cell and platelet antigens; likelihood of finding compatible blood:

- When blood is needed for a patient with an alloantibody, the likelihood of finding blood is equal to the likelihood of antigen-negative blood in the population. The likelihood of antigen-negative blood is equal to 1-antigen frequency. So, for example, if the patient has an anti-Jk^a (T2.20), then the likelihood of finding an antigen-negative unit is 1- 0.8 or about 0.2. This has some practical relevance, as it guides the laboratorian in deciding how many units to pull from the shelf in order to attempt to find a crossmatch-compatible unit. In this case, to have an even chance of getting one unit, I would want to pull 5 units from the shelf.

T2.19 Approximate Frequency of Antigens in USA Donor Population

Antigen	Frequency
K	10%
k	98%
Jk^a	80%
Jk^b	45%
Jk(a–b–)	Rare, except in Pacific Islanders
Fy^a	65% in whites, 10% in blacks
Fy^b	80% in whites, 20% in blacks
Fy(a–b–)	Rare in whites, 68% in blacks
A	45%
B	25%
AB	5%
D	85%
C	70% in whites, 30% in blacks
E	30%
c	80% in whites, 98% in blacks
e	98%
Le^a	20%
Le^b	70%
Le(a–b–)	5% in whites, 20% in blacks
M	80%
N	70%
S	50%
s	95%
Lu^a	10%
Lu^b	99%
Lu(a–b–)	rare
PL^{A1} (HPA-1a, GPIIIa)	98%
PL^{A2} (HPA-1b, GPIIIa)	30%
Bak^a (HPA-3a, GPIIb)	90%
Bak^b (HPA-3b, GPIIb)	60%

Assorted Blood Bank Take Home Points

T2.20 Red Cell Antigen Associations

Phenotype or Antibody	Association
Fy(a–b–)	Duffy antigen is the receptor for *P vivax* Duffy– confers resistance to *P vivax* and is more common in blacks
McLeod (Kell-null, Kx)	Chronic granulomatous disease. Acanthocytosis. Late-onset muscular dystrophy-like syndrome
Anti-P	Paroxysmal cold hemoglobinuria (PCH) Syphilis
Anti-I	*Mycoplasma pneumoniae* infection Lymphomas
Anti-i	EBV infection (infectious mono)
Anti-N	Renal dialysis
Acquired B phenotype	Colorectal carcinoma Intestinal obstruction Gram negative sepsis
Rh null (Bombay)	Hereditary stomatocytosis
Diego negative	Diego is an epitope on band 3 protein; Band 3 deficiency the cause of some cases of HS and HE
Gerbich negative (Leach phenotype)	Gerbich is an epitope on Glycophorin C A cause of HE

- When blood is needed for a patient with two or more alloantibodies, the calculation is similar; except the frequencies of antigen-negativities are multiplied. For example, if the patient has anti-Jk^a (frequency of antigen negative = 1–0.8 = 0.2) and anti-N (frequency of antigen negative = 1–0.7 = 0.3), then the frequency of Jk^a and N-negative blood is 0.2 × 0.3 = 0.06. So about 16 units will have to be crossmatched to find one compatible.

Bibliography

Adams RJ, McKie VC, Hsu L, Files B, Vichinsky E, Pegelow C, Abboud M, Gallagher D, Kutlar A, Nichols FT, Bonds DR, Brambilla D, Woods G, Olivieri N, Driscoll C, Miller S, Wang W, Hurlett A, Scher C, Berman B, Carl E, Jones AM, Roach ES, Wright E, Zimmerman RA, Waclawiw M. Prevention of a first stroke by transfusions in children with sickle cell anemia and abnormal results on transcranial doppler ultrasonography. *N Engl J Med* 1998; 339(1): 5-11.

Aygun B, Padmanabhan S, Paley C, Chandrasekaran V. Clinical significance of RBC alloantibodies and autoantibodies in sickle cells patients who received transfusions. *Transfusion* 2002; 42: 37-43.

Blanchette VS, Kühne T, Hume H, Hellmann J. Platelet transfusion therapy in newborn infants. *Transfus Med Reviews*. 1995; IX: 215-230.

Branch DR, Petz LD. Detecting alloantibodies in patients with autoantibodies. *Transfusion* 1999; 39: 6-10.

Brand A. Immunologic aspects of blood transfusions. *Transpl Immunol* 2002; 10: 183-190.

Brecher ME, Ed. *Technical Manual, 15th ed.* Bethesda: American Association of Blood Banks, 2005.

Burns KH, Werch JB. Bacterial contamination of platelet units. *Arch Pathol Lab Med.* 2004; 128: 279-281.

Castro O, Sandler SG, Houston-Yu P, Rana S. Predicting the effect of transfusing only phenotype-matched RBCs to patients with sickle cell disease: theoretical and practical implications. *Transfusion* 2002; 42(6): 684-690.

Choi PT, Yip G, Ouinonez LG, Cook DJ. Crystalloids vs colloids in fluid resuscitation: a systemic review. *Crit Care Med* 1999; 27:200–210.

Daniels G, Poole J, deSilva M, Callaghan T, MacLennan S, Smith N. The clinical significance of blood groups antibodies. *Transfus Med* 2002; 12: 287-295.

Domen RE, Hoeltge GA. Allergic transfusion reactions: an evaluation of 273 consecutive reactions. *Arch Pathol Lab Med.* 2003; 127: 316-320.

Domen RE. Policies and procedures related to weak D phenotype testing and Rh immune globulin administration. *Arch Pathol Lab Med.* 2000; 124: 1118-1121.

Dzik WH, Anderson JK, O'Neill EM, Assmann SF, Kalish LA, Stowell CP. A prospective, randomized clinical trial of universal WBC reduction. *Transfusion* 2002; 42: 1114-1122.

Fridberg MJ, Hedner U, Roberts HR, Erhardtsen E. A study of the pharmacokinetics and safety of recombinant activated factor VII in healthy caucasian and Japanese subjects. *Blood Coagul Fibrinolysis* 2005; 16(4):259-266

Fridey JL, Ed. *Standards for Blood Banks and Transfusion Services, 24th ed.* Bethesda: American Association of Blood Banks, 2006.

Gajic O, Moore SB. Transfusion-related acute lung injury. *Mayo Clin Proc* 2005; 80(6):766-770.

Garratty G, Dzik W, Issitt PD, Lublin DM, Reid ME, Zelinski T. Terminology for blood group antigens and genes—historical origins and guidelines in the new millennium. *Transfusion* 2000; 40: 477-489.

Garratty G, Petz LD. Approaches to selecting blood for transfusion to patients with autoimmune hemolytic anemia. *Transfusion* 2000; 42: 1390-1392.

Goodnough LT, Brecher ME, Kanter MH, AuBochon JP. Transfusion medicine: first of two parts. *NEJM.* 1999; 340: 438-447.

Goodnough LT, Lublin DM, Zhang L, Despotis G, Eby C. Transfusion medicine service policies for recombinant factor VIIa administration. *Transfusion* 2004; 44: 1325-1331.

Grocott MPW, Hamilton MA. Resuscitation fluids. *Vox Sang* 2002; 82: 1–8.

Hess JR. Update on alternative oxygen carriers. *Vox Sang* 2004; Suppl 2: S132-S135.

Bibliography

Hübel K, Dale DC, Engert A, Liles WC. Current status of granulocyte transfusion therapy for infectious diseases. *J Infect Dis* 2001; 183: 321-328.

Laupacis A, Brown J, Costello B, Delage G, Freedman J, Hume H, King S, Kleinman S, Mazzulli T, Wells G. Prevention of posttransfusion CMV in the era of universal WBC reduction: a consensus statement. *Transfusion* 2001; 41: 560-569.

Manci EA, Culberson DE, Yang Y-M, Gardner TM, Powell R, Haynes J Jr, Shah AK, Mankad VN. Causes of death in sickle cell disease: an autopsy study. *Br J Haematol* 2003; 123: 359–365.

Midathada MV, Mehta P, Waner M, Fink LM. Recombinant factor VIIa in the treatment of bleeding. *Am J Clin Pathol.* 2004; 121: 124-137.

Moise KJ. Management of Rhesus alloimmunization in pregnancy. *Obstet Gynecol* 2002; 100: 600-611.

Myhre BA, McRuer D. Human error—a significant cause of transfusion mortality. *Transfusion* 2000; 40: 879-885.

Pantanowitz L, Telford III SR, Cannon ME. Tick-borne diseases in transfusion medicine. *Transfus Med* 2002; 12: 85-106.

Przepiorka D, LeParc GF, Stovall MA, Werch J, Lichtiger B. Use of irradiated blood components. *Am J Clin Pathol.* 1996; 106: 6-11.

Ramasethu J, Luban MLC. T activation. *Br J Haematol* 2001; 112: 259-263.

Rebulla P. Revisitation of the clinical indications for the transfusion of platelet concentrates. *Rev Clin Exp Hematol* 2001; 5.3: 288-310.

Sacher RA, Kickler TS, Schiffer CA, Sherman LA, Bracey AW, Shulman IA. Management of patients refractory to platelet transfusion. *Arch Pathol Lab Med* 2003; 127: 409-414.

Sazama K, DeChristopher PJ, Dodd R, Harrison, CR Shulman IA, Cooper ES, Labotka RJ, Oberman HA, Zahn CM, Greenburg G, Stehling L, Lauenstein KJ, Price TH, Williams LK. Practice parameter for the recognition, management, and prevention of adverse consequences of blood transfusion. *Arch Pathol Lab* Med. 2000; 124: 61-70.

Schierhout G, Roberts I. Fluid resuscitation with colloid or crystalloid solutions in critically ill patients: a systematic review of randomised trials. *BMJ* 1998; 316:961-964.

Schiffer CA. Management of patients refractory to platelet transfusion. *Leukemia* 2001; 15: 683-685.

Schroeder ML. Transfusion-associated graft-versus-host disease. *Br J Haematol* 2002; 117: 275-287.

Silberman S. Platelets: preparations, transfusion, modifications, and substitutes. *Arch Pathol Lab Med.* 1999; 123: 889-894.

Silliman CC, Boshkov LK, Mehdizadehkashi Z, Elzi DJ, Dickey WO, Podlosky L, Clarke G, Ambruso DR. Transfusion-related acute lung injury: epidemiology and a prospective analysis of etiologic factors. *Blood.* 2003; 101: 454-462.

Silliman CC, Ambruso DR, Boshkov LK. Transfusion-related acute lung injury. *Blood* 2005; 105: 2266-2273.

Simpson J, Kinsey S. Paediatric transfusion. *Vox Sang* 2001; 81: 1-5.

Slichter SJ, and the Trial to Reduce Alloimmunization to Platelets Study Group. Leukocyte reduction and ultraviolet B irradiation of platelets to prevent alloimmunization and refractoriness to platelet transfusions. *N Engl J Med* 1997; 337: 1861-1869.

Slichter SJ, Davis K, Enright H, Braine H, Gernsheimer T, Kao K-J, Kickler T, Lee E, McFarland J, McCullough J, Rodey G, Schiffer CA, Woodson R. Factors affecting posttransfusion platelet increments, platelet refractoriness, and platelet transfusion intervals in thrombocytopenic patients. *Blood* 2005; 105(10): 4106-4114.

Smith JW, Weinstein R, Hillyer KL. Therapeutic apheresis: a summary of current indication categories endorsed by the AABB and the American Society for Apheresis. *Transfusion* 2003; 43:820-822.

Bibliography

Stowell CP, Levin J, Spiess BD, Winslow RM. Progress in the development of RBC substitutes. *Transfusion* 2001; 41: 287-299.

Task Force of the College of American Pathologists. Practice parameter for the use of fresh-frozen plasma, cryoprecipitate, and platelets. *JAMA.* 1994; 271: 777-781.

Toy P. Guiding the decision to transfuse: interventions that do and do not work. *Arch Pathol Lab Med.* 1999; 123: 592-240.

Spiess BD. Risks of transfusion: outcome focus. *Transfusion* 2004; 44:4S-14S

Wanko SO, Telen MJ. Transfusion management in sickle cell disease. *Hematol Oncol Clin N Am* 2005; 19: 803-826.

Wheeler CA, Calhoun L, Blackall, DP. Warm reactive autoantibodies: clinical and serologic correlations. *Am J Clin Pathol* 2004; 122: 680-685.

Chapter 3

Microbiology

Clinical Syndromes and Causative Agents

Urinary Tract Infection (UTI)

The term UTI encompasses asymptomatic bacteriuria, urethritis, cystitis, and pyelonephritis. UTIs are categorized clinically as complicated and uncomplicated; although agreement on the definition of these terms is not universal. Uncomplicated UTI often refers to those cases of cystitis that arise in essentially healthy young adult (nonpregnant) females without anatomic genitourinary anomalies. Some authors also include under this heading: pyelonephritis in healthy young adult females, cystitis in young adult males, and cystitis in healthy postmenopausal women. Essentially, the term is meant to imply a UTI that *will not result in serious sequelae* and that *will go away with treatment*. Thus, complicated UTI often refers to one arising in association with pregnancy, diabetes, stone, structural genitourinary anomalies, spinal injury, children, and males. The implication is an increased risk of complications: sepsis, chronic pyelonephritis, and treatment failure.

- In neonates, boys predominate. After about 50, a similar incidence is seen in men and women.

- Cystitis presents with dysuria, frequency, urgency, and, sometimes, hematuria. These symptoms, however, can be produced by noninfectious causes, such as stone, tumor, and upper tract bleeding; thus, documenting infection is necessary prior to instigating treatment. In children and adults UTI is more common in women.

- Pyelonephritis presents with flank pain, fever, nausea, and vomiting, often in association with the symptoms of cystitis. Again, this presentation may be produced by stone or papillary necrosis, and documentation of infection is important.

- There are persons with bacterial colonization of urine who do not manifest clinical symptoms (asymptomatic bacteriuria). Most require no treatment. The exceptions are: pregnant women and patients undergoing urologic instrumentation. Asymptomatic bacteriuria is diagnosed on the basis of:

  □ In asymptomatic women, 2 consecutive voided urine specimens with isolation of the same bacterial strain in quantitative counts of $>10^5$ colony-forming units per mL (cfu/mL).

  □ In asymptomatic men, a single voided urine specimen with isolation of a single bacterial species in a quantitative count of $>10^5$ cfu/mL.

  □ In men and women, a single catheterized specimen with a single bacterial species in a count of $>10^2$ cfu/mL.

Laboratory approach

- There are numerous surrogate markers for UTI. Hematuria microscopically detected or a positive urine dipstick for hemoglobin is a nonspecific but sensitive marker for UTI. A positive urine dipstick leukocyte esterase, reflective of pyuria, has a sensitivity of 70 to 95% and, though more specific than red cells, is still not specific. The dipstick nitrite test is positive whenever an organism capable of reducing nitrate to nitrite, such as a coliform, is present. In this test the specificity is quite high, but sensitivity is only about 50%. It is negative in the presence of *Staphylococcus saprophyticus* and *Enterococci*. In combination, the nitrite and leukocyte esterase tests are highly sensitive and specific. A bioluminescence assay is available that has a very high negative predictive value, thus permitting one to rapidly dispense with negative specimens. False negatives are mainly seen in candidal and enterococcal infections. Microscopic detection of pyuria or bacteriuria is highly suggestive of UTI; however, numerous causes of sterile pyuria are recognized. Recall that eosinophiluria is suggestive of acute interstitial nephritis and not of UTI.

- The most direct and informative test, however, continues to be culture. A sterile calibrated loop (1, 2, or $10\,\mu L$) is used to inoculate the agar plate. The bacterial count is calculated from the number of cfu on the plate after overnight incubation and the quantity of urine originally inoculated. In early studies validating the midstream urine, it was demonstrated that >95% of patients with acute pyelonephritis had $>10^5$ colony forming units per milliliter (cfu/mL); whereas, only <6% of asymptomatic patients had this degree of bacteriuria. This was accepted as the defining criterion for significant bacteriuria for many years. More recently, it has been suggested that lower bacterial counts may be important in particular circumstances, particularly in men and symptomatic women, when unusual organisms are present (fungi, fastidious bacteria), and in the so-called urethral (frequency-dysuria) syndrome. Patients with this syndrome may show no growth in routine media and should be investigated for other agents that cause non-specific urethritis, such as *Chlamydia trachomatis.* Lastly, almost any bacterial count from specimens obtained directly from the bladder (suprapubic aspiration), ureter, or kidney must be considered clinically significant. The Infectious Disease Society of America (IDSA) has revised its definition of cystitis to $>10^3$ colony-forming units per milliliter.

Specific agents

- *Escherichia coli* is the most common cause of UTI overall. About 80% of all community-acquired UTIs are due to *E coli,* particularly so-called UPEC (uropathogenic) strains.

- *Staphylococcus saprophyticus* is a very common cause in young sexually active women, and is responsible for perhaps 15% of community-acquired UTI.

- Other enterobacteriaceae—especially *Klebsiella* spp and *Enterobacter* spp— cause a significant number of the remaining cases.

- Many UTIs are culture negative; such cases are often due to *Ureaplasma urealyticum, Chlamydia* spp, or *Mycoplasma hominis.*

- *Corynebacterium* group D2 appears to be a significant cause of hospital-acquired UTI.

- Fungal UTI is mainly caused by *Candida* spp and associated with indwelling catheters or recent antibiotic therapy.

- Hemorrhagic cystitis due to adenoviruses, especially type 11, is most often seen in bone marrow transplant recipients.

Infectious Diarrhea

Differential diagnosis

- The most common cause of acute infectious diarrhea is a virus, especially noroviruses (calicivirus, Norwalk virus), enteric adenoviruses, and rotavirus. These agents account for at least 50% of community-acquired acute infectious diarrhea. In fact, if there is nothing unusual

in the history, such as hospitalization, antibiotic use, or travel, these agents cause 80-90% of cases. Viral agents tend to produce a brief (< 5 days) diarrheal illness, often accompanied by vomiting, at most mild fever, mild abdominal pain, no neutrophilic exudate in stool, and minimal blood. These patients often do not see a physician and when they do are treated supportively.

- After virus, the distant second-place finisher is *E coli* and other bacterial agents (*Salmonella, Shigella, Campylobacter, Vibrio*). Bacteria may cause inflammatory (colitic) or noninflammatory disease.

  - The typical causes of noninflammatory bacterial diarrhea are *Vibrio* spp, *E coli* (especially ETEC and EPEC), *C perfringens, S. aureus,* and *B. cereus.* Features that suggest a bacterial cause (as opposed to virus) include prolonged (>5 days) illness and fever.

  - Clinical features of bacterial inflammatory diarrhea are fever, bloody stool, severe abdominal pain, tenesmus, and neutrophils in stool. *C difficile,* long recognized as a cause of diarrheal illness in hospitalized patients, is an increasingly recognized cause of community-acquired diarrhea in outpatients. Note that patients who seek medical care represent a select group of patients who are more likely to have nonviral, non-ETEC, diarrhea caused by *C difficile, Salmonella, Campylobacter,* and *Shigella.*

  - Diarrhea with blood, especially *without* fecal neutrophils, suggests enterohemorrhagic (EHEC) *E coli* (O157:H7). This may also be seen with amebiasis (capable of destroying leukocytes).

- Protozoa (*Cryptosporidium, Giardia, Entamoeba, Microsporidia, Cyclospora, Isospora*) are the least common cause of acute infectious diarrhea in developed countries.

- Foreign travel alters the picture considerably. Most cases associated with travel to South and Central America are due to varieties of *E coli* (ETEC, EIEC); whereas travel to the far East is more often associated with *Campylobacter, Shigella,* and *Salmonella.*

- Diarrhea that develops during or shortly after hospitalization is most commonly due to *C difficile.* Community-acquired *C difficile* is now a serious consideration, particularly in elderly patients with a history of antibiotic use.

Specific agents

- *Escherichia coli* is a major cause of bacterial diarrhea. *E coli* O157:H7 (EHEC, STEC, VPEC) is acquired through the ingestion of undercooked processed (ground) beef and contaminated milk, fruit, and vegetables. Like other bacterial agents, O157:H7 may produce uncomplicated watery diarrhea, but in some cases it causes acute colitis with cramps, abdominal pain, and bloody diarrhea. Fever is usually at most mild, and often there are no fecal leukocytes (not always). The reason this bacterium has been the subject of much attention is its association with the hemolytic uremic syndrome (HUS). This appears to result from the presence in circulation of Shiga toxins and presents as the triad of microangiopathic hemolytic anemia, renal failure, and thrombocytopenia. HUS predominantly affects children under the age of 5; in fact, it represents a major cause of renal failure in this age group. The mortality rate is about 5%. The laboratory diagnosis (see bacteriology section, p212) requires the use of sorbitol-MacConkey agar, but there are ELISA assays for the Shiga toxin that can be performed on stool. Positive cases should be reported.

- *Salmonellae* (nontyphoidal species) are often contracted in association with animal contact—either live or in the form of food (milk, chicken, eggs). *Salmonella* is the most common cause of death from food-borne illness in the United States. Most infections produce only mild watery diarrhea, while others may take the form of a severe colitis. The real morbidity derives from a tendency to produce bacteremia, with a potential for seeding of bone, joints, vascular walls, heart, or brain. The very young and very old are at greatest risk for bacteremia, in addition to those with immunodeficiency, malignancy, diabetes, HIV infection, and indwelling prostheses.

- *Campylobacter jejuni* infection most often results from ingestion of contaminated food (chicken) or water. Diarrhea often lasts for more than 1 week. While usually not severe, complications such as bacteremia and severe colitis may occur. Furthermore, *C jejuni* is the most commonly identified cause of the Guillain-Barré syndrome, implicated in about 30% of cases. Type O:19 is most commonly associated with Guillain-

Barré. Another important complication of *C jejuni* is the development of a reactive arthropathy (so-called enteropathic arthritis), noted in persons with HLA-B27.

- *Vibrio*

  □ Cholera is a severe epidemic form of voluminous watery diarrhea that is very rare in the United States. The syndrome of cholera is caused principally by two serogroups of *V. cholerae:* serogroup O1 (*V. cholerae* O1) and serogroup O139. Noncholera (non-01 and non-139) strains may cause less severe gastroenteritis and/or wound infections. Cholera tends to occur in pandemics, related to a particular strain of *V. cholerae* (most recently El Tor from south and central Africa). *Vibrio* spp, including cholera and noncholera species, are commonly acquired in the United States from shellfish (especially oysters from the Gulf Coast) or rice. Clinically, cholera-related strains may produce illness ranging from very mild to very severe watery diarrhea of sufficient quantity to cause dehydration and death. Laboratory diagnosis requires plating on selective media such as thiosulfate citrate bile salt sucrose (TCBS) agar.

  □ *Vibrio parahaemolyticus,* like non-01, non-139 strains of *V cholerae,* can cause gastroenteritis and wound infections related to seafood or seawater. In fact, *V parahaemolyticus* is the most common cause of food-borne illness in Japan. *V parahaemolyticus* wound infection is seen when wounds are exposed to or acquired within seawater and can lead to severe septicemia, particularly in diabetics and alcoholics.

  □ *Vibrio vulnificus* can cause fatal food-borne infection in hosts with hepatic disease or immunodeficiency as well as wound infections, again related to seafood and seawater, respectively.

- *Yersinia enterocolitica* has been associated with infectious diarrhea and distal ileitis resembling acute appendicitis. Pathogenicity appears to relate to the presence within the bacterium of a particular plasmid (the pYV virulence plasmid) for which DNA-based assays are available. *Y. enterocolitica* is not among the more common causes of infectious diarrhea in the United States, but is very common in northern Europe. Infection frequently results from consumption of contaminated pork, but contaminated drinking water may also transmit infection. An HLA-B27-linked post-infectious arthritis may occur as with *Campylobacter* infection.

- *Shigella* is an agent that can spread quickly among close contacts, for example in day-care centers, nursing homes, and military barracks, due to the very small inoculum required for infection. While some infections may be mild, *Shigella* is a major cause of dysentery, with bloody stool, fever, and tenesmus.

- *Entamoeba histolytica* should be considered in prolonged diarrhea or in a recent traveler (or immigrant) who presents with bloody diarrhea. The organisms invade the colonic mucosa, to produce the characteristic flask-shaped ulcers, especially within the right colon. Colonic biopsies that contain ulcers or pronounced neutrophilic inflammation should be scoured for organisms. Stool microscopy has only about 50% sensitivity for *E histolytica* (and specificity is limited by the morphologically identical but nonpathogenic *E dispar*), but stool EIA has very high sensitivity and specificity.

- Viruses are the most common cause of infectious diarrhea in all age groups in the United States. Causes of pediatric viral gastroenteritis, in order of frequency, include: rotavirus (#1), enteric adenoviruses (serotypes 40, 41), coronavirus, and astroviruses. Norwalk virus (a Calicivirus) produces gastroenteritis at all ages, and is the most common cause of viral gastroenteritis in adults. The laboratory diagnosis of viral gastroenteritis is influenced by the fact that as a group these agents grow poorly in cell culture. Electron microscopy (of stool) has been used for diagnosis, with each virus having distinctive morphology; however, this modality is not always readily available. Rotavirus antigen can be detected in stool by either EIA or latex agglutination.

  □ Viral agents cause diarrheal illness that can be especially severe in infants and very young children. Rotavirus is especially common between 6-12 months of age. It is responsible for > 50% of cases of watery diarrhea in infants and very young children in the United States, and, worldwide, is a common cause of death in this age group. Nursing home outbreaks are an increasingly recognized problem. Outbreaks tend to occur during the cold weather months.

□ Caliciviruses that cause viral gastroenteritis include noroviruses (Norwalk-like viruses) and sapoviruses (Sapporo-like viruses). Norwalk is food-borne but can be transmitted from person-to-person, and tends to occur in outbreaks affecting large numbers of people simultaneously. This reflects the very low inoculum required for productive infection by Norwalk. Infection with Norwalk tends to have a prominent component of nausea and vomiting in addition to diarrhea.

□ Astroviruses get their name from a star-like appearance on electron microscopy. Diarrheal illness due to astrovirus affects primarily children younger than 4 years of age and has a seasonal—winter—peak.

□ Adenovirus serotypes 40 and 41 (enteric adenoviruses) are the cause of about 20% of pediatric viral gastroenteritis. There is no distinct seasonality, and the virus primarily afflicts children less than 4 years of age.

Infectious diarrhea in AIDS

- AIDS (and other forms of immunodeficiency) is characterized by infection with the common agents of infectious diarrhea as well as unique agents. With regard to the common agents, infection tends to be more severe, more prolonged, and require antibiotics.

- Agents somewhat unique to immunodeficient patients include cryptosporidium, cyclospora, microsporidia, isospora, CMV and MAI.

Laboratory evaluation

- In those presenting for laboratory evaluation, the approach includes stool examination and selective application of specialized techniques including EIA and culture.

- Stool microscopy has two purposes: (1) to determine whether leukocytes are present and (2) to look for ova and parasites.

- Assays for stool lactoferrin (a product of neutrophils) can substitute for a microscopic search for leukocytes.

■ Routine stool culture is capable of isolating a limited range of organisms: *Salmonella, Shigella, E coli,* and *Campylobacter.* Most labs routinely test for *E coli* O157:H7, and many labs now routinely test for *C difficile* in community-acquired diarrhea (and always in hospital-acquired cases).

Pneumonia

Differential diagnosis

■ The probable microbial agents differ with the circumstances under which the infection occurs—especially important are the underlying condition of the host (alcoholism, smoking, COPD, age, overall health **T3.1**) and whether acquired in-hospital or out. The most common causes of community-acquired pneumonia in immunocompetent, healthy, adults are *Mycoplasma pneumoniae, Chlamydia pneumoniae, Streptococcus pneumoniae,* and *Haemophilus influenzae.*

■ In elderly nursing home tenants, mycoplasma and chlamydia fall away from the list; *S pneumoniae, H influenzae,* aerobic gram-negative bacilli, and anaerobes become more common.

■ AIDS patients are particularly susceptible to bacterial and mycobacterial pneumonia when CD4 counts are moderately depressed. At very low CD4 counts, opportunistic infections due to pneumocystis, histoplasmosis, cryptococcus, penicillium, and coccidioides are common.

■ In hospitalized ventilated patients, the most common agents are: *S aureus, S pneumoniae, P aeruginosa, K pneumoniae, Serratia* spp, *Enterobacter* spp, *E coli,* and *fungi.*

Specific agents

■ *Streptococcus pneumoniae* (pneumococcus) is a very common cause overall of community-acquired and hospital-acquired pneumonia; an increased risk is associated with extremes of age, chronic alcoholism, dementia, HIV, and stroke. There have been increasing rates of penicillin-resistant pneumococci. Pneumococcus has been isolated in about a third of community-acquired pneumonias requiring hospitalization, and more than half of pneumonias *associated with bacteremia.* In fact, blood culture often provides the diagnosis of pneumococcal pneumonia. Since about 5%-10% of adults have pharyngeal colonization by *S pneumoniae,* sputum cultures produce an unacceptably high false-positive rate. Ideally, the culture diagnosis relies upon a specimen that bypasses the upper aerodigestive tract (ie, an invasive specimen or blood culture). A urinary antigen test has been developed that shows initial promise.

■ *Staphylococcus aureus* can produce more severe disease than most other agents of community-acquired pneumonia, tending to produce cavitary disease. Risk factors include prolonged hospitalization, old age, pre-existing lung disease, and recent antibiotic therapy. Methicillin-resistant strains should be suspected, particularly when the infection is hospital-acquired.

■ *Haemophilus influenzae* is isolated in about 10% of patients who require hospitalization for community-acquired pneumonia. Most isolates are non-typeable strains. Patients with COPD (airway type more than emphysematous) are at particular risk for *H influenzae* pneumonia. Other risk factors include the recent use of antibiotics or corticosteroids.

T3.1
Risk Factors for Agents of Pneumonia

Host factor	Agents suggested
COPD	*Hemophilus influenzae, Moraxella catarrhalis, Legionella pneumophila*
Alcoholism	*S pneumoniae,* anaerobes (aspiration), gram-negative aerobic bacilli
Neutropenia	Aerobic gram-negative bacilli
Animal exposure	*Coxiella burnetii* (cattle, cats), *Chlamydophila psittaci, Cryptococcus neoformans* (birds), *Histoplasma capsulatum* (bat or bird droppings), Hantavirus (mouse droppings), *Francisella tularensis* (rabbits)
Sandstorm exposure	Coccidioidomycosis
Bronchiectasis, cystic fibrosis	*Pseudomonas aeruginosa, Pseudomonas cepacia, Staphylococcus aureus*

- *Moraxella catarrhalis* is found to colonize the upper airways of about 5% of healthy adults, and lung disease promotes lower respiratory tract infection. Severe infection is seen predominantly in elderly patients with COPD, risk factors for aspiration, or congestive heart failure. Together, *H influenzae* and *M catarrhalis* are major causes of acute exacerbation in patients with COPD.

- *Legionella pneumophila* causes perhaps 5% of community-acquired pneumonia, but a much larger proportion of *fatal* community-acquired pneumonia. The infection is often acquired in association with an unusual exposure to aerosolized particles—construction-associated dust, hot tub, cooling systems. Severely affected patients usually have unhealthy lungs—smoking, COPD—or systemic illness—diabetes, hepatic insufficiency, renal insufficiency, hematolymphoid neoplasms, immunodeficiency, etc. Characteristic clinical features are high fever, *hyponatremia,* and neurologic manifestations. The laboratory diagnosis of *L pneumophila* is usually based upon culture; however, the urinary antigen assay is a rapid and reliable alternative.

- Aerobic gram-negative bacilli, such as *Pseudomonas aeruginosa,* are uncommon causes of community-acquired pneumonia, but they tend to be quite severe and to afflict those with underlying disease such as bronchiectasis, cystic fibrosis, and advanced malignancy. They are significant causes of hospital-acquired pneumonia, particularly ventilator-associated pneumonia. *P aeruginosa* produces severe necrotizing pneumonia, often associated with ARDS. In patients successfully treated, the organism *is rarely actually eradicated,* and most patients become chronic carriers, re-infecting themselves over time. *Serratia marcescens* and *Acinetobacter baumannii* have clinical and epidemiologic features similar to *Pseudomonas* spp.

- Anaerobes are generally acquired through *aspiration.* They often produce cavitary disease, abscess, and empyema. Since anaerobes are common in the oral cavity, the diagnosis of anaerobic lung infection must circumvent the upper airway; thus, the diagnosis relies upon transtracheal aspirates, transthoracic aspirates, or pleural (empyema) fluid. As a result, anaerobic lung infections are usually diagnosed and treated based upon clinical findings.

- *Mycoplasma pneumoniae* and *Chlamydia pneumoniae* cause atypical pneumonias, particularly in young adults. They cause the majority of community-acquired pneumonias that do not require hospitalization, often characterized by patchy, sometimes bilateral, infiltrates, a prolonged (weeks) dry cough, and extra-pulmonary manifestations. The diagnosis of *C pneumoniae* is facilitated by serology: detection of IgM in a titer of >1:16 or a 4-fold increase in IgG. The gold standard is culture, but this is not widely available. Serology for *M pneumoniae* is limited by a commonly delayed antibody response.

- Viral pneumonia

  □ Influenza viruses and RSV account for most cases of viral pneumonia. Parainfluenza viruses, metapneumovirus, and adenovirus cause additional infections. DFA testing panels may be performed on respiratory specimens in parallel with culture. Depending upon patient age, this panel may include influenza A, influenza B, RSV, parainfluenza, and/or adenovirus. *Specimen adequacy* is assessed based upon the number of ciliated epithelial cells. Note that while DFA provides rapid results, the sensitivity is about 20% below culture, so both techniques are valuable.

  □ Hantavirus pulmonary syndrome (HPS) was initially identified as an ARDS-producing illness in the Four Corners region of New Mexico, apparently caused by a member of the Bunyaviridae family, a Hantavirus that came to be named Sin Nombre Virus. The virus is carried by the deer mouse (*Peromyscus maniculatus*), which sheds virus into the environment, mainly in the form of infected feces. Humans are exposed to the virus through contact with this material and, in 1-2 weeks, develop a flu-like illness, a prodrome in which *thrombocytopenia* is commonly noted. Pulmonary edema develops, followed by hypotension, and additional peripheral blood findings: persistent thrombocytopenia, neutrophilia *without* toxic granulation, erythrocytosis (a reflection of hemoconcentration), and a population of immunoblastic lymphocytes that exceed a proportion of 10%. Eventually, a clinicopathologic picture of ARDS (DAD) develops within the lungs. There is at present a fatality rate of 30%-40%. A definitive diagnosis requires serologic detection of IgG and IgM anti-Hantavirus antibodies. The most recent cases of HPS have been reported in 5 states: Arizona, New Mexico, North Dakota, Texas, and Washington.

□ Severe acute respiratory syndrome (SARS) emerged in the Guandong Province of China and is attributed to a Coronavirus which is now called the SARS coronavirus (SARS-CoV). Human-to-human spread is common, and there is great risk for transmission to health care workers. Following an incubation period of 2 to 10 days, the infection produces a flu-like syndrome that leads to respiratory compromise clinicopathologically resembling ARDS (DAD). While SARS-CoV appears to grow well in cell culture (Vero E6 cell lines), real-time PCR, performed on nasopharyngeal specimens, is the preferred means of laboratory diagnosis.

Additional notes on the laboratory diagnosis of pneumonia

- Direct examination of sputum specimens by Gram stain has unclear value, depending largely upon the quality of the specimen.

- There has been much controversy over the issue of what constitutes adequate sputum for culture. Generally speaking, yield improves with more neutrophils and fewer squamous cells, but there is a range of what is considered acceptable. Nonetheless, many laboratories apply microscopic examination criteria to prescreen sputum specimens for adequacy.

- Whatever specimen is submitted, standard culture media for routine respiratory pathogens include 5% sheep blood agar, MacConkey, and chocolate agar. Chocolate agar is incubated in a hypercapneic environment to encourage the growth of *H influenzae*. Special media are required when *Legionella* or pertussis is suspected.

Infective Endocarditis (IE)

Differential diagnosis

- The microbial differential diagnosis of infective endocarditis depends largely upon the status of the underlying valve. Endocarditis should thus be viewed as three major clinical syndromes, each with its own differential diagnosis: infection of a previously normal native valve, infection of a previously abnormal native valve, and infection of a prosthetic valve.

□ Native valve endocarditis affecting a previously normal valve is due to infection by highly virulent organisms that rapidly destroy the valve, causing the clinical picture of acute bacterial endocarditis. The responsible agent is most often *S aureus*. Less common causes of acute bacterial endocarditis include enterococci and certain streptococci, especially *Streptococcus milleri*. Tricuspid endocarditis due to *S aureus* may be seen in IV drug abusers. Pneumococcal endocarditis is not seen much any more, but is a virulent form of acute bacterial endocarditis that historically formed part of Austrian's syndrome—the triad of endocarditis, meningitis, and pneumonia—seen in alcoholics.

□ Native valves with underlying structural damage can be infected by less virulent organisms. These organisms do not cause valve destruction; instead, they tend to form vegetations. The resulting syndrome is known as subacute bacterial endocarditis (SBE). In most cases, the basic valvular anomaly is due to rheumatic heart disease, most often affecting the mitral valve. Other cases are related to mitral valve prolapse, nodular dystrophic (age-related) calcification of the aortic valve, and congenital heart disease (eg, ASD, VSD, PDA, IHSS, and coarctation of the aorta). The clinical features derive from: infection itself (fever, constitutional symptoms); valve dysfunction (hemodynamic instability); emboli from the vegetation (Janeway lesions, Roth spots, strokes, renal dysfunction; Osler nodes); and immune stimulation (rheumatoid factor, circulating immune complexes leading to glomerulonephritis, etc). These infections are predominantly due to Viridans streptococci (*Streptococcus sanguis, Streptococcus mutans,* and *Streptococcus mitis*), group B streptococci, group D streptococci (*Streptococcus bovis*), Enterococci (*Streptococcus faecalis*) and other HACEK organisms.

□ Infection of prosthetic valves is most often due to *Staphylococcus epidermidis,* followed by *S aureus*. Cases arising a very long time after valve replacement tend to have a microbial differential diagnosis resembling that of SBE. Prosthetic valve infection sets up along the valve *suture ring,* leading to the possibility of dehiscence, dysrhythmia, and stenosis.

□ About 5-10% of cases of endocarditis are associated with negative blood cultures. The most common cause of *blood culture-negative endocarditis* (BCNE) is prior antibiotic therapy. Furthermore, causes of non-infectious endocarditis must be considered (Libman-Sacks endocarditis, nonbacterial thrombotic (marantic) endocarditis, carcinoid heart syndrome). The infectious agents that cause BCNE include *Coxiella burnetii, Bartonella, Chlamydia,* and *Legionella.*

Specific agents

■ While coagulase-negative staphylococci (*S epidermidis*) are uncommon causes of native valve endocarditis, they are a major cause of prosthetic valve and nosocomial endocarditis.

■ *S aureus* is the most common cause of acute bacterial endocarditis in native valves, and it is a major cause of prosthetic valve and nosocomial endocarditis. Furthermore, it causes the majority of right-sided (tricuspid) endocarditis in i.v. drug abusers. *S aureus* causes rapid destruction of the valve leaflets and the formation of abscesses in the valve ring and underlying myocardium. This produces a fulminant clinical picture with high fever, prostration, and in many cases hemodynamic collapse. Urgent surgical valve replacement is often required.

■ Streptococci, especially the viridans streptococci, are the most common causes of subacute bacterial endocarditis (SBE); however *S milleri* is known for its ability to cause acute endocarditis. As discussed later in this chapter, the α-hemolytic streptococci include *S pneumoniae* (not currently a common cause of endocarditis) and the viridans streptococci (including such common causes of SBE as *S sanguis, S mutans,* and *S salivarius*). Group D organisms, including the enterococci and *S bovis,* follow slightly in incidence and tend to affect an older age group. In series conducted in the first half of the 20th century, *S pneumoniae* was a major consideration in infective endocarditis, causing 10-20% of cases, and usually running a fulminant (acute endocarditis) course. Currently it is found in about 1% of cases. Many patients with pneumococcal infective endocarditis have traditionally been alcoholics, with concurrent meningitis and pneumonia (Austrian syndrome), and a very high rate of mortality. Enterococci represent the third most common cause of

infective endocarditis (after *Staphylococcus* and *Streptococcus*), responsible for 10-15% of cases.

■ *Bartonella* species, especially *B quintana* and *B henselae,* account for approximately 1% of all infective endocarditis cases and 10% of blood culture negative endocarditis (BCNE). The clinician must seek epidemiological clues when cultures turn up negative, such as homelessness and chronic alcohol use for *B quintana* infection and cat (kitten, usually) exposure for *B henselae.* Serology is probably the most useful confirmatory test for *Bartonella* endocarditis. High-titer (>1:800) IgG has a high predictive value (IgM is usually gone by the time of presentation). Culture is difficult but should be attempted. PCR testing on blood or excised heart valves may be attempted to confirm the diagnosis.

■ *Coxiella burnetii,* the causative agent of Q fever, causes about 3% of cases of infective endocarditis. *C burnetii* and *Tropheryma whipplei* in particular tend not to produce vegetations or other macroscopic clues to endocarditis. Microscopic sections may only show fibrosis, calcification, and a mononuclear infiltrate. As in the case of Bartonella, serology is the mainstay of clinical diagnosis. A very high IgG titer (>1:800) has high predictive value.

■ *Tropheryma whipplei,* like *Coxiella,* is likely to be missed clinically and pathologically. Histological findings, while including histiocytes, are not the classic findings of Whipple disease seen in other organs. Microbial staining can highlight the organisms, however.

■ Fungal endocarditis is increased in likelihood in immunodeficient patients, patients undergoing long-term antibiotic therapy, total parenteral nutrition, and i.v. drug abusers. *Candida* spp are the most common cause of fungal endocarditis, followed by *Torulopsis glabrata* and *Aspergillus* spp.

Laboratory approach to diagnosis

■ The diagnosis of endocarditis is based upon numerous clinical criteria and blood cultures (Duke criteria). In relatively stable patients (most of those with SBE), it is preferable to identify an organism prior to instigating antibiotic therapy; whereas in acute presentations empiric antibiotics are initiated immediately following the collection of blood for cultures.

- It is advised that blood cultures be performed in multiple. Three sets of blood cultures, drawn every 8 hours for the first 24 hours, each paired and of adequate volume (>10 cc, ideally 20-30 cc) is ideal.

  □ It is traditional teaching that blood cultures should optimally be drawn in the hour preceding a fever spike; most patients spike fever at about the same time every day, so that this is not as absurd as it might at first appear. However, the bacteremia in IE is relatively continual, and culture timing does not appear to alter yield for most organisms; furthermore, in acute endocarditis, a delay in obtaining cultures prior to initiating antibiotics is unacceptable.

  □ Paired cultures should be obtained (two separate sites, ideally opposite arms, with one aerobic and one anaerobic bottle at each site).

  □ There are several reasons to obtain more than one set of cultures when possible: (1) more cultures increase the likelihood of a positive culture, (2) positive cultures over two or more separate times *documents the continuous bacteremia that typifies endocarditis,* and (3) positive cultures over two or more separate times helps to justify that an organisms is not a contaminant (especially important in prosthetic valve endocarditis where *S epidermidis* is common).

  □ In modern automated blood culture systems using highly supportive media, most etiologic agents (including fastidious ones such as HACEK, *Brucella,* and *Francisella*) should produce a positive culture within 5 days. The recommended incubation of 3-4 weeks that many of us were taught was based upon traditional media using manual blood culture techniques.

  □ Fungal endocarditis is most commonly due to *Candida* spp, followed by *Torulopsis glabrata,* and *Aspergillus* spp. Fortunately, most blood cultures will support the growth of *Candida.* Recovery of other agents, including *Aspergillus,* requires special media, and many fungal agents are only diagnosed upon examination of the excised valve (or excised thromboemboli).

□ The identification of organisms such as *Bartonella* may require prolonged (>4 weeks) incubation. Identification of *C burnetii, T whipplei,* and *Chlamydophila psittaci* require unusual cell culture techniques, ideally utilizing a shell vial technique. Their isolation may require the culture of fresh surgical (valve) material.

□ The pathologist is likely to become involved directly in the case only upon examination of the excised valve. Gram staining of this material, particularly after a course of antibiotic therapy, can be somewhat misleading as antibiotic therapy *can alter the morphology of stained organisms.* Nonetheless, in blood-culture negative cases, histologic examination may be fruitful. Microbial stains (Gram, PAS, Steiner or Warthin-Starry) should be scrutinized; in some cases, immunohistochemical staining or PCR can facilitate the diagnosis of a suspected organism.

Meningitis

Differential diagnosis

- There are at least three major clinical syndromes produced by infection of the central nervous system: bacterial meningitis, aseptic (usually viral) meningitis, and encephalitis. Meningitis results from an inflammatory infiltrate within the meninges; whereas encephalitis refers to inflammation within the brain parenchyma. There are, of course, overlapping presentations (meningoencephalitis). The presentation of encephalitis is dominated by altered mental status. Bacterial and aseptic meningitis have similar clinical presentations (meningismus): headache, stiff neck, photophobia, fever, altered mental status, positive Brudzinski and Kernig signs. By definition, they are distinguished by microbial cultures, but they may be distinguished prospectively by the chemical and microscopic CSF findings.

  □ CSF in aseptic meningitis shows low-level leukocytosis (often <250 leukocytes per mL) with a predominance of mononuclear cells (especially lymphocytes). While the protein is moderately increased, the glucose is in the normal range.

□ In bacterial meningitis, there is marked leukocytosis with a predominance of neutrophils. The glucose is markedly depressed.

□ In encephalitis the CSF can vary between normal and findings typical of viral meningitis. The major exception is *herpes encephalitis, which can present with a bloody CSF, very high protein, and low glucose.*

■ Encephalitis is usually a viral illness but can be caused by other agents, notably the amebic organism *Naegleria fowleri.* The most common causes are herpes simplex type 1 (HSV-1), arboviruses (St. Louis encephalitis, California encephalitis, West Nile virus, Western equine encephalitis, Eastern equine encephalitis), HHV-6, mumps virus, measles virus, and varicella-zoster virus.

■ Aseptic meningitis is more common than bacterial meningitis and is most often due to a virus; however, it may be caused by mycoplasma, rickettsiae, mycobacteria, and parasites. The Enteroviruses (coxsackie A and B, echoviruses, poliovirus) are the most common cause of aseptic meningitis in all age groups, causing up to 70% of cases. Summer/Fall outbreaks are typical. Other viral causes of aseptic meningitis include herpes simplex virus (HSV), mumps virus, human immunodeficiency virus (HIV), and lymphocytic choriomeningitis virus (LCM).

■ Traditionally, the list of most common agents causing bacterial meningitis was topped by *H influenzae* type B; immunization has led to a major decline in *H influenzae* meningitis, and *S pneumoniae* is now the most common agent. Furthermore, since *H influenzae* was a major cause of childhood meningitis, the average age of patients afflicted has changed; previously a disease mainly of infants and young children, meningitis now peaks in young adults.

□ In neonates, group B streptococci, gram-negative aerobic bacilli (*E coli, Klebsiellae*), and *Listeria monocytogenes* are the most common causes of meningitis.

□ *Neisseria meningitides, S pneumoniae,* and *H influenzae* type B are the most common causes in infants and young children.

□ In adults, *S pneumoniae* is the most common, followed by *N meningitides.* In elderly adults, *N meningitides* is replaced by *L monocytogenes* in second place, followed by gram-negative aerobic bacilli.

Specific agents

■ Herpes simplex virus type 1 causes a form of encephalitis that is associated with *necrosis and hemorrhage within the anterior temporal lobes.* The presence of particular neurologic abnormalities—aphasia, olfactory and gustatory hallucinations, abnormal behavior—suggests HSV encephalitis, as does the finding of red cells in the cerebrospinal fluid. HSV encephalitis has a high fatality rate as well as a high rate of long-term neurologic deficits in survivors. When HSV-1 encephalitis is suspected, a rapid and reliable way to make the diagnosis is PCR, performed upon the cerebrospinal fluid.

■ Herpes simplex virus type 2 causes aseptic (viral) meningitis. CSF PCR is the best way to confirm this diagnosis.

■ HHV-6, the virus that causes exanthem subitum, is a common cause of viral encephalitis in children, and it is thought to contribute to many cases of febrile seizures in children. A rash that develops upon the breaking of a several-days-long high fever characterizes exanthem subitum. Most children recover without long-term sequelae.

■ The arboviruses, especially St. Louis and California (especially La Crosse) encephalitis viruses, are the most common causes of viral encephalitis in the United States. These agents are transmitted by mosquito and most commonly affect children. Characteristic clinical features include vomiting, hyponatremia, altered mental status, nystagmus, ataxia, and seizures. West Nile Virus, an arbovirus of the family Flaviviridae, causes encephalitis with the characteristic findings of weakness, paresis, and peripheral neuropathy. The virus, not found in the US prior to 1999, is found in birds. Mosquitoes transmit it from infected birds to humans. The best way to diagnose all of these arboviruses is serology.

■ Enteroviruses are the most common cause of aseptic (viral) meningitis. In particular, enterovirus meningitis occurs in the summer and fall. CSF PCR for enterovirus can help confirm the diagnosis.

- Lymphocytic choriomeningitis (LCM) virus is the most common cause of aseptic (viral) encephalitis in the winter and spring. LCM is acquired through exposure to the feces of infected mice. Infection with LCM during pregnancy may lead to serious visual or brain dysfunction in the fetus. The mumps virus used to be the most common cause of winter/spring aseptic meningitis, but immunization has altered this pattern in the United States. Occasional cases still arise in adolescents.

- *Haemophilus influenzae* was once the most common cause of bacterial meningitis, before the advent and wide application of immunization. Prior to immunization, it caused nearly 50% of cases; now it is responsible for about 5%. *H influenzae* is broadly divided into strains that do not possess an outer capsule (nontypeable strains) and strains that are encapsulated (typeable, based upon capsular proteins). The typeable strains are further divided into six serotypes, with *type b* being responsible for most cases of meningitis (prior to the widespread application of immunization). Nontypeable *H influenza* strains are the cause of an increasing proportion of meningitis, particularly in adults. The organism gains entry into the meninges usually following an untreated upper respiratory infection—otitis media, sinusitis. The fatality rate is around 5%.

- *Neisseria meningitides* serotypes B, C, and Y cause a large number of cases of bacterial meningitis. The bacterium is easily spread from person-to-person, leading to localized outbreaks—eg, in schools, barracks, and dormitories. Meningococcal meningitis is a very common cause of bacterial meningitis in children and young adults (ages 2-18 years). Persons with terminal complement deficiencies (C5, C6, C7, C8, C9 and properdin) are at particularly high risk. The case fatality rate is between 10 and 15%. In addition to the usual findings of bacterial meningitis, *N meningitides* infection is often associated with a petechial rash, first appearing on the trunk and lower extremities. In some patients the lesions coalesce, forming large ecchymoses (purpura fulminans); this finding is associated with a poor outcome.

  - *Pneumococcus* spp are now the most common cause of bacterial meningitis, causing about 50% of cases.

Furthermore it has for some time represented the most serious form of bacterial meningitis—producing the highest rates of mortality and long-term neurologic deficits. Mortality from pneumococcal meningitis ranges from 16% to 37% and neurological sequelae are estimated to occur in 30-52% of survivors.

- *Listeria monocytogenes* is responsible for about 10% of cases of bacterial meningitis overall, with a fatality rate of 15-30%. It is especially *common at the extremes of age:* younger than 1 month or older than 70 years of age. Other risk factors are corticosteroid therapy, transplant, diabetes mellitus, HIV infection, and iron overload.

- *Cryptococcus neoformans* is the most common cause of fungal meningitis. The organism is found mainly in dirt and bird droppings. Cryptococcal meningitis is common in patients with HIV infection.

- Group B streptococcus (*S agalactiae*) is a common cause of meningitis in neonates, especially because asymptomatic carriage in the vagina is common in pregnant women.

- Aerobic gram-negative bacilli (*Klebsiella* spp, *Escherichia coli, Serratia marcescens, Pseudomonas aeruginosa, Salmonella* spp) are important causes of bacterial meningitis in neonates, the elderly, and those with head trauma.

- Amebic meningoencephalitis is most often due to *Naegleria fowleri* and *Acanthamoeba. Naegleria,* the etiologic agent of primary amebic encephalitis (PAE), is acquired from fresh water sources, usually after swimming or diving in bodies of fresh water. Death generally occurs within 2 to 3 days from the onset of symptoms. *Acanthamoeba* causes granulomatous amebic encephalitis.

Laboratory evaluation

- Blood and CSF should be obtained for culture.

- Chemistry and cell count studies, performed on CSF, should be used to guide the differential diagnosis. Findings in the CSF that are typical of bacterial meningitis include a low glucose concentration (< 45 mg/dL), a high protein concentration (> 500 mg/dL), and a high white blood cell count (> 1000/mL), predominantly neutrophils. CSF lactate, procalcitonin, and

CRP have show promise in distinguishing bacterial from viral meningitis.

■ Gram stain of the CSF may quickly reveal the type of organism present. CSF gram staining, when the more common organisms are involved, has a sensitivity of 80-90%. The sensitivity falls below 50% for gram-negative bacilli and *L monocytogenes.*

■ Latex agglutination tests are available for performance on CSF. These tests are based upon reagents containing antibodies to specific bacteria and can be performed quickly. Assays are available and reliable for *H influenzae* type b, *S pneumoniae, Streptococcus agalactiae* (group B strep), and *N meningitides.*

Prosthetic Joint Infections and Other Clinical Syndromes (T3.2)

■ Studies on the topic of prosthetic joint infection have applied the following criteria for the diagnosis: growth of the same microorganism in two or more cultures of synovial fluid or periprosthetic tissue, purulence of synovial fluid or periprosthetic tissue, acute inflammation on histological examination of periprosthetic tissue, or presence of a sinus tract.

■ The most commonly involved organisms are coagulase-negative staphylococci (30-40%), *S aureus* (10-20%), mixed flora (10%), streptococci (10%), gram-negative bacilli (5%), enterococci (5%), and anaerobes (2-4%).

■ Some organisms (coagulase-negative staphylococci, *Propionibacterium acnes*) can represent either contaminants or pathogens and may have to be interpreted in the light of other laboratory findings.

■ Infections can be classified as early (developing <3 months after implantation), delayed (3 to 24 months), or late (>24 months), each representing roughly a third of cases.

   □ Early infections are typically related to organisms implanted at the time of surgery. Early infections present in fairly pronounced fashion—abrupt onset of joint pain, effusion, erythema and warmth over the implant site, fever, and, sometimes, overlying cellulitis or sinus tract formation—and are usually related to more virulent organisms such as *S aureus* and gram-negative bacilli.

   □ Delayed infection also is caused by organisms implanted during surgery, but less virulent ones—such as coagulase-negative staphylococci and *P acnes.* Delayed infection presents more subtly with implant loosening or persistent joint pain, symptoms that are difficult to distinguish from non-infectious joint failure.

   □ Late infections are usually the result of hematogenous spread of organisms from skin, respiratory tract, teeth, or urinary tract.

■ Radiographic studies can be helpful in diagnosing joint infection, including serial plain radiographs (looking for subperiosteal new bone and sinus tracts), arthrography (to detect implant loosening), nuclear scintigraphy (detects inflammation), and PET.

■ Laboratory studies are usually nonspecific; however a synovial fluid leukocyte count and differential, using cut-offs of 1700/mL and 65% neutrophils, has a fairly high sensitivity (about 95%) and specificity (about 90%).

■ Cultures of periprosthetic tissue provide the final word in most cases, but their sensitivity ranges from 65-95%. To optimize sensitivity, cultures from at least 3 separate sites should be taken.

■ Cultures do not address the need for intraoperative decision-making, however; so a great deal of hope has been placed in intraoperative consultation with frozen section examination. Surgical management may include débridement with retention of the prosthesis, one-stage exchange (single surgical procedure to remove old and insert new prosthesis) or two-stage exchange (removal of old prosthesis and periprosthetic tissue with cultures, postsurgical antibiotics, and second surgery to implant new prosthesis). Intraoperative histologic examination of periprosthetic tissue, in studies using cut-offs varying from 1 to 10 neutrophils per high power (400×) field, has demonstrated a sensitivity >80% and a specificity >90%. However, the interobserver variability is high, and inflammation may be patchy. Gram staining of synovial fluid and periprosthetic tissue has a high specificity (>95%) but a fairly low sensitivity (<30%).

T3.2
Clinical Syndromes and Causative Agents

Syndrome		Causative Agents (Most Common Listed First)
Bacteremia in patients with colon cancer		C septicum, S bovis
Bacterial meningitis	Neonatal	S agalactiae (Group B streptococcus), E coli
	Infants and young children	S pneumoniae, N meningitidis, H influenzae
	Young adults	S pneumoniae, N meningitidis, H influenzae
	Elderly adults	S pneumoniae, N meningitidis, H influenzae, L monocytogenes
Fungal meningitis		Cryptococcus
Viral (aseptic) meningitis		Enteroviridae (Coxsackie, Echovirus, Enterovirus)
Viral encephalitis		Alphaviridae (Eastern & Western Equine encephalitis) Flaviviridae (St Louis Encephalitis) Herpes simplex virus type 1
Infection following dog-bite		Capnocytophaga canimorsus, Pasteurella multocida Staphylococcus intermedius
Mycobacterial skin infection		M fortuitum-chelonae, M marinum, M haemophilum, M ulcerans, M leprae
Pseudomembranous colitis		C difficile
Toxic shock syndrome		S aureus
Botryomycosis		S aureus, P aeruginosa
Juvenile periodontitis		Actinobacillus actinomycetemcomitans
Ulceroglandular fever		Francisella tularensis
Glanders		Pseudomonas mallei
Melioidosis		Pseudomonas pseudomallei
Rocky mountain spotted fever		Rickettsia rickettsiae
Visceral larva migrans (VLM)		Toxocara canis/cati
Cutaneous larva migrans (CLM)		Ancylostoma braziliensis
Bacterial cellulitis	Most common overall	S pyogenes (Group A streptococci)
	Animal bite-associated	Pasteurella multocida
	Fresh water-associated	Aeromonas hydrophila
	Salt water-associated	Vibrio vulnificus
Dermatitis associated with whirlpools		P aeruginosa
Bacterial pharyngitis		S pyogenes (Group A streptococci), C diphtheriae
Whooping cough		Bordatella pertussis
Acute epiglottitis		H influenzae type B (HITB)
Chancroid		Haemophilus ducreyi
Lymphogranuloma venereum (LGV)		C trachomatis
Bacterial ('septic') arthritis	children & adults, monoarticular	S aureus
	young adults, polyarticular	N gonorrhea
Croup (acute laryngotracheobronchitis)		Parainfluenza virus, serotypes 1-3
Viral pneumonia	Infants/children	Respiratory syncytial virus (RSV)
	Adults	Influenza A (orthomyxovirus)

Clinical Syndromes and Causative Agents>Prosthetic Joint Infections and Other Clinical Syndromes

T3.2
Clinical Syndromes and Causative Agents (continued)

Bacterial pneumonia	Community-acquired	*S pneumoniae, L pneumoniae, H influenzae, S aureus, M pneumoniae*
	Chronic alcoholics	*K pneumoniae*
	Cystic fibrosis	*P aeruginosa*
	'Atypical' or 'walking' pneumonia	*Mycoplasma pneumoniae, Chlamydia pneumoniae*
	Nosocomial pneumonia	*E coli, P aeruginosa, S aureus, L pneumoniae*
Tinea versicolor		*Malassezia furfur*
Bacterial peritonitis	Spontaneous (cirrhosis with ascites)	*S pneumoniae*
	Secondary (ruptured bowel)	Mixed: *E coli*, enterococci, *B fragilis*, other anaerobes
Gastroenteritis	With short incubation period (1-8 h)	*S aureus, B cereus*
	Fried rice	*B cereus*
	Traveler's diarrhea	*E coli (ETEC)*
	Hamburgers in fast food restaurants	*E coli (EHEC)*
	Antibiotic-associated colitis	*C difficile*
	Viral	Rotavirus, Norwalk virus, enteric adenoviruses
Osteomyelitis		*S aureus*
Necrotizing fasciitis		Usually polymicrobial: *Streptococcus pyogenes* and anaerobes such as *Bacteroides fragilis*
Undulant fever	Pig-associated	*Brucella suis*
	Goat-associated	*Brucella melitensis*
	Dog-associated	*Brucella canis*
Rabit fever or deer-fly fever (Tularemia)		*Francisella tularensis*
Plague		*Yersinia pestis*
Carrion disease or verruga peruana (Bartonellosis)		*Bartonella bacilliformis*
Uterine infection following septic abortion		*Clostridium perfringens*
Leprosy (Hansen disease)		*Mycobacterium leprae*
Rat-bite fever		*Streptobacillus moniliformis*
San Joaquin Valley fever		*Coccidiodes immitis*
Superficial (noninvasive) mycoses	Dermatophytosis (Tinea capitis, Tinea cruris, etc.)	*Epidermophyton, Microsporon,* & *Trichophyton* spp
	Black piedra	*Piedraia hortae*
	White piedra	*Trichosporon beigelii*
	Tinea versicolor	*M furfur*
	Tinea nigra palmaris/plantaris	*Phaeoannelomyces werneckii*
Cutaneous & subcutaneous mycoses	Sporotrichosis	*Sporothrix shenckii*
	Chromoblastomycosis	*Phialophora, Cladosporium, Fonsacea*
	Lobomycosis	*Loboa loboi*
	Phaeohyphomycosis	*Exophiala jeanselmei, Phialophora, Wangiella dermatitidis*
	Sporotrichosis	*Sporothrix schenckii*
	Eumycotic mycetoma	*Exophiala, Wangiella, P boydii (scedosporium)*
	Rhinosporidiosis	*Rhinosporidium seeberi*

T3.2
Clinical Syndromes and Causative Agents (continued)

Rhinoscleroma	*Klebsiella rhinoscleromatosus*
Actinomycotic mycetoma (Madura Foot)	*Actinomyces, Nocardia, Streptomyces*
Measles	Rubeola virus
Erysipelas	*S pyogenes* (Group A streptococci)
Erysipeloid	*Erysipelothrix rhusiopathiae*
German measles	Rubella virus
Chicken pox	Varicella zoster virus
Impetigo	*S aureus*
Labial herpes	Herpes simplex virus type 1
Genital herpes	Herpes simplex virus type 2
Roseola infantum (exanthem subitum)	Human herpes virus 6
Fifth disease (erythema infectiosum, slapped-cheek disease)	Parvovirus B19
Chagas disease	*Trypanosoma cruzi*
African sleeping sickness	*Trypanosoma brucei*
Adiaspiromycosis	*Chrysosporium parvum*
Fungal external otitis	*Aspergillus niger*
Subacute sclerosing panencephalitis (SSPE)	Measles virus (reactivation)
Hand-foot-mouth disease	Coxsackie A
Viral myocarditis	Coxsackie B
Progressive multifocal leukoencephalopathy (PML)	JC Virus
Scarlet fever	*S pyogenes* (Group A streptococci)
Acute mastitis	*S aureus*
Postsplenectomy sepsis	*S pneumoniae*

Vectors (T3.3)

Virology

Laboratory Methods

Cell cultures The primary method for diagnosing most viruses is viral isolation in cell culture. Exceptions are many and include EBV, arboviruses, and rubella for which serology is the primary method and rotavirus and rhabdovirus for which antigen detection is the primary method. Most viruses can replicate in cell culture; however, turn-around-time is not ideal.

■ **Cell cultures are of three types:** cell cultures, cell lines, and established cell lines.

▫ Primary cell cultures are what you get if you culture a minced organ. These cells can be maintained in culture for a limited time with repetitive changes of the supporting fluid. An example is primary monkey kidney (PMK).

▫ Once cells are transferred or subcultured, a primary cell culture becomes a secondary cell culture or cell line. These are usually diploid. After a limited number of transfers (usually around 50), cell lines become exhausted and will no longer replicate. Examples of cell lines include human diploid fibroblasts (HDF) and MRC-5.

▫ However, individual cells may acquire an unlimited ability to replicate, and cell lines that continue to proliferate after having been transferred at least 70 times are considered established cell lines (and are often heteroploid). Established cell lines are often obtained from human malignancies; eg, HEp-2 is derived from laryngeal carcinoma, and HeLa is derived from cervical carcinoma. Uninfected diploid cell lines are morphologically fibroblastic and consist of long slender parallel cells. Uninfected

T3.3
Vectors

Organism	Vector	Comments
Plasmodium spp	Mosquito (*Anopheles*)	
Babesiosis	*Ixodes* tick	*Ixodes dammini* in the Eastern US, *I. pacificus* in the Western US, *I. ricinus* in Europe.
Leishmania spp	Sandfly (*Phlebotomus*)	
B burgdorferi	*Ixodes* tick	*Ixodes dammini* in the Eastern US, *I. pacificus* in the Western US *I. ricinus* in Europe, *I. persulcatus* in China. The natural reservoir is the white-footed mouse, but in endemic areas, deer are an important reservoir.
B recurrentes	Human body louse	
Trypanosoma cruzi	Reduviid bug	
Trypanosoma brucei	Tsetse fly	
Wucheria bancrofti	Mosquito	
Brugia malayi	Mosquito	
Loa loa	*Chrysops* (mango) fly	
Mansonella spp	Biting (*Culicoides*) midges	
Onchocerca volvulus	Blackfly (*Simulian*)	
Dirofilaria immitis	Mosquito	
Schistosoma spp	None	Direct penetration of skin by free-swimming cercaria.
Taenia solium	None	Ingestion of infected *pork* leads to intestinal infestation. Ingestion of *eggs* (usually from infected food-preparer) leads to cysticercosis.
R. rickettsiae	Tick	
R. prowazekii	Louse	
R. tsutsugamushi	Chigger	
R. typhi	Flea	
B henselae	Kitten	
R. conorii	Tick	
R. akari	Mite	
E chaffeensis	Lone Star Tick (*Amblyomma americanum*)	
E phagocytophilia	Deer Tick	
B bacilliformis	Sandfly	
B quintana	Louse	
C burnetii	None	Inhalation.
Fasciola hepatica	None	Ingestion of freshwater plants (*water cress*)
Francisella tularensis	Deerfly	Natural reservoir is small rodents such as rabbits.
Brucella spp	None	Natural reservoir is cattle (*B abortus*), goats (*B melitensis*) & pigs (*B suis*). Contracted from close contact (abattoir workers) or ingestion of infected milk.

Virology>Laboratory Methods

T3.4
Routine Cell Culture

Virus	PMK	Hep2	HDF	Notes
Enterovirus	+++	+	+++	.Angular, tear-shaped, cells
Influenza Mumps Parainfluenza	+++	–	+	If minimal to no CPE - confirm with hemadsorption
Adenovirus +	+	+++	+	Grape-like clusters
RSV				Syncytia
VZV CMV	–	-	+++	Slow, Focal clusters of CPE (plaques)
HSV1 and 2	+/–	+	+++	Rapid (1-2 days), sweeping CPE
Polio				Slow, random, focal CPE
Coxsackie B	+	+	–	Focal swollen cells
Coxsackie A Echovirus	+	–	+	Focal swollen cells

established cell lines morphologically appear as polygonal epithelioid cells.

□ Cell cultures vary in their susceptibility to become infected by different viruses **T3.4**. Specimens should be inoculated onto an array of cell cultures, selected according to the source of the specimen and the most likely agents for that source.

■ **Contamination of culture media** is most commonly due to *Mycoplasma* spp or Simian viruses. *Mycoplasma* contamination results in poor cell growth and inhibition of viral infection. Simian viral contamination may result in an false-positive hemadsorbtion; this problem is the reason for running parallel control hemadsorption tests on uninoculated tubes.

T3.5
Cell Culture Characteristics of Selected Viruses

Virus	Notes on cell culture
Adenovirus	Grape-like clusters of rounded cells on Hep2.
RSV	Syncytia in Hep2 cells (syncytia can be produced in various cell types by measles, parainfluenza, and mumps viruses).
HSV	CPE within 1-3 days on Hep2 and HDF.
EBV	Does not grow in routine cell culture. EBV proliferates only in B lymphocytes. Lymphocyte cultures take 4 weeks. Viral serology is the preferred method.
Influenza & Parainfluenza	Often display no CPE but can be detected in cell culture by hemadsorption.
	Performed by adding red cells to the cell culture, or the hemagglutination inhibition test; performed by adding antiviral immunoglobulin prior to adding red cells. Influenza and parainfluenza grow only on PMK (producing little to no visible CPE).
CMV	Infects mainly HDF.
VZV	Infects mainly HDF.
Parvovirus	Grows only on erythroid precurser cell lines.
Coxsackie A virus	Inoculated into suckling mice which are then observed for flaccid paralysis.

Virology>Laboratory Methods

T3.6
Viral Histology

Virus	Nuclear inclusions	Cytoplasmic inclusions	Syncytia	Notes
Influenza	−	−	−	
RSV	−	−	+	
HSV	+	−	+	Cowdry bodies
Adenovirus	+	−	−	
CMV	+	+	−	
Measles	+	+	+	Warthin-Finkeldey giant cells
Rabies	−	+	−	Negri bodies

■ In routine cell culture, a virus is detected by visual examination of cultures for viral *cytopathic effect* (CPE) with a phase-contrast microscope. Viruses **T3.6** can be provisionally identified based on (1) the morphology of the CPE, (2) the types of cells displaying CPE, and (3) the time from inoculation to detection of CPE. For example, HSV shows CPE usually within 3 days of inoculation, while RSV, CMV, and VZV may require 2 weeks. Influenza and parainfluenza viruses do not ordinarily induce CPE; however, they express hemagglutinins with which they can adsorb guinea pig RBCs to the surface of the culture cells. This forms the basis for the hemadsorption test.

■ A modification of the cell culture is the **shell vial technique.** This method is most commonly employed in respiratory virus panels. Cell cultures within a small vial overlaid with a coverslip are inoculated and centrifuged to bring virus into contact with the cells. After a short incubation (less than 3 days) the coverslip is removed and stained with antiviral antibody tagged with a fluorescent dye.

Serology (detection of circulating antibody) is helpful in the detection of current or past viral infection, particularly when isolation of the pathogen is difficult. A single

positive IgM antibody can be considered diagnostic in many circumstances. Paired sera taken seven to 10 days apart are recommended for diagnosis based upon IgG, although a single sample is acceptable for screening purposes. With paired samples, a fourfold or greater rise in IgG titer, between the acute and convalescent samples, is considered diagnostic of infection. Thus, the diagnostic usefulness of serologic tests is limited and often retrospective. Occasionally, serology is used for determining an individual's immune status; eg, to confirm hepatitis B vaccination or prior infection with varicella.

☐ In general elevated IgM titers or rising IgG titers (4-fold) are indicative of acute infection.

☐ Usually virus-specific IgM is detectable during the first week of a primary infection; the IgM becomes undetectable within 1-4 months.

☐ Virus-specific IgG begins to emerge 1-2 weeks into a primary infection. It usually peaks between 4-8 weeks; subsequently, it declines continually but usually remains detectable for life.

☐ In secondary infection (reactivation or new infection with the same virus), there may or may not be a re-emergence of IgM; and IgG, usually detectable from the start, increases for the next 4-8 weeks.

☐ Serologic techniques are numerous and include older systems (complement fixation, hemagglutination inhibition, and single radial hemolysis) as well as new ones (RIA, EIA, Western blot, and recombinant immunoblot assay (RIBA)).

Direct antigen detection. Enzyme-linked immunosorbant assay (EIA), latex agglutination, and direct fluorescent antibody (DFA) techniques are available. DFA

T3.7
Viral Classification

	DNA viruses	RNA viruses
Nonenveloped	Parvoviridae	Caliciviridae
	Adenoviridae	Papovaviridae
	Picornaviridae	Reoviridae
Enveloped	Herpesviridae	(all the rest)
	Poxviridae	Arenaviridae, Bunyaviridae, Coronaviridae,
	Hepadnaviridae	Flaviviridae, Filoviridae, Orthomyxoviridae,
		Paramyxoviridae, Togaviridae, Rhabdoviridae,
		Rhabdoviridae

provides the opportunity to directly observe the specimen and thereby determine that cells are present in the sample and which cells display reactivity (analogous to FISH).

Histology. Conventional light microscopy is useful for the detection of several viruses, particularly those with characteristic inclusions **T3.6**. Ultrastructural morphology (electron microscopy) allows recognition of several viral types. Some examples of highly characteristic viruses are illustrated below. Some enteric viruses (rotavirus, enteric adenovirus, Norwalk, astroviruses, and calicivirus), which do not grow readily in cell culture, may be identified this way.

Molecular techniques. Polymerase chain reaction (PCR) and in-situ hybridization (ISH) may be used for direct detection of viral nucleic acid. FISH is often applied to the histologic identification of HPV (cervical biopsies), CMV (lung biopsies), HSV (skin biopsies), and parvovirus B19 (marrow). Direct DNA (genomic) sequencing with PCR and branched (bDNA) amplification is commonly employed in the monitoring of patients with HIV and HCV infection.

Viruses (T3.7)

Human Herpes viruses (HHV) T3.8

- Herpes Simplex Virus (HSV)

  □ HSV type 1 is associated with gingivostomatitis, pharyngitis, keratoconjunctivitis, herpes labialis (cold sores), occasional skin infections (herpetic whitlow), and herpes encephalitis. Immuno-compromised persons are at risk for herpetic esophagitis, tracheobronchitis, pneumonia, and hepatitis. Herpes encephalitis, accounting for 15 % of all viral encephalitides, is characterized by bilateral hemorrhagic necrosis of the anterior poles of the temporal lobes. The CSF usually shows a pleocytosis, elevated protein, and numerous red blood cells. HSV1 is transmitted by saliva. Most primary infections occur before puberty. Some primary infections are asymptomatic, while others produce a painful gingivostomatitis, affecting the oral cavity diffusely, associated with fever and constitutional symptoms. The virus ultimately infects and achieves dormancy within the nuclei of trigeminal ganglia. Occasionally there is reactivation leading to localized lesions of the mouth or lips.

T3.8
Human Herpes Viruses

Herpes virus	Latency	Clinical Disease	
		Acute	**Reactivation**
HSV 1	Dorsal root ganglia	Acute gingivostomatitis Pharyngitis Skin infection (herpetic whitlow)	Herpes labialis Herpes encephalitis
HSV 2	Dorsal root ganglia	Genital herpes Skin infection (herpetic whitlow)	Genital herpes Herpes meningitis
CMV	Histiocytes	Mononucleosis-like syndrome Disseminated infection in neonates and immunocompromised hosts.	Disseminated infection
VZV	Dorsal root ganglia	Varicella (chicken pox)	Zoster (shingles)
EBV	B-cells	**T 3.9**	**T 3.9**
HHV-6	T-cells	Roseola (exanthem subitum)	Unknown
HHV-8	Unknown	Unknown	Kaposi sarcoma Primary body cavity lymphoma

□ HSV type 2 is the cause of genital herpes, occasional skin infections, and herpes meningitis (does not typically cause encephalitis). HSV type 2, like HSV1, produces primary, latent, and recurrent infection, with dormancy being established in sacral ganglia. Interestingly, HSV-2 seropositivity can be found in about 20% of the population, but only about 2% of the population suffers from genital herpes.

□ HSV type 2 is also the cause of congenital and neonatal herpes. Congenital herpes, implying *in utero* infection resulting from transplacental viremia, is rare in comparison with neonatal herpes. Neonatal herpes results from HSV transmission from mother to child during passage through an infected birth canal. In nearly half of these cases, there is no history of genital herpes. The severity of neonatal HSV-2 ranges from a few skin lesions to encephalitis, chorioretinitis, and sepsis. The American College of Obstetricians and Gynecologists (ACOG) recommends cesarean delivery for pregnant women with prodromal symptoms or active genital HSV lesions.

□ While cell culture is still considered the definitive method for the diagnosis of HSV1 and HSV2, direct DNA probes are becoming more widespread. HSV1 and 2 characteristically grow rapidly in almost any cell culture, with the exception of PMK. CPE that sweeps across the culture monolayer is usually detectable by day 2 or 3. The cells display rounded enlargement (ballooning) with occasional syncytia. A DFA test (culture cells are transferred to a glass slide and stained with fluorescent-tagged HSV antibodies) is confirmatory. An increasingly popular alternative is the shell vial technique, in which centrifugation is used to promote virus-culture cell interaction. This technique does not result in visible CPE; however, a DFA stain will usually be positive after one day.

□ A Tzanck smear is prepared by directly smearing material obtained from a lesion onto a glass slide, followed by Giemsa staining. If typical HSV CPE is observed, the diagnosis can be made. The technique has a sensitivity of 60-70%. Negative Tzanck smears should therefore be followed by culture.

□ DNA techniques, including PCR and hybrid capture signal amplification, appear as specific as culture and more sensitive.

□ Serology has limited utility in the diagnosis of HSV 1 and 2.

■ **Varicella-zoster virus** (VZV)

□ Primary VZV infection is the cause of childhood varicella (chicken pox). Though chicken pox in childhood is generally benign, it may be complicated by life-threatening pneumonia in healthy adolescents and adults.

□ Pregnant women and immunocompromised individuals are at risk for serious disseminated infection. Furthermore, infected pregnant women can transmit the virus transplacentally, leading to congenital varicella.

□ Congenital varicella is diagnosed when there is evidence of maternal varicella infection during pregnancy, skin lesions on the newborn that have a dermatomal distribution, and serologic evidence of infection in the newborn (either IgM or persistent IgG beyond 7 months). The incidence and severity of congenital varicella *depend upon the timing of maternal infection.* When a woman is infected during pregnancy, the overall incidence of congenital varicella is around 1-5%. The incidence is lowest when maternal infection occurs in the 1st trimester, higher in the 2nd, and highest in the 3rd. So-called perinatal varicella arises when maternal infection occurs within a few days of delivery. The likelihood of perinatal varicella in this instance is around 50-60%. Perinatal varicella can be quite severe, and before the availability of antiviral agents, the mortality was 15 to 30%. The CDC recommends the administration of varicella zoster immunoglobulin (VZIG) to infants born to a mother who develops a rash attributable to varicella between 5 days before and 2 days after delivery. VZIG may be augmented by i.v. acyclovir.

□ Reactivation of VZV is the cause of zoster (shingles). Herpes zoster presents as a dermatomal vesicular rash that is often quite painful. Reactivation of latent infection in the geniculate ganglion of the facial nerve is the cause of Ramsay

Hunt syndrome—presenting as otalgia, unilateral facial paresis, vertigo, hearing loss, and tinnitus. This syndrome is rare in the United States.

- Cytomegalovirus (CMV)

  □ Primary CMV infection, in the immunocompetent older child or adult, is either asymptomatic or causes a mononucleosis-like syndrome.

  □ In immunocompromised persons and neonates, primary CMV infection can cause pneumonia, hepatitis, retinitis, or disseminated disease.

  □ In allograft recipients, CMV infection commonly presents as a mononucleosis-like syndrome with fever and leucopenia. This may lead to infection within particular organs, especially the lungs, GI tract (eg, CMV colitis), liver, or kidneys. Interestingly, CMV tends to set up infection within the transplanted organ. In fact, CMV is thought to contribute to chronic rejection.

  □ In HIV infection, CMV becomes a major problem when CD4 counts are quite low (<100-200 cells per mL). CMV retinitis, encephalitis, and nephritis, while reported in transplant recipients, are much more common in HIV patients.

□ CMV is the most common congenital infection in the United States. Neonatal CMV results from transplacental infection and is most likely to occur when a pregnant woman experiences primary CMV infection during gestation. In its most severe form (cytomegalic inclusion disease—CID) it manifests with low birth weight, microcephaly, intracerebral calcifications, hepatosplenomegaly, jaundice, chorioretinitis, thrombocytopenia, petechial rash, and purpura. Only 30% of pregnancies with *primary* CMV infection result in congenital CMV, and only 10% of congenital CMV is severe as described above. In survivors of congenital CMV, the most common long-term problem is *sensorineural hearing loss*. Reactivation infection during pregnancy results in a much lower incidence (<1%) of transplacental transmission.

□ The rate of seropositivity (seroprevalence) of CMV infection increases with age, but rates differ substantially worldwide. In some parts of Africa, the seropositivity rate can reach 90% by the age of 10; whereas in the United States, the seropositivity rate at age 10 is about 20%. Even within the U.S. rates differ with socioeconomic status.

□ The diagnosis of CMV may be made by serology (positive IgM or 4-fold rise in IgG), direct antigen detection (DFA on peripheral blood leukocytes),

T3.9
Clinical Syndromes Caused by EBV

Disease	Stage of Infection	Notes
Infectious mononucleosis	Primary	Mainly in adolescents and young adults
X-linked lymphoproliferative disorder Primary Males affected	Hepatitis Primary Mainly older adults	Burkitt lymphoma Latent Nearly 100% of endemic BL in African children and 25% of sporadic BL, especially in HIV- infected adults
Hodgkin lymphoma	Latent	EBV in 50-70% of cases
Primary effusion lymphoma	Latent	EBV in 70% of cases (HHV8 in 100%)
Lymphomatoid granulomatosis	Latent	
Post-transplant lymphoproliferative disorder (PTLD)	Latent	>95% EBV positive
Oral hairy leukoplakia	Latent	In HIV infection; EBER negative
Nasopharyngeal carcinoma	Latent	Nearly 100% EBV positive in Chinese and
		Inuit populations; 75% EBV positive in US

PCR (on any body fluid or tissue), histology (characteristic inclusions), or culture.

■ **Epstein-Barr virus** (EBV)

□ EBV is transmitted in saliva. Uncommonly, it may be transmitted through blood transfusion or solid-organ transplantation. About 90% of people world-wide are infected with EBV. There are two genomic types of EBV—EBV1 and EBV2. It seems that these do not differ in disease association, but EBV1 is the predominant type in the West; whereas, EBV1 and EBV2 are evenly distributed elsewhere.

□ EBV enters the body through the pharyngeal mucosa and subsequently *infects B lymphocytes via the C3d receptor (CD21).* Reacting to the virus, CD8+ *T-lymphocytes are responsible for the peripheral blood atypical lymphocytosis* that is seen. The site of EBV latency is the B lymphocyte. The EBV genome persists in episomal form within a small population of B cells, where it usually causes no additional effects. Persistent salivary viral shedding may occur, and in some cases latency and reactivation are associated with clinical disease **T3.9**.

□ Primary infection with EBV is usually subclinical but may take the form of infectious mononucleosis (IM). Early asymptomatic childhood infection is common; in affluent populations, EBV infection tends to occur in late childhood or adolescence. Liver function tests (LFTs) are frequently (50%) elevated in EBV infectious mononucleosis. The classic IM presentation, seen primarily in adolescents, includes sore throat (pharyngitis), lymph node enlargement, tonsillar enlargement, and fever. In primary infection of older adults these findings are less likely; instead, hepatitis and jaundice

become more common. As in other herpes virus infections, latency ensues.

□ X-linked lymphoproliferative disorder (Duncan disease) is a manifestation of acute disease and refers to fulminant primary EBV infection that is frequently fatal and appears confined to males of rare kindreds. The mechanism of death is usually hepatic necrosis, associated with a pronounced T/NK cell infiltrate. In other cases, affected individuals have manifested hemophagocytosis, agammaglobulinemia, and B-cell lymphoma. The underlying genetic defect is found in the *SH2D1A* (aka SAP) gene that is normally expressed in T and NK cells. The SAP protein is a transmembrane signaling protein that becomes involved in the usual course of the immune reaction to viral infection. In those harboring this mutation, for as yet unknown reasons, EBV in particular results in uncontrolled activation of T/NK cells.

□ The traditional diagnostic criteria for infectious mononucleosis are *Hoagland criteria:* a leukocytosis consisting of >50% lymphocytes and >10% atypical lymphocytes, fever, pharyngitis, and adenopathy, and a positive serologic test. These criteria are quite restrictive, and many patients routinely diagnosed with infectious mono do not qualify. However, numerous other causes of sore throat with fever and adenopathy must be considered: streptococcal pharyngitis, pharyngitis due to other viruses (CMV and HIV), etc. And other causes of a mononucleosis syndrome must be considered: toxoplasmosis, CMV, dilantin, etc.

□ The laboratory diagnosis of EBV is primarily serologic **T3.10, F3.1**, based on the fact that *EBV induces production of antibodies including anti-i, rheumatoid factor, ANA, and the Paul-Bunnell **het-***

T3.10
EBV Serology

Stage	Heterophile	IgM Anti-VCA	IgG Anti-EA	IgG Anti-VCAgG	Anti-EBNA
Uninfected	–	–	–	–	–
Early Acute	–/+	+	–	+	–
Acute	+/–	+	+	+	–/+
Convalescent	–	–	+	+	+
Remote	–	–	+	-/+	+

erophile antibodies. Heterophile antibodies are IgM antibodies that have an affinity for sheep and horse red cells. They emerge during the first week of symptoms, 3-4 weeks after infection, and return to undetectable levels by 3 to 6 months.

☐ Antibody with strong affinity for beef erythrocyte antigens, uninhibited by adsorption with guinea pig kidney antigen (the differential absorption test), is specific for acute EBV infection. This test was developed into a rapid latex agglutination test (Monospot test).

☐ Heterophile antibody is fairly specific but *insensitive,* being present in 80% of infected teens and adults, 40% of all infected children, and only 20% of infected children under 4. Sometimes heterophile antibodies arise in non-EBV infections, such as the Forsmann antibody. Conditions sometimes associated with a false positive monospot test include HIV, lupus, and lymphoma.

☐ Subsequently, multiple specific EBV serologic markers were developed, including the IgG/IgM anti-viral capsid antigen (anti-VCA), EBV early antigen (EBV-EA), and EBV nuclear antigen (EBNA). These have very high sensitivity (>94%) and specificity (>95%) for EBV infectious mononucleosis. Following infection, the first marker **T3.10** to appear is IgM anti-VCA. IgM anti-VCA becomes undetectable after acute infection but re-emerges with reactivation. IgG anti-VCA emerges shortly after the IgM and slightly before

the heterophile antibody. IgG anti-EBNA and IgG anti-VCA persist indefinitely.

☐ In tissue sections, there are many ways to demonstrate EBV cellular infection.

● In situ hybridization with EBV-encoded RNA (EBER) can be performed on histologic sections or cytologic preparations, permitting determination of the EBV status in cells of interest. For example,
in Hodgkin lymphoma, EBER is localized to the nuclei of Reed-Sternberg cells, with little to no expression in the background small lymphocytes. EBER is positive in all EBV-related tumors (oral hairy leukoplakia is the only EBV-related lesion that is negative for EBER by ISH). In hyperplastic lymphoid tissue during infectious mononucleosis, EBER is expressed in a large number of lymphocytes. In the lymph nodes of patients with latent EBV infection, EBER is expressed in a very small percentage (about 0.1%) of lymphocytes. EBER
is used to support the diagnosis of post-transplant lymphoproliferative disorder (PTLD). It is expressed in about 50% of Hodgkin lymphomas and a large percentage of nasopharyngeal carcinomas, T/NK lymphomas of the nasal type, and endemic-type Burkitt lymphoma.

● In situ hybridization with the BamHIW sequence of EBV DNA. This provides excellent sensitivity, since the BamHIW sequence is

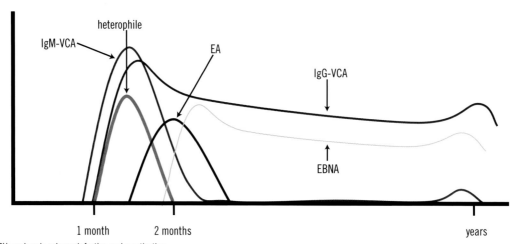

F3.1 EBV serology in primary infection and reactivation

repeated 11 times throughout the EBV genome; thus, it is preamplified.

- LMP1 immunohistochemistry performs nearly as well as EBER in situ hybridization in many settings—Hodgkin lymphomas, infectious mononucleosis, and PTLD; however, there continues to be discordance between the results of the two assays in other EBV-associated lesions. LMP1 staining is cytoplasmic and membranous. LMP1 IHC rarely produces a false positive result; false positives may result from nonspecific staining in plasma cells and eosinophils. However, when positive in the cells of interest, there is excellent correlation with EBER ISH. Thus a positive LMP1 is useful, but a negative one may need to be confirmed with EBER ISH.

- **HHV 6** is the etiologic agent of roseola infantum (fourth disease, Duke disease, exanthem subitum) in infants and toddlers. Fully-developed roseola manifests in only about 10% of those with acute HHV 6 infection, however, the remaining children displaying a nonspecific febrile illness. HHV 6 has been found to be highly neurotropic and is one of the causes of viral encephalitis. Due to its combined propensity to produce fever and CNS infection HHV 6 is responsible for a significant proportion of childhood febrile seizures. A more recently described herpes virus, HHV 7, appears to have clinico-pathologic features similar to HHV 6.

- **HHV 8** has come to be known as the Kaposi sarcoma–associated herpes virus (KSHV). It is associated with all clinical variants of *Kaposi sarcoma,* in addition to primary effusion lymphoma (PEL) and the subset of *multicentric Castleman disease seen in HIV+ patients.* The diagnosis of KSHV relies on molecular methods (either FISH or PCR), immunohistochemical staining (LANA-1 expression, in a speckled nuclear pattern, is the hallmark of cells harboring KSHV), or serology (IFA, ELISA, or Western Blot).

Adenovirus Adenoviruses are grouped into over 40 serotypes. Most of the respiratory infections are caused by the lower-numbered serotypes (1-14). Types 4 & 7 are associated with epidemic outbreaks of respiratory disease. Types 11 & 21 are associated with hemorrhagic cystitis. Types 40 & 41 are associated with childhood gastroenteritis.

Parvovirus Parvovirus is the cause of erythema infectiosum (slapped cheek disease; fifth disease). Primary maternal infection during gestation can lead to hydrops fetalis. Parvovirus B19 infects erythroid precursors and is responsible for aplastic anemia (aplastic crisis) in persons with chronic hemolytic states (such as sickle cell disease). Characteristic smudgy nuclear inclusions are seen in bone marrow biopsies. Parvovirus culture is not readily available, since it requires nucleated red blood cells.

Papovavirus

- Polyomaviruses include the JC virus and BK virus. Both are typically acquired in childhood and enter latency, supposedly within the brain and urothelium. If immunosuppression occurs, viral reactivation may lead to the development of *progressive multifocal leukoencephalopathy (PML) due to JC virus, or BK virus-induced hemorrhagic cystitis.* BK virus causes the appearance of so-called decoy cells in urine cytologic specimens: urothelial cells with a very high nuclear: cytoplasmic ratio that mimic the cells of urothelial carcinoma in-situ (CIS). Attention to the slight degeneration in these cells, the characteristic smudgy nuclear inclusions, and lack of the usual chromatin detail seen in CIS are the helpful clues to avoid this pitfall. Similar inclusions are seen within oligodendroglial cells in the demyelinative lesions of PML.

- Human papillomavirus (HPV)

  □ HPVs cause proliferative epithelial lesions (warts) in various locations T3.11. The incubation period after primary exposure is between 2-4 months. Common, plantar, and flat (juvenile) warts are acquired by direct contact; although, local abrasion or other trauma appears to enhance infectivity. Many forms of HPV (cervical, anal, and vulvar lesions) are sexually transmitted. In benign lesions, HPV DNA is **episomal** (extra-chromosomal); whereas, in malignant lesions, it is **integrated** into the host cell DNA. The viral **E6 & E7** genes are crucial for subsequent oncogenesis.

  □ Epidermodysplasia verruciformis is the condition in which the oncogenic potential of HPV was first noted. This is an autosomal recessive condition associated with a gene locus on chromosome 17 which seems to impair defenses against several specific HPV types. The lesions are found on the

Virology>Viruses

T3.11
Lesions Related to HPV

Lesion	HPV types (order of frequency)
Plantar wart	1, 2
Common wart	2, 1, 4 (HPV 7 in fish and meat handlers)
Flat (juvenile) wart	3, 10
Oral squamous papilloma	6, 11
Oral focal epithelial hyperplasia (Heck disease)	13, 32
Epidermodysplasia verruciformis	2, 3, 10, 5, 8
Laryngeal papillomas	6, 11
Condyloma acuminatum	6, 11
Low-grade cervical squamous intraepithelial lesions (LSIL)	6, 11
High-grade cervical squamous intraepithelial lesions (HSIL) Invasive cervical squamous carcinoma	16,18,31,33,35
Cervical adenocarcinoma in situ (AIS) Invasive cervical adenocarcinoma	18, 16

trunk and upper extremities, tend to be exophytic, and usually appear in the first decade of life. In young adulthood the lesions may undergo malignant transformation, invading as squamous cell carcinomas. Unlike other types of wart, epidermodysplasia verruciformis does not appear to be transmissible by contact with healthy subjects. Some of the implicated HPV types (especially HPV5) have been associated with psoriasis. Furthermore, lesions resembling epidermodysplasia verruciformis are sometimes seen in organ transplant recipients.

□ Recurrent respiratory papillomatosis (RRP) is caused by HPV 6 and HPV 11. There are two main clinical types: a juvenile-onset form, in which HPV is thought to be acquired during passage through the birth canal, and is more aggressive; and an adult form, thought to be sexually transmitted, in which papillomas are fewer. The papillomas arise most often on the true vocal cords. Malignant transformation is quite rare, but the lesions can be life-threatening because of airway obstruction, particularly in children. The juvenile form of RRP usually presents between the ages of 2-4 years. It is characterized by multiple papillomas that arise synchronously and serially. Affected children often require numerous, sometimes monthly, endoscopic resections. Adult-onset RRP is diagnosed most commonly between the ages of 20 and 40 years. Sometimes an HPV subtype is requested, as HPV 11 is associated with more aggressive disease than HPV 6.

T3.12
CDC Classification of Agents of Bioterrorism

Category A	Category B	Category C
Variola (smallpox)	Encephalitis viruses	Influenza viruses
Hemorrhagic fever viruses	*Brucella* spp	Nipah virus
Bacillus anthracis (anthrax)	*Burkholderia* spp	Hantavirus
Yersinia pestis (plague)	*Chlamydophila psittaci*	Rabies virus
Clostridium botulinum (botulism)	*Coxiella burnetii*	Yellow fever virus
Francisella tularensis (tularemia)	*Clostridium perfringens*	Drug-resistant TB
Yersinia spp (plague)	*Rickettsia prowazekii*	*Rickettsia conorii*
	Foodborne bacteria (eg, *Salmonella*)	
	Waterborne bacteria (eg, *Vibrio*)	

Virology>Viruses

T3.13
Hepatitis Viruses

Virus	Transmission	Incubation	Chronicity	Comments
HBV	Parenteral	15-150 days	10%	
HCV	Parenteral	30-150 days	50%	
HAV	Fecal-oral	15-30 days	0%	Most common viral hepatitis in US
HEV	Fecal-oral	15-42 days	<1%	20-30% fatality rate in pregnancy
HGV	Parenteral	Unknown	Unknown	

□ Anogenital HPV

- Benign squamous lesions (condyloma acuminata) of the anogenital region are usually associated with HPV 6 or HPV 11.

- Bowenoid papulosis is a condition that presents as multiple small (2-3 mm) pearly papules on the anogenital skin. Histologically, it resembles squamous cell carcinoma in situ (Bowen disease), but Bowenoid papulosis rarely results in invasive carcinoma. While histologically difficult or impossible to distinguish, true squamous cell carcinoma in situ (Bowen disease and erythroplasia of Queyrat) is usually easy to distinguish clinically. Bowenoid papulosis is caused by HPV 16.

- Together, HPV 16 and HPV 18 account for >70% of all malignancies in the anogenital region. The correlation is tightest with high-grade dysplasia and squamous cell carcinoma of the cervix, in which >98% of cases have detectable HPV. In fact, HPV is present in >95% of cervical adenocarcinomas and adeno-

carcinoma in situ. Outside the cervix, the rate of HPV detection in high grade and invasive squamous lesions varies from 80-95% for anal lesions to 30-40% for vulvar and penile lesions.

- Verrucous carcinoma (giant condyloma of Buschke and Lowenstein) is nearly always associated with HPV 6 or HPV 11.

Poxviruses DNA viruses that cause vesicular skin eruptions.

■ **Variola** causes smallpox which has been eradicated since 1977; however, stocks of the virus are maintained in labs throughout the world. Recently, there has been concern about smallpox as an agent of bioterrorism **T3.12**. The potential is significant, as variola can be easily acquired through aerosolized material, requires only a very small inoculum, and widespread immunization has not been practiced for some time. If this disease is suspected, samples should preferably be collected by someone who has been immunized. The best samples are scrapings, biopsy, or fluid from a skin lesion. Samples should be submitted to a specialized laboratory (eg, the CDC) that not only has the means

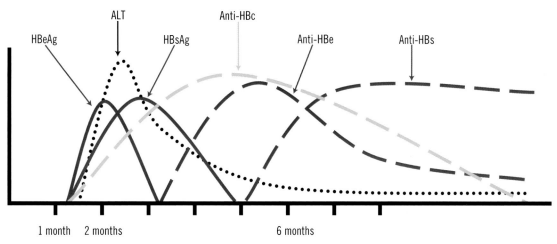

F3.2 Serologic patterns in acute HBV with resolution of infection

for making the diagnosis but also has biosafety level 4 capabilities. While there are characteristic light microscopic (viral inclusions called Guarnieri bodies) and electron microscopic findings, these lack specificity. Specific tests, including viral isolation in cell culture, DFA testing, and PCR are available.

- **Molluscum contagiosum virus** causes a vesicular eruption characterized by small waxy papules with central umbilication, single or multiple, located anywhere on the body but classically on the perineal skin. The lesions are quite characteristic histologically, with prominent **eosinophilic cytoplasmic inclusions** seen in lesional keratinocytes. If clinically confused with HSV, this confusion can carry over to the laboratory where in cell culture the virus can mimic the CPE of herpes. Unlike HSV, molluscum cannot be subcultured to subsequent cell cultures.

Hepatitis viruses T3.13

- **Hepadnavirus** (Hepatitis B virus—HBV)

  □ The HBV virus is a DNA virus whose intact virion is called the Dane particle. Important HBV viral markers include:

  - Hepatitis B surface antigen (HbsAg; Australia antigen), whose presence in serum *indicates active disease;* HBsAg would be expected to clear if infection is resolved and persist if infection is chronic.

- Hepatitis B e antigen (HBeAg) *indicates active viral replication.* In the hepatocyte, the genome of HBV can be present in two forms: as replicating virus or integrated into the host genome as a non-replicating form. HBeAg is only produced when the virus is in replicating form; thus, it can be used as a surrogate for HBV DNA production

- Antibody against hepatitis B core antigen (IgM and IgG anti-HBc) is present throughout the lifetime of somebody who has been infected with HBV. Its presence cannot be classify a patient as acute, resolved, or chronic. While IgM anti-HBc usually disappears after acute infection, it may persist for over a year; furthermore, in patients with chronic infection, IgM anti-HBc may re-appear in acute flares.

- Antibody against hepatitis B e antigen (anti-HBe) is found when HBe becomes negative. The presence of anti-HBe does not imply resolved infection or immunity.

- Antibody against surface antigen (HBsAb) *indicates resistance to infection.* It is found in immunized persons and those who have successfully cleared HBV infection.

□ Note: there is no circulating core antigen.

□ In acute hepatitis B infection **F3.2, T3.14** serologic markers begin to emerge between 2 to 10 weeks following exposure. *HBsAg appears first,* followed

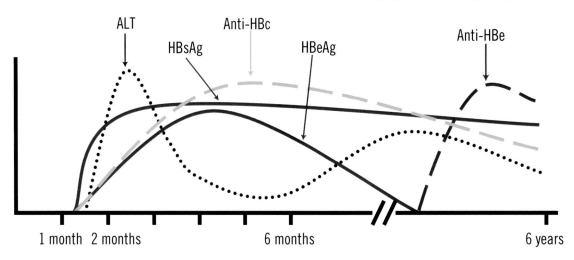

F3.3 Serologic patterns in acute HBV with development of chronic infection

Virology>Viruses

T3.14
HBV Serology

Clinical status	HBsAg	Anti-HBc	Anti-HBs
Neither prior infection nor immunization	–	–	–
Prior immunization	–	–	+
Acute HBV	+	+ (IgM)	–
Chronic HBV	+	+ (IgG)	–
Resolved HBV	–	+	+

by HBeAg and IgM anti-HBc. *HBV DNA is detectable in serum before HBsAg.* HBsAg becomes detectable before clinical symptoms appear. The development of antibodies (anti-HBs, anti-HBc) roughly coincides with the development of clinical symptoms. In the majority of patients, there is complete resolution of acute HBV infection. This is heralded by the emergence of anti-HBe and anti-HBs. Usually the latter developments somewhat follow the disappearance of HBsAg and HBeAg from serum. Anti-HBs therefore is indicative of resolved HBV hepatitis and implies life-long immunity.

□ With older less sensitive assays, there was a brief interval between disappearance of HBsAg and appearance of HBsAb, termed *the 'window' period.* The possibility of a false-negative serologic diagnosis of HBV infection existed during this period, unless IgM anti-HBc was measured. With present more sensitive assays, this window has narrowed considerably.

□ IgM anti-HBc emerges shortly after HBsAg and persists for many months. It is eventually replaced by *IgG anti-HBc, sometimes 18-24 months after infection.* Thus, IgG anti-HBc indicates past infection, either resolved (anti-HBs+) or in the chronic phase (HBsAg+). In patients who develop chronic HBV infection, IgM anti-HBc may re-emerge during acute flares.

□ There is a small group of patients who are found to *have only anti-HBc,* without HBsAg or anti-HBs. This may be seen in four scenarios: the **'window' period;** chronic HBV infection in which levels of HBsAg have fallen to undetectable levels; remote resolved HBV infection in which levels of anti-HBs have fallen to undetectable levels (common in HIV infection); and nonspecific false-positives. The presence of circulating HBV DNA in this setting is consistent with chronic HBV infection (with undetectably low HBsAg).

□ Chronic hepatitis B infection is defined by persistence of HBsAg after the acute phase (for more than 6 months) F3.3, T3.14. Persistent HBsAg without clinical hepatitis is called the chronic 'carrier' state. Chronicity develops in around 5% of healthy infected adults, 10% of immunocompromised adults, and up to *90% of neonates who have become infected transplacentally.* Chronic HBs antigenemia can be associated with polyarteritis nodosum (PAN). Hepatitis D virus (HDV) is capable of infecting hepatocytes with HBV DNA but not uninfected hepatocytes.

□ The HBV genome has several major gene regions: pre-S, S, C, P, and X. The pre-S genes encode the hepatocyte receptor–binding site. The S gene encodes surface antigen (HBsAg), a component of the viral envelope. The C gene encodes core antigen (HBcAg) and e antigen (HBeAg). The P gene encodes a DNA polymerase.

● The HBV genome can undergo mutation, altering the clinical features.

● One such mutation takes the form of so-called HBeAg-negative chronic hepatitis B. This is characterized by circulating HBV DNA, fluctuating aminotransferases, and a tendency towards fulminant hepatitis with liver failure. This form of hepatitis B results from mutations in the C or pre-C region, the most common mutation being an adenosine (A) for guanine (G) substitution at nucleotide position 1896 ($G_{1896}A$), leading to a premature stop codon that impairs synthesis of HBeAg.

- Mutations in the DNA polymerase gene often arise during treatment with lamivudine, resulting in decreased binding of lamivudine. These mutations may lead to abrupt progression of chronic hepatitis B in patients previously stable on treatment.

  □ Molecular assays

- There are three major applications of molecular assays in HBV: making the initial diagnosis of HBV, particularly when serology is equivocal; distinguishing replicative from nonreplicative chronic HBV infection; and monitoring therapy.

- With regard to diagnosis, HBV DNA can be detected approximately 3 weeks before HBsAg becomes detectable in serum. This lead-time is particularly useful to evaluate patients after an exposure (eg, a needle stick).

- The HBe antigen status is the traditional way to classify chronic HBV carriers as replicative or nonreplicative. Certain limitations in this approach—a tendency of HBe antigen to be undetectable in reactivation disease or to never appear in pre-core mutations—have made HBV DNA a more attractive analyte for this purpose. Currently, those with $>10^5$ copies of HBV DNA per mL are considered replicative.

- The response to therapy is monitored in several ways: (1) in the liver biopsy, a decrease in the histologic activity index (HAI) of ≥ 2 is considered a histologic response, (2) normalization of serum ALT is definitive of a biochemical

response, and (3) either a negative HBeAg or an undetectable HBV DNA level ($< 10^5$ copies/mL) is considered a virologic response.

- V of chronic HBV. Circulating HBV DNA can be found by PCR in a high percentage of patients with negative HBsAg and positive anti-HBs, anti-HBe, and anti-HBc. The significance of this is unclear at this time.

■ Hepatitis C virus (HCV)

□ HCV is an RNA virus from the Flavivirus family. It causes the vast majority of transfusion-associated viral hepatitis and the vast majority of what was previously called non-A, non-B hepatitis. About 55 to 85% people infected with HCV will develop chronic HCV infection. About 10-15% of those with chronic HCV will develop cirrhosis, usually after an illness of about 20 years. Those with cirrhosis due to HCV have a roughly 5% chance of developing hepatocellular carcinoma. The most powerful predictor of progression to cirrhosis is the finding of more-than-portal fibrosis (Ishak 3) on a liver biopsy. Extrahepatic manifestations of HCV infection include mixed cryoglobulinemia, glomerulonephritis, and aplastic anemia.

□ HCV infection has traditionally been diagnosed with EIA-based assays for anti-HCV antibodies, their presence indicative of infection. It is important to note that IgM and IgG anti-HCV cannot be reliably used to distinguish acute from chronic HCV infection; in fact, there is no reliable way to distinguish acute from chronic HCV infection and, for that matter, no compelling reason to do so. Most patients diagnosed with HCV, it is believed, are diagnosed with HCV in the chronic phase. The anti-HCV antibody test is now augmented by molecular assays for HCV RNA. While either a qualitative or quantitative HCV RNA test will suffice for this purpose, many clinicians request the quantitative test. Based upon these two assays, four sets of results are possible **T3.15**.

□ Chronic HCV develops in over 60% of infected patients. In some patients, the decision is made to treat, and the standard treatment presently is a combination of peginterferon alpha with ribavirin (PEGIFNa/RBV). The desired endpoint of treat-

T3.15
Possible Results of Hepatitis C Testing

Anti-	HCV	HCV RNA Interpretation
−	−	No infection
+	−	Probably not HCV infection; may represent recovery from acute HCV; retest for HCV RNA in several weeks
−	+	Probable early HCV infection; may also be seen rarely in chronic HCV infection, when patient is profoundly immunosuppressed, agammaglobulinemic, or on hemodialysis; retest for anti-HCV in several weeks
+	+	Infection

ment is a sustained virologic response (SVR), defined as undetectable HCV RNA *for a period of 24 weeks (6 months) after the end of treatment*. The most significant predictor of treatment response is the viral genotype: genotypes 2 and 3 have a high (70%) rate of response; genotype 1 has a low (40%) rate of response. Furthermore, the nature and duration of treatment is influenced by the genotype. The other genotypes—4 through 9—have not been sufficiently studied due to low prevalence.

☐ HCV genotyping may be performed on the basis of either molecular or serologic assays. The molecular assays involve direct sequencing of portions of the HCV genome (eg, the 5V noncoding region), hybridization with genotype-specific sequences, or RFLP analysis. Serologic assays detect serum antibodies against genotype-specific antigens. In the United States, the most common HCV genotype is 1 (about 80% of patients). Genotype 1 is further subdivided into 1a (about 60%) and 1b (about 20%), but to date, no significance has been assigned to these geno-subtypes. Genotype 2 represents about 20% of all infections, and genotype 3 about 5%.

☐ *Qualitative* assays for HCV RNA are based upon conventional PCR or transcription-mediated amplification (TMA) platforms. *Quantitative* assays for HCV RNA can be performed by real-time PCR (RT-PCR), transcription-mediated amplification (TMA), or branched DNA (bDNA). These techniques must be capable of detecting as little as 50 IU/mL, since this is the definition of a sustained virologic response. Furthermore, they must be equally sensitive to RNA from the different genotypes. The same testing platform should be used throughout treatment, since quantitative results are not directly comparable between methods.

☐ The liver biopsy remains important, particularly in making treatment decisions in patients infected with HCV genotype 1 or 4-9. Furthermore, the quantitative HCV RNA reflects neither the degree (grade) of hepatic inflammation nor the extent (stage) of hepatic fibrosis. And while HCV RNA is the best predictor of treatment response, it does not correlate, as histology does, with the likelihood of progressing to cirrhosis. Serial ALT measurements are only slightly better at predicting liver histology.

Most clinicians, therefore, continue to rely on the liver biopsy for assessing severity of liver disease, predicting prognosis, and deciding whether to treat.

■ **Hepatitis A virus (HAV)** is an RNA virus (a Picornavirus) that causes hepatitis usually associated with food-related outbreaks. It causes acute disease with relatively short incubation period, and chronicity is rare. However, a relapse of HAV occurs, usually proximate to the acute infection by no more than a few months, in around 5% of cases. Diagnosis of acute infection depends on demonstrating IgM anti-HAV which emerges early, slightly before the onset of symptoms. The presence of IgG anti-HAV may indicate acute or past infection, as it also emerges early but persists for life.

■ **Hepatitis E virus (HEV)** is an RNA virus with some clinical similarities to HAV: fecal-oral spread, rarely becomes chronic. Infection is rarely seen in the United states but is common in many pockets of the developing world, especially southeast Asia, northern Africa, and Mexico. HEV infection is more common in males, but it is more virulent in pregnant women, with a mortality rate approaching 30%. The diagnosis is made by detecting IgM anti-HEV in serum.

■ **Hepatitis G virus,** also called GBV-C virus, is an RNA virus belonging to the Flaviviridae family. Like HCV, it is transmitted by parenteral routes and leads to long-term chronic infection. Since its discovery, however, there has been no convincing evidence of its causing hepatitis. While the virus is present in 1-2% of the population and is known to infect hepatocytes for a very long time, it is not clear that it causes clinical disease.

■ Other viruses that cause hepatitis: EBV, CMV, HSV, yellow fever.

Orthomyxovirus

■ The virions have a lipid envelope containing several surface antigens. The dominant antigen is **hemagglutinin**. Hemagglutinin binds to sialic acid-containing receptors on respiratory epithelial cells and becomes expressed on the surface of infected cells. This expression forms the basis for the hemadsorption test. Only influenza A & B viruses and parainfluenza viruses are hemadsorption positive; such viruses are said to be "hemagglutinating viruses". Hemagglutinin (H) and neuraminidase (N) glycoprotein antigens form the basis for influenza virus identification (an isolate may be characterized H1N1, for example). H and N undergo periodic major antigenic changes and more frequent minor changes, while the other antigens are stable. Antigenic drift (minor changes) and shift (major changes) result in local annual outbreaks and worldwide outbreaks every 10 or 20 years, respectively. Currently, there are 15 H subtypes and 9 N subtypes. For the past several years, the major strains in circulation have been influenza A (H1N1), influenza A (H3N2), and influenza B. Birds, especially aquatic birds, serve as reservoirs for all subtypes.

- **Avian influenza** (H5N1) has been responsible for scattered pandemics in chickens, most recently in Southeast Asia. Hundreds of humans have become infected with H5N1, with a roughly 50% mortality rate. Unlike the more common influenza strains, H5N1 has affected predominantly children and young adults, with a median age of about 15 years. Infection rapidly produces patchy then diffuse lung opacity and an increased oxygen requirement; histologic findings of acute and organizing DAD have been found in autopsies. Lymphopenia is characteristic, without significant changes in the neutrophil count, erythrocytes, or platelets. The high mortality rate seems to be related to complete naivety to the H5 antigen and its tropism for non-ciliated epithelial cells of the lower respiratory tract. Tropism for the distal airways leads to an ARDS/DAD-like clinicopathologic picture and may explain the low rate of human-to-human transmission. Almost all human cases appear to result from exposure to sick birds (epizoonotic).

- **Influenza A** is more common than influenza B, and influenza A causes more serious disease. The influenza viruses cause annual outbreaks, usually during cold weather, with antigenic changes preventing the development of lifelong immunity. Influenza is usually heralded by the abrupt onset of fever, with myalgias, headache, sore throat and cough. Influenza B produces milder symptoms with a stronger gastrointestinal component, and characteristic features of calf myositis and ocular pain with movement. In the usual course of events, influenza resolves within 1 week; however, several complications may ensue: influenza pneumonia, secondary bacterial pneumonia (*S aureus*, *S pneumonia*, and *H influenza* most commonly), Reye syndrome,

myositis, myocarditis, and Guillain-Barre syndrome. Most deaths due to influenza are the result of secondary bacterial pneumonia.

- Diagnosis

  □ Culture is the gold standard diagnostic test, based upon a sample of nasopharyngeal secretions, sputum, or throat swabs. Conventional cell culture may require a week, but shell-vial techniques can provide a diagnosis within 2-3 days. The presence of virus in the culture may be confirmed by cytopathic effect, hemadsorption, immunofluorescent staining, or EIA.

  □ Direct fluorescent antibody (DFA) staining of nasopharyngeal secretions has a sensitivity of 80-90%. This test may also be performed on BAL fluid, sputum, or incubated cell-culture cells.

  □ Detection of influenza viral RNA can be performed using reverse transcriptase PCR. This can be done alone or as part of a multiplex PCR assay capable of detecting influenza A, influenza B, parainfluenza 1-3, and RSV.

  □ Serology can confirm influenza infection retrospectively, after study of acute and convalescent sera. The most commonly used serologic test to document influenza virus infection is hemagglutination inhibition (HI). This assay allows determination of the virus subtype and strain based upon specific antibodies.

- The treatment for severe cases of influenza A has been Amantadine (ineffective for influenza B). However, resistance is becoming widespread, and H5N1 strains appear to be resistant. Many resistant strains are susceptible to the neuraminidase inhibitors oseltamivir (Tamiflu) and zanamivir (Relenza).

Paramyxoviruses

- **Parainfluenza virus** 1 and 2 cause most cases of **croup** in children between the ages of 2 and 6, while parainfluenza virus 3 is the second most common cause (after RSV) of *respiratory bronchiolitis* ('viral pneumonia') in infants under age 2.

- **Measles (rubeola)** is the cause of classic measles, atypical measles (teenage patients who have received only one vaccination), and subacute sclerosing panencephalitis (SSPE). Measles is characterized by the classic prodrome of cough, coryza and conjunctivitis with or without Koplik spots followed by a descending rash beginning on the head. The most common complications of measles are **otitis media** (#1), pneumonia, myocarditis, and SSPE (rare). The first two of these complications are due to bacterial superinfection. *Appendicitis* may occur secondary to induced mesenteric adenitis or because of direct measles involvement of the appendix. Progressive fatal measles giant cell *pneumonia* occurs in immunocompromised hosts or in nutritionally deficient hosts. The characteristic histologic findings in lungs and appendices infected with measles virus include infected multinucleated cells with nuclear and cytoplasmic inclusions (Warthin-Finkledy giant cells). The risk of SSPE is approximately 0.001 % with a higher risk if measles is acquired at an early age, with an incubation period of 7 years. Vaccines have an SSPE risk of 0.0001 % with an incubation period of 3 years.

- **Mumps** virus causes parotitis, but only about 30% of affected individuals will have overt parotitis, 65% experience CSF pleocytosis, 10% will have clinical meningoencephalitis, 15% orchitis, and 5 % pancreatitis. 13 % of adults with mumps have myocarditis with S-T changes; some develop endocardial fibroelastosis.

- **Respiratory syncitial virus (RSV)** is the most common cause of lower respiratory tract infection (*pneumonia & respiratory bronchiolitis*) in infants and toddlers. RSV causes 90% of respiratory bronchiolitis in infants and almost half of lower respiratory tract infections in children. It is responsible for localized outbreaks, such as in day-care centers, where the attack rate can reach nearly 100%. Immunity to RSV is short-lived, and recurrence throughout childhood is the rule, though infections are progressively less severe with *bronchiolitis* uncommon after 12 months. RSV is also a cause of *croup*. Rapid diagnosis is important so that appropriate isolation precautions can be taken and so that aerosolized ribavirin can be initiated, the treatment of choice for severe RSV infection. Diagnosis can be made by rapid DFA or EIA techniques, performed on swab or secretions samples, or viral culture, with the highly characteristic formation of *syncytia in Hep2* cells. The difficulty in diagnosing RSV by culture is its

extreme fragility; specimen transport must be expeditious. Furthermore, RSV grows slowly in cell culture, often requiring over a week. Shell-vial techniques have ameliorated this somewhat. Nonetheless, as a result of these difficulties direct (DFA and EIA) techniques have proven as sensitive as culture for the diagnosis of RSV.

- **Metapneumovirus** is a recently identified virus that appears to be responsible for a significant proportion (up to 20%) of viral lower respiratory tract infections. It is capable of causing upper respiratory tract infections, lower respiratory tract infections (both bronchiolitis and pneumonia), and a flu-like illness. Growth has been slow on standard cell culture media, but both shell-vial techniques and RT-PCR offer more rapid diagnosis.

Picornaviruses (means small (pico-) RNA (rna) viruses).

- **Enteroviridae** (poliovirus, coxsackie A, coxsackie B, echovirus, enterovirus) enter the body via the GI tract. They are all capable of causing flu-like illness, gastroenteritis, and aseptic meningitis. Enteroviruses are the most common cause of *viral meningitis* (aseptic meningitis). RT-PCR is currently considered the gold standard for making the diagnosis of enterovirus in CSF. It demonstrates excellent sensitivity and same-day turnaround time. Cell culture should be performed as well, in case the PCR test is negative.

  □ **Poliovirus** causes the well-known neurologic infection based primarily upon destruction of spinal ventral horn motor neurons.

  □ **Coxsackie A** virus causes herpangina (painful oral infection) and hand-foot-mouth disease.

  □ **Coxsackie B** virus causes epidemic pleurodynia (the grippe), myocarditis, and pericarditis.

- **Rhinovirus** is considered the most common cause of the common cold. Culture is possible, but requires incubation at 32°C.

- **Hepatitis A** virus (Previously discussed).

Arboviruses. Viruses transmitted by arthropods were previously classified as arboviruses. They had in common a reservoir of mainly birds and the arthropod vector. Hence the name arthropod-borne (arbo) viruses. These viruses have now been dispersed into 4 families: bunya-, toga-, reo-, & rhabdoviruses. Not all the viruses within these families are arthropod-borne.

- **Family Bunyaviridae** includes hantaviruses (Sin Nombre, Black Creek, and Prospect Hill Hantaviruses), California encephalitis, and several hemorrhagic fever viruses (Crimean-Congo hemorrhagic fever virus, Rift Valley fever virus, LaCrosse virus).

  - □ **Hantavirus** is not acquired through an arthropod vector but rather through aerosolized rodent excreta. Hantavirus pulmonary syndrome consists of an often fatal (50%) acute respiratory failure characterized by histologic changes indistinguishable from diffuse alveolar damage.

  - □ **Hemorrhagic fever viruses** are numerous and not limited to the bunyavirus family. Not all hemorrhagic fever viruses are arboviruses. They share common manifestations including the sudden onset of fever, chills, severe epigastric pain, and the development of disseminated intravascular coagulation (DIC) with hemorrhagic manifestations. The hemorrhagic fever viruses are

    - ● **Bunyaviruses.** Crimean-Congo Hemorrhagic Fever (CCHF) virus, Rift Valley Fever virus, LaCrosse virus. Bunyaviruses are noteworthy for causing so-called hemorrhagic fever with renal syndrome (acute tubular necrosis).

    - ● **Togaviruses.** Flaviviruses (Dengue & Yellow Fever virus) and Togaviruses (Cikungunya virus)

    - ● **Arenaviruses.** Lassa fever virus

    - ● **Filoviruses.** Marburg & Ebola viruses

- **Family Togaviridae** includes the genus alphavirus (Eastern Equine, Western Equine, & Venezuelan encephalitis), flavivirus (St. Louis Encephalitis, dengue, yellow fever), and rubivirus (rubella virus). Most are agents of arthropod-borne encephalitis. Exceptions are yellow fever and rubella.

  - □ **Rubella virus** is biologically different from the others in this group. It is transmitted by person-to-person spread and causes a febrile illness with rash (German measles) which is only really consequential in pregnancy. *First-trimester infections* have the most serious fetal implications. Defects in first-trimester-infected neonates include sensorineural deafness, cataracts, glaucoma, microphthalmia, congenital heart disease (PDA), intrauterine growth retardation, and microcephaly. Hepatosplenomegaly, radiolucent bone lesions, and thrombocytopenia may occur. In affected adults, it is acquired by respiratory secretions and manifests as posterior cervical or suboccipital lymphadenopathy with a rash that first appears on the face and spreads down the body.

  - □ **Dengue & yellow fever** are transmitted by *Aedes aegypti* or *Aedes albopictus.* Dengue fever (breakbone fever) and yellow fever cause fever, chills, backache, jaundice, and hemorrhage in severe cases. Dengue hemorrhagic fever (DHF) is seen more commonly in children than adults and is more common after prior infection with another dengue virus serotype (of which there are 4). Yellow fever is viscerotropic for the heart, kidney, GIT, and liver. The most characteristic lesion of yellow fever is in the liver: extensive *midzonal* necrosis, Councilman bodies, microvesicular fatty metamorphosis, and absence of an inflammatory component.

- **Family Reoviridae** contains orbivirus and rotavirus. Rotavirus is the most common cause of viral gastroenteritis, other cases being due to Norwalk, enteric (serotypes 40 & 41) adenoviruses, calicivirus, and astrovirus.

- **Family Rhabdoviridae** includes rabies and vesicular stomatitis virus. In poorly controlled areas, dog and cats transmit 90% of rabies. In areas with good control of domestic rabies, most cases are the result of exposures to wolf, coyote, skunk, and raccoon. The histologic findings in the brain consist of **Negri bodies within Purkinje cells** of the cerebellum and hippocampus and Babes nodules, which are essentially microglial nodules. Antemortem diagnosis can be made by antigen detection in skin biopsy specimens from the nape of the neck.

Arenavirus. Lassa fever virus, Lymphocytic Choriomeningitis (LCM) virus, Machupo virus, & Sabia virus. Only LCM virus is located in the US. Virus particles contain host cell ribosomes in their interior, giving them a granular appearance. Arenaviruses are parasites of rodents which shed virus in their urine and feces—hamsters and house mice are the hosts to LCM virus. All have a viral prodrome followed by: hemorrhagic manifestations in all of them, hepatitis and myocarditis in Lassa fever, and meningitis in LCM.

Family Retroviridae comprises the human T-lymphotrophic viruses (HTLVs).

■ **HTLV-1**

  □ HTLV-1 is a retrovirus endemic in southern Japan, the Caribbean, southern Africa, and Brazil. There are pockets of relative prevalence in the southeastern United States. The virus is transmitted parenterally (iv drug use, transfusion, sexual contact) and transplacentally. Like HIV, the HTLV-1 virus infects CD4+ T lymphocytes. While acute infection may be asymptomatic, after a variably prolonged incubation period, the virus may cause neurologic or hematologic disease.

  □ Tropical spastic paraparesis (HTLV-1-associated myelopathy, Jamaican neuropathy) affects women infected with HTLV-1 about 3 times as often as men. The incubation period is much shorter than for ATLL, with some cases arising during acute infection. The disease tends to progress for 1-2 years then arrest, leaving affected individuals with a set of irreversible neurologic deficits. Histopathologically, demyelinating lesions are found in association with perivascular lymphocytic infiltrates, predominantly within the upper thoracic and lower cervical cord.

  □ Adult T-cell leukemia/lymphoma (ATLL) is the most common type of non-Hodgkin lymphoma in many HTLV-1-endemic parts of the world. The lifetime risk of ATLL is about 5% in people infected before the age of 20 years. The incubation period from the time of initial infection is 20-30 years. It presents with hepatosplenomegaly, jaundice, and weight loss. Peculiar features are hypercalcemia, a skin rash, high serum concentrations of free IL-2 receptor, and a pronounced sense of thirst. The neoplastic cells, having the characteristic "flower cell" morphology, express CD4 and CD25 (the IL-2 receptor).

  □ Diagnosis is similar to HIV—a screening ELISA followed by confirmatory Western blot or PCR. The proviral load (see below) appears to correlate with the likelihood of neurologic disease.

■ **HTLV-3 (HIV-1 & HIV-2)**

  □ **ELISA** is the principal method for HIV screening. The sensitivity for current HIV ELISA tests is > 99%. Anti-HIV antibodies are usually detectable within 6 to 8 weeks of infection; however, some patients seroconvert only after many months. So it is in these first weeks to months that most false negative ELISA tests occur (the window period). Because of passive transfer of maternal antibodies, the serologic diagnosis of neonatal HIV infection is not reliable. ELISA has suffered from insensitivity to HIV-2 and HIV-1 subtype O; however with recent improvements most, but not all, cases of HIV-2 and subtype O can be detected by current ELISA assays.

  □ Confirmatory testing is based generally on the **Western blot F3.4.** In this assay, a sample containing known HIV proteins is subjected to gel electrophoresis. The gel is then transferred (blotted) onto nitrocellulose paper, to which patient serum is added. After staining, visible bands reflect antibodies within the patients serum. The CDC has defined a positive HIV-1 Western blot as the presence of any two of the following bands: p24, gp41, gp120/160. If no bands are present, the test is considered negative. If one or more bands are present but not in a combination that meets criteria for positivity, then the test is considered indeterminate. The specificity of Western blot, when these criteria are rigorously applied, approaches 100%. Conventional Western blot results can give a false negative result in subtype O, and false-positive Western blots have been reported in hyperbilirubinemia; patients with HLA antibodies, autoantibodies, and polyclonal hypergammaglobulinemia. Patients who test as indeterminate should have a repeat test within 6 months. Those who are repeatedly indeterminate over 6 months and who have no risk factors can be considered negative. If there are risk factors and repeatedly indeterminate results, a nucleic acid-based test is advised.

□ The **p24 protein** is expressed very early in HIV infection, capable of reducing the width of the serologic 'window' by more than half. Serum p24 assays are based upon an antigen-capture ELISA platform, in which a solid substrate with attached anti-p24 antibody is washed over with patient sample (thus 'capturing' the p24). Enzyme-linked IgG is then added, and the reaction is measured colorimetrically. While the p24 assay has been used to diagnose pre-seroconversion HIV infection, the quantitative p24 level has been used for predicting prognosis (this has been supplanted by viral load testing).

□ The **CD4 count** has been used for some time to monitor disease progression. The count is determined by flow cytometry (see hematopathology chapter). Counts of circulating CD4+ T lymphocytes undergo pronounced diurnal variation, so specimens should be obtained at a consistent time of day. Furthermore, the CD4 count should be compared to age-appropriate reference ranges. Counts are monitored approximately every 6 months while the disease is stable and more frequently when treatment is being altered or there is illness. While CD4 counts are still instrumental in making treatment

decisions (eg, the decision to instigate PCP prophylaxis or define AIDS), the quantitative HIV RNA (viral load) is the preferred means of assessing response to anti-retroviral therapy.

□ **Detection of proviral DNA** can be used to confirm the diagnosis of HIV infection. Proviral DNA is the result of HIV RNA reverse transcription in to cDNA which then integrates into the host-cell genome. Its presence can be detected by PCR; however, the sensitivity of this assay is about 95% and the specificity 98%, both low by HIV-diagnosing standards.

□ **Quantification of circulating HIV RNA** (viral load) has become a mainstay in HIV management.

● Long-term outcome correlates extremely well with the viral load. The viral load has been found to be superior to the CD4 count for predicting disease progression; however, it appears that the combination of the two is superior to either in isolation. Furthermore, while viral load correlates very well with long-term (>10 years) prognosis, the CD4 count correlates better with short term

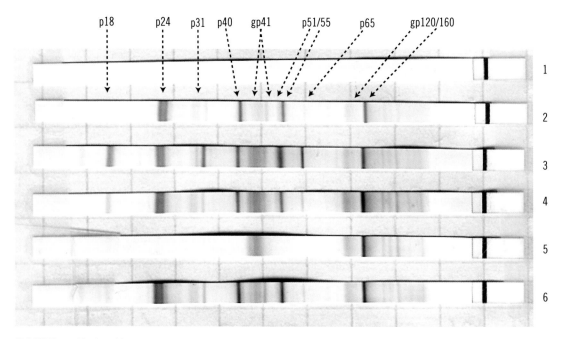

F3.4 HIV Western blot. Lane 1 is the negative control. Lane 2 is the weak positive control, and Lane 6 the strong positive control. Lanes 3-5 are patient samples testing positive.

(6 months) prognosis and susceptibility to infection.

- Transient increases in the quantitative HIV RNA (viral load) may occur following immune provocation; eg, following immunization. Up to a 0.3 log change can be attributed to nonspecific alteration in the quantitative HIV RNA; changes greater than 0.5 log are considered significant.

- The viral load is the primary variable used to determine when to initiate highly-active antiretroviral therapy (HAART), and it is the viral load that determines the efficacy of this treatment. The anticipated duration of viral suppression relate to both the rate of decline in viral load and the magnitude of the nadir.

- Three methods are currently available for measuring the HIV RNA (viral load): real-time PCR (RT-PCR), branched DNA (bDNA), and nucleic acid sequence-based amplification (NASBA). These methods have comparable analytic sensitivity and precision, but quantities cannot be directly compared between methods. An individual patient should be followed with a single method. In the RT-PCR assay, HIV-1 RNA and known standard RNA (a control of known copy number) compete for amplification within the same reaction chamber. First, the RNA is converted to cDNA by adding reverse transcriptase. Then a specific portion of the cDNA—within the gag gene—is amplified by PCR. Enzyme-linked oligonucleotide probes are added, one complementary for the HIV gag sequence and one for the RNA standard, and reaction product is measured. The ratio of reaction products determines the quantity of HIV RNA that is present. In the bDNA assay, complementary oligonucleotide is fixed to a solid substrate (microplate). The patient sample is added, capturing any HIV RNA present. Then a chemiluminescent enzyme-linked probes are added which are complementary to additional sequences of HIV RNA. The chemiluminescent signal is measured and compared to a known standard. The NASBA method is similar in concept to RT-PCR, except RNA is amplified instead of DNA.

□ *Detection of HIV infection shortly after a presumed* exposure may be very important, as there appears to be significant merit in the early administration of highly active antiretroviral therapy (HAART). Serology (ELISA and Western blot) are not useful in this setting, since antibodies do not reliably appear for many weeks. The p24 antigen seems to wane at various times during acute infection, leading to a suboptimal sensitivity of 89%. The best test in this setting may be HIV RNA quantification. HIV DNA detection may be just as good but has not been studied in the acute stage. The sensitivity of HIV RNA in acute infection is essentially 100%. However, the specificity is not 100%, and some false positives occur; as soon as feasible, a positive HIV RNA should be confirmed with ELISA and Western blot.

□ *Detection of HIV infection in neonates and infants* is sometimes difficult. ELISA and Western blot are not useful due to the persistence of transplacentally-acquired maternal antibodies. Furthermore, p24 antigen has a poor sensitivity in neonates and young infants, as low as 20% in the first month of life. PCR testing for HIV proviral DNA is the recommended test in this setting, but HIV RNA may be equally good. Umbilical cord blood should not be tested.

Parasitology

Laboratory Methods

- Parasites are usually not cultured, and diagnosis depends on direct examination. The use of an eyepiece micrometer is important, since the size of the observed forms is often key to identification.

- Both **wet mounts** and **stained slides** are examined. Wet mounts are good for looking for motile trophozoites and cyst forms. Detection of the latter is enhanced by adding a dilute iodide. General purpose stains include the trichrome, iron hematoxylin, and modified acid-fast stains. **Modified acid-fast stains may be positive in *cryptosporidium, cyclospora,* and *isospora.***

- **Genital pore injection.** Identification of *Taenia* spp is aided by injection of the genital pore with India ink to determine the uterine branching pattern. For example,

T solium has fewer than 13 lateral branches, *T saginatum* has more than 13, and *Dipylidium caninum* has two genital pores.

Specimens

- **Stool** This mainstay of parasitology requires the acquisition of semisolid to liquid stool, examination of direct wet mounts, stool concentration, and examination of permanent (fixed) stains. Three separately obtained specimens are required in order to exclude infection with any confidence. Specimens should be examined within 1 hour of collection, before disintegration of parasites can occur. Preservatives are available for specimens collected outside the hospital.

  □ The direct wet mount, wherein unconcentrated specimen is mixed with saline and examined, allows observation of motile organisms (protozoan trophozoites and helminth larvae).

  □ Concentration (by either sedimentation or flotation) enhances detection of protozoan cysts and helminth eggs.

  □ Fixed permanent stains are good for detection of protozoan trophozoites and cysts, the sensitivity of the aforementioned techniques being low for these forms. The most commonly used are the Wheatley trichrome and iron hematoxylin stains. Protozoa that are likely to be missed with these stains include: *Microsporidium, Cryptosporidium, Cyclospora,* and *Isospora*. The latter three require modified acid-fast stains (Kinyoun, DMSO, or

auramine-O), while *Microsporidium* may require direct examination of duodenal biopsies.

- **Duodenal Contents.** For the detection of duodenal infestation, such as *Giardia lamblia* or *Strongyloides stercoralis,* duodenal contents may need to be collected. For this purpose, there is the string technique, wherein one end of a string is swallowed; after several hours the string is pulled back, and the attached mucus is examined.

- **Cellophane tape.** Stool is a poor specimen for the detection of *Enterobius vermicularis* (pinworm). Instead, a strip of cellophane tape is applied to the perianal area before bedtime. As the adult worm migrates to the anus to deposit eggs during the night, some of the eggs will adhere to the tape. The tape can then be removed and applied to a slide for examination.

- **Blood Parasites** that may be detected in blood include: *Plasmodium* spp, *Babesia* spp, *Trypanosoma* spp, *Leishmania donovani,* and the microfilarial organisms (*Wuchereria bancrofti, Brugia malayi,* and *Loa loa*). Giemsa-stained thick and thin blood films are used to detect parasitemia. Thin films are the same as those used in routine blood smear review; thick films are prepared by concentrating blood is a small portion of the slide and lysing red cells. Thick films are good for screening, as they provide more blood per microscopic field; thin films are good for species identification. Sometimes buffy coat preparations are examined, particularly for the detection of *Leishmania donovani,* trypanosomes, and microfilariae. Identification of microfilariae in blood may require either filtration or concentration techniques.

T3.16
Amebae that Resemble *E histolytica*

Form	Characteristic	*E coli*	*E histolytica*	*E hartmanii*
Troph	Size	20-30 μm	20-30 μm	5-10 μm
	Motility	Nondirectional	Unidirectional	Unidirectional
	Ingested erythrocytes	Absent	Present	Absent
	Karyosome	Eccentric	Central	Central
	Nuclear chromatin	Clumped along nuclear membrane	Finely beaded along nuclear membrane	Finely beaded along nuclear membrane
Cyst	Nuclei	Up to 8	Never more than 4	Never more than 4
	Chromatoidal bars	Frayed ends	Rounded ends	Rounded ends

- **Sputum** may be examined for the detection of *Pneumocystis pneumoniae* or *Paragonimus westermanii*. In the case of pneumocystis, the yield from the examination of sputum is generally low and is only acceptably high in AIDS patients.

- CSF is examined in the case of suspected amebic encephalitis.

Serology has a limited role in parasitology. It can be useful to detect recent toxoplasmosis infection. It is mainly used for epidemiologic purposes.

Protozoa

Amebae (Sarcodinia) F3.5. *Unicellular organisms that are motile by pseudopodal extension.*

- **Intestinal amebae**

  □ ***Entamoeba histolytica*** is the primary pathogen in this group. Most others are nonpathogenic for humans but must be distinguished from it, particularly *E coli* and *E hartmanii,* its closest mimics. Features that distinguish these organisms are detailed in **T3.16**.

    - *E histolytica* trophozoites measure around 25 μm. **The nucleus is absolutely key for identification and is characterized by a small, central karyosome and finely beaded heterochromatin which is applied evenly to the inner nuclear membrane.** The cytoplasm may contain ingested red cells. Under direct examination in wet mounts, the trophozoites display progressive **unidirectional** motility. **Cyst** forms have up to (and no more than) **4 nuclei** and chromatoidal bodies with **smooth, rounded, ends.**

  - *E histolytica* is acquired through ingestion of cysts in contaminated food or water. Its distribution is worldwide. It is the main cause of intestinal amebiasis, a syndrome of protracted diarrhea due to infestation of the **colon.** It may lead to extraintestinal manifestations such as amebic abscess within the liver (**most common site of extraintestinal amebiasis**), spleen, or brain. Amebic abscesses are described as containing **anchovy paste**-like material. The lesion of intestinal amebiasis is the 'flask-shaped' ulcer in the colon, usually the **cecum.** Protracted infection may eventually lead to a napkin-ring lesion (ameboma) mimicking colonic adenocarcinoma.

- ***Entamoeba coli.*** The main features permitting distinction of *E coli* from *E histolytica* are its nondirectional motility, eccentric karyosome, clumped nuclear chromatin, frayed (splintered) chromatoidal bodies, and the presence of up to 8 nuclei in cyst forms. Furthermore, *E coli* trophs do not contain ingested red cells.

  □ ***Entamoeba hartmanii.*** This organism closely resembles *E histolytica*. The main feature distinguishing *E hartmanii* from *E histolytica* is its small size (5-10 μm).

  □ ***Entamoeba nana.*** *E nana* is easily recognized by its large knobby 'ball & socket' central karyosome. The cyst form has the same nuclei and lacks chromatoidal bodies.

  □ ***Iodamoeba butschlii.*** The quickest way to recognize *I butschlii* is the cyst's prominent iodine-staining vacuole. The trophozoite and cyst form, like *E nana,* have a large 'ball & socket' central karyosome, but the nuclear membrane is inconspicuous.

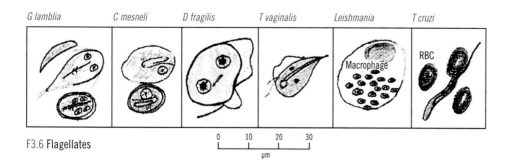

F3.6 Flagellates

■ Free-living amebae

□ *Naegleria fowleri*

- Its **trophozoites**, which can be found in CSF obtained by spinal tap or in perivascular locations in histologic sections of brain tissue, appear as typical amoebae with a central nuclear karyosome. The organism can be cultured on a lawn of inactivated *Escherichia coli*. A visible trail formed when the ameba moves across the plate ingesting the *E coli* is confirmatory.

- infection with this organism is associated with a classic history: fatal meningoencephalitis arising in children who have been swimming or diving in fresh-water pools. The organism infects the frontal lobe via the cribriform plate, and the infection is usually fatal within a matter of days.

- *Acanthamoeba* is the cause of **granulomatous amebic encephalitis (GAE)** and contact lens-associated **acanthamoebic keratitis.**

Flagellates (Mastigophora) (F3.6)

■ *Giardia lamblia*

□ *Giardia* **trophozoites** may be seen in stool specimens or small bowel biopsies. When viewed from the top, they are **kite-shaped** (or tear drop or pear-shaped) organisms that have a central axostyle running along their length. The flagella are not easily seen. From the side, the organisms are comma-shaped (or spoon-shaped). The cyst forms are oval, thick-walled, structures with **4 nuclei located along a central axostyle.** In wet mounts, the troph demonstrates a characteristic **falling-leaf** motility. In stool samples, *G lamblia* must be distinguished from nonpathogenic *Chilomastix mesnili*.

□ *Giardia* is the most common cause of protozoal gastroenteritis. It is particularly common in the Colorado Rocky Mountains, Leningrad, and Moscow. Infection is associated with day-care centers & backcountry hiking.

■ *Chilomastix mesnili* is a nonpathogenic organism that lacks an obvious central axostyle, has rotary motion, and has only anteriorly located flagella. The cyst form

has a **single** nucleus located adjacent to a **safety pin**-shaped structure.

■ *Dientamoeba fragilis.* These trophozoites appear as a round binucleate structure whose nuclei have a '**fractured'** (fragile) central karyosome. Another characteristic feature is the single flagellum which appears attached to the wall of the organism at several points. It is an occasional cause of diarrhea and anal pruritus, particularly in children. *Dientamoeba* and *Enterobius* (pinworm) co-infection is common.

■ *Trichomonas vaginalis.* Another vaguely pear-shaped organism which has a 2 nuclei located at the **anterior end** of a central axostyle. It characteristically has an **undulating membrane** that extends about halfway down the organism. *Trichomonas hominis* is a nonpathogenic organism that has a single nucleus located at the anterior end of a central axostyle. It has an undulating membrane that extends along the top of and all the way down the organism.

■ *Leishmania* spp

□ The organism can only be diagnosed by biopsy of infected tissue, most often skin or marrow. Careful scrutiny of smears or sections from infected tissue reveal multiple tiny 2-5 μm intracellular amastigotes within histiocytes T3.17. The amastigote is the stage that lacks an external flagellum, proliferates exclusively intracellularly, and is the only form seen in the human host. The organisms are visible in H&E or Giemsa stains as oval structures with a nucleus adjacent to the distinct transverse bar-like kinetoplast. While other small intracellular organisms must be considered in the morphologic differential diagnosis (histoplasmosis, toxoplasmosis, leishmaniasis), only *Leishmania* spp share the finding of a kinetoplast. The organism may be cultured

T3.17 Differential Diagnosis for Multiple Tiny 2-5 μm Organisms within Histiocytes

Organism	Comment
Leishmania	Kinetoplast
Histoplasma capsulatum	Budding
Toxoplasma	Somewhat curved, mostly extracellular
Trypanasoma cruzi	Kinetoplast

on Novy-MacNeal-Nicolle medium. Culture is significantly more sensitive than visual detection and permits species identification. In culture (as well as within insect vectors), the promastigote form is observed.

☐ Acquired from the sandfly (genuses *Phlebotomus* and *Lutzomyia*). The resulting clinical disease varies with species as follows.

- Old-world leishmaniasis, associated with *L tropica, L major,* and *L aethiopica,* most often results in a solitary cutaneous lesion (oriental sore) that is self-limiting. *L aethiopica* may disseminate to other cutaneous sites, producing multiple lesions. Old-world cutaneous leishmaniasis is seen principally around the Mediterranean (southern Europe, northern Africa, Middle East), and it was seen in troops returning from deployment in Kuwait. In this latter setting, the visceral dissemination was often noted.

- Old-world leishmania is usually caused by *L donovani* which results in widespread systemic disease (visceral leishmaniasis or kala azar) associated with hepatosplenomegaly and bone marrow infection. *L donovani* infections are found in Africa, India, Asia, and the Middle East. Furthermore, some cases of cutaneous leishmaniasis may disseminate (*L aethiopica*, for example, is prone to this complication).

- New-world leishmania, caused most often by *L mexicana,* also leads to a self-limiting solitary cutaneous lesion (chiclero ulcer of the ear lobe). This disease is seen in South America and in localized parts of Texas.

- New-world leishmaniasis caused by *L braziliensis* leads to a form of disease known as mucocutaneous leishmaniasis, characterized by persistent cutaneous and mucosal lesions. This form of disease is seen in South and Central America.

■ *Trypanasoma* spp

☐ Trypomastigotes can be found in the peripheral blood. In African trypanosomiasis, they may also be found in lymph node aspirates or cerebrospinal fluid. In American trypanosomiasis, they may be seen in aspirates of chagomas, lymph nodes, or infected tissue. Those of *T cruzi* measure about 20 μm and are C- or S-shaped. Those of *T brucei* appear as 30 μm delicately curved structures with an undulating flagellum that is attached along its length, ending in a whip-like tail. A roughly central kinetoplast is usually evident, larger in *T cruzi* than *T brucei*. Finding peripheral blood trypomastigotes is more common in the acute phase than in chronic infection and can be aided by examination of the buffy coat. In chronic infection, tissue biopsy may be necessary. The organism can be cultured on Novy-MacNeal-Nicolle medium.

☐ *T. cruzi* is the cause of Chagas disease (American trypanosomiasis), which is a leading cause of congestive *heart failure* in South and Central America. It can also infect the muscularis of the distal esophagus, resulting in *achalasia*. It is acquired from the reduviid (kissing) bug, whose inoculation site (Chagoma), when present about the eye, is called Romaña sign.

☐ *T. brucei* is the cause of African sleeping sickness (African trypanosomiasis), which is an acute febrile illness often resulting in death. It is acquired from the tsetse (glossina) fly. Cases in eastern Africa are associated with *T brucei rhodesiense,* and cases in western Africa are associated with *T brucei gambiense.*

Ciliates (*Ciliophora*). There is only one ciliate to know: *Balantidium coli* **F3.7**. Anytime you see an organism with cilia uniformly covering its surface, it is probably the trophozoite of *B coli*. It measures approximately 50 to 70 μm and has a kidney bean-shaped macronucleolus. The cyst form has cilia that can be seen beneath the outer cyst wall, measures 40 to 60 μm, and has the characteristic kidney bean-shaped macronucleolus.

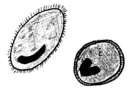

F3.7 *Balantidium coli*

Coccidia (Sporozoa) F3.8

- **Cryptosporidium parvum.** In small intestinal biopsies, *cryptosporidium* is recognized as dome-shaped, 8 to 15 µm, basophilic structures that appear to be adherent to the enterocyte brush border. In actuality, the organism is located within an apical vacuole and is actually intracellular. In stool samples, the *weakly acid-fast eggs* appear as fairly non-descript 5 micron oval structures. Like *I belli, Cryptosporidium* is a major cause of protracted diarrhea in immunocompromised hosts, especially those with AIDS. In developed countries, cryptosporidium is responsible for about 2% of diarrheal illness in immunocompetent persons; about 15% in AIDS. In developing countries, it causes about 10% of cases in immunocompetent persons, and about 25% in AIDS. *Cryptosporidium* may also ascend the biliary tree to cause strictures.

- **Isospora belli.** In small intestinal biopsies, *Isospora* appears as thin elliptical structures interposed between adjacent enterocytes. In stool samples, the weakly acid-fast eggs measure 15 to 30 µm in length, 2 to 5 µm in width, and appear as elliptical structures with one (unsporulated) or two (sporulated) sporocysts.

- **Microsporidium** (*Enterocytozoon bieneusi* & *Septata intestinalis*). In small intestinal biopsies, microsporidia appear as numerous tiny intracellular organisms within the apical aspect of enterocytes. Definitive diagnosis in biopsy specimens required electron microscopy. In stool samples, 1 to 1.5 µm spores may be found in the trichrome stain.

- **Cyclospora** (*Cyclospora cayetanensis*). Infection with this recently recognized organism is seen only during certain months of the year, essentially disappearing in-between these times. It is found principally in Nepal, Peru, Haiti, and Guatemala. The organism appears to be acquired from ingestion of contaminated fruit and leafy vegetables. It infects the small bowel and produces a highly characteristic syndrome: several days of fever accompanied by severe, watery, diarrhea, followed by an extended period of anorexia and fatigue associated with significant weight loss. Small bowel biopsies show active inflammation. The organisms appear in biopsies or concentrated stool as 8 micron spheres that are *acid-fast* by modified techniques (Kinyoun) and auto-fluorescent.

- **Sarcocystis** appear as hour glass-shaped eggs with two sporocysts. Acquired from beef or pork, *Sarcocystis* leads to self-limited gastroenteritis in humans.

- **Toxoplasma gondii**

  □ The diagnostic forms are found in imprints and sections of infected tissue such as brain, heart, retina, or lymphoreticular tissue. The **tachyzoite** is a small, curved, 3 to 5 µm, free (extracellular) form of the organism. When numerous organisms are packed into the cytoplasm of a histiocyte, this pseudocyst form of the organism is called a **bradyzoite** and must be distinguished from other small intracellular organisms (histoplasmosis, leishmaniasis, trypanosomiasis). Giemsa is good for demonstrating the organism in tissue. PCR has proven extremely useful in the diagnosis of CNS and systemic infections. Serology, based usually upon an EIA platform, is the most common way to make the diagnosis of toxoplasmosis. Anti-toxo IgM establishes the diagnosis of congenital and acute infection, but false-positive reactions and a tendency for IgM to persist for months limit the specificity. Since exposure to toxoplasma is widespread, anti-toxo IgG is very common. Still, rising or very high (>1:1024) IgG titers suggest recent infection. Furthermore, the presence of low-level IgG suggests prior infection

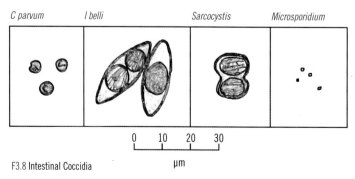

F3.8 Intestinal Coccidia

and suggests that a pregnant woman is at little risk the neonatal complications of a new infection.

☐ The cat is the definitive host. Infection is acquired through ingestion of material contaminated with cat feces containing eggs.

☐ The recently infected child or adult may develop a mononucleosis-like syndrome characterized by fever and posterior cervical lymphadenopathy.

☐ About 15% of women of childbearing age have been previously infected with toxoplasmosis. Prior infection can be confirmed by serology for IgG against *T gondii*. These gestations are safe from intrauterine toxoplasmosis infection. When primary infection is acquired during pregnancy, there may be transplacental spread. When maternal infection occurs *in the first trimester, there is a risk of fetal loss. If infection occurs in late pregnancy, there is a risk of fetal CNS infection.* CNS infection centers around the retina and ventricles, with the residual effect of periventricular calcification and chorioretinitis.

☐ Immunocompromised patients are at great risk for CNS toxoplasmosis.

■ *Plasmodium* spp (malaria)

☐ There are four major species that cause malaria: *P falciparum, P vivax, P ovale,* & *P malariae.* All are spread by the anopheline mosquito. Malaria infection presents with fever, anemia, and splenomegaly. The symptoms tend to be paroxysmal, with an individual paroxysm lasting 6-12 hours, correlating with intermittent intravascular hemolysis. A paroxysm begins with shaking chills, followed by high fever, followed by profuse sweating and defervescence. Hemosiderinuria and hemoglobinuria are the reason for the appellation 'blackwater fever'. Some clinical features are species-specific:

● Fever spikes every 48 hours (tertian fever) characterize *P ovale, P vivax,* and *P falciparum.*

● *P malariae* produces febrile spikes every 72 hours (quartan fever).

● Due to its lethality and every other day fever, *P falciparum* is also called 'malignant tertian malaria.' *P vivax* & *P ovale* are known as 'benign tertian malaria.'

● Nephrotic syndrome is associated with *P malariae.*

● CNS involvement is associated with *P falciparum.*

● True disease relapse is seen only with *P vivax* & *P ovale.*

● Recrudescence is possible with any of the species.

● *P vivax* and *P ovale* infect younger erythrocytes. This is the reason infected erythrocytes appear enlarged. *P malariae* infects older erythrocytes, and *P falciparum* infects any erythrocyte.

☐ After a mosquito obtains blood from an infected host, the time required for the organism to mature into an infective (sporozoite) form is 8-21 days. The sporozoites injected into a host by the sting of a mosquito go directly to the liver where they proliferate (this phase is called exoerythrocytic schizogony), rupture, and release of merozoites into the bloodstream. These infect red cells to initiate the phase of erythrocytic schizogony. True disease *relapse* (*P vivax* and *ovale*) results from the harboring of latent sporozoites (called hypnozoites) within the liver. *Recrudescence* (*P falciparum* and *malariae*) results from a rebound of persisting (though depleted to levels that are undetectable) blood forms to clinically detectable levels. Neither transfusion-transmitted infection nor transplacental infection is associated with relapse, no matter what organism is involved.

☐ Malaria is largely confined to that part of the globe located between latitudes 45 degrees North and 40 degrees South. All except *P ovale* are widely distributed, with most cases of *P ovale* being located in western Africa.

☐ Certain host features may confer a degree of protection:

● Hemoglobin S trait (HbSA) is protective against *P falciparum.*

- Duffy blood group antigens mediate attachment of *P vivax*. Duffy negative individuals are protected from *P vivax*.

- Glucose-6-phosphate dehydrogenase (G6PD) deficiency protects against all *Plasmodium* spp.

▢ Malaria is diagnosed **T3.18** by examination of peripheral blood films, where red cells infected with the organisms can be found. The ideal time to obtain a specimen is immediately preceding the next anticipated fever spike. There are several forms of the organism:

- **Trophozoites** (ring forms), are the most numerous form to be seen in peripheral blood films and consist of a ring like structure, occupying <½ the red cell, with 1 or at most 2 nuclei. The trophozoite is the growing form of the organism. Early ring forms are tiny, and they become progressively enlarged and amoeboid as they mature, eventually developing into a schizont.

- Any mononuclear structure occupying >½ the red cell is a **gametocyte,** which is usually a large amoeboid structure that nearly fills the entire erythrocyte. All mature stages of the organism may be associated with hematin pigment, not seen in immature organisms (ring forms), found within the structure of the organism. This is distinct from Schüffner stippling, which is seen within the red cell, outside the organism.

- Multinuclear structures are **schizonts,** which usually appear as intra-erythrocytic wads of several (number depends on species) **merozoites,** each with its own nucleus. The schizont eventually ruptures the cell, releasing merozoites and beginning a new cycle.

▢ *P falciparum* is potentially lethal and must be identified when present. To do this, know these morphologic features of *P falciparum* malaria

- Only early ring forms and gametocytes are usually seen within peripheral blood erythrocytes

- Ring forms may have double chromatin dots

- Multiple ring forms may be seen in a single erythrocyte

- Accolé, marginal, or appliqué forms may be seen

- Schizonts and developing (enlarging) ring forms are not usually seen

- Gametocytes are banana-shaped

- Infected red cells are not enlarged when compared to uninfected cells in the same smear. If these features are seen in the blood smear, alert the clinician that you suspect *P falciparum*

▢ *P vivax* and *P ovale* are morphologically very similar to one another, and the distinction of between them is not of major importance. *P ovale* is fairly rare, it being confined to limited regions of Western Africa. The morphologic features of *P vivax /ovale* are

- Infected erythrocytes are slightly enlarged compared to uninfected erythrocytes in the same smear

- Schüffner dots may be present

- All stages of developing organism are seen—early rings, developing (enlarging) rings, schizonts, gametocytes

- Gametocytes are amoeboid in shape, **not** banana-shaped

- Schizonts have 12 to 14 nuclei

- *P ovale* is associated with fimbriated erythrocytes

▢ *P malariae* has the following features

- Infected erythrocytes are not enlarged

- No Schüffner dots

- All stages of developing organism are seen

- Schizonts have 6-12 nuclei

- Coarse malarial pigment may be present

T3.18
Features of the Plasmodia Species

Species	Stages	Size of infected red cell	Shüffner stippling	Troph	Gametocyte	Hematin pigment	Number of nuclei in schizont
P falciparum	Rings forms, gametocytes	Normal	Absent	Smallest, sometimes multiple, sometimes marginal (appliqué), often a double chromatin dot	Crescent-shaped banana body	Black	Rarely seen
P malariae	All	Normal	Absent	Small, dense cytoplasm, rare band froms	Rounded	Dark brown	6-12 (Average 8)
P vivax	All	Enlarged	Present	Small, some may become ameboid	Rounded	Light brown	12-24 (Average 16)
P ovale	All	Enlarged, some oval and fimbriated	Present	Small, some with large chromatin mass	Rounded	Dark brown	6-14 (Average 8)

- Occasional **band form** trophozoites are seen

  □ Mixed infections are encountered in up to 5% of cases, most often due to mixed *P falciparum* and *P vivax.*

■ *Babesia microti*

  □ Trophozoites (ring forms) are usually multiple within red cells in peripheral blood, often forming **tetrads** or Maltese cross arrangements. Unlike malaria, extraerythrocytic ring forms are present, and neither pigment, schizonts, nor gametocytes are seen.

  □ Most cases, particularly those in the Eastern US where it is most common, are caused by *B microti.* Some are caused by by Babesia WA-1 (Western US) and Babesia divergens (Europe).

  □ The organism is acquired from the tick *Ixodes dammini* (same as Lyme disease) in the Eastern US, *Ixodes pacificus* in the Western US, and *Ixodes ricinus* in Europe.

  □ Infection results in a **nonperiodic** fever and hemolysis. The severity varies, and fatal disease may be seen in splenectomized or immunodeficient individuals. In addition to hemolytic anemia, leukopenia and abnormal liver function tests are characteristic findings. **Coinfection with flavivirus and Lyme disease is common.**

■ *Pneumocystis carinii*

  □ **Diagnostic forms.** The **trophozoites** may be found in lung sections, bronchoalveolar lavage specimens, or sputum. They appear as 5 to 8 μm **concave discs** when their walls are stained with GMS, but in Wright-Giemsa, which does not stain the wall, they appear as 2 to 5 μm structures with a negatively staining space around them. In H&E or Pap stains, the organisms are not seen at all, but there is a characteristic **'frothy' exudate** which suggests the organisms presence.

  □ Acquired by airborne dissemination. Currently the organism primarily affects immunocompromised hosts, particularly AIDS patients, in whom PCP continues to be the most common AIDS-defining illness. It causes pneumonia with bilateral (butterfly) pulmonary infiltrates. Uncommonly, extrapulmonary infection can be seen. Historically, mainly in malnourished adults, the infection has been associated with a plasma cell pneumonitis.

Metazoa

Nematodes (round worms) (F3.9)

■ *Trichuris trichiura* (whipworm)

  □ The **adult** worm measures up to 5 cm and has a **whip-like anterior end.** The male has a coil posteriorly. The **egg** is brownish and looks like a **barrel with corks** at both ends.

□Infection results from ingestion of eggs and causes intestinal (cecal) infestation which may be asymptomatic. Some cases present with dysentery-like manifestations, and heavy infestations may produce **rectal prolapse** in young children. Dual infection with *Ascaris lumbricoides* may be seen.

■ *Ascaris lumbricoides*

□The **adult worm** is characterized by being **really** big: up to 35 cm. The male has a terminal curvature which the female lacks. In feces, the egg is around 60 μm, **bile-stained,** and its thick hyaline shell has a **rough, mammillated, exterior.** Those that have lost the external mammillated shell (decorticate eggs) may resemble hookworm eggs.

□Infection results from ingestion of eggs which hatch in the intestine, giving rise to larvae that penetrate the mucosa and enter the bloodstream to be carried to the lungs. There, they mature, are expectorated and swallowed, eventually to infest the duodenum. During migration through the lung, the larvae may provoke a Loeffler syndrome (transient pulmonary infiltrates with eosinophilia). Duodenal infestation may be asymptomatic or result in abdominal discomfort, obstruction, cholangitis, or appendicitis. Typically, worms inhabit the bowel for around 1 year then are spontaneously expelled.

■ *Necatur americanus* & *Ancylostoma duodenale* (Hookworms)

□Adult hookworms measure about a cm in length. The **mouthparts** of the two hookworms differ: *N americanus* has **cutting plates;** *A duodenale* has **teeth.** The side-view of both hookworm larvae look essentially the same. They also look similar to *S stercoralis* larvae but are distinguished by having a **long buccal cavity** and **indistinct genital primordium.** In feces, the **eggs** of these two hookworms are indistinguishable from one another and from the eggs of *S stercoralis*. They have a thin translucent wall that encloses a morula-like cluster of several spherical embryos.

□The largest number of infections worldwide are found in Asia and sub-Saharan Africa. Coastal regions are the preferred location for this organism,

since larvae enjoy the sandy soil. *N americanus* can be found in the United States. *A duodenale* does not occur in the United States. Infection results from penetration of skin by larvae. Often this takes place in the feet, resulting in a localized pruritic lesion (ground itch). The larvae enter the circulation, trespass the lungs (sometimes associated with Loeffler syndrome), are expectorated and swallowed. Intestinal (small bowel) infestation may persist for years, often leading to **iron deficiency anemia.** *Ancylostoma braziliense* is a zoonotic hookworm that, rather than proceeding through skin into the circulation, results in cutaneous larva migrans.

■ *Strongyloides stercoralis*

□Adult females measure about 3 mm and can be found burrowed into the intestinal crypts. The **egg** is identical to the hookworm egg but is not usually found in stool; instead, eggs hatch in the bowel, and the organism appears in feces as rhabditoid larvae.

□The **larvae** are very similar to hookworm larvae but have a **short buccal groove** and **prominent genital primordium.**

□Duodenal aspirates or string test specimens may be helpful when stool examination is negative.

□In addition to being found in many tropical and subtropical regions throughout the world, *S stercoralis* is found in the southeastern US.

□Infection results from penetration of skin, often the feet, by larvae. These circulate to and migrate through the lungs, a trespass often associated with Loeffler syndrome. Intestinal (duodenal) infestation results from swallowing larvae. These mature into adult females that burrow into the intestinal crypts and begin to produce eggs. The eggs hatch within the small intestine, and mature into rhabditoid larvae which are passed into stool (eggs are usually not seen in stool). Rhabditoid larvae mature in the environment into filariform larvae capable of penetrating skin.

□In some instances, particularly in a weakened (eg, malnourished) host, larvae mature into infective forms while still within the bowel; these are capable of penetrating the bowel wall,

Parasitology>Metazoa

T3.19
Filaria

Organism	Sheath	Tail nuclei	Periodicity of microfilariae in blood	Adult found in
Wuchereria bancrofti	+	None	Nocturnal	Lymphatics
Brugia malayi	+	2 discontinuous	Nocturnal	Lymphatics
Loa loa	+	Continuous row	Diurnal	Subcutis
Mansonella perstans	−	Continuous row	None	Body cavities
Onchocerca volvulus	−	None	Not found in blood	Subcutis

circulating through the lungs and re-infecting the duodenum, a condition called **autoinfection.** Autoinfection results in long-term carriage, a state that is often asymptomatic or characterized by persistent eosinophilia, and sometimes by the formation of linear urticaria (larva currens). However, in immunocompromised hosts, autoinfection can lead to *hyperinfection,* a deadly complication in which larvae penetrate the bowel wall and disseminate widely via the bloodstream. Hyperinfection often presents as pneumonia with gastroenteritis and sepsis.

■ *Enterobius vermicularis* (pinworm, oxyuriasis) **T3.19**

◻ The **adult worm has a bent & pointed (pin-like) tail.** In cross sections, such as may be seen in histologic sections of bowel, the adult worm has characteristic **lateral alae.** The **egg** is characterized as a thin-walled 30 to 50 µm oval with one side flattened. The egg is **not** routinely found in stool specimens, necessitating a **cellophane tape test.**

◻ Pinworm is the most common helminthic infection in American children. Infection is acquired from ingestion of eggs and results in intestinal (cecal) infestation. Nocturnal migration of the adult to lay eggs in the perianal region may result in a clinical presentation of nocturnal anal pruritus, vaginitis, and/or enuresis. Appendicitis (look for cross sections of adult worms with lateral alae in appendectomies) is an occasional complication.

■ **Filaria**

◻ **Microfilaria,** usually found in peripheral blood, are the diagnostic forms of this group of organisms. The presence or absence of a sheath and the pattern of nuclei in the tail are the main features which allow distinction of the various species **T3.19, F3.10**.

◻ Microfilaria that can be found in blood

● *W bancrofti* and *B malayi* are acquired through the bite of a mosquito.

● *Loa loa* is acquired from the mango (*Chrysops*) fly.

● Both *W bancrofti* and *B malayi* infest the lymphatics, leading to lymphadenitis and lymphedema (elephantiasis).

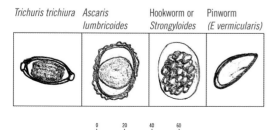

F3.9 Nematode eggs

Trichuris trichiura *Ascaris lumbricoides* Hookworm or *Strongyloides* Pinworm (*E vermicularis*)

Wuchereria bancrofti *Brugia malayi* *Loa loa* *Mansonella perstans* *Onchocerca volvulus*

F3.10 Microfilaria

- *Loa loa* inhabits subcutaneous and conjunctival locations.

- All are shed into and can be found in the blood at periodic intervals, especially at night (blood should be drawn between 2 and 4 am).

  □ Microfilaria not found in blood

  - *M perstans* is acquired from the biting midge (*Culicoides*) and inhabits body cavities such as the pleura.

  - *O volvulus* is acquired from the *Simulium* black fly and infects subcutaneous and conjunctival locations, leading to the formation of nodules and/or blindness. Microfilariae, rather than circulating in the blood, migrate continuously through the skin and eye, resulting in dermatitis, keratitis, and corneal opacity. It is the leading cause of blindness in Central Africa and parts of Central America.

  - *Dirofilaria immitis* is acquired from a mosquito and infects the lungs, where the organisms are found in granulomatous nodules.

- **Trichinella spiralis**

  □ Encysted larvae seen on histologic sections of infected skeletal muscle are typically spiraled.

□ Acquired by consumption of undercooked infected pork. Results in infection of the skeletal muscle by encysted larvae, leading to myositis and weakness.

- **Toxocara canis & cati**

  □ The organism is rarely provided or recovered for examination. Diagnosis is usually clinical with or without serology.

  □ *T canis* and, to a lesser extent, *T cati* are the principle causes of visceral larva migrans (VLM) and ocular larva migrans (OLM). The syndrome typically affects children who ingest soil contaminated with cat or dog feces. The organism, incapable of completing its life cycle in humans, wanders throughout various organs. This produces a syndrome of hypereosinophilia, hepatosplenomegaly, and pneumonitis.

- **Anisakiasis** is acquired from ingestion of raw fish such as sushi. The organism penetrates the GI tract and sets up permanent residence in the bowel wall. Endoscopic biopsy may disclose an eosinophil-rich granuloma containing the nematode.

Trematodes (*flukes*) T3.20, F3.11

- **Fasciola hepatica**

  □ The **adult** is a flattened worm with a cephalic cone that distinguishes it from *F buskii*. At 100 to 150 μm, the **egg** is about the largest seen in human parasitology. It is oval with a thin shell and an unshouldered operculum (which resembles a hatch door). The egg is identical to that of *F buskii*.

T3.20
Operculated Eggs

Organism	Shoulder	Size (μm)	Abopercular knob
Clonorchis sinensis	+	30	+
Diphylobothrium latum	−	60	+
Paragonimus westermani	+	90	−
Fasciola hepatica/ Fasciolopsis buskii	−	150	−

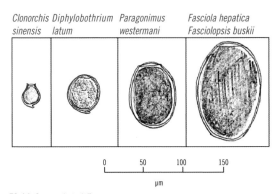

F3.11 Operculated Eggs

□ Acquired by ingestion of freshwater plants (water cress). Results in infestation of the **bile ducts** with eventual biliary fibrosis.

■ *Fasciolopsis buskii*

□ The **adult** is a flattened worm with a pointed, but not conical, cephalad. The **egg** is identical to *F hepatica.*

□ Like *F hepatica,* is acquired by ingestion of freshwater plants. Found in China primarily. Results in infestation of duodenum and bile ducts.

■ *Clonorchis sinensis*

□ The **adult** has a snout-like cephalad. The **egg** is oval and tiny, measuring 10 to 20 μm, and is characterized by a **shouldered operculum** with a small abopercular knob.

□ Acquired through ingestion of undercooked freshwater fish. Found in the Orient. Results in chronic biliary tract infestation, leading to biliary fibrosis. Is a risk factor for cholangiocarcinoma.

■ *Paragonimus westermanii*

□ The egg is oval, 75 to 125 μm, and has a shouldered operculum.

□ Acquired by ingestion of undercooked shellfish. Results in lung infestation with pulmonitis.

■ *Schistosoma* (**bilharziasis**)

□ The eggs **F3.12** may be detected in stool, urine (*S haematobium*), or tissue (with a surrounding granulomatous and fibrous reaction). They are oval, 75 to 150 μm, and have spines as follows: *S hematobium* has a terminal spine, *S mansoni* has a lateral spine,

S hematobium   S mansoni   S japonicum

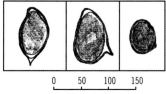

F3.12 Schistosomes

and *S japonicum* has a small, knob-like, spine. The small size and blunt spine of *S japonicum* allows it to sometimes disseminate within the host. Adult schistosomes look like a snake in a canoe; that is, the female (snake) resides within the male (canoe). **F3.12**

□ Schistosomes are acquired by penetration of the skin (swimmer's itch) by free-swimming, fork-tailed, circariae found in *snail-infested water.* They eventually make their way into the mesenteric and pelvic blood vessels. During egg-laying, there may be a systemic febrile illness (Katayama fever), caused by circulating immune complexes. Over time, the tissue reaction to eggs can lead to localized visceral dysfunction.

□ *S mansoni* is found mainly in Africa, especially the Nile delta. The adult worms infect the *hepatic portal vasculature and the inferior mesenteric vessels.* Eggs are passed into the intestine but also deposited in the periportal hepatic parenchyma. Reaction to deposited eggs can lead to so-called pipestem fibrosis and eventual cirrhosis.

□ *S hematobium* is found in Africa and the Middle East. The adult worms infect the *veins of the bladder* and deposit eggs into the bladder wall, leading to hematuria and irritative bladder symptoms. Long-term infection may result in *squamous cell carcinoma of the bladder.* A terminal urine specimen (the last 10-20 mL passed) is ideal for detection of *S hematobium.* The specimen is best collected around mid-day (greatest shedding) or following exercise. The eggs of *S intercalatum* closely resemble those of *S hematobium*; however, *S intercalatum* produces intestinal schistosomiasis, and the eggs are seen in feces instead of urine.

□ *S japonicum* is found in the Philippines, China, and SE Asia. Like *S mansoni,* it infects the liver, leading to cirrhosis. *S japonicum* rarely disseminates to the brain and spinal cord. *S mekongi,* in many respects similar to *S japonicum,* is found in Cambodia and Laos.

Parasitology>Metazoa

Cestodes (tapeworms) F3.13

- *Taenia saginata* (beef tapeworm)

  □ The diagnosis is usually made by finding eggs in stool. The egg, which is identical that of *T solium,* is 30 to 40 µm, spherical, has a **thick radially striated wall,** and **contains 3 pairs of hooks.** The finding of such eggs is reportable as '*Taenia species*' only. Further characterization relies upon examination of the **scolex** or proglottids. The scolex (the head structure by which the worm attaches to the bowel) has **4 suckers** and a smooth surface (**unarmed rostellum**). Each **proglottid** (tapeworm segment) is elongated and has >**13** lateral uterine branches.

  □ While common in South and Central America, *T saginata* is rare in North America. It is acquired by ingestion of encysted organisms (cysticerci) in beef. This results in intestinal (small bowel) infestation by the adult worm. The eggs of *T saginata* are not infectious to humans; thus, unlike *T solium,* cysticercosis due to *T saginata* does not occur.

- *Taenia solium* (pork tapeworm)

  □ The egg is identical to that of *T saginatum.* The **scolex** has **4 suckers** and many tiny hair-like hooks on its surface (**armed rostellum**). Each **proglottid** is short and has <**13** lateral uterine branches. The

encysted larval form (as seen in neurocysticercosis) consists of a spherical cyst measuring roughly 1 cm. The wall of the cyst measures up to 200 µm in thickness. An invaginated scolex with a double row of hooklets (which are acid-fast and birefringent) is the key finding.

  □ This organism is occasionally seen in the U.S., most commonly in a recent immigrant. **Intestinal infestation** results from ingestion of **encysted organisms (cysticerci)** in 'measly' pork. This situation is very similar to infection with *T saginata.* **Cysticercosis,** a condition in which cysts, containing larvae, are found in the brain and elsewhere, **results from ingestion of eggs,** with any kind of food, usually due to a food-preparer who is actively shedding in stool.

- *Diphyllobothrium latum* (fish tapeworm)

  □ The diagnosis is usually made by finding eggs in stool. The **egg** is a 60-70 µm oval structure with a smooth shell and an **unshouldered operculum** (like a hatch door) at one end. A small **abopercular** (located on the other end from the operculum) **knob** is seen. This egg is to be distinguished from that of *P westermanii* which has a shouldered operculum (small swellings rise up on either side of the operculum). The **scolex** looks like an elongated almond with **longitudinal grooves.** Each **proglottid** is characteristically **much wider than it is long** and contains a coiled uterus.

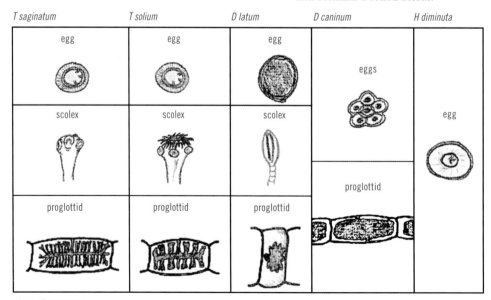

F3.13 Tapeworms

☐ *D latum* is somewhat unusual in that it is found in temperate zones—Scandinavia, Russia, Canada, and northern US, and Alaska. It is acquired through ingestion of poorly-cooked freshwater fish, resulting in intestinal infestation. In some cases, infection **is complicated by vitamin B$_{12}$ deficiency.**

■ *Hymenolepsis nana* **(dwarf tapeworm)**

☐ The **egg** has an inner shell and an outer shell with a wide space in between. The inner shell has two polar thickenings, pairs of filaments that look like **tiny bows**. The egg of *H diminuta* is similar but lacks the little bows. The adult worm is very small (2 to 4 cm).

☐ *H nana* is the most common cestode recovered in the US. Intestinal infestation follows ingestion of contaminated water or food; the usual contaminant being rodent droppings. Person-to-person spread may occur.

■ *Dipylidium caninum*

☐ The egg looks like other tapeworm eggs, except that they tend to occur in globular packets of 5 to 6 eggs enclosed by a thin membrane. The proglottid has a double genital pore, one exiting out of each side.

☐ The tapeworm commonly infects cats and dogs, but occasionally infects humans, especially children.

■ *Echinococcus* spp

☐ The protoscolices of the larvae can be found in hydatid cyst fluid and appear as extremely short

☐ Acquired when ingesting food contaminated with eggs from the stool of an infected dog, the definitive host. Sheep & cattle are intermediate hosts; thus, the infection is commonest in sheep and cattle-raising areas. Results in the formation of cysts in various organs, particularly the liver. One or several unilocular hydatid cysts are seen in *E granulosis,* while multilocular cysts are seen with *E multilocularis.* Polycystic hydatid cyst disease is seen with *E vogeli.* Hepatic cysts may rupture through the diaphragm, giving rise to pulmonary cysts.

Parasitology Take Home Points

Dual infections

■ *Ascaris* & *trichuria*

■ Pinworm & *D fragilis*

■ *Babesia,* Lyme disease, & flavivirus
■ Lepromatous leprosy & *Strongyloides* hyperinfection

Falling leaf motility *G lamblia*

Progressive motility *E histolytica*

Parasites in culture
■ Amoebae: bed of *E coli*
■ Hemoflagellates: Novy-MacNeil-Nicolle medium

T solium
■ Eat cysts: get intestinal infestation
■ Eat eggs: get cysticercosis

Skin/eye infestation: *Loa loa, Onchocerca volvulus*

Capable of person-to-person spread: *E vermicularis, H nana*

Parasitic infections in immunodeficient patients

■ T-cell (cellular) immunodeficiency is the usual basis for immune susceptibility to parasitic infection (eg, AIDS, post-transplant immunosuppression, steroid therapy, and inherited T-cell defects). Many infections (toxoplasmosis) are more common in T-cell immunodeficiency; others are not more common but are more severe (*Strongyloides*). Patients with AIDS have difficulty eradicating certain infections (cryptosporidium, isospora, cyclospora, microsporidia) from the bowel and suffer protracted diarrhea that may lead to a wasting syndrome. *Microsporidium* may disseminate in these patients.

■ B-cell (humoral) immunodeficiency forms the basis for susceptibility to *Giardia*.

■ Splenectomy, while not increasing the incidence of babesiosis, markedly increases its severity.

Mycology

Laboratory Methods

Direct examination

- **Calcofluor white** is a fluorochrome that selectively binds to the cellulose in fungal cell walls. It is a popular direct examination technique for fungal screening. After 10% KOH digestion of a drop of specimen, a drop of calcofluor white is added. The slide is then examined under fluorescence. The organisms, whether yeasts or hyphae, fluoresce bright white. As a general guideline, the detection of hyphae is usually indicative of clinical infection. Yeasts may be normal flora, and are only indicative of infection when obtained from normally sterile sites.

- **India ink** is used for the identification of *Cryptococcus neoformans,* particularly in CSF, where its sensitivity is only around 50%. A small amount of India ink is added to a drop of CSF on a slide. The slide is examined for the yeasts which appear as round and narrow-necked budding areas of India ink clearing.

- In tissue sections, most fungi are not seen in routine H&E-stained sections. The exception are the endogenously pigmented (dematiaceous) molds. For identification of most fungi, special stains are needed. Commonly, either a gormori methenamine silver (GMS) or periodic acid schiff (PAS) is used.

Fungal culture. For general purpose cultures, several media are typically incubated simultaneously, including Brain Heart Infusion (BHI) agar, Sabouraud agar, and Inhibitory Mold Agar. Cultures are incubated at

T3.21
Special Fungal Culture Techniques

Culture conditions	Purpose
Cornmeal agar with Tween 80	Good for visualizing yeast morphology
Overlay with olive oil	*Malssezia furfur*
Ascospore agar	Identification of *Saccharomyces* spp
Potato dextrose agar with 1% glucose	Pigment development of *Trichophyton rubrum*
Potato flake agar	Pigment development of *Trichophyton rubrum*
Czapek-Dox agar	Identification of *Aspergillus* spp
Trichophyton agars	Differentiation of *Trichophyton* spp
Bird (niger) seed agar	Demonstration of melanin in *Cryptococcus neoformans*
Brain-heart infusion with 5% SBA	Growth of dimorphic fungi

25-30°C for 4 to 6 weeks. Specific culture techniques may be applied either for initial isolation or for differentiation. **T3.21**

Identification of a fungal isolate (**T3.22**)

- The first clue is the colony morphology: yeasts form small creamy colonies; molds make larger fuzzy colonies. *Yeasts* are unicellular organisms, many of which display budding, and molds are multicellular organisms which form hyphae.

- A large, fuzzy colony usually indicates the presence of a mold. The major considerations in the differential diagnosis are the hyaline septate molds, pigmented (dematiaceous) septate molds, aseptate molds, and dimorphics. Note that the dimorphic fungi will present in the labora-

T3.22
Classification of Fungi

Yeasts			Dimorphics	Molds		
Coccoid	Coccoid with pseudohyphae	Arthroconidia	*Histoplasma* *Blastomyces* *Coccidioides* *Sporothrix* *Paracoccidioides*	Septate		Aseptate
				Hyaline	Dematiaceous	
Cryptococcus *Torulopsis* *Rhodotorula* *Malassezia* *Saccharomyces*	*Candida* spp	*Trichosporon* *Geotrichum*		*Aspergillus* *Fusarium* *Pseudoallescheria* *Dermatophytes* *(Epidermophyton, Microsporum, Trichophyton)* *Penicillium* *Paecillomyces*	*Alternaria* *Bipolaris* *Cladosporium* *Exophiala* *Fonsecaea* *Phialophora* *Wangiella*	*Zygomycetes* *(Cunninghamella, Mucor, Rhizomucor, Rhizopus)*

tory as a mold; dimorphism (with yeast conversion) or an exoantigen test will distinguish these from other molds. Once dimorphic fungi have been excluded, speciation of molds is carried out by considering four major characteristics— rate of growth, type of hyphae, pigmentation, and type of sporulation. Rapidly growing molds that cover the dish (lid lifters) suggest zygomycetes. Dimorphics tend to be extremely slow growing, sometimes requiring the full 6 weeks to develop. Other molds fall somewhere in between. The two major types of hyphae are septate hyphae and the aseptate, ribbon-like hyphae of the zygomycetes. In addition, septate hyphae may be pigmented (dematiaceous) or nonpigmented (hyaline). Sporulation is perhaps the most pivotal feature of all and provides the basis for instant pattern recognition of the various molds.

■ A small, smooth, bacterial-like, creamy colony usually indicates the presence of a yeast. The morphology of organisms grown on Cornmeal Tween 80 agar usually serves as the basis for initial categorization of an unknown yeast isolate. A small number of biochemical tests further clarifies this category.

■ The rate of growth is a clue to the identity of a fungal isolate. Dimorphic and dematiaceous fungi are slow growers, requiring over a week to make visible colonies. Rapidly growing colonies, especially if rapid growth is observed after prolonged incubation, are suspicious for a contaminant; however, several pathogenic fungi are notoriously rapid growers: most yeasts, *C immitis*, *Aspergillus* spp, *Scedosporium apiospermum*, and *Zygomycetes* ('lid lifters').

■ Cycloheximide is present in several commonly used isolation media (eg, Mycosel agar). Many contaminating species are completely inhibited by cycloheximide, and a few specific pathogens may be completely inhibited by cycloheximide: *Zygomycetes, Aspergillus* spp, and *C neoformans*. Uninhibited, slow, progressive, growth in the presence of cycloheximide is typical of many fungal pathogens. A mold slowly growing in the presence of cycloheximide suggests a dimorphic fungus or, in the appropriate setting, a dermatophyte.

■ Biochemical tests are used predominantly for yeasts but have a limited role in identification of molds. These are further discussed in relation to particular organisms.

□ Assimilation tests assess the ability of an isolate to use a particular carbohydrate as its sole source of carbon or its ability to use nitrate as its sole source of nitrogen. These assimilation assays are incorporated into the commercially available identification systems in widespread use.

□ Stimulations tests assess the sensitivity of an isolate to growth stimulants such as inositol and thiamine. Growth in the presence of stimulant is compared to growth in its absence. This sort of test is of particular importance in identifying *Trichophyton* spp.

□ The phenol oxidase test is used to aid in the identification of *C neoformans,* which is capable of oxidizing diphenolic compounds (caffeic acid, dopamine, dopa) to produce a pigment. Traditionally, the reagent used for this test was caffeic acid, obtained from niger seed (the Staib test).

□ The urease test is another assay used to identify *C neoformans.* It is especially useful in respiratory specimens, in which *Cryptococcus* (pathogenic and produces urease) may need to be distinguished from *Candida albicans* (upper respiratory contaminant, *usually* not pathogenic, does not produce urease). Urease production can be determined by inoculating Christensen urea agar; a pH indicator present in the agar changes color if the organism can produce ammonium from urea. Rapid versions of this test are also currently available. Urease production is not entirely specific for *C neoformans* and may be seen in other yeasts: *Rhodotorula* spp, *Trichosporon beigelii,* and *Candida krusei.* Furthermore, it is used in the distinction of dermatophytes, particularly the differentiation of *Trichophyton mentagrophytes* (produces urease) from *Trichophyton rubrum* (does not produce urease).

■ In order to identify the dimorphic fungi, one must demonstrate the capacity of the organism to convert from mold to yeast (ie, one must demonstrate dimorphism). Fungal cultures are routinely incubated at a temperature (25-30°C) in which dimorphics grow as a hyphal form (a mold); however, if then incubated at 37°C the dimorphics will grow as (convert to) yeasts (the tissue form). While many of the dimorphics undergo yeast conversion easily, some will need a little coaxing. *Histoplasma capsulatum* needs to be plated on BHI with blood, and *B dermatitidis* needs BHI or cottonseed agar for optimal conversion. *C immitis* is virtually never successfully converted, though this is possible with specialized media.

■ In many laboratories, the exoantigen test has replaced yeast conversion. This is a test for fungal antigens that is performed on culture material (not on clinical specimens). An extract is prepared from the fungal isolate, and this is reacted with species-specific antisera.

■ Serologic testing is available for many of the dimorphic fungi and aspergillus. The latter assay is particularly useful in evaluating patients with suspected aspergilloma or allergic bronchopulmonary aspergillosis.

■ Antigen detection techniques, performed directly upon clinical specimens, first found widespread application in the diagnosis of *Cryptococcus* in CSF. Detection of cryptococcal antigen in CSF is diagnostic of cryptococcal meningitis with a sensitivity is around 90-95% and can be enhanced by pretreatment with pronase.

■ DNA-based testing is available for some of the more common dimorphic fungal infections (eg, *H capsulatum* and *C immitis*). These tests are based upon labeled oligonucleotide probes complementary to segments of fungal species-specific ribosomal RNA (rRNA).

Isolate Growing *in vitro* as a Mold: Dimorphic Fungi and Molds

Dimorphic fungi **F3.14, T3.25**

■ *Histoplasma capsulatum*

☐ In tissue sections, *H capsulatum* typically presents as a granuloma, often necrotizing. The organisms are found **within histiocytes** where they are seen as 2 to 5 μm yeasts with narrow-based budding. Their bundling within histiocytes makes them appear to be encapsulated (pseudocapsules).

☐ In initial fungal cultures, they are very slow-growing molds which look exactly like the mold Sepedonium: hyaline hyphae with intermittent

T3.23
Histoplasma capsulatum

	var. capsulatum	*var. duboisii*
Geography	Worldwide. In the US, found in Ohio & Mississippi river valleys.	Africa
Disease	Pulmonary & mediastinal ± reticuloendothelial dissemination	Pulmonary & mediastinal ± dissemination to skin and bones
Culture	Hyaline septate mold with lollipop-like smooth microconidia and spiked macroconidia	Indistinguishable from *var. capsulatum*
Tissue	2-5 μm budding yeasts	10-15 μm thick-walled budding yeasts

F3.14 Dimorphic Fungi

small smooth lollipoplike microconidia and occasional **spiked macroconidia.** The latter are extremely helpful but may be absent in early cultures and are more a **feature of mature cultures.** Thus, young cultures may mimic the 'birds-on-a-wire' appearance of *T rubrum* or the 'lollipop' appearance of *B dermatitidis* and others. This makes yeast conversion and/or exoantigen tests very important.

▢ The yeast form of *H capsulatum* consists of uniform 2 to 5 μm spherical structures with narrow-based budding. *H capsulatum var duboisii* is contrasted to the usual-type *H capsulatum var capsulatum* in **T3.23**.

▢ Histoplasmosis is most prevalent in the **Ohio and Mississippi River valleys** where it is found in soil contaminated by feces from **chickens,** other birds, and **bats.** *H capsulatum var duboisii* is found in Africa.

▢ Histoplasmosis may present as pulmonary nodules, chronic sclerosing mediastinitis, hepatosplenomegaly, or lymphadenopathy. Like most dimorphics, it is acquired through inhalation, results in an initial pulmonary infection which may be asymptomatic or flu-like, and then may disseminate. Disseminated histoplasmosis typically involves the reticuloendothelial system and is often easily diagnosed in

bone marrow biopsies. The small subcapsular granulomata that are found commonly in spleens most often represent healed histoplasmosis.

■ *Coccidioides immitis*

▢ In tissue sections *C immitis* is seen within granulomata as giant 50 to 200 μm spherules with thick hyaline walls that enclose hundreds of tiny 2 to 5 μm **endospores.** They are often visible on H&E-stained sections, and are easily found within touch imprints of granulomata. The spherules may be confused with *Rhinosporidium seeberi* and *Prototheca wickerhami*. However, the classic clinical presentations differ, with *R seeberi* typically presenting as an exophytic nasal lesion and *P wickerhami* an olecranon bursitis. Sometimes the endospores are seen spilling from the spherules, and individual endospores may be confused with *H capsulatum*. In contrast to like-sized *H capsulatum* yeasts, they do not bud.

▢ In culture, the mold form of *C immitis* grows readily (usually in about 7 days) and is found microscopically as mycelia formed of easily-separated **barrel-shaped arthroconidia.** Like *Histoplasma,* conversion to the yeast form in vitro is difficult and not generally relied upon for diagnosis.

▢ *Coccidioides* has recently been divided into *C immitis* (California isolates) and *C posadasii* (elsewhere isolates) which produce indistinguishable clinical features. It is prevalent in arid desert regions, especially the San Joiquin desert, where it is responsible for Valley Fever. *Coccidioides* is acquired through inhalation of environmental arthroconidia, initially involves the lung, then disseminates to the skin, mainly, but can involve viscera.

▢ The primary risk factor for *Coccidioidomycosis* is being in an endemic area. This risk is compounded by inhalation of soil—sandstorms, excavations, et cetera. Compromise of the immune system predisposes infected persons to dissemination, and for some reason those with blood group B and those in certain ethnic groups (Filipino and African American) are at greater risk for dissemination. Pregnancy in the third trimester is another risk factor for severe disease.

T3.24
Mold Forms with Lollipop-like Conidiophores (Species Distinguishing Features)

B dermatitidis	Very slow-growing (10-30 days). Mold form shows thick-walled yeasts with broad-based budding.
Paracoccidioides brasiliensis	Very slow-growing. Mold form shows mariner's wheel configuration.
H capsulatum	Very slow growing. Mold form (mature colonies) also has spiked macroconidia. Exoantigen test.
Scedosporium & Chrysosporium	Rapidly growing (2-4 days). Cannot be converted to yeast form.
Sepedonium	Rapidly growing. Mold also shows presence of larger spiked macroconidia (indistinguishable from mold form of *H capsulatum*).

T3.25
Summary of Dimorphic Fungi

Species	Yeast form	Mold form	1° infection	2° (disseminated) infection
H capsulatum	2-5 μm Narrow-based budding	Hyphae with periodic lollipop-like microconidia and spiked macroconidia	Lung	Reticuloendothelial system Splenic granulomas Sclerosing mediastinitis
C immitis	50-200 μm spherules with 2-5 μm (nonbudding) endospores	Barrel-shaped arthroconidia	Lung	Skin & Viscera
B dermatitidis	8-12 μm Broad-based budding	Hyphae with lollipops	Lung	Skin & Bone
S schenckii	2-5 μm Elongated (cigars) with narrow-based budding	Daisy heads	Skin	None
P braziliensis	10-15 μm Mariner's wheel budding	Hyphae with lollipops	Lung	Reticuloendothelial & gastrointestinal

□ *Coccidioides* is a risk to laboratory personnel and can be contracted from laboratory specimens.

■ ***Blastomyces dermatitidis***

□ In tissue sections, *B dermatitidis* appears as fairly uniform, 8 to 12 μm yeasts with **broad-based budding.**

□ In culture, the mold is identical to the mold *Chrysosporium* which has hyphae with intermittent **lollipoplike smooth conidia T3.24**. Yeast conversion is often possible. The mold form of Blastomyces must be distinguished from Sepedonium (identical to the mold form of *H capsulatum), Paracoccidioides, Scedosporium, and Chrysosporium* spp, all of which produce 'lollipops'.

□ *Blastomycosis* has a geographic distribution similar to *Histoplasmosis,* but instead of chickens and bats, it is found in **dogs.**

□ It initially infects the lung, and disseminated infection most often involves the **skin and bones.** Rare primary cutaneous blastomycosis has been called Gilchrist disease.

■ ***Sporothrix schenckii***

□ In tissue sections, *S schenckii* appears as 2 to 5 μm elongated, cigar-shaped, yeasts with narrow-based budding, usually seen in a background of purulent inflammation.

□ In cultures, the mold form consists of hyphae with **daisy head**-like conidia.

□ Unlike other dimorphics, *S schenckii* is not usually acquired by inhalation. Instead, it is a subcutaneous mycosis, traumatically introduced into the skin, most often the hand or arm, classically by the puncture of a **rose thorn.** *S schenckii* is found in nature as a saprophyte upon dead vegetation. A localized infection with suppuration results, leading to localized lymphangiitis, manifesting as a chain of nodules proceeding up the extremity (lymphocutaneous sporotrichosis).

□ A subcutaneous mycosis is a fungal infection that develops at the site of a puncture wound. These tend to be prolonged, persistent, and slowly progressive infections. The main fungal subcutaneous infections are: sporotrichosis, chromoblastomycosis, mycetoma, lobomycosis, rhinosporidiosis, and subcutaneous phaeohyphomycosis.

□ In immunocompromised hosts the organism may disseminate, especially to bone (disseminated sporotrichosis).

□ In chronic alcoholics there have been descriptions of an inhalational form of Sporotrichosis resembling that associated with other dimorphics.

■ *Paracoccidioides braziliensis* (**South American blastomycosis**)

□ In tissue sections, the diagnostic form is the 10-15 μm yeast with circumferential budding, giving the appearance of a mariner's wheel. In cultures, the mold is indistinguishable from *Blastomcyces dermatitidis.*

□ Found in Central and South America. Inhalation of spores leads to pneumonitis. After initial lung infection, disseminated infection involves the reticuloendothelial system, bowel, and liver. In an alternate form of Paracocidioidomycosis, ulcerative lesions are found in the mucosa of the mouth and nose.

Hyaline septate molds

■ **Dermatophytes (F3.15)**

□ Dermatophytes are identified based on characteristic morphology, especially after incubation on DTM. They grow in culture as wooly white-tan colonies. *Trichophyton rubrum* is particularly distinctive in that it produces a **red pigment** that diffuses into the agar. Microscopically, these species appear as hyaline molds that produce either microconidia or macroconidia or both. Macroconidia are key for the diagnosis of the first three species, while microconidia are key for the other three.

□ Rapid diagnosis of dermatophytes can be made, with KOH-stained scrapings (KOH prep). This does not permit species identification, which is not always necessary.

□ *Microsporum canis* macroconidia are spindle-shaped structures with pointed and somewhat upturned ends and transverse septae.

□ *Microsporum gypseum* macroconidia are oval-shaped structures with blunt ends and transverse septae.

□ *Epidermophyton floccosum* macroconidia are club-shaped structures with transverse septae. Microconidia are never produced.

□ *Trichophyton rubrum* tear-shaped microconidia are spaced along the hyphae, giving a **birds-on-a-wire** appearance.

□ **Trichophyton mentagrophytes** microconidia are arranged in grape-like clusters, and occasional spiral hyphae may be seen. *T mentagrophytes* has the ability to penetrate hair shafts (endothrix), unlike *T rubrum.*

□ **Trichophyton tonsurans.** The key feature that makes *T tonsurans* distinctive is the marked size and shape **variability** of its microconidia.

● Dermatophyte infection may take many forms, including: tinea capitis, tinea corporis (ringworm), tinea cruris, tinea pedis, and tinea unguium (onychomycosis).

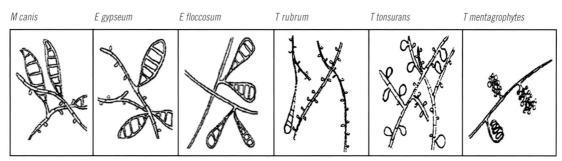

| M canis | E gypseum | E floccosum | T rubrum | T tonsurans | T mentagrophytes |

F3.15 Dermatophytes

- A distinction is made between a cutaneous mycoses (infections of the epidermis and dermis with an associated inflammatory response) and superficial mycoses (colonization of the superficial stratum corneum, without a host response).

- There are three clinical forms of *tinea pedis:* interdigital (web spaces), moccasin (plantar), and vesiculobullous. Onychomycosis may accompany any of these presentations.

- *Tinea corporis* (ringworm) presents as an erythematous round patch with a raised advancing edge.

- *Tinea cruris* (jock itch) presents as a pruritic patch in the groin area, characteristically sparing the scrotum and penis (in contrast to *Candida* which involves the scrotum and base of penis).

- *Tinea capitis* may only present as a pruritic patch, but may also present with alopecia, hair breakage (black dot alopecia), or a kerion. Certain fungi may invade the hair shaft; the pattern of invasion may be ectothrix (arthroconidia seen on the outside of the hair shaft, with destruction of the cuticle—seen in *M canis, M gypseum,* and *T verrucosum*), or endothrix (arthroconidia seen within the hair shaft, cuticle intact—*T tonsurans*).

- *Onychomycosis* (*tinea unguium*) is an infection of the nail plate or nail bed. While most commonly due to a dermatophyte (*Trichophyton* spp most commonly), it may be cause by other fungi. Onychomycosis is particularly common in diabetics and those with HIV infection. HIV infection in particular may cause what is an unusual presentation in healthy individuals—proximal subungual onychomycosis. Most healthy persons with onychomycosis have the distal subungual form, most commonly caused by *T rubrum.*

  □ Candidal skin infection, including Candidal onychomycosis, is unusual. It is seen most often in the setting of chronic mucocutaneous candidiasis (see chapter 6).

- Conidia arising from conidiophores that end in a **swollen vesicle** (fruiting head): *Aspergillus* spp.

  □ In tissue sections, *Aspergillus* spp **F3.16** are recognized as hyaline septate molds with characteristic 45° dichotomous branching. However, this appearance is not specific for aspergillosis and can represent any of the hyaline molds. The histologic differential should also include such things as *Penicillium, Scedosporium* (*P boydii*), *Fusarium,* etc. The diagnostic fruiting heads of *Aspergillus* are common in cultures, but they are not typically seen in tissue. The exception is whenever *Aspergillus* grows in an air-filled space (such as a fungus ball).

  □ On routine fungal media, *Aspergillus* is rapidly growing and produces characteristic colonies having a distinct margin and white apron. *Aspergillus* spp are identified based on characteristic morphology, especially after growth on Czapek agar.

  □ *A fumigatus* colonies are blue-green with a distinct white apron. Its microscopic morphology is notable for conidiophores that terminate in a swollen vesicle having a **single row** of phialides, each of which gives rise to a chain of conidia, that cover **only the top** of the vesicle. Care must be taken not to confuse *A fumigatus* with the hyalinohyphomyces having branching chains of conidia (*Penicillium,* etc.).

| A fumigatus | A flavus | A niger | A terreus |

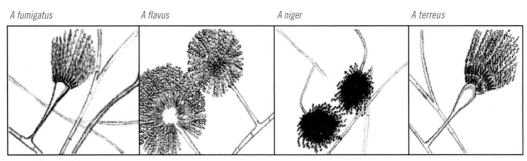

F3.16 *Aspergillus* spp

□ *A niger* has conidia so heavily pigmented that additional details cannot normally be seen. Its cultures have a blackened surface, due to its pigmented conidiophores, **but the reverse side is yellow-gray.** This contrasts with cultures of dematiaceous molds which are pigmented **front and back.**

□ *A terreus* looks superficially like *A fumigatus,* but it has **two rows of phialides** (bisereate). A. terreus colonies are characteristically **cinnamon buff** to orange.

□ *A flavus* has **circumferential phialides** and resembles a lollipop.

□ The most common human isolate is *A fumigatus* which may cause invasive infection anywhere in the body but is most commonly associated with some variety of pulmonary disease. The type of pulmonary disease depends on host factors. An otherwise immunocompetent individual with cavitary disease, such as from old tuberculosis, is prone to develop the saprophytic form of aspergillus, an **aspergilloma (fungus ball),** which is a noninvasive colonization by the mold form. The upper lobes are most commonly involved. Fruiting heads may be seen in fungus balls. **Allergic bronchopulmonary aspergillosis (ABPA)** is a condition in which *Aspergillus* mold colonizes the airway, without invasion, and elicits a marked allergic response characterized by mucus impaction, peripheral eosinophilia, and reactive airways. The inflammatory response can be sufficiently severe to cause hemoptysis and eventual bronchiectasis. While this form of aspergillus is often seen in patients with an atopic history, there is an increased incidence of the cystic fibrosis (CFTR) mutation in this condition. The diagnosis can be supported with tests for serum anti-*Aspergillus* IgE. Allergic sinonasal aspergillosis (allergic fungal sinusitis) is a related condition which can be diagnosed on the basis of sinus curreting histology: inflamed sinonasal mucosa and eosinophil-permeated mucin containing fungal hyphae. In addition to *A fumigatus,* *A flavus* is a common cause of ABPA. An individual with honeycomb lung, emphysema, or other structural lung disease, who is coincidentally receiving steroid therapy, is prone to develop **semi-invasive pulmonary aspergillosis,** also called chronic necrotizing pulmonary aspergillosis, in which the mold colonizes cavitary regions of the emphysematous lung parenchyma and invades superficially into the surrounding lung tissue. An immunosuppressed host is susceptible to invasive bronchopulmonary aspergillosis (IBPA), a very serious condition in which the mold invades the pulmonary parenchyma and may disseminate. *Aspergillus* (and *mucormycosis*) is unique for its propensity to invade vessel walls (angioinvasion) and give rise to tissue infarctions, characteristically associated with tissue calcium oxalate deposition.

□ *Fungal sinusitis,* like *Aspergillus* infections in the lung, comes in several varieties. These include allergic fungal sinusitis (most common), mycetoma/fungus ball, chronic invasive fungal sinusitis, and acute/fulminant invasive fungal sinusitis. Allergic fungal sinusitis, is characterized by copious mucin containing abundant eosinophils and Charcot-Leyden crystals (so-called allergic mucin) and noninvasive fungal hyphae. This form of sinusitis may be associated with various fungal species, including *Alternaria* spp, *Bipolaris* spp, *Curvularia* spp, and *Aspergillus* spp. Mycetoma/ fungus ball displays abundant, noninvasive, tightly packed fungal hyphae, without allergic mucin. These are most commonly *Aspergillus* spp. Chronic invasive fungal sinusitis is associated with tissue granulomas and fungal hyphae. Lastly, acute fulminant fungal sinusitis shows fungal vascular invasion.

□ Otitis externa due to aspergillus is most commonly caused by *A niger.*

■ **Hyalinohyphomyces** The remainder of the hyaline molds can be grouped as hyalinohyphomyces **F3.17** due to their shared clinical significance. Hyalohyphomycosis is a term that refers to invasive fungal infections caused by hyaline-septate molds that have not been further speciated. When the species is known as a result of culture, a more specific term can be applied. These agents can be distinguished in the microbiology laboratory by the morphology of their conidia, beginning with observing whether the conidia occur singly, in clusters, or in branching chains.

□ **Conidia occuring in clusters:** *Acremonium, Gliocladium, Fusarium. Acremonium* species are characterized by long, hair-like conidiophores bearing clusters of tiny conidia. *Gliocladium* spp have highly distinctive branching phialides that bear clusters of spherical conidia, resembling a golf ball held at the end of outstretched fingertips. *Gliocladium* colonies typically produce a wall-to-wall lawn of green growth, without an apron. *Fusarium* is characterized not only by microconidia borne in clusters at the ends of conidiophores, but more recognizably by its fusiform macroconidia. In tissue sections, *Fusarium* may superficially resemble a dichotomous branching organism such as *Aspergillus*, but on closer inspection, its hyphae branch at right (90°) angles. Its colonies are typically red top and bottom.

☐ **Conidia occuring in branching chains:**
Penicillium, Paecilomyces, Scopulariopsis. Penicillium marneffei is the most common clinically significant isolate, characterized by a broom-like arrangement of branching phialides that give rise to chains of conidia, **superficially** resembing *A fumigatus.* Their colonies also resemble those of *A fumigatus,* having green coloration and a white apron. *Paecilomyces* species are notable for terminal conidiua which appear larger than the rest in the chain. Lastly, *Scopulariopsis brevicaulis* is characterized by branching phalides, each of which bears one to several large, rough-walled, lemon-like conidia.

☐ **Conidia occuring singly:** *Scedosporium, Beuveria, Sepedonium, Chrysosporium. Scedosporium* (aka *Pseudoallescheria boydii*) cannot easily be distinguished from *Aspergillus* species in tissue sections, a distinction of clinical importance due to differing antibiotic regimens. In culture, however, they are

easily distinguished, as both *Scedosporium* & *Chrysosporium* species have single, pear-shaped, conidia borne lollipop-like from simple conidiophores. This resembles the mold form of *B dermatitidis. Scedosporium* (*P boydii*) cultures are characteristically house-mouse grey with tiny water droplets upon their surface. *Sepedonium* species also have singly borne *conidia,* but the individual conidia are spiked. The morphologic features are indistinguishable from the mold form of *H capsulatum. Beuveria* is characterized by tiny conidia borne singly from the ends of branching and slightly bent (geniculate) conidiophores.

☐ This group of organisms is known for causing such things as mycotic keratitis, onychomycosis, and eumycotic mycetoma.

☐ *Chrysosporium parvum* is the etiologic agent of Adiaspiromycosis, a unique form of pulmonary infection that is characteristically asymptomatic and self-limited. Histologically, one finds granulomata with concentric fibrosis around one or two large (200 to 400 μm) thick-walled (20 to 40 μm) spherules. The organism does not replicate in human tissues and is therefore relatively benign.

☐ *Fusarium* spp cause a spectrum of infections, including superficial infection (keratitis, onychomycosis, sinusitis), invasive infection, catheter-tip infection, and disseminated infection. Disseminated infection is seen almost exclusively in immunocompromised patients—particularly those with impaired cell-mediated immunity or neutropenia.

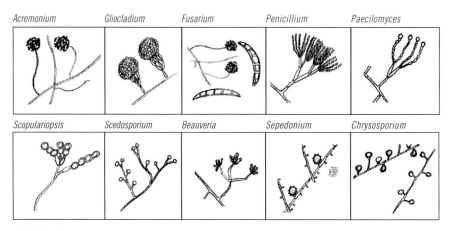

F3.17 Hyalinohyphomyces

Fusarium species have recently become major opportunistic pathogens in burn wounds. Airborne infection can lead to pulmonary infection, and it appears that a combination of factors—fusarium in the hospital water supply and showering—may conspire to cause this in immunocompromised patients. Skin manifestations are common in disseminated fusariosis, and fungemia, a very uncommon manifestation of disseminated fungal infection due to other species, is very strikingly common in fusariosis. In fact, there is a high frequency of positive blood cultures.

☐ Many of the hyalohyphomyces—*Scedosporium, Paecilomyces, Acremonium*—can be found in soil, saprophytic upon decaying vegetation. *Scedosporium apiospermum*, in addition to causing various localized infections after penetrating trauma, is a cause of disseminated infection after near-drowning accidents. It is the most common cause of eumycotic mycetoma in the US. Pulmonary involvement and disseminated infection are common, like fusariosis, in immunocompromised patients, especially transplant recipients.

Pigmented (dematiaceous) molds

■ Dematiaceous molds **F3.18** in general can be recognized by the characteristic **front-and-back** pigmentation of their colonies due to endogenously pigmented hyphae. The first two groups below (conidia with septa) are relatively rapid-growers, while the last group is a short list of disparate slow-growers. In tissues, there are no features that permit distinction to the genus

level, but endogenous pigmentation is a clue to the presence of a dematiaceous mold.

☐ **Conidia with transverse septa:** *Bipolaris, Drechslera, Exserohilum, Helminthosporum, Curvularia.*

- *Bipolaris* is characterized by oval transversely septated conidia that arise from bent (geniculate) conidiophores. Bipolaris gets its name from the production of germ tubes from both ends of the conidia in saline mounts incubated for 12 to 24 hours.

- The genus *Drechslera* produces similar conidia but is distinguished from *Bipolaris* by its lack of production of bipolar germ tubes in saline incubation; instead, it produces germ tubes along the sides of the conidia.

- *Exserohilum* also somewhat resembles bipolaris, except that its condia are longer and thinner.

- *Helminthosporium* has a highly characteristic bottle brush-like arrangement of side-by-side conidia.

☐ *Curvularia* is easy to recognize, since its transversely septated condia curve slightly.

☐ Conidia with **transverse & longitudinal septa:** *Alternaria, Ulocladium, Stemphilium.*

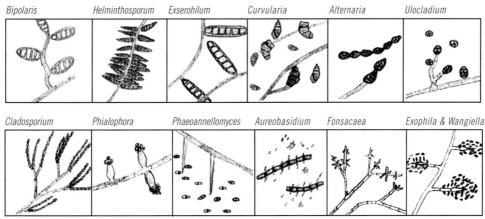

Bipolaris   Helminthosporum   Exserohilum   Curvularia   Alternaria   Ulocladium

Cladosporium   Phialophora   Phaeoannellomyces   Aureobasidium   Fonsacaea   Exophila & Wangiella

F3.18 Dematiaceous molds

- *Alternaria* spp produce chains of transverse & longitudinally septated (muriform—resembling a brick wall) conidia which have alternating blunt and pointed ends.

- *Ulocladium* is characterized by oval muriform conidia borne singly on bent (geniculate) conidiophores.

- *Stemphilium* conidia somewhat resemble those of ulocladium but are borne upon straight conidiophores.

☐ **Slow-growing dematiaceous molds** This group of organisms grows very slowly, eventually producing a small darkened colony with a fuzzy surface.

- *Cladosporium carrionii* is characterized by long chains of conidia arising from dematiaceous hyphae.

- *Phialophora* spp produce **flask-shaped** phialides that give rise to bunches of tiny spherical *conidia*.

- *Fonsacaea pedrosi* produces sequential phialides with sporulation that give the appearance of a wooden coat rack.

- *Exophila jeanselmei* and *Wangiella dermatitidis* are virtually indistinguishable and both produce characteristic pointed conidiophores that give rise to bunches of tiny spherical conidia.

- *Aureobasidium pullulans* forms large dark hyphae that break up into arthroconidia, with perpendicular translucent (non-pigmented) oval conidia.

- *Phaeoannellomyces wernickii* hyphae give rise to pointed conidiophores with bunches of two-celled *conidia* with dividing 'scars'.

☐ The first two groups (septated conidia) produce superficial cutaneous infections but may also cause mycotic keratitis, eumycotic mycetoma, and invasive disease.

☐ *Phialophora, Cladosporium carrionii,* and *Fonsecaea pedrosoi* are the principle causes of chromoblastomycosis, a subcutaneous mycosis associated with prominent pseudoepitheliomatous hyperplasia of the overlying epidermis. In histologic sections, chromoblastomycosis is characterized by there being, in addition to pigmented hyphae, yeasts that are septated in more than one plane (muriform) known as "Medlar bodies" or "Copper pennies." Chromoblastomycosis is found in tropical and subtropical areas, particularly where shoes are not regularly worn. The organisms gain entrance through puncture wounds, so infections tend to be found on the lower extremities. Lesions are usually solitary and may take the form of verrucous lesions (due to pseudoepitheliomatous hyperplasia), nodules, or massive tumors.

☐ Mycetoma (Madura foot, Maduromycosis), is another form of subcutaneous infection in which a sometimes cystic subcutaneous nodule is formed, which is usually associated with 'sulfur granules' and often with a draining sinus tract to the skin. Like chromoblastomycosis, it is usually the result of a puncture wound. It may be due to fungi (eumycotic mycetoma) or bacteria (actinomycotic mycetoma). The causes of eumycotic mycetoma include *Madurella, Exophiala, Wangiella,* and *P boydii (Scedosporium)*. Actinomycotic mycetomas are due to *Actinomyces, Nocardia,* and *Streptomyces* species.

Aseptate molds (Zygomycetes): *Rhizopus, Mucor, Absidia*

- A rapidly growing gray-brown mold that grows from wall to wall without producing any kind of margin (a 'lid lifter') is suggestive of one of the zygomycetes **F3.19**. (Note: a slower-growing wall-to-wall green lawn suggests *Gliocladium* species.) The hyphae are broad and ribbon-like. In culture, they give rise to two diagnostically useful structures: sporangia and rhizoids.

  ☐ *Rhizopus* produces rhizoids and sporangiophores that arise **nodally** (directly over the rhizoids). Their sporangia are prominent spherical structures full of tiny spores which tend to collapse when mature, resembling a **collapsed umbrella.**

  ☐ *Absidia* also produces rhizoids but its sporangiophores arise **internodally** (between rhizoids). Their sporangia resemble those of *Rhizopus* but do not collapse.

☐ *Mucor* spp do not produce rhizoids. Their sporangia are large spherical structures that tend to fall apart, releasing their numerous spores.

☐ *Cunninghamella* spp produce spherical vesicles from which spherical sporangioles arise directly via delicate connections.

☐ *Circinella* spp have sporangia on the ends of curved (circinate) sporangiophores.

☐ *Syncephalastrum* species are characterized by chains of spores that radiate from a spherical vesicle, producing a daisy-head-like structure somewhat resembling A. flavus.

■ Zygomycetes may produce several forms of infection: rhinocerebral, endobronchial, invasive pulmonary, gastric, and cutaneous. Mucormycosis is an environmental organism that only infects when the victim is severely compromised. In the classic scenario, the rhinocerebral mucormycosis affects persons suffering from **diabetic ketoacidosis,** but this and other forms of zygomycosis may arise in other immunocompromising states such as acute leukemia is often the predisposing influence. Like *Aspergillus* species, the zygomycetes characteristically **invade vessel walls** and produce parenchymal infarction.

Beware incorrectly identifying one of the **branching filamentous bacteria** (*Actinomyces, Nocardia, and Streptomyces*), that easily grow on fungal culture media, as a fungus. Their 'hyphae' are much thinner than any mold.

Yeast Identification (F3.20)

A small, smooth, bacterial-like, creamy colony usually indicates the presence of a yeast.

■ Formation of **pseudohyphae** on Cornmeal Tween 80 Agar is consistent with *Candida* spp. Furthermore, chlamydospore formation on Tween 80 is highly species-specific for *C albicans.*

■ Formation of **arthroconidia:** *Geotrichum* or *Trichosporon.* Of these, *Trichosporon* spp are urease positive.

■ **No hyphae formed:** *Cryptococcus, Rhodotorula,* or *Saccharomyces. Cryptococcus* is urease + and phenoloxidase +, while *Rhodotorula* is urease + but phenoloxidase −. *Saccharomyces* is inert in both of these tests.

The germ tube test. Yeasts are suspended in serum and incubated at 37°C **for 2 hours** (it is essential to limit incubation time to 2 hours, since other organisms may begin to form germ tubes after prolonged incubation). A wet mount is prepared and examined for the formation of germ tubes—hyphae that begin to form directly from the wall of a yeast cell and that, in contrast to early pseudohyphae, have parallel walls that show **no constriction at the juncture with the yeast cell.** A positive test for germ tubes can identify *C albicans* with 90% sensitivity and around 100% specificity.

The **urease test** is typically performed using Christensen agar, but other more rapid formats are currently available. Urease + fungi include: *Cryptococcus, Rhodotorula, Candida krusei,* and *Trichophyton mentagrophytes.*

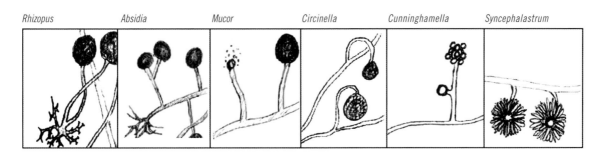

| Rhizopus | Absidia | Mucor | Circinella | Cunninghamella | Syncephalastrum |

F3.19 **Zygomycetes**

The **phenol oxidase** test is also used to identify *Cryptococcus.* Phenol oxidase is an enzyme that converts various amines to the pigment melanin, and it is contained in the cryptococcal cell wall. The phenol oxidase test is traditionally carried out by incubating organisms in **bird seed agar (niger seed agar)** which contains the substrate caffeic acid (3,4 dihydro cinnamic acid). *Cryptococcus* has the ability to turn **caffeic acid** into the pigment melanin.

One must suspect *Malassezia furfur* in order to successfully culture it, since this organism must be incubated at 35°C, and **overlaid with olive oil** as a source of long-chain fatty acids.

Notes on specific yeasts

- *Candida* spp

   □ *C albicans* is by far the most common candidal isolate. Its cultures are noteworthy for the formation of filamentous extensions (**'feet', 'spider colonies'**) around the edges of older colonies.

   □ The organisms in tissue sections and culture are round to oval 3 to 5 μm budding yeasts with accompanying pseudohyphae. True septate hyphae are occasionally encountered.

   □ In cornmeal agar, characteristic blastoconidia and chlamydospores are diagnostic for *C albicans.* The tight clusters of blastoconidia are arranged at set intervals along the length of pseudohyphae, and chlamydospores are found at the termini of pseudohyphae.

   □ Asymptomatic colonization is the usual form taken by *C albicans.*

□ In immunosuppression, pregnancy, diabetes, or treatment with broad-spectrum antibacterials, clinical infection may be seen. Mucocutaneous infection is the most common form of infection in these settings, but visceral involvement can occur as well. *C albicans* and *Torulopsis* (previously *candida*) *glabrata* are common causes of urinary tract infection.

□ An inherited condition known as **chronic mucocutaneous candidiasis** is characterized by a *Candida*-specific immunodefiency, characterized by protracted superficial candidal infections of skin, nails, oral cavity and pharynx. Many also have endocrinopathies such as hypoparathyroidism and adrenal insufficiency. A late-onset type is associated with thymoma.

- *Cryptococcus neoformans*

   □ Despite numerous species within the genus, the main pathogens are *C neoformans* and *C gattii.* Previously, *C gattii* was considered a variety of *C neoformans,* but these have now been placed in separate species. *C neoformans* is the cause of most infections in the US; however, *C gattii,* previously confined to tropical zones, has now been reported as an increasing cause of infection in North America.

   □ In histologic sections, cryptococci present as yeasts that **range in size** from 3 to 15 μm, bud, and usually have even spacing due to a thick polysaccharide-rich capsule that contains the enzyme phenoloxidase. The polysaccharide is the basis for positivity with **mucicarmine and alcian blue,** and phenoloxidase reacts with **Fontana-Masson** stains.

   □ **India ink** cannot penetrate the cryptococcal capsule, and this leads to the appearance of the organisms as budding ghosts in India ink prepara-

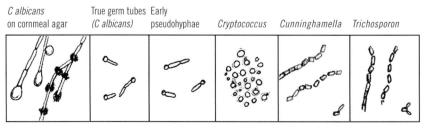

| *C albicans* on cornmeal agar | True germ tubes (*C albicans*) | Early pseudohyphae | *Cryptococcus* | *Cunninghamella* | *Trichosporon* |

F3.20 **Yeasts**

tions. India ink is particularly useful for finding the organisms in CSF. The sensitivity is about 80% in HIV-associated cryptococcal meningoencephalitis, but only about 40% sensitive in non-HIV-associated infection.

☐ In interpreting yeasts in tissue sections, one should recall that cryptococcus can mimic several of the yeasts, since it (a) can range from 3 to 15 μm in size, (b) forms buds that, due to the presence of a capsule may be interpreted as narrow- or broad-based, and (c) can exist as capsule-deficient forms. The key feature to observe in tissues is the **size variability** of cryptococci. Thus, although small capsule-deficient yeasts may resemble *H capsulatum,* large encapsulated yeasts may resemble *B dermatitidis,* etc, the wide spectrum of sizes present will betray the identity of *C neoformans.*

☐ The cryptococcal capsular polysaccharide antigen can be detected in either serum or body fluids (CSF). Latex particles coated with antibodies against cryptococcal capsular antigen form the basis for this test, providing performance significantly better than India ink. The sensitivity and specificity are both >95%.

☐ In cultures, the organisms grow as yeasts surrounded by even spaces (due to the capsule) which do not form pseudohyphae in cornmeal agar. A characteristic feature is the capability of *C neoformans* to grow at 37° C in culture. In fact, this ability combined with its ease of cultivation results in the frequent appearance of *C neoformans* in bacterial cultures.

☐ *C neoformans* is urease + & phenoloxidase +.

☐ *C neoformans* is acquired from inhalation of infected soil, particularly soil contaminated with bird excreta (eg, pigeon, chicken). *C gattii* appears to be associated with trees, especially eucalyptus trees. *C neoformans var grubii* is the most common isolate worldwide. *C neoformans var neoformans* is commonly seen in Europe and the US. *C gattii,* appears increasingly relevant for two reasons: it is appearing increasingly outside the tropics, and seems capable of causing infection in immunocompetent hosts.

☐ The lungs are the portal for cryptococcal entry and the most common site of primary infection. Pulmonary infection may be mild and asymptomatic, flu-like, or take the form of severe pneumonia. Well-defined single or multiple nodules are the most common radiographic presentation.

☐ *Cryptococcus* may disseminate, particularly to the **brain and bone.** In suspected CNS infections, cryptococcosis can be reliably diagnosed in CSF by India ink preparations or cryptococcal antigen tests.

☐ HIV infection is the primary setting for cryptococcal infection. With the advent of HAART treatment, the incidence of cryptococcal infection in HIV has fallen substantially in the US. An increasing proportion of infections is being observed in other forms of immunodeficiency—such as organ transplant recipients.

■ *Trichosporon* & *Geotrichum* spp

☐ In cornmeal agar, *Trichosporon* and *Geotrichum* yeasts form arthroconidia. They can be distinguished on two bases:

☐ Pseudohyphal extensions extend from one corner of the rectangular arthroconidia of Geotrichum, resembling a **hockey stick,** whereas, two pseudohyphae extend from adjacent corners of Trichosporon, resembling **rabbit ears**

☐ Trichosporon species are **urease +,** *Geotrichum* species are not

☐ *Trichosporon beigelii* is the causative agent for white piedra.

■ *Rhodotorula*

☐ Cultures of *Rhodotorula* have red colonies. Microscopically, yeasts are observed. Pseudohyphae **are not** produced on cornmeal agar.

☐ Rarely significant clinically.

■ *Malassezia furfur*

☐ In KOH preps of skin scrapings and in histologic sections of affected skin, *M furfur* appears as short hyphae and spherical yeasts. This "spaghetti and meatballs" or "meatballs and frankfurters" appearance distinguishes it from the usual hyphae-only appearance of typical dermatophytes. In culture, *M furfer* grows as yeasts in just a few days on Sabouraud medium when appropriately cultured: 35°C & overlaid with olive oil.

- *M furfur* is associated with two forms of clinical infection

- Causative agent for *tinea versicolor* where the typical meatballs and franks morphology is seen in KOH preps of skin scrapings

- Causative agent in total parenteral nutrition-related *sepsis*

Mycology facts

The birdseed agar substrate is **caffeic acid;** the enzyme detected is **phenol oxidase.**

A fungus with a **beer-like odor:** *Saccharomyces*

A fungus with **feet** around edge of a yeast-like colony: *Candida*

Colonies with red **pigment:** *Rhodotorula, Penicillium marnefii, Fusarium*

If *Malassezia furfur* is suspected, cultures should be overlaid with **olive oil.**

Parenchymal infarction and angioinvasion: *Aspergillus* & *Zygomycosis*

Lobomycosis *Loboa loboi,* a fungus that does not grow in culture, is the causative agent of this South American cutaneous infection which results in enlarging verrucous skin lesions that must be treated by excision. Histologically, the dermis contains the yeasts which are around 10 to 12 μm and characteristically arranged in chains ('string of beads') that occasionally branch.

Prothecosis *Prototheca wicherhamii* is not a fungus and is possibly the only **algae** that causes human infection. Two types of infection have been recognized, both following some kind of penetrating skin trauma: cutaneous infection and olecranon bursitis. Distinctive endosporulating cysts (which look like a hub cap) are the diagnostic finding.

Bacteriology

Laboratory Methods

T3.26
Characteristic Gram-Stain Morphologies

Organism	Gram stain morphology
Enterobacteriaceae	(−) straight barrel-shaped rods
Streptococcus pneumoniae	(+) lancet-shaped diplococci
Neisseria	(−) kidney-shaped diplococci
Bacillus	(+) thick sporeforming bacilli
Clostridia	(+) thick sporeforming bacilli
Listeria	(+) small bacilli
Corynebacteria & Propionibacteria ("diphtheroids")	(+) small bacilli in "Chinese letters"
Vibrio	(−) curved rods
Campylobacter	(−) curved, S- or corkscrew- shaped rods. Pairs look like seagulls.
Yersinia pestis	(−) rods with safety pin appearance
Legionella	(−) coccobacilli in tissue
Cardiobacterium hominis	(−) highly pleomorphic bacilli when grown on BCYE: lollipop, dumbbell, and teardrop shapes
Nocardia	(+) branching, filamentous, bacilli
Actinomyces	(+) branching, filamentous, bacilli

Specimens

- Routine **aerobic and anaerobic cultures** can be performed on a wide variety of specimens. Specimens for anaerobic culture should be transported to the lab immediately, if possible, in anaerobic containers. Specimens transported anaerobically can still be used for aerobic cultures as well. The following sites normally harbor indigenous anaerobic flora and should not be cultured for anaerobes: stool, skin, oropharynx, vagina, and urethra.

- **Blood** culture bottles are ideally inoculated with **>10 mL of blood.** Inoculation of less than 5 mL has been shown to markedly reduce yield. The optimal number of blood cultures in a 24 hour period is 3. The sensitivity of 3 blood cultures is around 99.9%. Two or fewer blood cultures in 24 hours is significantly less sensitive. Greater than 3 does not improve sensitivity. When a patient is initially suspected of having bacterial sepsis, two separate blood cultures, drawn greater than 30 minutes apart from separate sites, are recommended. Otherwise, blood cultures are spaced about 8 hours apart.

- **Stool.** A single stool culture is usually adequate for an immunocompetent patient with acute enteritis. *C difficile* stool cultures are unreliable in hospitalized patients, since colonization is so common in this population. In this setting, *C difficile* **toxin assays** are preferred.

- **Throat.** Throat swabs are usually routinely cultured only for **group A streptococci.** If clinical suspicion is high for *C diphtheri*a or *N gonorrhea,* then cultures can be directed for those.

T 3.27
Additional Bacterial Stains

Organism	Stain
Haemophilus influenza in CSF	methylene blue stain
Nocardia	modified acid fast stain
Spirochetes	dark field examination
Corynebacterium diphtheria	Loeffler methylene blue (metachromatic granules)
Legionella	silver stain (Dieterle)

- **Urine.** Urines are cultured quantitatively. .

- **CSF.** Culture can be performed on CSF, which is a normally sterile site. Also, most labs can perform rapid antigen tests for the more common agents of meningitis.

- **Swabs.** For *N gonorrhea* do not use cotton-tipped applicators, as cotton is toxic to the organism. Transport and culture as soon as possible.

Direct examination

- **Gram staining** is routinely performed on all specimens from sterile sites. **T3.26**

  □ The gram stain is **not very sensitive,** and the sensitivity of culture is several times greater.

  □ **Crystal violet** stains the bacterial peptidoglycan cell wall. Iodine acts as a 'mordant'. **Gram-positive** organisms, that have a thick peptidoglycan cell wall, retain their crystal violet stain during the decolorization step. **Gram-negative** organisms, with their thin and attenuated cell walls, lose the crystal violet. **Safranin** is added as a counterstain. Alternatively, **basic fuchsin** can be used to counterstain weakly stainining organisms such as *Legionella.* **Note that older colonies of gram-positive organisms may stain as gram-negative due to degradation of their cell walls.** Over-decolorization can have the same result. Thus, if even some of the organisms in a smear are gram-positive, then the organism is best interpreted as gram-positive. This is because it would be extremely unusual for a gram negative to anomalously stain as a gram-positive, while, for the reasons stated, gram-positive may stain as gram -negative.

  □ **Gram staining procedure**

  - *Heat-fix* a smeared slide

  - *Crystal violet* for 20 seconds, then wash with tap water

  - *Gram iodine* for 20 seconds, then wash with tap water

  - *Decolorize,* then wash with tap water

- **Safranin** for 20 seconds, then wash with tap water

  - Air-dry

- **Acid-fast stains**

  □ These stains are based on the ability of *Mycobacteria* and certain other organisms to retain the red dye **carbol fuchsin** despite acidic decolorization. The basis for *Mycobacteria's* acid-fastness is the **mycolic acid** in their cell walls.

  □ In the usual **Ziehl-Neelsen** technique, heat is used to aid penetration of the carbol fuchsin. A strong acid, 3% HCl, is used for decolorization. The counterstain is methylene blue.

  □ In the Kinyoun ('cold') technique, heat is not applied.

  □ In the Fite (modified acid-fast) technique, a weaker acid, such as 1% H_2SO_4, is applied instead of hydrochloric acid for decolorization. Bacteria that are not acid-fast by the Ziehl-Neelsen technique, such as *Nocardia* and *M leprae,* may be acid-fast with Fite.

  □ An alternative to acid-fast stains for mycobacteria is the **fluorescent auramine-rhodamine stain.** This is more sensitive than acid-fast stains but nonspecific. Positive auramine-rhodamines must be confirmed with an acid-fast stain.

  □ AFB + organisms include: *Mycobacteria, Nocardia, Cryptosporidium, Microsporidium, Isospora, Sarcocystis, Legionella micdadei, Rhodococcus equi, Saccharomyces.*

- Other stains useful in direct examination **T3.27**.

Culture media **T3.28**, **T3.29**, **T3.30**

- **Blood agar.** Most pathogens can grow on blood agar, which is used for initially culturing most specimens. Sheep blood is most commonly used (SBA). Sheep blood may inhibit the growth of *Haemophilus.*

- **Chocolate agar** is the result of heating blood agar until the blood lyses. This frees factors required by certain species, especially *Haemophilus.*

- **Campy-BAP.** Used for selective isolation of *Campylobacter.*

- **Buffered charcoal yeast extract (BCYE) agar.** Used for isolation of *Legionella.*

- **Thayer-Martin agar.** Used for the isolation of *Neisseria* spp.

- **MacConkey agar.** Selective and differential medium for Enterobacteriaceae and related gram-negative bacilli. growth of gram-positives and many fastidious organisms is inhibited by bile salts. Lactose is the sole carbohydrate.

  □ **Red colonies**: *Escherichia, Klebsiella, Enterobacter* (strong lactose fermenters)

  □ **Pink colonies:** *Citrobacter, Providencia, Serratia, Hafnia*

  □ **Colorless colonies:** *Proteus, Edwardsiella, Salmonella, Shigella*

- **Eosin methylene blue (EMB) agar.** Like MacConkey, contains inhibitory substances (in this case aniline dyes) for gram positives and serves as a selective and differential medium.

  □ **Green-black-purple colonies:** *Escherichia, Klebsiella, Enterobacter, Serratia, Hafnia, Citrobacter, Providencia*

  □ **Colorless colonies:** *Proteus, Edwardsiella, Salmonella, Shigella*

- **Salmonella-Shigella (SS) agar** A highly selective agar which inhibits the growth of most coliforms. The high bile salts concentration and sodium citrate inhibit all gram positive bacteria and many gram negatives. Lactose is the sole carbohydrate.

  □ **Red colonies** Any lactose fermenters that manage to grow

  □ **Colorless colonies** *Shigella*

Bacteriology>Laboratory Methods

T3.28
Selective Agar for Gram-Negative Enteric Organisms

Selective Agar	Color of Fermenters	Nonfermenters
EMB	green-purple	clear
MacConkey	red-pink	clear
XLD	yellow	red
HE	yellow-orange	green
SS	red	clear
TCBS	yellow	clear

T3.30
Characteristic Odors in Culture

Organism	Peculiar Odor
Pseudomonas aeruginosa	grapes
Proteus	burned chocolate
Eikenella	bleach
Alkaligenes	freshly cut apples
Nocardia	musty basement
Bacteroides	acrid

T 3.29
Culture Procedures for Specific Organisms

Organism	Culture procedure
Haemophilus	Chocolate agar, SBA with staph streak, or colistin nalidixic acid (CNA) agar in moist environment with increased CO_2 (3%-5%)
Shigella from stool	Hektoen enteric agar, XLD agar, and Salmonella-Shigella (SS) agar
Staphylococcus aureus from mixed cultures such as stool	Colistin nalidixic acid (CNA) agar, mannitol salt agar (MSA), or phenylethyl alcohol (PEA) agar, all of which inhibit the growth of gram negatives.
Gardnerella vaginalis	Human blood agar is preferred
Campylobacter jejuni from stool	Inoculation of selective media such as Campy-BAP, in microaerophilic conditions (5% oxygen, 10% carbon dioxide, 85% nitrogen), and high incubation temperature (42° C)
Corynebacterium diphtheria	Inoculate Loeffler serum glucose medium, cystine telurite agar (Tinsdale agar), and 5% SBA.
Clostridium difficile	Inoculate CCFA (cycloserine-cefoxitin fructose-eggyolk agar).
Bordatella pertussis	Inoculate Bordet-Gengeou or Regan-Lowe agar in carbon dioxide-enriched environment at 35° C.
Legionella	Buffered charcoal yeast extract (BCYE) agar. Growth on BCYE but not cystine-deficient media is presumptive evidence of Legionella. The only other consideration is F. tularensis.
Salmonella typhi from stool	Wison-Blair bismuth sulfite agar
Neisseria	Modified Thayer-Martin, Martin-Lewis, or New York City media in CO_2 incubater or candle extinction jar at 35° C
Vibrio cholera	Thiosulfate-citrate bile sucrose (TCBS) agar is selective for V cholera. The recovery of yellow colonies (sucrose fermentation) is presumptive evidence of V cholera. Non-sucrose fermenting colonies of V parahemolyticus and V vulnificus are green.
Yersinia enterocolitica	Cefsulodin irgasan novobiocin (CIN) agar. Grows optimally at room temperature.
Clostridium difficile	Cycloserine cefoxitin eggyolk agar.
Streptobacillus moniliformis	Organism is inhibited by sodium polyanethol sulfonate in blood culture bottles and must be anticoagulated with citrate. Incubate at 35° C in a candle jar or CO_2 incubator. In broth, the organisms grow as 'puff balls'.
Brucella	The specimen of choice is bone marrow, although blood may also yield positive cultures. Biosafety level 3. Culture should be inoculated in Castaneda bottles, in which a slant of agar is partially submerged in a broth ('biphasic agar'). Should be inoculated at 35° C for 6 weeks with frequent blind subcultures to chocolate and blood agar.
E coli 0157:H7	Sorbitol MacConkey Medium. Sorbitol negative colonies are presumptively identified as 0157:H7.

□ **Colorless colonies with black center** *Salmonella*

■ **Hektoen-enteric (HE) agar** Serves the same purpose as SS agar.

□ **Salmon-pink to orange colonies** Fermenters

□ **Green colonies** *Shigella*

□ **Green colonies with black center** *Salmonella*

■ **Mannitol salt agar (MSA)** Is inhibitory towards most gram negative organisms. Can be used to isolate *S aureus* from mixed cultures.

Culture temperature. The optimal temperature for initial plating is usually 37°C. *Pseudomonas fluorescens* and *Mycobacterium marinum* grow optimally at 25°C to 30°C, while *Campylobacter* species tend to grow well at 42°C. *Listeria monocytogenes* is unique in that it grows at 37°C but displays its characteristic motility only at 25°C.

Biochemical tests

■ **Catalase** is an enzyme that converts hydrogen peroxide to water and oxygen. To peform the catalase test, a few drops of 3% hydrogen peroxide is added to a colony. Rapid and sustained effervescence indicates the presence of catalase. Ideally this test should be done from a medium that does not contain blood. The catalase test is often the first test used to initially categorize a gram positive isolate. It can differentiate Micrococcaceae (+) from streptococci (-). Micrococcaceae includes *Staphylococci* and the less clinically relevant *Micrococci*.

■ **Furazolidone susceptibility.** This is one of the tests used to distinguish *Staphylococci* from the other Micrococcaceae. *Staphylococci* are susceptible while *Micrococci* are not.

■ **Coagulase.** The coagulase test is used to distinguish *S aureus* (coagulase positive) from other staphylococci (coagulase negative). Coagulase is a protein with prothrombinlike activity capable of converting fibrinogen into fibrin. Two test formats are used

□ The **slide test** looks for **bound** coagulase. Bacterial clumping on the surface of a slide upon addition of rabbit plasma indicates the presence of bound coagulase.

□ The **tube test** looks for **free** coagulase and is substituted for the more rapid slide test when insufficient numbers of colonies are present to make a dense emulsion or when the slide test is negative at 30 seconds. Examination of the tube at **both** 4 and 20 hours is necessary, since certain strains produce a fibrinolysin, which will dissolve any coagulum that forms, giving a false-negative result if only examined at 20 hours. Others produce a delayed reaction that will give false-negative results if examined only at 4 hours.

■ **Novobiocin susceptibility.** This is one of the tests used to distinguish among coagulase negative staphylococci. *S saprophyticus* is the common novobiocin resistant species, and *S epidermidis* is susceptible. Thus, coagulase negative staphylococci that are novobiocin resistant can be presumptively identified as *S saprophyticus*.

■ **Bacitracin & TMP-SXT.** Susceptibility to bacitracin and TMP-SXT provides an easy method for presumptive differentiation of β-hemolytic streptococci. Group B streptococcus is resistant to both, while group A streptococcus is resistant to TMP-SXT but sensitive to bacitracin. Other β-hemolytic streptococci are susceptible to both.

■ **6.5% NaCl tolerance.** To separate group D enterococci from group D non-enterococci, the salt tolerance test is performed. *Enterococcus* spp will be salt tolerant, whereas group D organisms (*S bovis*) will not.

■ **CAMP test.** This test is used to presumptively identify group B b-hemolytic streptococci. The test was first described by Christie, Atkins, and Munch-Peterson (hence the name CAMP). It is based on the fact that the hemolytic activity of the β-hemolysis of *S aureus* is enhanced by an extracellular protein (CAMP factor) produced by group B streptococci.

■ **PYR test.** The PYR (pyrrolindonyl-b-naphthylamide) test is used to identify group A and group D streptococci. It can replace the bacitracin and salt tolerance tests, respectively. Aminopeptidase produced by these bacteria hydrolyzes PYR which, in the presence of a detection reagent, yields a red color change.

■ **Bile-esculin test.** Enterococci & and group D non-enterococci (*S bovis*) can grow in 40% bile and hydrolyze esculin. To perform the test, a bile-esculin agar slant is streak-inoculated and incubated for 24 hours. Diffuse blackening of more than half the slant indicates esculin hydrolysis.

- **Bile solubility.** *S pneumoniae* (pneumococci) are soluble in bile (deoxycholate).

- **Optochin** (P-disk) selectively inhibits *S pneumoniae* (pneumococci).

- **Cytochrome oxidase.** The immediate development of a blue color after a colony is smeared on a reagent-impregnated strip or after reagent is added to a colony indicates oxidase activity. The reagent, *p*-phenylenediamine, is oxidized by cytochrome oxidase, forming iodophenol blue. All Enterobacteriaceae are oxidase negative. *Vibrionaceae, Aeromonas, Neisseria, Pseudomonas, Campylobacter* & *Pasteurella* are oxidase positive.

- **Indole.** The immediate development of a red color after the addition of Kovac or Ehrlich reagent (*p*-dimethylaminocinnamaldehyde) indicates the presence of indole, the product of bacterial tryptophanase which cleaves tryptophan into indole, pyruvate, and NH_4. Lactose +, indole + colonies appearing after 24 hours on MacConkey agar, particularly on isolates from the urinary tract, are presumptively identified as *E coli*.

- **Methyl red test.** Only two pathways are used by bacteria to metabolize pyruvate: resulting in mixed acid *or* butylene glycol production. Mixed acid production (strong acid production) results in a pH below 4.4 which is the indicator point for methyl red. Species that are methyl red negative are Voges-Proskauer positive and vice versa.

- **Voges-Proskauer.** The pathway that metabolizes pyruvate to butylene glycol instead of mixed acid gives off acetyl methyl carbinol (acetoin) as a by-product. When KOH is added, the acetoin is converted to diacetyl which reacts with a naphthol to produce a red color. Among enterobacteriaceae, the Klebsiellae (*Klebsiella-Enterobacter-Hafnia-serratia*) are VP positive while all others are MR positive.

- **Nitrate reduction.** Certain organisms can reduce nitrates to nitrites. The presence of nitrites can be detected by adding a-naphtylamine and sulfanilic acid

with the formation of a red color. However, the reduction of nitrate to nitrite is only the first step in the case of some bacteria that go on to produce N_2 gas. Thus, if a red color does not develop upon addition of reagent, then either nitrate has not been reduced or nitrite has been further processed to other compounds such as N_2. A small quantity of zinc is then added to reduce any residual nitrate; production of a red color after zinc is added thus indicates that nitrate was never reduced in the first place, and confirms a negative nitrate reduction test. **All enterobacteriaceae demonstrate nitrate reduction.** This test is also used in differentiating members of the *Hemophilus, Neisseria,* and *Branhamella* genera.

- **Urease.** In this test, organisms that produce urease hydrolyze urea releasing ammonia producing a pink-red color. Stuarts broth is heavily buffered, requiring large quantities of ammonia to induce a color change. Stuarts broth, therefore, is virtually selective for *Proteus.* Christensens broth contains less buffer and is accordingly less specific. It detects rapid urea splitters (*Proteus*) which turn the entire medium red, and slow urea splitters (*Klebsiella*) which turn only the slant red.

- **Hugh-Leifson OF medium.** Most conventional media designed to detect acid production from fermentation are not suitable for the study of "nonfermenters" which either do not grow or produce too weak an acid to convert the pH indicator. Hugh-Leifson OF medium is formulated to increase growth of such organisms and increase sensitivity for acid production. Two tubes are incubated: one exposed to air, and the other overlaid with mineral oil. Acid production is detected in the medium by the appearance of a yellow color. Oxidative organisms produce acid only in the open tube, and fermenting organisms produce acid in both tubes. Nonsaccharolytic bacteria are inert in both tubes.

- **Flagellar stain** T3.31. Most motile bacteria possess flagella. The Leifson staining technique is most commonly employed for this test. Flagella are classified as: (1) polar monotrichous—single polar flagellum (2) polar multitrichous (3) subpolar (4) lateral (5) peritrichous—flagella arranged around cell. This test is used among the nonfermenters.

- **Esculin hydrolysis.** Esculin hydrolysis is used primarily as a differential characteristic to distinguish *Pseudomonas* spp.

- **String test.** When colonies of *V cholera* are mixed in a drop of 0.5% sodium deoxycholate on a slide, they produce a viscous suspension that can be drawn into a string with an inoculating loop. This string becomes more tenacious with time in contrast to other vibrios that may give an initial string reaction that diminishes within 60 seconds. Thus, *V cholera,* with the exception of the el Tor biotype, can be distinguished from non-cholera vibrios.

- **Staph streak test.** *Haemophilus* spp may grow as pinpoint colonies around colonies of *S aureus,* a phenomenon called satellitism. This is due to the ability of *S aureus* to synthesize V factor, and to release X factor by lysing blood. A colony of possible *Haemophilus* spp can be subcultured to an SBA plate and streaked as a lawn. A single streak of *S aureus* is made through the inoculum. After overnight growth in a CO_2-enriched environment, the *Haemophilus* colonies may be observed within the hemolytic area adjacent to the staphylococcal growth. This is presumptive evidence that an unknown isolate is a *Haemophilus* spp.

- **CHO utilization tests for *Neisseria*.** An organism growing on selective media, suspected of being a *Neisseria* species, is further delineated by CHO utilization tests to distinguish *N gonorrhea, N meningitidis,* & *N lactamica.* Traditionally, cysteine-tryptic digest semi-solid agar (CTA) is used for this purpose. The battery includes CTA-glucose, CTA-maltose, CTA-sucrose, & CTA-lactose. A color change from red to yellow indicates production of acid. Results are interpreted as follows. An organism that is glucose positive is *N gonorrhea.* One that is maltose positive is *N meningitidis.* Lactose positive is *N lactamica.* An organism that is negative for all sugars is *M catarrhalis.*

- **Superoxol test.** Superoxol is a helpful test for the rapid presumptive diagnosis of *N gonorrhea.* Superoxol is 30% hydrogen peroxide (not the 3% solution routinely used for the catalase test). *N gonorrhea* strains rapidly produce brisk bubbling. *N meningitidis* produces weak, delayed bubbling.

- **Tests for X/V factor T3.32.** X factor (hemin) and V factor (NAD) requirements are used to classify various *Haemophilus* spp. Filter paper disks or strips impregnated with these factors are placed on the surface of a factor-deficient medium such as brain-heart infusion agar. Organisms are then inoculated onto this medium.

- **DNAse** *Moraxella catarrhalis* is the only gram-negative coccus that produces DNAse. This allows for its distinction from *Neisseria.*

Specific Bacteria: Key Characteristics

Gram-positive cocci. Once the obligate anaerobes (Peptococcus and Peptostreptococcus) have been excluded, the remaining pathogenic organisms, for practical purposes, include only *Staphylococci* and *Streptococci.* The first test to distinguish among these, besides the gram stain morphology, is the **catalase test.**

- **Anaerobes**

  □ Peptostreptococcus

  □ Peptococcus

T3.31
Flagellar Characteristics

Organism	Flagellar staining
Bordatella	Peritrichous
Flavobacterium	Nonmotile
Pseudomonas aeruginosa	Polar monotrichous
Pseudomonas cepacia	Polar multitrichous
Acinetobacter	Nonmotile
Xanthomonas	Polar muititrichous
Moraxella	Nonmotile

T3.32
Tests for X/V Factor

Organism requires	Species
X & V factors	H influenzae, H haemolyticus, H aegyptius
V factor only	H parainfluenzae, H parahaemolyticus, H aphrophilus
X factor only	H ducreyi

- **Catalase-positive**, gram-positive *cocci* in clusters, pairs, or tetrads: *Staphylococci*. These are divided into coagulase positive and coagulase negative *Staphylococci*. The latter are usually only further classified in urine specimens. Coagulase-positive *Staphylococcus*, for practical purposes, equals *S aureus*. However, *S intermedius*, *S hyicus*, & *S delphini* are uncommon isolates that are also coagulase positive. *S intermedius* is isolated from dog-bite infections.

  □ *S aureus*. Distinguished from other staphylococci by being uniquely coagulase-positive, β hemolytic, and DNAse-positive.

  □ *S saprophyticus*. Produces white chalky colonies and is the only coagulase-negative staphylococcus that is novobiocin resistant.

  □ *S epidermidis*. Coagulase-negative and novobiacin-sensitive

- **Catalase-negative**, gram-positive cocci in chains: *Streptococci*. Over the years, these organisms have been categorized according to hemolytic ability (α, β, or γ), pathogenicity (pyogenic, viridans, or enterococcal), or surface antigens (Lancefield). For practical purposes, streptococci are initially subclassified according to hemolysis—whether they produce complete (β), incomplete (α), or no (γ) hemolysis. **β-hemolytic** colonies are either group A (*S pyogenes*), group B (*S agalactiae*), or uncommonly fall into a miscellany of organisms in groups C, F, and G. **α-hemolytic** colonies are either *S pneumoniae* or a group of miscellaneous organisms called viridans streptococci. **γ-hemolytic** colonies are either group D streptococci (which includes both Enterococci and non-Enterococci) or viridans streptococci. Serotyping for Lancefield group antigens can be carried out as a confirmatory test of any presumptive isolate.

  □ β hemolysis

    - *S pyogenes* (group A *streptococci*): β hemolysis, bacitracin (A-disk) sensitive, PYR hydrolysis +

    - *S agalactiae* (group B streptococci): β hemolysis, **CAMP test +**, hippurate hydrolysis +

    - Group C, F, and G: non-group A or B streptococci which form minute β hemolytic colonies

  □ **Group D**

    - *E faecalis* & *E faecium* (Group D Enterococci): Bile-esculin positive, γ-hemolytic, 6.5% NaCl tolerant, PYR hydrolysis-positive

    - *S bovis* (Group D non-Enterococci): Bile-esculin-positive, γ-hemolytic, no growth in 6.5% NaCl, PYR hydrolysis-negative

  □ *S pneumoniae* α-hemolytic, bile soluble, Optochin (P-disk) sensitive. Pathogenic strains have an antiphagocytic capsule that results in smooth colonies. Rough colonies lack the capsule and are nonpathogenic.

  □ *S mutans, S salivaris, S sanguis, S mitis, S anginosus* (Viridans streptococci) γ- or α-hemolytic colonies that are bile-esculin negative and Optochin (P-disk) resistant.

- **Catalase-negative, vancomycin-resistant, gram-positive cocci in chains** *Streptococcus*-like organisms (*Leuconostoc* & *Pediococcus*)

Gram-negative cocci

- **Anaerobes: Veilonella**

- **Oxidase-positive, catalase-positive, nonmotile, gram-negative, kidney-bean shaped diplococci:** *Neisseria*. Like *Moraxella* spp (below), these organisms are fastidious and require prompt incubation in a CO_2-rich environment at 35°C. Chocolate agar with several antibiotics to inhibit indigenous flora (such as Thayer-Martin agar) is most commonly used for isolation. Avoidance of cotton-containing swabs is crucial in sample collection. In direct examination of clinical specimens (eg, urethral swabs), organisms often appear as **intracellular** diplococci.

  □ *N gonorrhea:* Ferments glucose only, superoxol test-positive

  □ *N meningitidis:* Ferments glucose & maltose

  □ *N lactamica:* Ferments glucose, maltose, and lactose

■ Oxidase-positive, catalase-positive, non motile, **DNAse** -positive, gram negative, kidney-bean shaped diplococci, whose colonies display the hockey puck sign (colonies are hard to emulsify and can be pushed across the agar): *Moraxella catarrhalis.*

Gram-positive bacilli. One way to initially classify gram positive bacilli is by their gram stain morphology. A group of gram-positive rods appearing as beaded, often branching, filamentous chains include *Actinomyces* & *Nocardia* (and *Mycobacteria*). *Actinomyces* are non-acid-fast and anaerobic, while *Nocardia* are weakly acid-fast and aerobic. Gram-positive rods with so-called diphtheroid morphology include *Corynebacterium, Listeria,* and *Propionibacterium.* The remaining gram-positive bacilli, which are nonbeaded and nondiphtheroid, are classified according to whether they form spores and are anaerobic. Obligately anaerobic spore-formers are *Clostridia.* Nonanaerobic spore-formers are *Bacillus.* Nonspore-formers are *Lactobacilli* (anaerobic) or *Listeria* (aerobic).

■ **Anaerobic gram-positive bacilli**

☐ **Spore formation** *Clostridia*

● ***C perfringens*** Double zone of hemolysis, lecithinase-positive, stormy fermentation of milk

T3.33
Taxonomy of the Enterobacteriaceae

Family (Tribe)	Genus & Species
Escherichieae	***Escherichia:*** *E coli* **Shigella:** *S sonnei, S flexneri, S dysenteriae, S boydii*
Edwardsiellae	*Edwardsiella tarda*
Salmonellae	***Salmonella:*** *S enteritidis, S typhi, S paratyphi, S cholerasuis*
Citrobactereae	*Citrobacter freundii*
Klebsiellae	***Klebsiella:*** *K. pneumoniae* **Enterobacter:** *E aerogenes, E cloacae* **Hafnia:** *H alvei* ***Pantoea:*** *P agglomerans* **Serratia:** *S marcescens*
Proteae	***Proteus:*** *P vulgaris, P mirabilis* ***Morganella:*** *M morganii* ***Providencia:*** *P stuartii*
Yersinieae	*Yersinia enterocolitica*

● ***C botulinum.*** Toxin production

● ***C tetani*** Motility, toxin production, terminal spores

● ***C septicum***

● ***C difficile***

☐ **Non-spore formers**

☐ ***Actinomyces*** Branching filamentous bacteria that are non-acid-fast

● ***Bifidobacteria*** have bifid ends

● ***Propionibacterium.*** Diphtheroid morphology, propionic acid production

● ***Lactobacillus***

■ **Aerobic gram-positive bacilli**

☐ **Spore-formers** *Bacillus.* On Gram stain, *Bacillus* species are large, square-ended bacilli, with spores, that often form chains. With the notable exception of *B anthracis,* they are motile.

● *B anthracis.* No hemolysis, nonmotile, penicillin sensitive. Medusa-head colonies on SBA. Cell wall contains a ***poly-D-glutamyl polypeptide.*** Produces a 3-part toxin (edema factor, protective antigen, and lethal factor).

● *B cereus* β-hemolytic, motile, penicillin sensitive. Causes food poisoning associated with boiled rice.

☐ **Non-spore formers**

● ***Listeria monocytogenes.*** β-hemolytic, tumbling motility (umbrella motility) at room temperature, catalase-positive, bile-esculin-positive. Isolation is enhanced if tissue is kept at 4°C for several days prior to culture (cold enrichment). *L monocytogenes* appears to preferentially infect pregnant women and older immunocompromised individuals. Causes a transient febrile illness in pregnancy that may eventuate in premature birth. Infants born to infected women may devel-

op 'granulomatosis infantisepticum', characterized by abscesses in many organs including lung, brain, liver, kidney, bone, soft tissue, and skin that are typical suppurative abscesses and not true granulomata. In immunocompromised adults, meningitis is common.
About 10% of infected individuals have a marked peripheral **monocytosis.**

- *Erysipelothrix.* H$_2$S production on TSI agar

- *Nocardia* weakly acid-fast, thin branching filamentous rods. Can use paraffin as sole carbon source. Colonies are dry and chalky and have a characteristic 'musty basement' odor. Nocardia species may be isolated from bacterial, fungal, or mycobacterial cultures.

- *Streptomyces*

- *Rhodococus* is weakly acid-fast

- *Corynebacterium diphtheria.* Club-shaped gram positive rods with diphtheroid morphology. Contain metachromatic granules when stained with methylene blue. Produces a toxin that, in addition to local effects on the throat, causes myocarditis and neuropathy.

- *Corynebacterium jeikeium.* Metallic sheen in colonies grown on SBA, resistant to everything except vancomycin. Cause infections of immunocompromised hosts and of prosthetic devices.

Gram-negative bacilli. Once obligate anaerobes (*Fusobacterium, Bacteroides,* etc) have been excluded, the gram-negative bacilli are initially classified by their growth characteristics on MacConkey agar. The Enterobacteriaceae are organisms that grow robustly on MacConkey. These organisms are further subdivided by their ability to ferment lactose. The so-called fastidious organisms that do not grow well on MacConkey are a confusing hodge-podge of different species that must be grown on special media.

- ■ **Anaerobic gram-negative bacilli**

  - □ *Bacteroides*

  - □ *Porphyromonas/Prevotella:* production of a brown-black pigment, brick-red fluorescence.

  - □ *Fusobacteria*

- ■ **Growth on MacConkey, glucose fermentation-positive, nitrate-positive, oxidase-negative, catalase-positive:** Enterobacteriaceae. The Enterobacteriaceae are a large group of organisms that can be difficult to sort out. **T3.33** Some benchmark characteristics to remember.

  - □ **Strong lactose fermenters:** *Escherichia, Klebsiella.*

  - □ **Phenylalanine deaminase (PDA)-positive:** *Proteus, Morganella, Providencia* (all Proteae).

  - □ **Nonmotile:** *Shigella, Klebsiella.* **Yersinia** **are non motile at 37°C, but motile at 22°C.**

  - □ **Hydrogen sulfide (H$_2$S)-positive:** *Salmonella, Edwardsiella, Citrobacter, Proteus*

  - □ **Voges-Proskauer (VP)-positive:** *Klebsiella, Enterobacter, Hafnia, Serratia* (all Klebsielleae).

  - □ **Methyl red (MR)+** :the opposite of VP.

  - □ **The Kligler Iron Agar & Triple Sugar Iron (KIA/TSI) slants.** Recall that these are test tubes with agar that contains proteins, sugars, and a phenol red indicator. The sugars are present in a 10 g of lactose to 1 g of glucose ratio. The phenol red indicator is yellow when the pH is below 6.8 and red when above 6.8. The organism is inoculated by stabbing all the way to the bottom of the tube then streaking the surface. The organism undergoes aerobic growth on the slant and anaerobic growth in the deep (or butt). Its ability to ferment the sugars in the medium is evidenced by lowering of the pH (yellowing of the indicator). The slants are interpreted at 24 hours. A bacterium that ferments glucose but not lactose will produce, after 8 hours, an acidic (yellow) slant and acidic (yellow) deep. However, oxidative metabolism of proteins (which can only take place in the oxygen rich environment of the slant) will turn the slant back to alkaline (red) by 24 hours. Organisms that ferment lactose, since it is present in the agar in such high quantities, will overcome this protein alkalinization and maintain a yellow slant until 24 hours. Any gas or

H_2S production in the deep implies prior fermentation and is interpreted as acidic. After 24-hour incubation, results are interpreted as follows

- *Alkaline slant/alkaline deep (K/K):* Enterobacteriaceae excluded. Possibilities include nonfermentative bacteria such as *Pseudomonas, Eikenella, Moraxella, Campylobacter.*

- *Alkaline slant/Acid deep (K/A):* Glucose fermented, lactose not fermented. Possibilities include *Shigella, Serratia, Providencia, Yersinia.*

- *Alkaline slant/Acid deep, with H_2S production (K/A/ H2S+):* Glucose fermented, lactose not fermented, production of H_2S. Possibilities include *Salmonella, Edwardsiella, Citrobacter,* & *Proteus.*

- *Acid slant/Acid deep (A/A):* Lactose fermenters. Possibilities include *Eschericia.*

- *Acid slant/Acid deep, with gas production (A/A/Gas+):* Lactose fermenters that produce gas. Possibilities include *Klebsiella* and *Enterobacter.*

□ ***Proteus.*** Any urease + isolate should be considered a member of the family Proteae, which includes *Proteus, Morganella,* and *Providencia.* Members of this family are also uniformly PDA-positive. Proteus species produce H_2S and grow in colonies appearing either as a thin film or as a wavelike spreading of the organism across large portions of the plate, due to **swarming motility.** *P mirabilis* is the most common isolate from this genus. It causes urinary tract infections (UTI) and, due to its production of urease, can promote alkalinization of the urine and precipitation of staghorn calculi.

□ ***Shigella*** Most common cause of shigellosis in developed countries such as the US: *S sonnei.* In underdeveloped contries: *S flexneri.* Shigella infection requires the smallest inoculum of any form of bacterial gastroenteritis—only about 100-200 bacteria. Shigella, like EHEC discussed below, can cause hemolytic uremic syndrome (HUS). The laboratory characteristic to remember about Shigella is that it is negative for almost everything except methyl red. It is lactose-negative, does not

produce gas or H_2S, Voges-Proskauer -, Indole -, Citrate -, PDA -, and non-motile. It is methyl red +.

□ ***Yersinia*** is selectively isolated using 'cold enrichment', in which a specimen is stored at 4°C for 2 weeks prior to culturing. A unique feature is that most *Yersinia* infections are zoonotic. Humans are accidental hosts.

□ ***Y enterocolitica*** causes enterocolitis in places with colder climates. It characteristically centers upon the terminal ileum and can cause the misdiagnosis of appendicitis. *Y. enterocolitica* is responsible for most cases of **blood transfusion-related sepsis.**

□ ***Y pseudotuberculosis*** is an uncommon cause of disease, but is noteworthy because it produces necrotizing granulomata histopathologically resembling tuberculosis.

□ ***Y pestis*** causes plague. Sylvatic plague is that variety which is found in nonurban settings and is carried by squirrels, field rats, and domestic cats. Urban plague is found in densely populated areas and is carried by rats.

□ ***Citrobacter*** A genus closely resembling *Salmonella,* including citrate positivity. It differs mainly from Salmonella in the ONPG reaction, which is positive for Citrobacter.

□ ***Edwardsiella*** is a great mimicker of *Salmonella* and *E coli* due to its similar biochemical reactions. It differs from *E coli* only in its production of H_2S. It is distinguished from *Salmonella* with a positive indole test. It is unique in many respects, including: its proclivity to infect persons with iron overload, and coinfection with *E histolytica.*

□ ***Escherichia.*** Members of this genus are presumptively identified when an Enterobacteriaceae organism is lactose fermenting and indole-positive. Close mimickers of the Escherichiae include *Shigella* which differs only in being nonmotile and *Edwardsiella* that is H_2S-positive.

- *ETEC* (enterotoxigenic *E coli*) causes infection of the small intestine resulting in secretory diarrhea with clinical manifestations indistinguishable from cholera. It is the main cause of 'traveler's diarrhea'. It produces toxins similar to the cholera toxin, the so-called heat-stable and heat labile enterotoxins which stimulate guanylate and adenylate cyclase, respectively.

- *EIEC* (enteroinvasive *E coli*) causes invasion of the colon and a clinical dysentery similar to that caused by *Shigella*.

- *EPEC* (enteropathogenic *E coli*) causes gastroenteritis in infants in underdeveloped countries.

- *EHEC* (enterohemorrhagic *E coli*) elaborates a verotoxin (shiga-like toxin) which inhibits protein synthesis, causing damage to enterocytes. Once released into the blood stream, the shiga-like toxin causes damage to endothelial cells. EHEC has gained notoriety for its association with hemolytic uremic syndrome (HUS), after the production of a hemorrhagic colitis. HUS develops in about 10% of infected children, about 5-12 days after the onset of diarrhea. The EHEC serotype O157:H7 is the most commonly implicated in this syndrome. Its identifying laboratory characterisitic is its inability to ferment sorbitol. Suspected cases are incubated onto both regular MacConkey and a special MacConkey containing 1% sorbitol instead of lactose. A bacterium capable of fermenting lactose of regular MacConkey (grows as yellow colonies) but incapable of fermenting 1% sorbitol (grows as clear colonies) is presumptively identified as EHEC. The major reservoir for EHEC is cattle, with ingestion of contaminated meat and milk being the most common route of infection. An emerging form of EHEC is O157:NM, found presently in Australia and Europe, and capable of causing HUS.

  - *EAggEC* (enteroaggregative *E coli*) causes infant diarrhea in underdeveloped countries.

☐ *Salmonella.* Salmonellosis is most commonly manifested as enteritis; however, certain species have the potential to produce bacteremia: *S cholerasuis, S paratyphi, S typhi.* This is particularly a problem in children. Typhoid fever, caused by *S typhi* or *S paratyphi,* is yet another possible consequence of Salmonella infection. In this syndrome, bacteria traverse the bowel wall and entrench themselves within reticuloendothelial cells of the liver, spleen, & gallbladder. From these organs, repeated bouts of bacteremia occur. From the gallbladder, the bowel is continually reinfected, leading to long-term shedding of the bacterium.

☐ *Klebsiella.* You know you are dealing with a member of the family Klebsielleae when the isolate is Voges-Proskauer-positive. Among the Klebsielleae, *Klebsiella* is unique in its lack of motility and the production of large mucoid colonies. Actually, *Klebsiella* and *Shigella* are the only nonmotile Enterobacteriaceae. Also called the 'Friedlander bacillus', *K. pneumoniae* causes lobar pneumonia, particularly in alcoholic males. *K. rhinoscleromatis* is the cause of rhinoscleroma, a condition in which dense collections of foamy histiocytes are found in the nasopharynx.

☐ *Serratia. S marcescens* is causes pneumonia and sepsis in hospitalized, debilitated patients. It is a notorious cause of nosocomial infections linked to a common source, often a medical device. A minority of strains produce a red pigment known as 'prodigiousum'.

■ **Growth on MacConkey, oxidase-positive, glucose fermentation:** nonenteric fermenters

☐ *V cholerae.* Sucrose-positive on TCBS (yellow colonies), string test-positive. El Tor biotype is distinctive for β-hemolysis, weak string test, & ability to agglutinate chicken erythrocytes. *Vibrio cholerae* is traditionally classified by somatic O antigens (more than 150 O types currently recognized), by biotype (classical and El Tor), or by serotype (Ogawa, Inaba, and Hikojima). Based upon O antigens, isolates are broadly characterized as *V cholerae* O1 (etiologic agents of most cases of cholera) and non-O1 *V cholerae*. Serogroup O139 has emerged as an additional significant cause of cholera in the Indian subcontinent.

☐ *V parahemolyticus:* sucrose-negative on TCBS (green colonies).

☐ *Aeromonas*

□ *Plesiomonas*

- **Growth on MacConkey, oxidase-positive, glucose nonfermenters:** nonfermenters.

  □ *Pseudomonas:* Oxidase-positve, motile by means of polar monotrichous flagellum, β-hemolytic, grape-like odor, green pyocyanin pigment, growth at 42° centigrade.

  □ *Xanthomonas maltophilia:* Oxidase-negative, motile by means of polar multitrichous flagella.

  □ *Acinetobacter:* Oxidase-negative, nonmotile, coccobacilli resembling *neisseria*.

  □ *Flavobacterium meningosepticum* Oxidase-positive, yellow colonies on sheep blood agar.

- **No growth on MacConkey, slow growth of pinpoint colonies on enriched media: fastidious organisms.**

  □ *F. tularensis:* slow-growing gram-negative coccobacillus that requires cysteine and cystine.

  - Tularemia is usually acquired from arthropods or exposure to infected animals, but some are the result of inhalation of contaminated dust. Tularemia has a high fatality rate. The presentation is nonspecific and flu-like (fever, chills, headache, pulmonary manifestations, fatigue), with cutaneous ulcers and lymphadenopathy. Tularemia is also known as rabbit fever and deer fly fever. Clinical presentations are variously described as ulceroglandular, oculoglandular, pneumonic, and typhoidal.

    - Serology is the most common way that the diagnosis is made, but often this requires paired sera, delaying the diagnosis. The organisms is difficult to culture, and the attempt creates a danger to laboratory personnel. But serology can take more than a week to confirm the diagnosis and there is cross-reactivity with other organisms. Recently, PCR assays have been developed for use in formalin-fixed, paraffin-embedded tissue, as well as direct clinical specimens, providing the opportunity for rapid and safe diagnosis.

□ *Francisella* is one of the agents considered a possible agent of bioterrorism.

□ *Brucella:* very slow-growing gram negative coccobacillus that is urease-positive, oxidase-positive, and catalase-positive. Catalase tests should be avoided because they may aerosolize the organism. The organisms is commonly isolated in Castaneda bottles, and biosafety level 3 precautions must be observed. *Brucella* spp can be isolated from blood, bone marrow, bone, and other tissues.

- The major source of infection is livestock, particularly cattle (*Brucella abortus*), goats and sheep (*Brucella melitensis*), and swine (*Brucella suis*). Rare cases are due to *Brucella canis,* acquired by exposure to dogs. The epidemiology of brucellosis in the US has changed from an occupational disease among livestock handlers and abattoir workers to a foodborne illness acquired by consumption of unpasteurized goat and cow dairy products. Airborne transmission is possible, raising the possibility of use as a bioterrorism agent. 50 to 60% of brucellosis infections in the US now occur in California and Texas, mostly among Hispanics.

- Upon entering the body, the organisms have tropism for the reticuloendothelial system. The clinical manifestations are largely nonspecific, but fever is invariable, lymphadenopathy, hepatosplenomegaly and inflammatory arthritis are common, and malodorous perspiration is considered nearly pathognomonic. Arthritis may

T3.34

Hemolysis and Growth Factor Characteristics

Species	Requires X-factor	Requires V-factor	Hemolysis
H influenzae	+	+	−
H parainfluenza	−	+	−
H haemolyticus	+	+	+
H parahaemolyticus	−	+	+
H aegyptius	+	+	+
H ducreyi	+	−	−

affect the appendicular joints as well as the sacroiliac joint and spine. Other manifestations include spontaneous abortion, hepatitis (with granulomas in biopsies), and endocarditis (a principal source of mortality).

- Infections commonly manifest nonspecific laboratory abnormalities: mild anemia, mildly depressed white blood cell counts with relative lymphocytosis, and abnormal liver function tests. The abnormalities in *B melitensis* infections are more severe, giving the greatest elevations in AST, ALT, and LDH, and tend to include thrombocytopenia.

- Relapses, usually within the first year, occur in about 10% of cases.

- Definitive diagnosis of brucellosis requires isolation of the bacterium from blood or tissue samples. The sensitivity of blood culture is low, just over 50%, and prolonged incubation may be required (traditionally up to 4 weeks in biphasic medium with periodic blind subcultures onto solid media were the standard of practice); although most become positive within 2 weeks. Bone marrow cultures have much higher yield.

- Serologic testing, traditionally involving the serum agglutination test, is considered positive when titers above 1:160 are found. However, the serum agglutination test is insensitive to *B canis* and cross reacts with *Francisella tularensis,* some *Escherichia coli* species, and *Vibrio.* ELISA assays have been developed that overcome many of the limitations facing the serum agglutination test and demonstrate superior sensitivity and specificity.

- Real-time PCR is most promising test at the present time.

□ *Bordetella:* growth in 2-4 days on Bordet-Gengeau or Regan-Lowe media, peritrichous flagella.

□ *Pasteurella:* a gram negative rod isolated from a likely source (animal bite) that is oxidase-positive, catalase-positive, and strongly indole-positive.

□ *Legionella:* no growth on MacConkey or SBA, but small whitish colonies in 2-5 days on BCYE medium (must exclude *F. tularensis* which shows the same growth characteristics).

□ *Campylobacter jejuni:* curved seagull-shaped gram-negative rods, 42° C growth on selective media (Campy-BAP), hippurate hydrolysis, oxidase-positive, catalase-positive. The hippurate hydrolysis test is key for distinguishing *C jejuni* from other *Campylobacter* spp.

□ *Capnocytophaga canimorsus:* requires high CO_2 for growth, gliding motility, finger-like extensions at margin of colonies. One of the agents of post-dog-bite soft tissue infections.

□ *Streptobacillus monoliformis*: puffball or cotton-ball-like colonies in broth. Causative agent of rat-bite fever.

□ *Haemophilus:* no growth on MacConkey or SBA, but small colonies on chocolate agar. The species are classified by hemolysis and growth requirements **T3.34**.

□ *Helicobacter pylori* is a gram-negative spiral bacillus that is the cause of the vast majority of cases of chronic gastritis and the ultimate cause of gastritis complications—peptic ulcer disease, gastric adenocarcinoma (predominantly the intestinal type), and gastric MALT lymphoma.

- *H pylori* prevalence varies with patient age, socioeconomic status, and ethnic group. Typically, incidence increases with age. Infection has lowest prevalence in upper socioeconomic groups. In the US, prevalence is about 50% in African Americans, 60% in Mexican Americans, and 26% in whites.

- *H pylori* infection is a chronic condition. There tends to be long latency before manifestations develop. Eradication is recommended for all patients with the infection, regardless of symptoms, in order to reduce the risk of malignancy. Interestingly, treatment of *H pylori* may result in enhanced gastric acid production (due to reversal of atrophic gastritis), leading to so-called unmasking of gastroesophageal reflux disease (GERD).

- The diagnosis may be made through numerous avenues:

- Serologic testing for IgG anti–*H pylori* becomes positive by 4 weeks after infection. Since most patients who present for testing have been infected for many years, the sensitivity of this test is quite good. Testing can be performed on urine as well as serum. Serology can remain positive for many years after eradication. A consequence of this is the uselessness of serology to confirm eradication.

- Urea breath testing can be used both to diagnose *H pylori* and confirm eradication. The patient ingests radiolabeled urea which, if *H pylori* is present, is converted by bacterial urease into radiolabeled CO_2.

- Stool antigen testing and stool culture are available.

- Histologic examination has the advantage of permitting not only detection of *H pylori*, but examination of the biopsy for premalignant changes (intestinal metaplasia, dysplasia). Additional tissue can be subjected to rapid urease testing or culture.

- Following treatment for *H pylori*, which has a high failure rate, confirmation of eradication is necessary. At least 4 weeks should elapse between cessation of treatment and confirmatory testing, to permit re-growth of residual bacteria; otherwise the false negative rate is unacceptably high. If a stool-based test is used for confirmation, 6 to 12 weeks should elapse.

□ *Tropheryma whippelii* has not been successfully cultured. The causative agent of Whipple disease, a systemic infection of the intestine, CNS, lymph nodes, spleen, and joints in which foamy histiocytes, packed with bacilli, are seen in tissues. A very peculiar feature of the disease is its propensity to mainly infect males (10:1 male:female ratio), usually white males aged 30 to 50. The organisms are

T3.35
Clinical Stages of Syphilis

Stage	Definition	Possible complications	Pathology
Incubation	Exposure to symptoms, usually 3 weeks (3-90 days)	None	None
Primary	Chancre, lasting 1-8 weeks	Regional lymphadenopathy, Jarish-Herxheimer reaction	
Secondary	Dissemination	Skin rash, condyloma lata, aseptic meningitis, hepatitis, arthritis, Jarish-Herxheimer reaction, Immune complex glomerulonephritis	
Early latent	Asymptomatic phase <4 years	Relapse	
Late latent	Asymptomatic phase >4 years		Two features common to all lesions: obliterative endarteritis and plasmacytic infiltrate.
Tertiary	Any of 3 complications ⇒	1. Neurosyphilis: meningovascular, parenchymatous, tabes dorsalis, general paresis, otitis, optic neuritis 2. Cardiovascular: aortic insufficiency and/or coronary artery stenosis 3. Gummatous: bones and/or skin	
Congenital	Transplacentally acquired syphilis	Chorioamnionitis, hepatosplenomegaly, skin rash, rhinitis (sniffles), periostitis, cytopenias, Clutton joints, saddle nose, sabre shins, Hutchinson teeth	

PAS+ but AFB negative in tissue, allowing distinction from *M avium-intracellulare* which produces a similar tissue reaction.

☐ *Calymmatobacterium granulomatis* is the causative agent of granuloma inguinale (Donovaniasis). Has been isolated on chicken egg yolk but will not grow on agar. Bacteria-containing phagocytic vacuoles within macrophages are called Donovan bodies.

Spirochetes. The spirochetal infections (*Treponema, Leptospira, Borrelia, Brachyspira*) have in common a triphasic course: initial manifestations at the site of inoculation (primary phase), systemic manifestations during dissemination (secondary phase), and manifestations at sites where organisms are harbored (latent phase). Diagnosis is usually serologic; however, direct visualization is sometimes possible.

■ *Treponema*

☐ **Treponemal species** are tightly coiled (8-15 coils) gram-negative microaerophilic organisms with characteristic flexing and bending motility.

☐ *T. pallidum* (subspecies pallidum): distributed worldwide; causes venereal syphilis.

☐ *T. pallidum* (subspecies pertenue): Africa, Asia, South America; causes Yaws.

☐ *T. pallidum* (subspecies endemicum): Africa, Asia, Middle East; causes endemic, non-venerial syphilis (Bejel).

☐ *T. carateum*: South America; causes Pinta.

☐ Clinical types/stages of syphilis **T3.35**

☐ Laboratory diagnosis **T3.36**. In direct material from clinical lesions, one may visualize the organism using darkfield microscopy, direct fluorescent antibodies, immunohistochemistry, or silver stains. Serologic tests are categorized as 'treponemal' or 'nontreponemal'. Treponemal tests are more specific and include FTA-ABS and MHA-TP. Nontreponemal tests are more sensitive in early syphilis and include RPR, TRUST, and VDRL. Nontreponemal tests are less sensitive in the later stages and tend to revert to negative when the disease is treated. Serum RPR is the screening test of choice for primary syphilis. CSF VDRL is the screening test of choice for excluding neurosyphilis.

■ **Borrelia**

☐ Microaerophilic, loosely coiled (5-8 coils), bacteria with corkscrew motility.

☐ *B burgdorferi* is the cause of Lyme disease. It is transmitted by the tick *Ixodes dammini* in the Eastern US where it is most prevalent. In the Western US, it is transmitted by *I. pacificus,* in Europe by *I. ricinus,* and in China by *I. persulcatus*. The natural reservoir is the white-footed mouse, but in endemic areas, deer are an important reservoir.

☐ Stages

● *Stage 1.* erythema chronicum migrans (ECM) skin lesion and hematogenous spread.

● *Stage 2.* Neurologic, cardiac, or joint involement. Neurologic involvement consists most commonly of Bell palsy, less commonly aseptic meningitis, with CSF lymphocytic pleocytosis and elevated protein. Cardiac involvement manifests usually as A-V block due to myocarditis.

T3.36
Sensitivities of Serologic Tests for Syphilis

Test	1° Syphilis	2° Syphilis	3° Syphilis	Treated Syphilis
Nontreponemal (RPR, VDRL, TRUST)	80%-100%	~100%	70%	40%-70%
Treponemal (FTA-ABS, MHA-TP)	70%-90%	~100%	~100%	97%

- **Stage 3.** Chronic arthritis, usually affecting the knees, or chronic encephalopathy.

■ Diagnosis

- **Serology.** Even in patients with symptoms of Lyme disease, false positives outnumber true positives, due to cross-reactivity with the antigens of spirochetes comprising the normal oral flora. False negatives are also common.

- **Culture.** Barber-Stoenner-Kelley (BSK) medium.

- **PCR**

□ Coinfection with *Babesiosis* and/or *Flavivirus* is common.

□ **B recurrentes** is the cause of relapsing fever. It is transmitted by the human body louse, Pediculosis humanis, in epidemics; and by Ornithodoros ticks in sporadic settings. Tick-borne relapsing fever is uncommon, however, since the tick resides at 7000-10,000 feet. The disease is diagnosed by ***demonstrating the Borrelia organisms in peripheral blood*** either by darkfield examination or with Wright-Giemsa stain in thick blood films. Note that *Borrelia burgdorferi* in Lyme disease **cannot** usually be seen in blood films.

■ *Leptospira interrogans*

□ Microaerophilic, tightly coiled (8-10), motile bacteria with hooked ends

□ *L interrogans* is the causative organism of leptospirosis, a multisystem zoonotic disease sometimes characterized by the triad of meningitis, hepatitis, and nephritis (Weil disease). Presentations may be icteric or nonicteric. Nonicteric disease characterizes mild infections with a very low mortality. Icteric leptospirosis is a severe disease with up to 15% mortality. In this syndrome, one may see acute renal failure, pancreatitis, thrombocytopenia, and pulmonary involvement. In the latter circumstance, intraalveolar hemorrhage is a common pathologic finding. The occurance of myocarditis is rare but carries a high mortality. Conjunctival suffusion is seen in the majority of patients, and

in the presence of scleral icterus it is said to be pathognomonic of Weil disease.

□ Histopathologically, leptospirosis is characterized by vasculitis, endothelial damage, and inflammatory infiltrates. The histopathology is most marked in the liver, kidneys, heart, and lungs. In the liver, there may be intrahepatic cholestasis, hypertrophy Küpffer cells, and erythrophagocytosis. The kidneys display interstitial nephritis. The heart may show lymphocytic myocarditis. In the lungs, pulmonary congestion and hemorrhage are common.

□ Humans are infected through contact with the urine of an infected animal, the usual portal of entry being abrasions or cuts in the skin or conjunctiva. Within the US, the highest incidence is found in Hawaii. Rats are the usual hosts for the species that affect humans (*L interrogans* serogroup icterohaemorrhagiae). Domestic animals, like humans, often act as accidental hosts, and direct contact with them is the most common source of occupational infections (farmers, veterinarians, abattoir workers, meat inspectors). Indirect contact with rats is an important source for sewer workers. In tropical regions, infection may be acquired from walking in bare feet.

□ Laboratory findings in severe leptospirosis include a peripheral leukocytosis, thrombocytopenia, elevated creatinine, hyperbilirubinemia (with lesser increases in transaminases and alkaline phosphatase). The organisms may be visualized in tissue by dark-field microscopy, immunofluorescence microscopy, or immunohistochemical staining.

□ Unlike other spirochetes, *Leptospira* grows well on laboratory growth media. Fletcher medium or Ellinghausen-McCullough-Johnson-Harris (EMJH) medium are primarily used. Growth in culture is possible but extremely slow, and cultures are retained for up to 13 weeks. Since organisms circulate only during the first stage of the disease, blood cultures should be taken as soon as possible after the patient's presentation. Other samples that may be cultured include CSF and urine (especially after the second week). All of that having been said, most cases of leptospirosis are diagnosed by serology.

■ *Brachyspira aalborgi*

☐ Though still controversial, this organism has been associated with intestinal spirochetosis.

☐ In colorectal biopsy specimens, the organisms are visible as a 'purple haze' of organisms lining the luminal surface of enterocytes. Closer inspection, especially on Steiner-stained slides, shows that the organisms stand on-end on the surface of enterocytes (but not goblet cells).

☐ The clinical significance of intestinal spirochetosis is controversial, and whether it is the cause of disease or an incidental finding remains unclear. *Brachyspira aalborgi* and another organism, *Brachyspira pilosicoli,* both anaerobic spirochetes,

appear to be associated with most cases. Infections are seen in both asymptomatic and symptomatic individuals, and a significant minority of these occur in the setting of HIV infection. Spirochetosis may be found in any part of the colon and does not tend to elicit significant inflammation

Chlamydiae. Obligate intracellular bacteria that cannot replicate outside cells or synthesize ATP. The organisms exist in two forms: the **elementary body** is a dense spherical form measuring 0.2 to 0.4 μm and is the **infective form,** capable of limited extracellular survival; the **reticulate body** measures 0.6 to 1.0 μm and is the **intracellular form.** The outer membrane of the bacterium contains the antigen known as major outer membrane protein (MOMP) which is used in diagnosis.

- *C trachomatis* is the **most common sexually-transmitted disease** (STD) in the US; moreover, in the form of trachoma it is considered the most common preventable cause of blindness worldwide. It causes several clinical syndromes, including trachoma, lymphogranuloma venereum (LGV), urethritis, epididymitis, prostatitis, proctitis, cervicitis, and neonatal infections (inclusion body conjunctivitis, pneumonitis, and otitis). Serotypes A, B, & C are responsible for trachoma. Serotype L is responsible for LGV, which produces stellate microabscesses in lymph nodes that are histologically indistinguishable from the lesion of cat scratch disease. Serotypes D-K cause the remaining infections. There are several diagnostic modalities:

  ☐ Presumptive diagnosis can be made from Wright-stained conjunctival smears/scrapings in which one sees cytoplasmic (reticulate body) inclusions in exfoliated cells.

  ☐ Cell culture, on McCoy cells for example, remains the gold standard.

  ☐ In most labs, direct fluorescence (DFA) or ELISA are employed. DFA allows direct visualization of the cellular constituents, and, since *C trachomatis* infects columnar epithelial cells, it is essential that these be present. The antibodies used in the assay are directed against MOMP.

  ☐ The most sensitive method for detection of *C trachomatis* is nucleic acid amplification.

T3.37
Rickettsial diseases

Disease	Organism	Vector
Rocky mountain spotted fever	*Rickettsia rickettsii*	Tick
Epidemic typhus	*Rickettsia prowazekii*	Louse
Scrub typhus	*Orientia* (previously *Rickettsia*) *tsutsugamushi*	Chigger
Murine typhus	*Rickettsia typhi*	Flea
Cat scratch disease	*Bartonella henselae*	Kitten
Bacillary angiomatosis	*Bartonella henselae*	Kitten
Boutonneuse fever	*Rickettsia conorii*	Tick
Rickettsialpox	*Rickettsia akari*	Mite
Human monocytic ehrlichiosis	*Ehrlichia chaffeensis*	Lone Star Tick (*Amblyomma americanum*)
Human granulocytic ehrlichiosis	*Anaplasma* (previously *Ehrlichia*) *phagocytophilia*	Deer Tick
Oroya fever bartonellosis	*Bartonella bacilliformis*	Sandfly
Verruga peruana	*Bartonella bacilliformis*	Sandfly
Trench fever	*Bartonella quintana*	Louse
Brill-Zinsser disease	*Rickettsia prowazekii*	None (Recrudescence of epidemic typhus)
Q fever	*Coxiella burnetii*	None (inhalation)

□ Serology has a limited role. It is mainly used to support a diagnosis of LGV or neonatal pneumonitis.

■ *C psittaci* (now called *Chlamydophila psittaci*), the causative agent of psittacosis, infects individuals in contact with some kind of bird, person-to-person spread being rare. The organism enters the body via the respiratory tract and then multiplies in the liver and spleen. It manifests primarily as pneumonitis. Diagnosis is usually based upon serology.

■ *C pneumoniae* (TWAR bacillus, now called *Chlamydophila pneumoniae*) causes so-called walking or atypical pneumonia. Diagnosis is usually serologic.

Rickettsiae T3.37. Several genera now comprise this family: *Rickettsia, Ehrlichia, Coxiella, Bartonella, Orientia, Anaplasma,* and *Neorickettsia.* They prefer to replicate intracellularly, but unlike chlamydiae, these organisms can survive for extended periods outside the cell. Rickettsial organisms target and infect **endothelial** cells. All rickettsial infections cause endothelial swelling and disseminated mononuclear vasculitis with intravascular thrombi. With the exception of *Coxiella,* all are transmitted by arthropod. It is important to remember that many of these diseases must be treated empirically. There are not readily available direct means of identifying the organisms, and serology is only fruitful (during the acute phase) in about 20% of cases.

■ **Rocky mountain spotted fever** has occurred in nearly every state, but is most common in the Southeast US where the tick *Dermacentor variabilis* is the reservoir and vector. Symptoms arise 2 to 14 days after exposure and consist of nausea, abdominal pain, fever, and a maculopapular rash beginning at the wrists and ankles. Renal failure, DIC, and CNS involvement ensue in severe cases. A fulminant form, seen in African American males with glucose-6-phosphatase deficiency, is rapidly fatal.

■ **Ehrlichiosis** is found mainly in North America. The causative organisms can be seen on Wright-stained blood films within intracellular vacuoles where they appear as mulberries or morulae. Both human monocytic ehrlichiosis (HME) and human granulocytic ehrlichiosis (HGE) present as acute febrile illnesses with thrombocytopenia, leukopenia, and elevated transaminases. One is much more likely to find organ-

isms in peripheral blood in HGE than HME, where the infected monocytic cells are more tissue-based.

■ *Coxiella burnetii* is the causative agent of Q fever, an occupational hazard for abattoir workers, farmers, and veterinarians.

□ Acute Q fever presents as a nonspecific flu-like illness with pneumonitis and sometimes hepatitis. Thrombocytopenia is present in 25% of cases, and hepatic enzymes are often elevated. The fatality rate is 1%-2%, often due to myocarditis. Granulomata can be found in the liver and bone marrow and have a classic fibrin-ring appearance.

□ Chronic Q fever most often takes the form of endocarditis. Usually there are no detectable vegetations, and blood cultures are negative. Q fever endocarditis is often fatal if untreated. It usually develops in people with underlying disease: valve disease or immunosuppression. Histologically, Q fever endocarditis is characterized by inflammatory cells admixed with foamy histiocytes (containing organisms)—fibrin-ring granulomas are not seen.

□ Recrudescence of Q fever may occur during pregnancy and often leads to premature birth, abortion, or neonatal death.

□ *C burnetii* is a pleomorphic gram-negative coccobacillus with small-cell variants (SCV) and large-cell variants (LCV) distinguishable by electron microscopy. The SCV survives well in the environment and is passively ingested by host monocytes; whereas, the LCV cannot survive in the environment but is capable of multiplying within monocyte phagolysosomes.

□ The diagnosis is based largely on serology, but serology has a large false negative rate in Q fever, and re-testing may be necessary. With regard to serology, it helps to know that *C burnetii* has two antigenic states: bacteria obtained directly from infected humans or animals are in phase I, while those obtained after several passes through embryonated eggs are in phase II. Oddly, the antibody response in acute human disease is primarily to phase II antigens, while antibodies to the phase I organism are elevated in chronic disease. For acute Q fever, a four-fold rise in paired sera gives the highest specificity, but sufficiently elevated single titers may also provide the diagnosis. PCR is highly sensitive when applied to tissue samples, such as heart valves, but is not useful for testing on blood. Histological findings are generally non-specific. Fibrin ring (doughnut) granulomas are the classic finding in Q fever hepatitis.

- *Bartonella* spp are numerous, but the most commonly associated with human disease are *B henselae, B bacilliformis,* and *B quintana.* Clinical syndromes classically associated with *Bartonella* include trench fever (*B quintana*), Oroya fever and Verruga peruana (*B bacilliformis*), cat-scratch disease and bacillary angiomatosis (*B henselae*).

  □ Trench fever was a major cause of sickness and death in World War I, and has recently been noted in homeless alcoholics. It is transmitted by the human body louse (*Pediculus humanus corporis*).

  □ Infection with *B bacilliformis* results in a bacteremia associated with hemolysis and spiking fevers (Oroya fever), seen predominantly in the Andean regions of South American countries, where the bloodsucking *Lutzomyia phlebotomine* sandfly is found. Some infected individuals develop a cutaneous manifestation (resembling bacillary angiomatosis) known as Verruga peruana. Unlike BA, these patients are not immunocompromised. The Oroya fever—Verruga peruana spectrum has been called Carrion disease.

  □ Cat scratch disease (CSD), due to *B henselae,* is characterized by lymphadenitis, usually at epitrochlear and/or axillary sites and unilateral, with or without an inflamed inoculation site. *B henselae* has its natural reservoir in cats and is transmitted to humans through a scratch or bite. Human-to-human transmission has not been documented. Usually a single lymph node site is involved, but in 10% of cases more than one site is affected. The affected site is most commonly the upper extremity (50%), including axillary and epitrochlear nodes, followed by cervical nodes (25%), inguinal nodes (15%), and preauricular nodes (5%). The eye is the most common nonlymphoid site of *B henselae* infection, resulting in (i) Parinaud oculoglandular syndrome, in which a granuloatous unilateral conjunctivitis results in ulceration of the conjunctival mucosa or,

less commonly (ii) Leber stellate neuroretinitis. *B henselae* appears to be the most common cause of both of these ocular conditions. With regard to laboratory diagnosis, it is useful to remember that many individuals, especially those with frequent contact with cats, have an IgG antibody titer of >1:64; thus, a high titer of IgG (>1:512) or an increasing titer (4 dilution change) must be shown to document infection. A positive IgM antibody is also indicative of acute infection. Culture is not very practical for this genus. Histologic sections display characteristic stellate microabscesses with palisading epithelioid histiocytes within which clumps of bacilli may be visualized with Warthin-Starry or Brown-Hopps stains (not as often as in BA). **Both LGV and tularemia may produce histologically similar lesions.**

  □ More recently, *Bartonella* spp have been associated with culture-negative endocarditis.

  □ In those with HIV, disseminated bartonellosis may occur. Alternatively, or in association with disseminated disease, HIV+ patients may develop bacillary angiomatosis (BA), within skin, lymph nodes, or viscera (sometimes called peliosis). Most cases are due to *B henselae,* but bone lesions are most often due to *B quintana.*

  □ The laboratory diagnosis of *Bartonella* spp is supported principally by serology and/or molecular methods. In culture, the organisms are quite fastidious. They sometimes grow as pleomorphic gram-negative bacilli in a CO_2-enriched environment, on enriched media, after prolonged periods of incubation. Several IFA and EIA tests have been developed to serologically diagnose *Bartonella* infection, and these may be the best way to make the diagnosis at present. There is tremendous cross-reactivity among *Bartonella* spp, however, and some cross-reactivity with non-*Bartonella* spp (*Coxiella burnetii, Chlamydia, Francisella tularensis*). Molecular assays have been developed that promise to significantly improve diagnostic accuracy, but it is unclear at this time which assay is best. PCR offers high sensitivity and specificity, rapid turnaround, and the capacity to identify *Bartonella* to the species level. Furthermore, it may be performed on both blood and tissue specimens.

Mycoplasma are pleomorphic bacteria which lack cell walls. Mycoplasma belong to the Mollicutes class. They are distinct from bacteria in that they lack a cell wall. Unlike viruses, they contain both DNA and RNA and can replicate in cell-free media. Unlike both bacteria and viruses, they have cell membranes containing sterols. The lack of cell wall makes them insensitive to β-lactam antibiotics and negative by gram stain. The most common site of extrapulmonary involvement is thought to be the CNS, manifesting most commonly as encephalitis.

- ■ *M pneumoniae* causes atypical pneumonia (walking pneumonia), sometimes associated with autoimmune hemolytic anemia due to the cold agglutinin IgM anti-I. Cold agglutinins appear by the end of the first week in around 50% of infected persons, and this can serve as a nonspecific diagnostic test. The organisms produce typical **fried-egg colonies** in culture. Serology is the primary means of diagnosis.

- ■ *Ureaplasma urealyticum* and *Mycoplasma hominis* cause **nongonococcal urethritis**.

Other Bacteriology Facts

Carriage rates T3.38

Bacteria that produce **H$_2$S**: *Salmonella, Proteus, Citrobacter, Edwardsiella*

Swarming motility: *P mirabilis, P vulgaris*

Motile gram-positive bacteria: *Listeria* (at 22°C), *Bacillus,* and (variably) *Corynebacterium*

Darting motility: *Campylobacter* & *Vibrio*

Motility only at 22°C: *Listeria* & *Yersinia*

Infection associated with marked **lymphocytosis** (with cleaved lymphocytes): *Pertussis*

Infection associated with marked **monocytosis:** *Listeria*

HACEK: Acronym for a group of organisms including *Hemophilus aphrophilus, Actinobacillus actinomycetem-comitans, Cardiobacterium hominis, Eikenella corrodens,* and *Kingella*. These organisms are united by their growth requirements and clinical associations. All are slow-growing, fastidious organisms that require 48 to 72 hours to grow in an enriched CO$_2$ environment on chocolate agar. Their growth is enhanced by X-factor. Clinically, they are associated with subacute endocarditis in persons with poor dental hygiene.

Bacterial infections that **resemble mycoses** clinically

- ■ *Actinomyces* & *Nocardia* *Actinomyces* spp are anaerobic bacteria that are non-acid fast. They infect **immuno-competent** hosts and produce localized infections. The most common isolate is *A. israelii. Nocardia* species are aerobic bacteria that are weakly acid fast and infect compromised hosts. *N asteroides* is the most common isolate.

    - □ *Actinomyces* spp are normal inhabitants of the oral cavity (tonsillar crypts). Three forms of clinical actinomycosis are commonly found, usually in immunocompetent individuals: actinomycotic mycetoma, cervicofacial, pulmonary, and pelvic. Cervicofacial actinomycosis usually follows some kind of dental problem and leads to a localized lesion with a draining sinus tract. Pulmonary infection follows aspiration of oral actinomyces. Pelvic actinomyces is associated with intrauterine devices (IUD).

T3.38
Carriage Rates

Organism	Carriage Rate
Staphylococcus aureus	20%-40%
Streptococcus pneumoniae	5%-70%
Group *B Streptococci* in pregnant women	20%-40%
Clostridium difficile	3% of normals, 30% of hospitalized adults, 50% of neonates
Neisseria meningitidis	20%-40%

□ *Nocardia* spp are not normal inhabitants and infect **immunocompromised** hosts. They cause actinomycotic mycetoma and infections of lung, CNS, and other sites.

- **Botryomycosis.** A chronic, localized infection of skin or soft tissue associated with nonfilamentous bacteria (when filamentous organisms are involved, often called actinomycotic mycetoma). Most commonly caused by *S aureus*, but may also be caused by *P aeruginosa*.

Recovered from respiratory infections in patients with cystic fibrosis (CF): *P aeruginosa*

Most frequent human **anaerobic** isolate: *B fragilis*

Staphylococci other than *S aureus* that are coagulase positive: *S intermedius, S hyicus, S delphini*

Acute rheumatic fever (ARF)

- ARF results from an autoimmune response to infection with group A streptococcus. Streptococcal M antigen is felt to be involved in the molecular mimicry that produces this response. Acute rheumatic fever (ARF) refers to the acute illness, and rheumatic heart disease (RHD) refers to the resulting chronic heart disease. ARF is a disease of childhood, and RHD is a disease of adulthood, initially presenting on average at 25-34 years of age. Mitral regurgitation is the predominant finding early in the disease, but mitral stenosis becomes progressively more common with increasing age.

- Only **pharyngeal** infection with group A streptococcus causes ARF (whereas poststreptococcal glomeru-

lonephritis may follow either pharyngeal or skin infections), and it appears that repeated infection is necessary to develop ARF and RHD.

- In addition to the Jones criteria **T3.39** for the diagnosis of ARF, initially proposed in 1944 and modified several times, WHO criteria now exist. The WHO criteria are somewhat less stringent, intended to diagnose and treat more cases of ARF in populations with a high incidence. In brief, they (1) allow as evidence of recent streptococcal infection a recent episode of scarlet fever, (2) do not require evidence of antecedent streptococcal infection in patients with either carditis or chorea; (3) with those exceptions apply the Jones criteria for episodes in patients without established RHD; (4) in patients with established RHD require only two minor criteria for the diagnosis.

Mycobacteria

Laboratory Methods

Direct examination of clinical specimens

- On routine gram stain, mycobacteria are either negative (gram ghosts) or visible as weakly gram-positive bacilli. They appear as ghosts in Wright-Giemsa stains as well.

- Mycobacteria are detectable by either acid-fast stains or auramine-rhodamine fluorochrome stains. The latter acts as a useful screening test, with high sensitivity and greater ease. It is thought, however, that these have lower specificity, and positive fluorescent stains should be confirmed by routine acid-fast stain.

- *M marinum* is characterized by broad bacilli with cross banding. Bacilli with a shephard's crook: *M kansasii.*

Culture-suspected mycobacteria may be cultured on both solid and broth media. Solid media include Lowenstein-Jensen and Middlebrook 7H11 agars. Broth systems are numerous.

- Any growth in a broth is stained with acid-fast stains. Positively staining organisms with cording are reported as presumptive *M tuberculosis.* Positively staining organisms without cording are reported as nontuberculous *Mycobacterial* spp.

T3.39

Jones Criteria (2 major criteria *or* 1 major + 2 minor *and* evidence of antecedent group A streptococcal infection [positive throat culture, positive rapid antigen test, or rising streptococcal antibody titer])

Major Criteria	Minor Criteria
Carditis	Arthralgia
Polyarthritis	Fever
Chorea (Sydenham)	Elevated ESR or CRP
Erythema marginatum	Prolonged PR interval
Subcutaneous nodules	

- Any growth in a broth can be subjected to NAP testing. NAP sensitive isolates are presumptively identified as *M tuberculosis*.

- Whereas traditionally it was visual inspection that disclosed an isolate on growth media, requiring weeks to develop, modern broth methods detect an isolate through the measurement of metabolic products (eg, CO_2 release). Some systems have fluorescent or colorimetric indicators that 'trip' when growth occurs, and an isolate can be detected sometimes in 1-2 weeks.

- Growth on Lowenstein-Jensen or Middlebrook agar

  □ **Rapid growers** (<7 days)

    - *Arylsulfatase-negative: nonpathogens.*

    - Arylsulfatase-positive, nitrate-positive: *M fortuitum.*

    - Arylsulfatase-positive, nitrate-negative: *M chelonae.*

  □ **Slow growers**

    - Nonphotochromogens

    - Niacin-positive: *M tuberculosis*

    - Niacin-negative: *M avium-intracellulare (MAI)* or *M bovis*

  □ Photochromogens: *M kansasii, M simiae, M asiaticum,* or *M marinum.*

  □ Scotochromogens: *M scrofulaceum or M gordonae.*

- The **Runyon** classification is used to classify nontuberculous (atypical) mycobacteria. *M tuberculosis* is not included in the classification but would fall under group III.

  □ **Group I** organisms that produce yellow carotene pigment when grown in light (photochromogens), include: *M kansasii, M simiae, M marinum,* and *M asiaticum. M szulgai* is a scotochromogen at 37° C and a photochromogen at room temp (22-24°C).

  □ **Group II** organisms that make yellow pigment in the absence of light (scotochromogens), include: *M scrofulaceum, M gordonae,* and *M flavescens. M szulgai* is a scotochromogen at 37°C and a photochromogen at room temperature (22-24°C).

  □ **Group III** organisms that do not make much pigment (non-photochromogens), include: *M avium-intracellulare (MAI), M haemophilium, M xenophi, M bovis.*

  □ **Group IV** Rapid growers, with or without pigment, including *M fortuitum* & *M chelonei.*

Nucleic acid amplification tests (NAAT)

- The NAATs amplify specific nucleic acid sequences using a nucleic acid probe. They combine the rapidity of direct smears with the sensitivity and specificity of culture.

- In the case of *M tuberculosis,* the CDC now recommends that AFB smear and NAAT be performed on the first sputum collected. If both are positive, then the diagnosis of pulmonary tuberculosis is made. If the smear is positive and the NAAT is negative, the CDC recommends testing the sputum for inhibitors (by adding lysed *M tuberculosis* to the sample and repeating the NAAT assay). If inhibitors are not detected, then testing is repeated on additional samples. If the sputum is repeatedly AFB-positive with negative NAAT, then the diagnosis of non-TB mycobacterial infection is made. When the AFB stain is negative but the sputum is NAAT-positive, additional samples should be tested. If the sputum is repeatedly NAAT-positive but AFB-negative, then a diagnosis of pulmonary tuberculosis is made.

Important Species T3.40

Mycobacterium tuberculosis (MTB)

- **Key characteristics** include: NAP test+, cording+, Niacin+, formation of bird nest colonies on Middlebrook 7H-10, "Ruff buff" colonies, catalase negative.

- **Cord factor** is believed to be a virulence factor and is responsible for the cord-like arrangement of organisms grown in broth.

■ **Clinical features**

  □ Tuberculosis is spread from person to person by respiratory droplets.

  □ Primary infection is respiratory and may lead to resolution (>90%), tuberculous pneumonia, or miliary tuberculosis. The latter outcomes are seen primarily in infants and immunocompromised individuals. Most primary cases are asymptomatic and become latent; cell-mediated immunity manages to control the infection by localizing it into caseating granulomatous lesions (Ghon complex), most often in the upper lobes.

  □ Eventually, around 5% to 10% of immunocompetent individuals and a larger number of immunocompromised individuals develop active (relapsed) TB, which is usually pulmonary but may be extrapulmonary or multi-organ (kidneys, bone, meninges, etc).

  □ Diagnosing active TB is of paramount importance, since the disease is often fatal and is easily spread person-to-person. The diagnosis of active tuberculosis is most often made with direct stains for acid-fast bacilli, culture, or nucleic acid amplification tests (NAAT). The tuberculin skin test has limited value in the setting of active TB, due to inadequate sensitivity and specificity. An initial effort is usually made to make the diagnosis on the basis of expectorated sputum. Three samples on three separate days are submitted for AFB smear and culture. In resource-poor regions—regions in which TB is often widespread—the cost of culture may be prohibitive, and much reliance is placed upon sputum smear microscopy. This approach may miss as many as half of cases. Furthermore, many of these populations have a high rate of HIV infection, and smear-negative TB is particularly prevalent in HIV patients. In patients incapable of producing an adequate sputum sample, sputum induction may be attempted. In patients with repeatedly negative sputum, invasive sampling is often undertaken, in the form of bronchoscopy or gastric lavage. Culture is far more sensitive than direct smears, allow species identification, and allows susceptibility testing; however, its value is limited by the prolonged incubation required.

  □ Diagnosing (and treating) latent TB provides the only hope for eventual disease eradication. This is much more challenging than diagnosing active TB, since patients are asymptomatic and not actively expectorating organisms. The tuberculin skin test is fraught with difficulties. Tuberculin is a filtrate of tuberculosis broth culture whose manufacture was refined over time to create purified protein derivative (PPD), in wide use today. PPD, a precipitate of tuberculosis culture supernatant, contains a large number of antigens, some of which are shared with other mycobacteria; thus, a positive PPD may signify past infection with a nontuberculous mycobacterium or vaccination with BCG. Anergy, for example due to HIV infection, is a common cause of false-negative results. Poor standardization of test application and interpretation further compound these problems. There is no alternative test at this time.

Mycobacterium avium-intracellulare (**MAI**)

  ■ Is second to *M tuberculosis* in frequency in the US

  ■ MAI usually enters via the GI tract. It then disseminates and localizes mainly to the reticuloendothelial system.

  ■ Unlike TB, MAI does not always cause caseating granulomata, and the classic histologic picture is instead sheets of foamy macrophages, closely resembling Whipple disease.

M scrofulaceum

  ■ Causes cervical lymphadenitis in children (scrofula) characterized by confluent, matted, lymph nodes having caseating granulomata. *M tuberculosis* is itself a common cause of the scrofula presentation.

T3.40
Important Mycobacterial Species

Site	Most common *Mycobacteria* spp
Lung	*M tuberculosis, M kansasii, MAI, M xenopi*
Lymph node	*M tuberculosis, M scrofulaceum, MAI*
Skin & soft tissue	*M ulcerans, M fortuitum, M chelonei, M marinum*
GI	*M tuberculosis, MAI*

M kansasii causes pulmonary disease primarily in persons with underlying pneumoconioses.

Mycobacteria causing skin & soft tissue infections.
M ulcerans, M fortuitum, M chelonei, and *M marinum.*
This is a group of mycobacterial organisms united by the lack of a primary pulmonary phase and their tendency to cause infection following penetrating trauma. *M marinum* is associated with freshwater fish and causes localized cutaneous infection with secondary lymphadenitis clinically resembling sporotrichosis. Its growth is enhanced with 25°C incubation. *M ulcerans* causes indolent, necrotizing cutaneous lesions (Buruli ulcer).

M leprae

- **Cause of leprosy (Hansen disease).** 3rd leading cause of blindness worldwide.

- In the US, found in Hawaii, Texas, Louisiana (where it is found in armadillos).

- Cardinal sign: Hypoesthetic skin lesions & prominence of peripheral nerves.

- **Lepromatous vs tuberculoid leprosy.** These polar forms of leprosy are joined by a range of indeterminate forms which can progress in either direction. The **anergic** (**lepromatous**) form of leprosy, characterized by widespread skin involvement (mostly on cool skin surfaces), is notable for larger numbers of acid-fast bacilli and sheets of foamy histiocytes identifiable within lesions. This form of infection may be complicated by *Strongyloides* superinfection. The **tuberculoid** form is characterized by one to several localized lesions containing noncaseating granulomata having few to no identifiable acid-fast organisms.

Agan BK, Dolan MJ. Laboratory Diagnosis of Bartonella Infections. *Clin Lab Med* 2002; 22: 937–962.

Albrich WC, Kraft C, Fisk T, Albrecht H. A Mechanic With A Bad Valve: Blood-Culture Negative Endocarditis. *Lancet Infect Dis* 2004; 4: 777–784.

Alkalay AL, Pomerance JJ, Rimoin DL. Fetal Varicella Syndrome. *J Pediatr* 1987; 111: 320-323.

Archibald LK, Banerjee SN, Jarvis WR. Secular Trends In Hospital Acquired Clostridium Difficile Disease In The United States, 1987–2001. *J Infect Dis* 2004; 189: 1585–1589.

Atkins BL, Athanasou N, Deeks JJ, Crook DWM, Simpson H, Peto TEA, McLardy-Smith P, Berendt AR. Prospective Evaluation of Criteria For Microbiological Diagnosis of Prosthetic-Joint Infection at Revision Arthroplasty. J Clin Microbiol 1998; 36: 2932-2939.

Avidor B, Varon M, Marmor S, et al. DNA Amplification For The Diagnosis Of Cat-Scratch Disease In Small-Quantity Clinical Specimens. *Am J Clin Pathol* 2001; 115:900–909.

Bangham CRM. HTLV-1 Infections. *J Clin Pathol* 2000; 53:581–586.

Barenfanger J, Drake CA. Interpretation of Gram Stains for the Nonmicrobiologist. *Lab Med.* 2001; 7: 368-375.

Barlow K, Tosswill J, Clewley J. Analysis And Genotyping Of PCR Products Of The Amplicor HIV-1 Kit. *J Virol Methods* 1995; 52: 65–74.

Bartlett JG, Dowell SF, Mandell LA, File TM, Jr, Musher DM, Fine MJ. Practice Gidelines for the Management of Community-Acquired Pneumonia in Adults. *Clinical Infectious Diseases.* 2000; 31:347-382.

Beigel JH, Farrar J, Han AM, et al. Avian Influenza A (H5N1) Infection in Humans. *N Engl J Med* 2005; 353(13): 1374–1385.

Carapetis JR, McDonald M, Wilson NJ. Acute Rheumatic Fever. *Lancet* 2005; 366: 155–168.

Caserta MT, Mcdermott MP, Dewhurst S, Schnabel K, Carnahan JA, Gilbert L, Lathan G, Loftus GK, Hall CB. Human Herpesvirus 6 (HHV6) DNA Persistence and

Bibliography

Reactivation in Healthy Children. *J Pediatr* 2004; 145: 478-484.

Centers for Disease Control and Prevention. Hantavirus pulmonary syndrome—five states, 2006. *MMWR Morb Mortal Wkly Rep.* 2006; 55: 627-629.

Chavez-Bueno S, McCracken, GH, Jr. Bacterial Meningitis in Children. *Pediatr Clin N Am* 2005; 52: 795– 810.

Chen X-M, Keithly JS, Paya CV, LaRusso NF. Cryptosporidiosis. *N Engl J Med* 2002; 346(22): 1723-1731.

Chevaliez S, Pawlotsky J-M. Use of Virologic Assays in the Diagnosis and Management of Hepatitis C Virus Infection. *Clin Liver Dis* 2005; 9: 371– 382.

Chng WJ, Lai HC, Earnest A, Kuperan P. Haematological Parameters in Severe Acute Respiratory Syndrome. *Clin Lab Haem* 2005; 27:15-20.

Cleghorn FR, Manns A, Falk R, et al. Effect Of Human T-Lymphotropic Virus Type I Infection On Non-Hodgkin's Lymphoma Incidence. *J Natl Cancer Inst* 1995; 87: 1009–1014.

Cohen A, Wolf DG, Guttman-Yassky E, Sarid R. Kaposi's Sarcoma-Associated Herpesviruses: Clinical, Diagnostic, and Epidemiological Aspects. *Critical Reviews in Clinical Laboratory Sciences* 2005; 42(2): 101–153.

Daar E, Little S, Pitt J. Diagnosis of Primary HIV-1 Infection. *Ann Intern Med* 2001; 134: 25–29.

Drosten C, Gunther S, Preiser W, et al. Identification of a Novel Coronavirus in Patients With Severe Acute Respiratory Syndrome. *N Engl J Med* 2003; 348(20): 1967–1976.

Duchin JS, Koster FT, Peters CJ, et al. Hantavirus Pulmonary Syndrome: A Clinical Description Of 17 Patients With A Newly Recognized Disease. *N Engl J Med* 1994; 330:949-955.

Enright AM, Prober CG. Herpesviridae Infections In Newborns: Varicella Zoster Virus, Herpes Simplex Virus, And Cytomegalovirus. *Pediatr Clin N Am* 2004; 51: 889–908.

Enders G, Miller E, Cradock-Watson J, et al. Consequences Of Varicella And Herpes Zoster In Pregnancy: Prospective Study Of 1739 Cases. *Lancet* 1994; 343: 1548–1551.

Fihn SD. Acute Uncomplicated Urinary Tract Infection in Women. *N Engl J Med.* 2003; 349: 259-266.

Fihn SD. Clinical Practice. Acute Uncomplicated Urinary Tract Infection in Women. *N Engl J Med* 2003; 349: 259–266.

Fine MJ, Smith MA, Carson CA, et al. Prognosis and Outcomes of Patients With Community-Acquired Pneumonia. *JAMA* 1996; 275: 134–141.

Franks TJ, Chong PY, Chui P, et al. Lung Pathology of Severe Acute Respiratory Syndrome (SARS): A Study of 8 Autopsy Cases From Singapore. *Hum Pathol* 2003;34(8):743–748.

Goodgame R. A Bayesian Approach to Acute Infectious Diarrhea In Adults. *Gastroenterol Clin N Am* 2006; 35: 249-273.

Goodgame RW. Emerging Causes Of Travelers Diarrhea: Cryptosporidium, Cyclospora, Isospora, And Microsporidia. *Curr Infect Dis Rep* 2003; 5: 66–73.

Gopal R, Ozerek A, Jeanes A. Rational Protocols For Testing Faeces In The Investigation Of Sporadic Hospital-Acquired Diarrhoea. *J Hosp Infect* 2001; 47: 79–83.

Graham JC, Galloway A. The Laboratory Diagnosis of Urinary Tract Infection. *J Clin Pathol* 2001; 54: 911–919.

Granville L, Chirala M, Cernoch P, Ostrowski M, Truong LD. Fungal Sinusitis: Histologic Spectrum and Correlation with Culture. *Hum Pathol* 2004; 35(4): 474-481.

Gratz NG. Emerging and Resurging Vector-Borne Diseases. *Annu Rev Entomol.* 1999; 44: 51-75.

Guerrant RL, Gilder TV, Steiner TS, Thielman NM, Slutsker L, Tauxe RV, Hennessy T, Griffin PM, DuPont H, Sack RB, Tarr P, Neill M, Nachamkin I, Reller LB, Osterholm MT, Bannish ML, Pickering LK. Practice Guidelines for the Management of Infectious Diarrhea. *Clinical Infectious Diseases.* 2001; 32:3431-350.

Bibliography

Guleria R, Nisar N, Chawla TC, Biswas NR. Mycoplasma pneumoniae and Central Nervous System Complications: A Review. *J Lab Clin Med* 2005; 146(2): 55-63.

Gutierrez Y, Bhatia P, Garbadawala ST, Dobson JR, Wallace T, Carey TE. *Strongyloides stercoralis* Eosinophilic Granulomatous Enterocolitis. *Am J Surg Pathol* 1996; 20(5): 603-612.

Haque R, Huston CD, Hughes M, Houpt E, Petri WA. Amebiasis. *N Engl J Med*. 2003; 348: 1565-1573.

Harris KR, Dighe AS. Laboratory Testing for Viral Hepatitis. *Am J Clin Pathol*. 2002; 118: S18-25.

Hoagland RJ. Infectious Mononucleosis. *Prim Care* 1975; 2: 295-307.

Hotez PJ, Brooker S, Bethony JM, Bottazzi ME, Loukas A, Xiao S. Hookworm Infection. *N Engl J Med* 2004; 351(8): 799-807.

Houpikian P, Raoult D. Blood Culture-Negative Endocarditis in a Reference Center: Etiologic Diagnosis of 348 *Cases. Medicine* 2005; 84(3): 162-173.

Hovelius B, Mardh PA. Staphylococcus Saprophyticus as a Common Cause of Urinary Tract Infections. *Rev Infect Dis* 1984; 6: 328–337.

Hughes RA, Cornblath DR. Guillain-Barre syndrome. *Lancet* 2005; 366: 1653–1666.

Jones TD. The Diagnosis of Acute Rheumatic Fever. *JAMA* 1944; 126: 481–484.

Karch H, Tarr PI, Bielaszewska M. Enterohaemorrhagic Escherichia coli in Human Medicine. *International Journal of Medical Microbiology* 2005; 295: 405-418.

Kass EH. Bacteriuria and The Diagnosis of Infections of the Urinary Tract. *Arch Intern Med* 1957; 100: 709–714.

Kessler HH, Sanker B, Rabenau H, et al. Rapid Diagnosis Of Enterovirus Infection By A New One-Step Reverse Transcription-PCR Assay. *J Clin Microbiol* 1997; 35: 976.

Koneman Ed., *Color Atlas and Textbook of Diagnostic Microbiology*

Koteish A, Kannangai R, Abraham SC, Torbenson M. Colonic Spirochetosis in Children and Adults. *Am J Clin Pathol* 2003; 120: 828-832.

Kravetz JD, Federman DG. Toxoplasmosis in Pregnancy. *Am J Med* 2005; 118: 212-216.

Lamps LW, Havens JM, Sjostedt A, Page DL, Scott MA. Histologic and Molecular Diagnosis of Tularemia: A Potential Bioterrorism Agent Endemic to North America. *Modern Pathology* 2004; 17: 489–495.

Larsen SA, Steiner BM, Rudolph AH. Laboratory Diagnosis And Interpretation Of Tests For Syphilis. *Clin Microbiol Rev* 1995; 8: 1-21.

Levett PN. Leptospirosis. *Clin Microbiol Rev* 2001; 14(2): 296–326.

Magill AJ, Grogl M, Gasser RA, et al. Visceral Infection Caused by Leishmania tropica in Veterans of Operation Desert Storm. *N Engl J Med* 1993; 328: 1384.

Maguina C, Garcia PJ, Gotuzzo E, et al. Bartonellosis (Carrion's disease) in the Modern Era. *Clin Infect Dis* 2001;33:772–779.

Marchand E, Verellen-Dumoulin C, Mairesse M, et al. Frequency Of Cystic Fibrosis Transmembrane Conductance Regulator Gene Mutations And 5T Allele In Patients With Allergic Bronchopulmonary Aspergillosis. *Chest* 2001; 119(3): 762–767.

Marr KA, Carter RA, Boeckh M, et al. Invasive Aspergillosis In Allogeneic Stem Cell Transplant Recipients: Changes In Epidemiology And Risk Factors. *Blood* 2002; 100(13): 4358–4366.

Massei F, Gori L, Macchia P, Maggiore G. The Expanded Spectrum of Bartonellosis in Children. *Infect Dis Clin N Am* 2005; 19: 691-711.

McDonald JR, Olaison L, Anderson DJ, Hoen BM, Miro JM, Eykyn S, Abrutyn E, Fowler VG, Habib G, Selton-Suty C, Pappas PA, Cabell CH, Corey GR, Marco F, Sexton DJ. Enterococcal Endocarditis: 107 Cases From The International Collaboration On Endocarditis Merged Database. *Am J Med* 2005; 118: 759-766.

Bibliography

Mead PS, Slutsker L, Dietz V, McCaig LF, Bresee JS, Shapiro C, et al. Food-Related Illness and Death in the United States. *Emerg Infect Dis* 1999; 5(5): 607–625.

Moscona A. Neuraminidase inhibitors for influenza. *N Engl J Med* 2005; 353(13): 1363–1373.

Nafziger SD. Smallpox. *Crit Care Clin* 2005; 21: 739-746.

Nagai M, Usuku K, Matsumoto W. Analysis Of HTLV-I Proviral Load In 202 HAM/TSP Patients And 243 Asymptomatic HTLV-I Carriers: High Proviral Load Strongly Predisposes To HAM/TSP. *J Neurovirol* 1998; 4:586–593.

Orth G, Favre M, Majewski S, et al. Epidermodysplasia Verruciformis Defines A Subset Of Cutaneous Human Papillomaviruses. *J Virol* 2001;75: 4952-4953.

Pappas G, Akritidis N, Bosilkovski M, Tsianos E. Brucellosis. *N Engl J Med* 2005; 352: 2325-2336.

Pawlotsky JM. Use and Interpretation of Virological Tests for Hepatitis C. *Hepatology* 2002; 36(Suppl 1): S65–S73.

Peiris JS, Yuen KY, Osterhaus AD, et al. The Severe Acute Respiratory Syndrome. *N Engl J Med* 2003; 349(25): 2431–2441.

Podzorski RP. Molecular Testing in the Diagnosis and Management of Hepatitis C Virus Infection. *Arch Pathol Lab Med* 2002; 126: 285–290.

Poutanen SM, Simor AE. Clostridium Difficile–Associated Diarrhea In Adults. *CMAJ* 2004; 171: 51–58.

Powderly WG, Stanley Jr SL, Medoff G. Pneumococcal Endocarditis: Report Of A Series And Review Of The Literature. *Rev Infect Dis* 1986;8:786-791.

Queiroz-Telles F, McGinnis MR. Subcutaneous Mycoses. *Infect Dis Clin N Am* 2003; 17: 59–85.

Ramoz N, Rueda LA, Bouadjar B, et al. Mutations In Two Adjacent Novel Genes Are Associated With Epidermodysplasia Verruciformis. *Nat Genet* 2002;32: 579-581.

Ramzan NN. Traveler's Diarrhea. *Gastroenterol Clin North Am* 2001; 30: 665–678.

Rebucci C, Cerino A, Cividini A, et al. Monitoring Response To Antiviral Therapy For Patients With Chronic Hepatitis C Virus Infection By A Core-Antigen Assay. *J Clin Microbiol* 2003; 41: 3881–3884.

Ronald A. The Etiology of Urinary Tract Infection: Traditional and Emerging Pathogens. *Am J Med* 2002; 113(Suppl 1A): 14S–19S.

Ross AGP, Bartley PB, Sleigh AC, Olds GR, Li Y, Williams GM, McManus DP. Schisotosomiasis. *N Engl J Med* 2002; 346(16): 1212-1220.

Salkin I, Graybill JR. Nucleic Acid Amplification Tests for Tuberculosis. *MMWR Morb Mortal Wkly Rep* 2000; 49(26): 593–594.

Sander A, Berner R, Ruess M. Serodiagnosis Of Cat Scratch Disease: Response To Bartonella henselae In Children and a Review Of Diagnostic Methods. *Eur J Clin Microbiol Infect Dis* 2001; 20: 392–401.

Schuachat A, Robinson K, Wenger JD, Harrison LH, Farley M, Reingold AL, et al. Bacterial meningitis in the United States in 1995. *N Engl J Med* 1997; 337: 970–976.

Shlim DR. Cyclospora cayetanensis. *Clin Lab Med* 2002; 22: 927–936.

Sigurdardottir B, Bjornsson OM, Jonsdottir KE, et al. Acute Bacterial Meningitis In Adults: A 20-Year Overview. *Arch Intern Med* 1997; 157: 425-430.

Spangehl MJ, Masri BA, O'Connell JX, Duncan CP. Prospective Analysis of Preoperative and Intraoperative Investigations for the Diagnosis of Infection at the Sites of Two Hundred and Two Revision Total Hip Arthroplasties. *J Bone Joint Surg Am* 1999; 81: 672-683.

Steingart KR, Henry M, Ng V, Hopewell PC, Ramsay A, Cunningham J, Urbanczik R, Perkins M, Aziz MA, Pai M. Fluorescence Versus Conventional Sputum Smear Microscopy For Tuberculosis: A Systematic Review. *Lancet Infect Dis* 2006; 6: 570–581.

Steketee RW, Abrams EJ, Thea DM, et al. Early Detection of Perinatal Human Immunodeficiency Virus Type 1 Infection Using HIV RNA Amplification and Detection. *J Infect Dis* 1997; 175: 707–711.

Bibliography

Svenungsson B, Lagergren A, Ekwall E, et al. Enteropathogens In Adult Patients With Diarrhea And Healthy Control Subjects: A 1-Year Prospective Study In A Swedish Clinic For Infectious Diseases. *Clin Infect Dis* 2000; 30: 770–778.

Taylor GP, Tosswill JHC, Matutes E. A Prospective Study Of HTLV-I Infection In An Initially Asymptomatic Cohort. *J Acquir Immune Defic Syndr* 2000; 22:92–100.

Tigges S, Stiles RG, Roberson JR. Appearance of Septic Hip Prostheses on Plain Radiographs. *Am J Roentgenol* 1994; 163: 377-380.

Trampuz A, Hanssen AD, Osmon DR, Mandrekar J, Steckelberg JM, Patel R. Synovial Fluid Leukocyte Count and Differential for the Diagnosis of Prosthetic Knee Infection. *Am J Med* 2004; 117: 556-562.

Trampuz A, Steckelberg JM, Osmon DR, Cockerill FR, Hanssen AD, Patel R. Advances in the Laboratory Diagnosis of Prosthetic Joint Infection. *Rev Med Microbiol* 2003; 14: 1-14.

Troy SB, Rickman LS, Davis CE. Brucellosis in San Diego: Epidemiology and Species-Related Differences in Acute Clinical Presentations. *Medicine* 2005; 84(3):174-187.

Ugolini V, Pacifico A, Smitherman TC, et al. Pneumococcal Endocarditis Update: Analysis Of 10 Cases Diagnosed Between 1974 And 1984. *Am Heart J* 1986; 112: 813-819.

Weisfelt M, van de Beek D, Spanjaard L, Reitsma JB, de Gans J. Clinical Features, Complications, And Outcome In Adults With Pneumococcal Meningitis: A Prospective Case Series. *Lancet Neurol* 2006; 5: 123–129.

Wiwanitkit V. Hematologic Manifestations of Bird Flu, H5N1. *Infection Infect Dis Clin Pract* 2006; 14: 9–11.

Workowski KA, Levine WC. Sexually Transmitted Diseases Treatment Guidelines 2002. *MMWR Morb Mortal Wkly Rep* 2002: 51 RR-7:18-30.

Zerr DM, Frenkel LM, Huang H-L, Rhoads M, Nguy L, Del Beccaro MA, Corey L. Polymerase Chain Reaction Diagnosis Of Primary Human Herpesvirus-6 Infection In The Acute Care Setting. *J Pediatr* 2006; 149: 480-485.

Zimmerli W, Trampuz A, Ochsner PE. Prosthetic-Joint Infections. *N Engl J Med* 2004; 351(16): 1645-1654.

Chapter 4

Hematopathology

Methods

Measurement of Total Hemoglobin

Most commonly, hemoglobin is measured by the cyanohemoglobin (hemiglobin cyanide) method, in which hemoglobin is converted to hemiglobin cyanide (HiCN), whose concentration is measured by spectrophotometry. To carry out this conversion, blood is dissolved in a solution of potassium ferricyanide and potassium cyanide which oxidizes the hemoglobin to hemiglobin (Hi; methemoglobin) and then converts it to hemiglobin cyanide, (HiCN). The solution's absorbance at **540 nm** reflects the amount of hemoglobin originally present. This method detects all forms of hemoglobin (Hb, HbO_2, Hi, HbCO) **except sulfhemoglobin** (SHb). The hemoglobin concentration (Hb) is usually stated in terms of g/dL.

Red Blood Cell Indices

Manual techniques

- The hematocrit (Hct) can be measured directly by centrifuging a tube of whole blood. The ratio of the packed red cell column height to the total height is the hematocrit. This method has been adapted for small samples (micromethods) using a tube with an internal bore of 1mm. Blood is drawn up into the microtube through capillary action, centrifuged, and measured to calculate the hematocrit. The Hct is a unitless value, as the units cancel out in its calculation.

- Erythrocytes (as well as leukocytes and platelets) can be counted manually to give the RBC count, through the use of a hemocytometer. RBC counts may be given in terms of cells per mm^3 (eg, $5.5 \times 10^6/mm^3$), per μL (conventional units), or per L (SI units).

- When the Hct and RBC count are determined manually, the remaining red cell indices can be calculated:

  - MCV = Hct × 1000 / RBC. The result is stated in femtoliters (fL). One fL = $1 \mu L^3 = 10^{-15}$ L.

  - MCHC = Hb / Hct.

Automated techniques

- On most automated instruments, the red cell count (RBC), mean corpuscular volume (MCV), and red cell distribution width (RDW) are measured directly (as is the total hemoglobin). The instrument then calculates the other indices, such as hematocrit.

- There are at least three different methods used by automated instruments to count cells: impedance (counts any particle of given size), optical methods—forward and side light scatter (can to a certain degree distinguish one particle of a given size from another), or combination of impedance and light scatter.

- The red blood cell count (RBC)

  - When determined by impedance counting, the cells are suspended in a conductive diluent and passed one-by-one through an aperture across which a current is flowing. A cell within the aperture causes a momentary increase in electrical resistance (impedance). Voltage, a product of resistance and current ($V = I \times R$), increases when the resistance increases.

  - The instrument interprets a momentary increase in voltage as a single cell. The amount of voltage change is proportional to the size of the cell.

  - The instrument is instructed to count particles measuring between 36 and 360 fL as red cells. Of course leukocytes, which are within this size range, will be counted as erythrocytes, but their relative number is so small (usually) that their effect is typically negligible.

- MCV and RDW

  - Red blood cells passing through the aperture come in a range of sizes (volumes), distributed in a roughly Gaussian curve. The mean of this distribution is taken as the mean corpuscular volume (MCV).

  - The variance in the curve is the red cell distribution width (RDW).

- The rest of the red cell indices can be calculated as follows:

  - Hematocrit (Hct) = MCV × RBC

□ Mean corpuscular Hb concentration (MCHC) = Hb / Hct × 100

Leukocyte Indices

Total leukocyte count. Automated leukocyte counts can also be carried out by impedance counting (the Coulter principle). Red blood cells are lysed, and the remainder is subjected to counting. Particles larger than 36 fL are counted as leukocytes. Interferences are minimal, as the red cells have been lysed, and platelets usually measure less than 35 fL.

Leukocyte differential. A 3-dimensional scatterplot can be generated by performing 3 simultaneous measurements on each cell that passes the aperture: impedance (volume~size), conductivity (cell complexity), and side-angle light scatter (cytoplasmic granularity). This "VCS" technology allows identification of 5 populations: neutrophils, lymphocytes, monocytes, eosinophils, and basophils. Using forward and side-angle light scatter can also resolve most leukocyte populations (**F4.1**).

Platelets

Platelets can also be counted by electrical impedance. Particles measuring between 2 fL and 20 fL are counted as platelets. In a manner analogous to the MCV, the mean platelet volume (MPV) is also determined.

Erroneously low platelet counts may result from a clotted specimen, large platelets, clumped platelets (problem in heparinized patients, sometime spontaneous, both due to EDTA-antibody interactions, both show platelet agglutination on peripheral smear).

Reticulocytes

All techniques for the differentiation of reticulocytes from mature red cells are based upon the abundance of RNA (ribosomal RNA) in the reticulocyte.

Techniques for enumerating reticulocytes include manual counting by light microscopy, optical light scatter, and flow cytometry. In the first two methods, red cells are stained with a supravital dye (eg, new methylene blue or azure B) which highlight residual cytoplasmic RNA. In flow cytometry, the cells are stained with an RNA-specific fluorochrome. The result is given as a percentage of total red cells.

Automated techniques are much more precise than manual methods. Furthermore, the automated techniques can subdivide reticulocytes into mature and immature fractions.

Reticulocytes are slightly larger than mature red blood cells (thus pronounced reticulocytosis can raise the MCV). The very immature reticulocyte contains mitochondria, numerous ribosomes, and Golgi bodies, and it is still in the process of making hemoglobin. Transferrin receptors are still present on the surface, and these forms are normally not released into the circulation. After about 48 hours of further maturation, a reticulocyte that has much less RNA is released into the circulation. The relative age of a reticulocyte can be determined from its RNA content.

The absolute reticulocyte count is calculated by multiplying the percent reticulocytes by the red blood cell (RBC) count. The corrected reticulocyte count (CRC) takes into account spuriously increased reticulocyte percentages due to a low Hct. The reticulocyte production index (RPI) reflects the fact that in anemia, reticulocytes are released earlier from the marrow and therefore have a longer maturation time than normal to mature

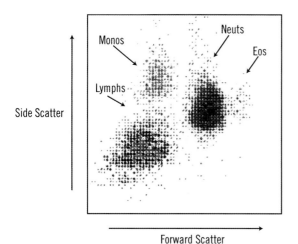

F.4.1 Automated leukocyte differential, based upon light scatter.

243

into red cells. The correction factor is 1.0 when the Hct is normal, 2.0 when Hct is 30, and 3.0 when Hct is 15.

$$CRC = \% \text{ retics} \times Hct/45$$

$$RPI = CRC \times 1/\text{Correction factor}$$

$$\text{Absolute retic count} = \% \text{ retics} \times RBC \text{ count}$$

Detection of Normal and Variant Hemoglobins

Rapid detection of sickling hemoglobin

- The hemoglobin solubility (dithionate) test detects insoluble forms of hemoglobin within a lysate of blood. In this test, red cells are lysed in sodium dithionate buffer with saponin. After several minutes, marked turbidity indicates a positive screen. Note that this test detects free hemoglobin with altered solubility. The test should be interpreted as indicative of sickling hemoglobin, but it says nothing in particular about the genotype and may be positive in SS, SA, SC, SD, and C_{harlem}. This test may be negative when the concentration of HbS is too small; eg, in neonates.

- The sickling (metabisulfite) test detects red cells with sickling hemoglobins. In this test, whole blood is subjected to metabisulfite, which encourages cells containing HbS to sickle. A smear is then examined microscopically for sickling. Like the solubility test, this test does not give genotypic information and may be positive in SS, SA, SC, S-other, and C_{harlem}. The test requires at least 10% HbS to be positive. Thus, it may not be positive in neonates or those very aggressively transfused.

Detection of fetal hemoglobin (HbF)

- The acid elution technique may be used to detect red cells containing HbF, in support of a diagnosis of hereditary persistence of fetal hemoglobin (HPFH) or fetomaternal hemorrhage. In an acid buffer, HbA elutes from red cells, but HbF does not. Cells with persistent eosinophilia following acid elution contain HbF.

  □ Two patterns may be seen: heterocellular (some RBCs contain HbF but others do not) and pancellular (all RBCs contain HbF).

  □ The pancellular pattern is characteristic of most types of hereditary persistence of fetal hemoglobin (HPFH).

  □ Other examples of elevated HbF are heterocellular (eg, thalassemia).

- A quantititative assay for HbF is based upon the principal that HbF is resistant to alkali denaturation (in 1.25 Molar NaOH). HbA is denatured and precipitated out; the optical density of the remaining supernatant reflects the quantity of HbF.

- HPLC is also a highly accurate method of HbF quantitation (see below).

Hemoglobin electrophoresis **F4.2a, F4.2b**

- Routine hemoglobin electrophoresis is performed by placing a sample of lysed blood on cellulose acetate at pH 8.6 (alkaline electrophoresis). The gel is subjected to electromotive force, fixed, and stained.

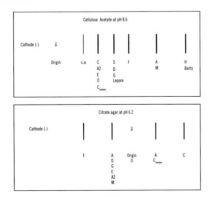

F4.2a The expected electrophoretic destination of the more common hemoglobin variants on cellulose acetate at pH 8.6 (above) and citrate at pH 6.2 (below).

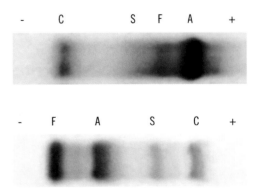

F4.2b The expected electrophoretic destination of the more common hemoglobin variants on cellulose acetate at pH 8.6 (above) and citrate at pH 6.2 (below).

- The normal adult has mostly hemoglobin A which is a fast-moving hemoglobin found near the anode. A small amount (less than 3%) of slower-moving hemoglobin A2 is detectable, seen in the C band. Carbonic anhydrase is also seen, near the origin.

- A fast hemoglobin is one that migrates beyond A on the alkaline gel, and this may represent HbH or HbBarts.

- When a band is present in the S region, its identity can be confirmed by the sickle screen; if negative, this may indicate D, G, or Lepore.

- When A2 or F appear increased, a more reliable quantitative assay should be performed to obtain an exact amount.

- Thalassemia, being a *quantitative* defect in production of entirely normal hemoglobins, does not produce abnormal bands on the electrophoresis. Instead, β-thalassemia is diagnosed by the presence of *'thalassemic indices'* (*increased RBC count, low MCV*) and a quantitatively increased Hb A2. α-thalassemia has 'thalassemic indices' and normal Hb A2.

- True hemoglobinopathies are due to production of structurally abnormal hemoglobin molecules that usually produces a distinct band on electrophoresis. The identity of most, but not all, abnormal hemoglobins can often be determined by routine electrophoresis, particularly when supplemented with some clinical information and CBC data. When there is uncertainty, electrophoresis on citrate agar at pH 6.2 (acid electrophoresis) produces a different set of electrophoretic positions which, in combination with the alkaline gel, can help identify an abnormal band.

High pressure liquid chromatography (HPLC) F4.3

- Alkaline electrophoresis is widely available and capable of separating common hemoglobin variants, such as HbA, HbF, HbS, and HbC; however, it does not separate HbS from HbD, HbG, and HbLepore nor does it resolve HbC, HbA2, HbO-Arab, and HbE. Acid electrophoresis is needed for clarifying these variants, but does not help to separate HbD from HbG and HbLepore or HbE from HbO-Arab. The list of possible misinterpretations due to very rare variants is quite long. Lastly, electrophoresis does not permit accurate quantitation of A2 or F, requiring an additional assay for this purpose.

- HPLC is a technique that employs a pump to provide the high pressure needed to push a sample (the 'mobile phase') through a column at a much greater rate than could be obtained by gravity alone. A column is a steel cylinder into which are packed numerous small particles (the 'stationary phase') such as silica gel beads. Individual molecules exit the column (elute) at different rates, depending upon their particular properties. As a molecule elutes, a light source produces a deflection on a spectrophotometer that is proportional to the concentration of that molecule in the original sample. Thus, HPLC can give information about the identity of a hemoglobin molecule (when correlated with known rates of elution) and its percentage in the sample.

Molecular methods (PCR). 1%-2% of variant hemoglobins detected by HPLC or gel electrophoresis cannot be definitively identified. The DNA sequence of a

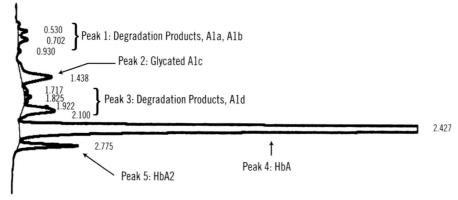

F4.3 High pressure liquid chromatography (HPLC) of blood lysate. This is an example of a normal study. When abnormal peaks are present, their time of elution is compared, on published charts, to known times of elution to determine their identity.

hemoglobin gene can be determined to characterize the exact genotype for a given individual. While this is sometimes useful in adult evaluations, it holds special promise in prenatal diagnosis—since one can analyze any sample of fetal tissue, and actual fetal blood need not be obtained.

Histochemistry and Cytochemistry

Wright stain is a Romanowsky-type metachromatic stain made by mixing methylene blue dye with eosin and alcohol. Basic components of the cell, such as hemoglobin, attract the acidic portion of the stain, eosin, and are said to be eosinophilic. Acidic cell components, such as nucleic acids, take up the basic dye components, methylene azure, and stain blue or purple. pH must be carefully controlled through the use of a buffer. If the pH is too acidic, the stain will take on a pinkish tint, and nuclear structures will be poorly visualized. A basic pH will cause all intracellular constituents, nuclei, etc. to be blue-black in color, with poorly defined structure.

Cytochemical stains for typing blasts T4.1

- Myeloperoxidase (MPO) stains the primary (azurophilic) granules indicative of granulocytic differentiation. It is negative in lymphoblasts, erythroblasts, monoblasts, and megakaryoblasts. Fine dusty positivity may be seen in monoblasts. Thus, a negative MPO in the early evaluation of uncharacterized blasts does not necessarily imply lymphoid leukemia. MPO *degrades quickly in wet specimens,* but is stable in smears for up to a month.

- Sudan black B (SBB) stains lipid material found in granulocytic and monocytic cells.

T4.1
Cytochemical Stains in Myeloblasts

Type	PAS	SBB	MPO	CAE	NSE	Auer rods
M0	–	–	–	–	–	rare
M1	–	+	+	+	–	50%
M2	–	+	+	+	–	50%
M3	–	+	+	+	–	95%
M4	–	+	+	+	+	64%
M5	–	–	–	–	+	0
M6	+	+	+	–	–	50%
M7	+	–	–	–	+/–	rare

- Chloroacetate esterase (CAE) is found only in the granulocytic series. Monocytes and lymphocytes are negative.

- Nonspecific esterases (NSE) include alpha naphthyl acetate esterase and alpha naphthyl butyrate esterase. They stain cells of the monocytic series and, to variably lesser extents, megakaryocytic, lymphocytic, granulocytic, and erythroid series. Monocyte NSE activity is *inhibited by sodium fluoride (NaF).*

- Periodic acid Schiff (PAS) is positive in most lymphoid and some myeloid blasts. In ALL, it shows "block" positivity, often encircling the nucleus in a "rosary bead" fashion. In AML, when positive, it is usually a diffuse, granular hue of positivity.

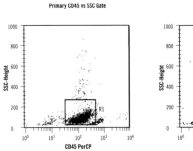 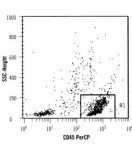 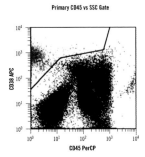

F4.4 Examples of flow gating. The plot on the left has CD45 (x-axis) versus side-scatter (y-axis), and the selected gate is the blast population (CD45 dim, low side-scatter). The middle plot also has CD45 versus side-scatter, with gating around lymphocytes (bright CD45, low side-scatter). The plot to the right has CD45 (x-axis) versus CD38 (y-axis), permitting plasma cell gating (CD45 negative, CD38 bright).

■ The vacuoles in the blasts of L3 ALL stain positively with the oil red O stain.

Leukocyte alkaline phosphatase (LAP) score.

■ Leukocyte alkaline phosphatase (LAP) hydrolyzes the substrate naphthol AS-biphosphate to form a colored product.

■ Bands and neutrophils are scored on the intensity of cytoplasmic staining from 0 to 4+ until 100 cells are counted. The number resulting from the sum of the 100 values is reported as the LAP score.

■ Normal adults score in the range of 40-120. Patients with CML generally have a decreased LAP score (0-15). Other instances with a low LAP score include paroxysmal nocturnal hemoglobinuria, some myelodysplastic syndromes, congenital hypophosphatasia, and neonatal septicemia (LAP paradoxically decreased). Elevated levels (>180) are seen in leukemoid reaction, non-CML myeloproliferative disorders, glucocorticoid administration and the third trimester of pregnancy.

Detection of fetal red cells.

■ The acid elution (Kleihauer-Betke) test is based upon the principle that Hb A can be eluted out of alcohol-fixed red cells with buffered citric acid. Hemoglobin F remains inside red cells under these conditions and can be stained with eosin.

■ Two patterns may be seen: heterocellular (some RBCs contain Hb F but others do not) and pancellular (all RBCs contain Hb F). The pancellular pattern is characteristic of most types of hereditary persistence of fetal hemoglobin (HPFH). Other examples of elevated Hb F are heterocellular (eg, fetomaternal hemorrhage, thalassemia).

Immunophenotyping

Flow cytometry

■ The specimen is distributed among several tubes. Into these are added various fluorochrome-labeled antibodies against cell surface antigens. The 'stained' cells are run through the flow cytometer so that only one cell at a time passes through the counting chamber.

■ As a cell passes through the chamber multiple parameters are obtained: size (forward light scatter - FLS), nuclear complexity/cytoplasmic granularity (90° light scatter or side scatter (SSC)), and the intensity of fluorochrome on the cell surface.

■ Fluorochromes are substances that absorb light (from a laser in this case) at a certain wavelength and emit it at a different wavelength. This difference in absorbed and emitted wavelength is essential so that one can simultaneously detect both the original wavelength (to determine size and complexity characteristics of the cell) and the fluorochrome-emitted wavelength (to determine antigen expression), and this difference is called the Stokes shift. Common fluorochromes include fluorescein isothiocyanate (FITC) and phycoerythrin (PE), but there are many.

■ Compensation is something that is done by the flow cytometer's computer. When more than one fluorochrome is used, there is usually some overlap between their emission spectra, so-called 'bleeding-over.' Compensation errors—over- or undercompensation—are a potential source of error.

■ Gating, in which cells of interest are digitally selected for consideration, is the key first step in flow interpretation **F4.4.** For example, if one seeks to examine lymphocytes in a sample, one would "gate" around those which have low side scatter and strong CD45 expression on a graph of CD45 expression vs side scatter. Alternatively, one could gate around those having low side and forward scatter on a graph of SSC vs FSC. Plasma cells can be selected out of a mixed population (eg bone marrow) with CD45 vs CD38 gating, wherein the plasma cells have very low CD45 and very high CD38 expression.

Immunohistochemistry uses nonfluorescence-based enzymatic chromagen production to allow visualization of antibody binding to corresponding surface and cytoplasmic antigens. Not all antibodies used for fresh tissue flow cytometry are available for tissue or cytologic immunohistochemistry.

Expected immunophenotypes of hematopoietic cells

■ Hematopoietic stem cells have dim CD45 expression, allowing blast gating with relative ease. As they differentiate, CD45 expression changes, with lymphocytes and

T4.2
B- and T-cell Maturation Sequences

B-cell stage	Definition	T-cell stage	Definition
Lymphoid stem cell	CD34+, TdT+, HLA-DR+	Lymphoid stem cell	CD34+, TdT+, HLA-DR+
Pro-B cell	CD34+, TdT+, HLA-DR+, CD19+, CD10+, Ig H chain rearranging	Prothymocytes	CD34+, TdT+, CD2+, CD7+
Pre-B cell	CD34 -, TdT -, HLA-DR+, CD19+, CD10+, CD20+, Cytoplasmic μ heavy chains, Ig light chain rearranging	Immature / Common thymocytes	CD34-, TdT+, CD1+, CD2+, cytoplasmic CD3+ (surface CD3-), CD5+, CD7+, CD4 and CD8+,TCR rearranged
B cell	All of the above plus surface Ig, CD21+, CD22+	Mature thymocyte	All of the above, except: TdT– and CD1–. Surface CD3 becoming +, CD4 or CD8+
Plasma cell	Loss of B-cell markers (CD19–, CD20–) and cytoplasmic (not surface) Ig+.	Mature T cell	All of the above, except surface CD3+

monocytes having bright expression, granulocytes an intermediate intensity, and erythrocytes almost none.

■ B Lymphocytes **T4.2.** The earliest B-cell precursors express CD34, TdT, CD38, dim CD45, CD10, and CD19. By the time IgM is expressed, all of the above are lost except CD19. At this same time, there is surface expression of CD20, CD22, CD79, and CD40. CD38 is expressed again in activated B cells. The normal blood and tissue T:B ratio is 2-6:1. When B cells mature into plasma cells, they lose CD45 and most pan-B antigens (CD19, CD20, CD22, CD40, surface Ig). They keep CD79a and acquire stronger CD38 and CD138. Often they express CD10 as well as the myeloid antigens CD13 and CD33.

■ T lymphocytes **T4.2.** The earliest T-cell precursors (prothymocytes) express CD34, TdT, HLA-DR, CD38, dim CD45, CD2, and CD7 and have cytoplasmic CD3. Note that CD7 is not lineage-specific, and it is expressed in normal and many neoplastic myeloid cells. As they mature, T cells begin to express CD5, CD1, surface CD3 (coincides with expression of surface TCR), and CD4, and CD8, with progressive diminution of CD34, TdT, CD1, and HLA-DR. Later, selection leads to loss of either CD4 or CD8, coincident with the loss of CD1. Therefore, there is a stage of T-cell maturation in which the cell is both CD4–, CD8–, followed by a period of both CD4+, CD8+, with eventual expression of either one or the other. In the normally functioning immune system the CD4:CD8 cell ratio is 2:1. CD38 is

re-expressed upon T-cell activation. The vast majority of mature T-cells have TCRs with αβ light chains (noncovalently associated with the antigen CD3). γδ T cells represent a small (3%-5%) population of overall T cells, but a large proportion of dermal, intestinal, and splenic T cells.

■ NK cells. A subset of lymphocytic cells that bear *neither* the TCR nor immunoglobulin, lack surface CD3 (CD3 negative by flow cytometry, may express cytoplasmic CD3 by immunohistochemistry), and are positive for CD16 and CD56. CD16 is the receptor for the Fc portion of γ heavy chains (FcgR).

■ Granulocytes. The myeloblast expresses CD34, HLA-DR, CD38, CD117, CD13, and CD33. Promyelocytes are negative for CD34 and HLA-DR, continue to express CD13 and CD33, and acquire CD15. Metamyelocytes acquire CD11b.

■ Monocytes. The monocyte derives from the myeloblast. In the promononocyte stage, there is loss of CD34 and expression of CD11b and CD15. With additional maturation, there is expression of CD64 and CD14.

Antigens

■ Alk. Expressed in anaplastic large cell lymphomas (ALCL) that are t(2;5)+.

- Bcl-1 (cyclin-D1, PRAD-1). Expressed by neoplastic mantle cells.

- Bcl-2, in normal and reactive lymph nodes, is expressed only by mantle cells and the small number of mantle cells that normally permeate the follicle center (this number is increased in follicular lysis). Bcl-2 is expressed by most low-grade B-cell lymphomas and many high-grade B-cell lymphomas. Expression in follicular lymphoma decreases with grade, varying from >95% in grade 1 to 75% in grade 3. Bcl-2 is useful in distinguishing neoplastic from reactive germinal centers, but not useful to distinguish FL from other B-cell lymphomas. In this latter regard, CD10 is preferable. Bcl-2 is not expressed by Burkitt lymphoma, and can be helpful to separate Burkitt from Burkitt-like lymphomas.

- Bcl-6 is strongly expressed in normal germinal center B-cells. It is also is expressed in a limited series of lymphomas—Burkitt lymphoma, follicular lymphoma (FL), nodular lymphocyte predominant Hodgkin lymphoma (NLPHL), and a subset of diffuse large B-cell lymphoma (DLBCL). In DLBCL, bcl-6 overexpression has been associated with a translocation involving the bcl-6 gene on chromosome 3q and the IgH gene on 14q.

- CD1a is expressed by Langerhans cells, dendritic reticulum cells, interdigitating reticulum cells, and cortical thymocytes.

- CD2 is expressed by T lymphocytes and NK cells, even from a very early stage.

- CD3 is expressed by T lymphocytes (mature non-neoplastic and neoplastic) but not expressed by very immature T lymphocytes, $\gamma\delta$ T cells, or NK cells. Cytoplasmic expression precedes surface expression and may be detectable by immunohistochemistry (eg, in immature T cells and NK cells) when surface expression is not detected by flow cytometry.

- CD4 is expressed by a subset of T lymphocytes, specifically, T_{helper} cells. It is also expressed by monocytic and dendritic cells. The normal CD4:CD8 in blood and tissue is anywhere from 2-6:1. CD4+/CD8+ co-expressing T cells are normally only found in the thymic cortex. CD4–/CD8– T cells are not normal and probably neoplastic. The majority of T-cell lymphomas and leukemias are CD4+.

- CD5 is expressed by normal and neoplastic T cells (not expressed by very immature T cells) and a small, normally inconspicuous, B cell subset. Occasionally, patients have increased (polyclonal, benign) circulating CD19+/CD20+/CD5+ B cells, particularly in rheumatoid arthritis. CD5 co-expression in B cells is the hallmark of small lymphocytic lymphoma/chronic lymphocytic leukemia (SLL/CLL) and mantle cells lymphoma (MCL). CD5 is sometimes lost in T cell lymphoma/leukemia.

- CD7 is expressed by normal and neoplastic T cells and NK cells. Its loss is a common form of aberrant phenotype in T cell lymphoma/leukemia. Sometimes expressed in AML (about 10% of cases—especially M4/M5).

- CD 8 is expressed by the CD4-negative subset of T lymphocytes and neoplastic NK, $T_{cytotoxic}$ and $T_{suppressor}$ cells.

- CD10 (CALLA) is the characteristic antigen of follicle center B lymphocytes, and it is expressed by both normal and neoplastic follicle center cells. CD10 is also present on B-cell acute lymphoblastic leukemia (B-ALL), and some proliferations of neoplastic plasma cells.

- CD11b (MAC-1) is found on monocytes and granulocytes, and the neoplastic B cells of hairy cell leukemia (HCL).

- CD11c (C3r) is normally expressed by monocytes and granulocytes. Among neoplasms of small B cells, CD11c expression is distinctive for CLL/SLL and HCL.

- CD13 is a marker of granulocytic cells and precursors. In acute leukemia, it is expressed in AML M1, M2, M3, M5, and M6.

- CD14 is a marker of monocytic cells and a variable marker of monocytic precursors. It is often (but not uniformly) expressed in AML M4 and M5. It is also expressed in >85% of CLL and FCL.

- CD15 (Leu-M1) is expressed in mature monocytes and granulocytes, Reed-Sternberg cells, and most adenocarcinomas. CD15 immunohistochemistry in Reed-Sternberg cells is somewhat unreliable, and positivity, when present, is often limited to faint golgi-zone staining. In the setting of AML, it indicates a maturing phenotype; for example, it is strongly expressed in acute promyelocytic leukemia

(APML, M3). Its absence is a distinctive feature of the neoplastic cells in anaplastic large cell lymphoma (ALCL).

- CD16 is expressed by normal and neoplastic NK cells and granulocytes.

- CD19 is expressed by B cells from the pre-B stage onward. While expressed by normal plasma cells, expression is typically lost in neoplastic plasma cells. CD19 is quite often weakened and sometimes lost in follicular lymphoma (FL). It may be present on some cases of AML, especially AML with t(8;21)(q22;q22).

- CD20 is expressed on the surface of maturing B cells just after the appearance of CD19 and before CD22. It is not expressed by plasma cells, Reed-Sternberg cells (except in NLPHD), or anaplastic large cell lymphoma (a CD20+, CD30+ lymphoma is classified as a diffuse large cell lymphoma according to WHO). Furthermore, CD20 *expression by CLL/SLL is distinctively dim.* FMC-7 is an antibody that recognizes a particular conformation of CD20. Cells with weak CD20 (CLL/SLL) tend to be FMC-7-negative. Cells with bright CD20 (most other B-NHLs) tend to be FMC-7+.

- CD22 is expressed by normal and neoplastic B cells; this being the latest antigen acquired in B cell maturation, CD22 is seen in only a small percentage of B-ALL.

- CD23 (the IgE receptor) is instrumental in the immunophenotypic distinction of CLL (positive) from MCL (negative).

- CD25 (the IL-2 receptor) is expressed by activated lymphoid cells (T and B) and the neoplastic cells of hairy cell leukemia and adult T cell leukemia/lymphoma (ATCL). In fact, soluble IL-2 receptor is usually elevated in the serum of patients with ATCL.

- CD30 (Ki-1; Ber-H2) is found on normal plasma cells, immunoblasts (such as in viral (EBV) lymphadenopathy) and NK cells. CD30 expression is the hallmark of Reed-Sternberg cells. It is also found on anaplastic large cell lymphoma (ALCL) and embryonal carcinoma. Expression of CD30 is a characteristic feature of mediastinal-type diffuse large B cell lymphoma.

- CD33 is expressed by normal and neoplastic myeloid and monocytic cells. It is usually positive in AML M1—M5.

- CD34 is a marker of immature mesenchymal cells; it is expressed by normal and neoplastic endothelial cells, immature myeloid cells, gastrointestinal stromal tumors, dermatofibrosarcoma protuberans (DFSPs), chloromas, and solitary fibrous tumors.

- CD38 expression in nonneoplastic settings is confined to *activated* T and B cells and plasma cells. Its expression is common in B- and T- cell neoplasms as well; however, expression in CLL/SLL is limited to a subset of cases with more aggressive clinical features.

- CD40 is expressed by normal and neoplastic B cells.

- CD41/CD61 are markers of normal and neoplastic megakaryocytic cells.

- CD43. Expressed by normal and neoplastic T cells. Under-expressed in Wiskott–Aldrich syndrome. Anomalously expressed on B cells in majority of cases of MCL, SLL, and some cases of MZL (not commonly seen in FCL).

- CD45 (leukocyte common antigen, LCA) is found in nearly all normal and neoplastic leukocytes. However, dim to absent CD45 (usually with strong CD34) is the immunophenotypic signature of myeloblasts, and dim to absent CD45 (with strong CD38) is indicative of plasma cells. Furthermore, CD45 is not expressed in Reed-Sternberg cells (except NLPHD).

- CD45-RO (UCHL-1) is expressed by normal and neoplastic T cells.

- CD56 is expressed by normal and neoplastic NK cells, plasma cells, and neural cells.

- CD57 (Leu-7) is expressed by a subset of normal and neoplastic NK cells and most neural cells.

- CD59 is present on nearly all human cells. Decreased (along with CD55—DAF) cell surface expression is a feature of the affected clone in paroxysmal nocturnal hemoglobinuria (PNH).

- CD68 is expressed by macrophages and histiocytes, but its specificity is poor.

- CD79a is expressed by normal and neoplastic B cells and plasma cells.

- CD99 (p30/32, mic-2; O-13) was initially thought to be specific for PNET/Ewing; however, it is now known to be expressed in lymphoblastic lymphomas, granulosa cell tumors, synovial sarcoma, rhabdomyosarcoma, solitary fibrous tumor, and others.

- CD103 is a very sensitive and specific marker for hairy cell leukemia (HCL).

- CD117 (c-kit) is a tyrosine kinase whose gene is found on chromosome 4q12, adjacent to PDGFRA. It is expressed by the so-called interstitial cell of Cajal (the precursors of GI stromal tumors), melanocytes (particularly junctional), seminomas, progenitor myeloid cells (AML, CML) and mast cells (mastocytomas).

- CD138 is a plasma cell marker. Within hematolymphoid proliferations, CD138 is a very specific marker of plasma cell differentiation; however, CD138 is positive in a wide range of epithelial and mesenchymal proliferations.

- Clusterin expression, in a discrete golgi pattern, appears to be unique to anaplastic large cell lymphoma (ALCL). Cytoplasmic staining may be seen in several epithelial neoplasms and occasional Hodgkin lymphomas. In addition, strong cytoplasmic reactivity is noted in megakaryocytes.

- Epithelial membrane antigen (EMA) is expressed by plasma cells, ALCL, NLPHL, and T-cell rich B-cell lymphoma (TCRBCL).

- Fascin is expressed by RS cells and dendritic reticulum cells.

- FMC-7. See CD20.

- HLA-DR is expressed by monocytic cells, B cells, and activated T cells. As the *earliest marker of B-cell differentiation,* it is expressed in most B–ALLs, and usually not in T–ALL. Furthermore, HLA-DR is expressed in most AML subtypes; notably *not* expressed in AML M3 (APML).

- Light chains (κ or λ) are expressed on the surface of most mature B cells and in the cytoplasm of most plasma cells. They are absent on the surface of most B-ALL, but present in Burkitt (L3) lymphoma/leukemia.

Conventional cytogenetics. After a brief cell culture, cells are arrested in metaphase and examined visually. This is extremely useful to detect structural chromosomal aberrations such as t(9;22), but the sensitivity of this technique is relatively low (see Chapter 7).

Molecular Techniques

Lymphocytes

- B and T cells undergo somatic gene rearrangements in order to produce the genes that will ultimately encode their respective immunoglobulin (Ig) and T-cell receptor (TCR) proteins. For example, a primitive B cell begins life with its genes in a *germline* (embryonic) configuration. In the germline configuration, the segments of DNA that will encode the Ig heavy (IgH) chain are all found on chromosome 14 but separated by considerable distances. These separate segments of DNA are called V, D, J and C (for variable segment, diversity segment, joining segment, and constant segment). Analogously, the germline κ light chain gene segments, on chromosome 2, consist of separately located V, J and C segments (no D), and the germline λ light chain gene segments, on chromosome 22, also are V, J, and C. All these segments become linked closely enough together to produce a functional protein following *gene rearrangement.*

- In B cell maturation, the IgH genes rearrange first, followed by the κ light chain genes. If the κ rearrangement is nonproductive, then λ rearranges. Finally, with all the rearranging complete, the cell begins to make immunoglobulin in its cytoplasm (cIg+). Later, it will incorporate this immunoglobulin into its cell membrane (sIg+) and will be defined as a mature B cell.

- The process is similar for T cells.

- A *clonal* rearrangement is supportive of a diagnosis of neoplasia. The finding of only *germline* genes with no clonal rearrangements is indicative of (i) a benign lymphoid proliferation, (ii) a lymphoid neoplasm composed of very early lymphoid cells, eg, some cases of ALCL, or (iii) nonlymphoid neoplasm.

- A couple of conditions are worth noting. First, for unclear reasons, a number of B-cell neoplasms will display, in addition to rearrangement of Ig genes, rearrangement of TCR genes (lineage infidelity). A number of T cell neoplasms will do the same. Second, clonal populations can be detected where no neoplasm exists, particularly in immunocompromised individuals. In general, a clone representing >1-5% of cells is required for a confident diagnosis of malignancy. This threshold happens to be the lower limit of detection for Southern blot hybridization.

- *Southern blot hybridization (SBH) with Restriction fragment length polymorphisms (RFLP).* Radiolabeled probes for the IgH gene, Igκ gene, and TCRβ gene are applied to an agarose gel that contains DNA which has been (i) extracted from the cells of interest, (ii) cut with restriction enzymes (EcoRI, BamHI, HindIII) and (iii) electrophoresed. The resulting clonal band (restriction fragment), if any, is then displayed on an autoradiograph. A lymphoid neoplasm will show a strong clonal band. The DNA from a polyclonal process will show only germline bands, the many individual rearranged genes not hybridizing strongly enough in any one spot to display a band.

- *Polymerase chain reaction* (PCR) **T4.3.** Either ethidium bromide or probe is added to a gel which contains DNA that has been (i) extracted from the cells of interest (ii) amplified in a mixture of primers, nucleotides, and DNA polymerase put through a heat cycler, and (iii) electrophoresed. The primers are responsible for the specificity of this technique, as they anneal preferentially to the genomic areas of interest, usually sequences known to lie on either side of the target gene. At the end of this process, if the target gene is present, there will be a dark blot corresponding to the known size of the gene. PCR is preferred for detecting many, but not all, chromosomal

translocations. In particular, the t(11;14) translocation of MCL is poorly suited for detection by PCR.

- *Fluorescence in-situ hybridization (FISH)* **T4.4.** Interphase FISH is well suited for detecting most oncogene translocations. In particular, detection of the bcl-1, bcl-2, bcl-6, and c-myc translocations is most sensitive by FISH.

Diseases of Red Blood Cells

Cytoskeletal Disorders

Hereditary spherocytosis (HS)

- Hereditary spherocytosis (HS) was also known as hereditary hemolytic jaundice. Its cardinal features are chronic hemolysis, jaundice, and splenomegaly.

- In the United States the incidence is about 1 in 5000.

- While most families display autosomal dominant inheritance, about ¼ show autosomal recessive or other forms of inheritance. This variation derives from the fact that HS can be caused by any one of several defects in cytoskeletal proteins, including band 3, protein 4.2, spectrin, and ankyrin. A deficiency in any of these components can lead to the cytoskeletal instability that underlies HS.

- The plurality of underlying molecular defects contributes to clinical heterogeneity, with phenotypes ranging from mild to severe. HS may present early, as neonatal jaundice, or it may present in late childhood with splenomegaly and mild anemia. While anemia in some cases, is quite severe, in most cases it is mild and well-compensated. Some patients require splenectomy, which usually results in clinical remission. As HS patients age, they are at risk for pigmented gallstones.

T4.3
Southern Blot (SBH) vs Polymerase Chain Reaction (PCR)

	SBH	**PCR**
Specimen	Substantially larger than PCR, fresh or frozen	Minute quantities, fresh, frozen, or paraffin
Time needed	48 hrs	1-2 weeks
Sensitivity (for B-cell clonality)	0.001% of all cells in sample	1%-5% of all cells in sample
Specificity (for B-cell clonality)	60%-80%	>95%

T4.4
Detection of bcl-1 by Various Modalities

Method	**Sensitivity (%)**
FISH	>95
Cytogenetics	80
Southern blot	70
PCR	40-50

Diseases of Red Blood Cells>Cytoskeletal Disorders

- HS is the most common red cell disorder in persons of Northern European descent.

- Splenomegaly is common. In fact, in all chronic hemolytic disorders *except sickle cell disease,* splenomegaly is common.

- The most characteristic CBC abnormality is an increased MCHC. The MCV and MCH are usually normal but variable. The peripheral blood film shows numerous spherocytes, lacking in central pallor. There is usually an elevated reticulocyte count. While spherocytes are typically smaller than normal red cells, the MCV may be low, normal, or high, owing to reticulocytosis.

- Typical of extravascular hemolysis, the lactate dehydrogenase (LDH) and bilirubin are elevated.

- Either the osmotic fragility or autohemolysis test may be used for screening.

  □ The **osmotic fragility test** is performed by incubating the red cells in incrementally hypotonic NaCl solutions and measuring the degree of hemolysis.

T4.5
Molecular Genetic–Hematologic Disease Associations

Disease or Gene	Chromosome	Comment
Immunoglobulin heavy (IgH) chains	14	
κ light chains	2	
λ light chains	22	
T cell receptor (TCR)	7	
Acute myelogenous leukemia (AML-M1)	t(9;22)	20% of cases
Acute promyelocytic leukemia (APML)	t(15;17)(q22lq12-21)	Retinoic acid receptor (17) translocated to PML gene (15q); 90%
Chronic myelogenous leukemia (CML)	t(9;22)(q34;q11)	Breakpoint cluster region (bcr) on 22; abl on 9; makes abnormal tyrosine kinase
Chronic myelomoncytic leukemia (CMML)	t(5;10)(q33;q21)	Minority of cases
Chronic eosinophilic leukemia (CEL)	T(5;12)(q33,p13)	PDGFRβ, and TEL
Chronic lymphocytic leukemia (CLL)	del(13q), del(11q), +12, del(17p)	Only about 20% have a normal karyotype
Lymphoplasmacytic leukemia (LPL)	t(9;14)(p13;q32)	Pax-5 and IgH
MALT lymphoma	t(11;18)(q21;q21)	API2 and MLT
Mantle cell lymphoma (MCL)	t(11;14)(q13;q32)	bcl-1 (PRAD-1; Cyclin D1) gene (11) translocated to Ig gene (14)
Diffuse large B-cell lymphoma	t(3;14)(q27;q32)	bcl-6/IgH
Follicular lymphoma (FL)	t(14;18)(q32;q21)	bcl-2 gene (18) translocated to Ig gene (14)
Anaplastic large cell lymphoma (ALCL)	t(2;5)(p23;q35)	ALK and NPM
Burkitt lymphoma	t(8;14)(q24;q32), t(2;8), and t(8;22)	c-myc gene (8) translocated to Ig gene (14), κ gene (2), or λ gene (22)
β-globin chains (β, δ, γ)	11	2 copies of each per cell
α-globin chains (α, ζ)	16	4 copies of each per cell
Myelodysplasia	−5, −5q, −7, −7q, or −8	Most commonly seen are complex abnormalities involving one or more

Spherocytic cells hemolyze more readily in hypotonic saline than normal cells; however, this test merely serves to identify the presence of spherocytes from any cause.

□ The **autohemolysis test** is performed by incubating the red cells at 37°C for 48 hours and measuring hemolysis. HS cells autohemolyze more readily than normal, but this can be ameliorated by incubating with excess glucose as an energy source.

■ When confronted with spherocytes in the a peripheral smear, the differential diagnosis includes immune-mediated hemolysis and HS. Usually a direct antiglobulin test (DAT) and low MCV will identify the former.

Hereditary elliptocytosis (HE)/hereditary ovalocytosis

■ An autosomal dominant disorder due most commonly to defective formation of spectrin tetramers.

■ By definition, >25% of circulating red cells are elliptocytes, defined as cells twice as long as they are wide. Elliptocytes, usually less than 25%, may be seen in association with iron deficiency anemia, megaloblastic anemia, myelodysplasia, and myelophthisis.

■ There are three types:

□ The common type is found mostly in African Americans; the heterozygotes have mild or no hemolysis, while the homozygotes have moderate to severe anemia. A variant of common HE is hereditary pyropoikilocytosis (HPP), which is characterized by unusual sensitivity of red cells to heat. In vitro incubation of HPP red cells at 45°C leads to hemolysis; whereas normal red cells can withstand up to 49°C. It is most common to see HPP as a transient finding in neonates with common HE; HPP as a permanent aberration is rare.

□ The **spherocytic type** results from double heterozygosity for HS and HE.

□ The **stomatocytic type,** also known as Southeast Asian ovalocytosis (SAO), is a common finding in Malaysia. It is due to a band 3 protein defect and confers protection against *P. vivax* malaria.

Hereditary stomatocytosis (HSt)

■ A group of autosomal dominant disorders in which red cells have an elongated, mouth-like, central pallor.

■ Stomatocytosis is associated with abnormal Na/K permeability.

■ There are at least two main types: a more severe hydrocytotic (overhydrated) type in which red cells take on extra water; and a less severe xerocytotic type in which they lose water.

□ Significant stomatocytosis, macrocytosis, moderate to severe hemolysis, and a low (24-30%) MCHC characterize the hydrocytosis syndromes. The membrane protein Stomatin is decreased.

□ The xerocytosis syndromes have normocytic red cells characterized morphologically by spiculated dessicocytes, mild stomatocytosis, and target cells. As seen in HS, the MCHC is increased. The gene for xerocytic HSt has been mapped to 16q23-q24.

■ HSt syndromes have a marked tendency towards *thrombosis following splenectomy,* so therapeutic splenectomy is generally avoided (and usually unnecessary). Post-splenectomy thrombotic manifestations have included DVT, pulmonary embolism, and pulmonary hypertension.

■ Stomatocytosis is also a feature of the Rh_{null} red cell phenotype.

Enzyme Disorders

Glucose-6-phosphate dehydrogenase (G6PD) deficiency

■ Even in normal circumstances, reticulocytes have significantly more G6PD activity than older red cells. The most common forms of G6PD deficiency are associated with an accentuation of this pattern, in which red cell G6PD is exceptionally fragile and short-lived. G6PD is involved in the production of NADPH, which maintains glutathione, and consequently other proteins, in the reduced state when erythrocytes are subjected to an oxidant stress. When Hb becomes oxidized, it precipitates as Heinz bodies. When red cells bearing Heinz bodies pass through the spleen, they are targeted by sinusoidal macrophages. Sources of oxidant stress are medications, fava beans (hemolysis associated with ingestion of fava beans is called favism), and infection.

- There is a high prevalence of G6PD deficiency in Africa, southern Europe, the Middle East, Southeast Asia, and Oceania. Because G6PD deficiency is an X-linked disorder, the main clinical manifestations are seen in males. In areas where G6PD deficiency is prevalent, homozygous females will also be affected. There are two main types of disease-causing mutation—Mediterranean ($G6PD_{Med}$) and African ($G6PD_{A-}$). The main difference is that the $G6PD_{Med}$ mutation is much more severe, due to the fact that even very young red cells are depleted of G6PD. The steady-state enzyme activity in $G6PD_{Med}$ is around 10% of normal. In the $G6PD_{A-}$ type, which we see much more commonly in this country, young red cells (reticulocytes) maintain adequate G6PD levels for longer, and the steady-state G6PD activity is in the range of 20-60%.

- The consequences of these differences are two-fold. First, the rise in enzyme concentrations caused by reticulocytosis may cause G6PD activity to appear to be within the normal range if the $G6PD_{A-}$ patient is tested while actively releasing reticulocytes (immediately after a hemolytic episode). Second, the presence of young red cells imposes a limitation on the extent of hemolysis in $G6PD_{A-}$, a limitation that is not available to those with $G6PD_{Med}$.

- G6PD deficiency affects 12% of African Americans, most of whom have the milder African-type allele.

- Following oxidant exposure, the peripheral smear shows poikilocytosis, spherocytosis, Heinz bodies (with supravital dyes such as methyl violet, crystal violet, or brilliant cresyl blue), bite cells, and blister cells.

- Tests for G6PD deficiency

  □ The ascorbate cyanide test is performed by adding ascorbate cyanide to the patient's red cells. G6PD deficient red cells are more sensitive to this sort of oxidant stress than normal cells.

  □ The fluorescent spot test is performed by incubating red cells with NADP and G6P and measuring the production of NADPH (which fluoresces).

  □ Because, in most forms of the disease, G6PD is abundant in younger red cells, older cells are selectively destroyed during acute hemolytic episodes. In the days following a hemolytic crisis, the surviving red cells have normal G6PD activity; therefore, testing during this time may yield falsely negative (normal) results. Repeat testing in >3 months should confirm the diagnosis in these individuals.

Pyruvate kinase (PK) deficiency

- PK deficiency is usually a recessively inherited condition. A myelodysplastic syndrome or acute myeloid leukemia may rarely result in acquired PK deficiency. The disease is worldwide in distribution with no profound geographic predilections; however, a relatively high frequency is found in Northern Europe and Pennsylvania Amish.

- PK catalyzes the rate-limiting step in the Embden-Meyerhoff (glycolysis) pathway, which is the main generator of ATP in red cells. A by-product of the glycolytic pathway is the conversion of NADH to NAD. PK deficiency leads to ATP depletion, impaired ion pumps, red cell dehydration, and finally hemolysis.

- PK deficiency causes chronic hemolysis at a relatively constant rate, producing the usual manifestations of chronic hemolysis—gallstones, jaundice, and splenomegaly—but the severity differs from one patient to the next. **Echinocytes** (dessicocytes) are the classic peripheral smear finding, but these appear in large numbers only after splenectomy. The benefit of splenectomy is well established.

- The autohemolysis test is positive, but unlike HS, does not correct with the addition of glucose. It does normalize with the addition of ATP. A fluorescent spot test is performed in which red cells are incubated with NADH (which fluoresces) to check for conversion to NAD (which does not).

Miscellaneous Disorders

Congenital dyserythropoietic anemia (CDA)

- CDA type II is by far the **most common** in this uncommon group of red cell disorders. It is recessively inherited and characterized by **multinucleate erythroid precursors** and a **positive acidified serum** test, hence

255

the alternate designation: hereditary erythroblast multi-nuclearity with positive acidified serum (HEMPAS).

■ There is an important distinction between the positive acidified serum (Ham) test in CDA type II and that seen in paroxysmal nocturnal hemoglobinuria (PNH). Lysis in CDA type II is observed in heterologous serum only; whereas that in PNH is seen in autologous **and** heterologous serum. The positive Ham test in CDA II is due to an abnormal red cell antigen to which one, third of normal individuals have an antibody.

■ An exceptionally high density of **i antigen** is observed on the red cells.

Paroxysmal nocturnal hemoglobinuria (PNH)

■ This is an **acquired** clonal red cell disorder. The defect is acquired at the level of a hematopoietic stem cell, and the affected clone, initially small, has a set of intrinsic defects. Over time, this clone expands to ultimately dominate the red cell population and variable proportions of the white cell and platelet populations. All of anomalies intrinsic to this clone appear to spring from a single molecular defect—decreased glycosyl phosphatidyl inositol (GPI) anchors. The GPI anchor is a protein whose function it is to attach an array of proteins to the cell surface. Many of the GPI-anchored proteins function to deflect destruction by the immune system (*Schistosoma mansoni,* for example, incorporates host GPI into its own cell membrane as a means of defense against the host immune system). The initial step in GPI synthesis is encoded by the phosphatidyl inositol glycan class A (*PIG-A*) gene located on the X chromosome. PNH is currently thought to the result of various *PIG-A* mutations.

■ Classically, though not usually, patients are described as having episodic hemolysis especially at night. Affected individuals more commonly develop a chronic normocytic, normochromic anemia. Over time, transient thrombo- and leukopenias develop. Eventually, there may be evolution to aplastic anemia and/or acute myelogenous leukemia.

■ The affected red cells display a set of characteristic abnormalities, including diminished cell-surface **decay-accelerating factor** (DAF, CD55), decreased membrane inhibitor of reactive lysis (MIRL, CD59), decreased acetylcholinesterase (AchE), decreased CD16, and decreased CD48.

■ Affected red cells are hypersensitive to complement-mediated lysis, as demonstrated in the **sucrose hemolysis test**, and the acidified serum (Ham) test.

□ The **sucrose hemolysis test** is performed by incubating the patient's red cells in serum and isotonic sucrose (which promotes complement binding). Enhanced hemolysis in comparison with control red cells is consistent with PNH.

□ The **acidified serum (Ham) test** is performed by incubating the red cells in heterologous and homologous serum that has been acidified (activating complement). Enhanced hemolysis in both types of sera is consistent with PNH.

■ Flow cytometry can demonstrate diminished CD59 and CD55 on the surfaces of leukocytes and platelets as well as red cells. When patients are studied serially by flow cytometry, the abnormal red cell population may initially be small in proportion. It expands with successive studies as the disease progresses.

■ Leukocyte alkaline phosphatase (LAP score) is decreased.

■ The bone marrow is hypercellular in early PNH, but evolution to aplastic anemia and/or acute myelogenous leukemia is common.

Sideroblastic anemia

■ The term sideroblastic anemia denotes a group of disorders unified by the presence of anemia and ringed sideroblasts in the bone marrow aspirate.

■ The peripheral blood usually shows a hypochromic anemia that is microcytic, normocytic, or macrocytic. Microcytic presentations are more common in inherited forms of sideroblastic anemia, while macrocytosis more often is seen in acquired forms. The classic finding is a bimodal red cell volume distribution. A form of basophilic stippling, due to iron-containing Pappenheimer bodies, may be observed.

■ The bone marrow shows, in addition to ringed sideroblasts, increased iron stores and erythroid hyperplasia. There may be a degree of dyserythropoiesis.

■ The serum iron concentration is elevated, transferrin percent saturation is high, and ferritin is high. Often, due to intramedullary hemolysis associated with ineffective erythropoiesis, there is hyperbilirubinemia, high LDH, and a drop in the serum haptoglobin.

- Sideroblastic anemia, particularly hereditary forms, must be distinguished from hereditary hemochromatosis, since both produce a clinical picture of iron overload. The low hemoglobin (and low MCV) should help in this distinction.

- Causes

  □ Acquired forms include a clonal stem cell defect (a form of myelodysplasia called refractory anemia with ringed sideroblasts), medications (isoniazid, chloramphenicol, chemotherapy), irradiation, and alcohol. Rare forms of acquired sideroblastic anemia include Pearson syndrome (sideroblastic anemia with pancreatic insufficiency) and copper deficiency. *The vast majority of acquired cases are in fact associated with a clonal stem cell defect.* This typically presents in older adults with macrocytic, hypochromic anemia. The bone marrow aspirate shows >15% ringed sideroblasts. Cytogenetic studies find a chromosomal anomaly in 25%-50% of cases.

  □ Inherited forms are rare and usually display XLR inheritance. Some inherited sideroblastic anemias can be overcome with large doses of pyridoxine (B$_6$). The responsible gene is most often *ALAS2,* found on the X chromosome, in which a large number of different mutations have been found. Inherited sideroblastic anemia usually manifests initially in childhood, and while organ dysfunction due to iron overload may occur in any of the sideroblastic anemias, it is particularly common in this form. The MCV is usually low, and the RDW is usually high, with a distribution that may be bimodal.

Pure red cell aplasia

- Causes

  □ Acquired pure red cell aplasia: thymoma and infection with parvovirus B19.

  □ Congenital pure red cell aplasia: the Blackfan-Diamond syndrome.

- Parvovirus B19 may cause transient arrest of red cell production in healthy children and adults without serious consequences. Infection usually lasts about 2 weeks, and in those with a normal red cell life span of 120 days, this may be barely noticed. However, in those with chronic hemolytic anemia, a transient arrest of erythropoiesis may be catastrophic. The virus infects erythroid progenitor cells, causing a maturation arrest at the pronormoblast stage. Marrow examination finds numerous giant pronormoblasts, a reduction of the more mature forms, and viral nuclear inclusions.

- Transient erythrocytopenia of childhood (TEC) is a self-limiting disorder arising in previously healthy children, 1 to 4 years of age, in which there is a temporary arrest in erythropoiesis. The peripheral blood shows reticulocytopenia and a normochromic, normocytic anemia. Often there is thrombocytosis. The marrow is hypocellular due to erythroid hypoplasia. The etiology in at least some of the cases appears to be parvovirus B19.

- Congenital pure red cell aplasia (Blackfan-Diamond Syndrome) is a rare, constitutional red cell aplasia, which usually becomes evident by the age of 5 years. Leukocytes and platelets are unaffected. Erythroid precursors in the marrow are typically low or absent. The i antigen is often over-expressed on red cells, and the Hb F is increased (in contrast to TEC in which these are normal). About 75% of patients respond to corticosteroids.

- Acquired pure red cell aplasia usually affects adults. Over half of cases are associated with a thymoma (especially the spindle cell/medullary type). Other cases are associated with collagen vascular disease, lymphoproliferative disorders of large granular lymphocytes, or medications. Pure red cell aplasia has been increasingly seen as a complication of erythropoietin therapy. Anti-erythropoietin antibodies are detected in many of these cases.

Fanconi anemia

- Fanconi anemia (FA) is one of many inherited disorders that may lead to aplastic anemia. Others: dyskeratosis congenita, Schwachman-Diamond syndrome, reticular dysgenesis, Down syndrome, and familial aplastic anemia. Some inherited syndromes cause aplasia of only a single cell line, such as Kostman syndrome (neutropenia), Blackfan-Diamond syndrome (anemia), and thrombocytopenia-absent radii (TAR) syndrome (thrombocytopenia).

■ Fanconi anemia is an inherited (autosomal recessive) chromosomal breakage syndrome.

　□ Fanconi anemia (FA) often manifests initially with congenital anomalies, including abnormal skin pigmentation (café au lait spots, hypo- and hyperpigmentation), skeletal anomalies (abnormal radii, hypoplastic thumb, scoliosis), renal anomalies (horseshoe kidney), short stature, microphthalmia, and mental retardation. Up to 1/3 of those with FA display none of these abnormalities.

　□ Over time aplastic anemia develops in most patients, usually by the age of 10. Often anemia (or thrombocytopenia) exists in isolation for a period before pancytopenia fully develops.

　□ In those who do not succumb to the complications of marrow failure, clonal hematopoietic defects develop, including MDS and AML. The predominant type of AML has monocytic differentiation (M4 or M5). There is an increased incidence of epithelial malignancies as well, including cutaneous malignancies, hepatocellular carcinoma, gastric carcinoma, and others.

■ The diagnosis is confirmed with cytogenetic studies displaying an increased propensity for spontaneous-chromosomal breakage. In particular, cells of patients with FA are hypersensitive to clastogenic agents such as diepoxybutane and mitomycin C. In fact, this hypersensitivity has made it necessary to apply altered (weakened) preconditioning regimens prior to bone marrow transplant. Other chromosomal breakage syndromes are xeroderma pigmentosum (XP), ataxia telangiectasia (AT), Bloom syndrome (BS), and Cockayne syndrome.

Hemoglobin Disorders

Normal hemoglobins T4.6

Structurally abnormal hemoglobins (hemoglobinopathies)

■ HbS (β6glu→val)

　□ The allele that encodes HbS (the sickle cell gene) has persisted in parts of the world in which falciparum malaria is prevalent. In the United States, the vast majority of those carrying the gene are African American. The prevalence of sickle cell trait (genotype SA) is about 10% among African Americans.

□ Sickle cell disease (homozygous HbS, SS)

● The clinical manifestations associated with sickle cell disease are not limited to those with the SS genotype, being more or less similar in sickle cell-$\beta°$-thalassemia, SC disease (HbSC), and sickle cell-β^+-thalassemia.

● Sickled red blood cells result from the abnormal polymerization of deoxygenated hemoglobin S. These cells have a shortened survival in the blood, with an average lifespan of 17 days (normal is 120 days).

● The electrophoresis in SS shows >80% HbS, 1%-20% HbF, 1%-4% HbA2, and 0% HbA.

● The peripheral smear shows numerous sickled cells (in addition to the SS genotype, sickled cells may also be seen in S- β−thalassemia, S-C, S-D, and C_{Harlem}). The metabisulfite sickling test, based on the principle that metabisulfite promotes Hb deoxygenation, is positive. The dithionate solubility test (Sickledex), in which lysed red cells are incubated with dithionate that precipitates HbS, is also positive.

● Hb F, present at birth, has an inhibitory effect on Hb S polymerization; thus, the manifestations of sickle cell disease are not apparent until Hb S levels increase beyond 50%—usually at about 6 months of age. Likewise, in patients with combined sickle cell disease-hereditary persistence of fetal hemoglobin (SS-HPFH) clinical manifesta-

T4.6
Normal Hemoglobins

Hemoglobin	Components	Role
HbA	$\alpha_2\beta_2$	Major adult Hb
HbA2	$\alpha_2\delta_2$	Minor adult Hb
HbF	$\alpha_2\gamma_2$	Major late fetal Hb
Hb$_{Gower1}$	$\varsigma_2\varepsilon_2$	Major early fetal Hb
Hb$_{Gower2}$	$\alpha_2\varepsilon_2$	Minor early fetal Hb

tions are milder than in SS. The lower intra-ery-throcyte concentrations of Hb S associated with α-thalassemia also lessen the hematologic and clinical manifestations of disease.

- Cells that remain sickled despite re-oxygena-tion—irreversibly sickled cells (ISCs)—are noted in the peripheral blood smears of patients with sickle cell disease. Theoretically, sickled cells should return to their normal shape upon expo-sure to atmospheric oxygen. Thus, sickled forms on the peripheral blood smear are by definition ISCs. The ISC percent is more or less constant in an individual and does not appear to predict or reflect episodic crises; however, it does seem to be correlated inversely with that patient's red cell survival.

▢ Clinically, sickle cell disease is characterized by chronic hemolytic anemia and recurrent crises.

- Thrombosis is thought to contribute significantly to the clinical expressions of sickle cell disease. For example, it is known that patients with SS, even in intercritical periods, have elevated levels of prothrombin fragments 1+2, d-dimer, fib-rinopeptide A, and factor V. Similarly, their platelets are hypersensitive in vitro.

- Aplastic crises are due to a transient arrest of ery-thropoiesis and are characterized by an abrupt drop in hemoglobin, reticulocytes, and red cell precursors in the marrow. Although these episodes typically last only a few days, the level of anemia may be severe. Parvovirus B19 accounts for nearly 70% of aplastic crises in children.

- Splenic sequestration crisis presents as worsening of anemia in association with an enlarged, tender spleen. These episodes often occur during a viral illness. Children (whose spleens have not yet undergone fibrosis) and adults with SC disease or sickle cell-β+-thalassemia are most susceptible.

- Worsening of anemia in a more slowly progressive fashion than that seen in aplastic and sequestra-tion crises may be due to progressive renal insuffi-ciency (with decreasing erythropoietin) or super-vening iron/folate/B$_{12}$ deficiency.

- Hyperhemolytic crisis presents as a sudden exac-erbation of anemia in association with profound reticulocytosis and hyperbilirubinemia. This complication has been associated in many patients with concomitant G6PD deficiency.

- Acute pain crisis (acute painful episode) is thought to be due to a vasoocclusive event within bone. These episodes often follow exposure to cold, dehydration, infection, or alcohol consumption. The acute chest syndrome presents with dyspnea, cough, chest pain, and fever. One may find tachypnea, leukocytosis, a pulmonary infiltrate on chest x-ray, and progressive hypoxia. This syndrome is thought to be related to either vasoocclusive events or bacterial pneumonia.

- Patients with sickle cell disease, as a result of numerous transfusions, are prone to develop alloantibodies, with associated immediate and delayed hemolytic transfusion reactions. A para-doxical worsening of anemia following transfu-sion is sometimes observed. The mechanism for this is unclear, but it has been theorized that it results from 'innocent bystander' destruction of host red cells in the presence of a minor antigen incompatibility.

- Infections are a major source of morbidity and mortality, made worse by the functional asplenia that is so common in sickle cell disease. *S. pneu-moniae* infections, including pneumococcal sep-sis, pneumonia, meningitis, and arthritis, are the most common overall. Other common infections include *Salmonella, Haemophilus* (HITB), and *M pneumoniae.*

- Neurologic complications are frequent, manifest-ing as transient ischemic attacks (TIAs), cerebral infarcts, cerebral hemorrhage, cord infarction, sensorineural hearing loss, and meningitis. Approximately 1 in 3 patients with sickle cell dis-ease will have an angiographic appearance of moyamoya disease (segmental arterial stenoses with 'puff of smoke' collaterals).

- Acute hepatic cell crisis (right upper quadrant syn-drome) manifests as progressive jaundice, elevated LFTs, and a tender, enlarged liver. This usually

259

resolves within 2 weeks, but it may progress to liver failure. Chronic nonspecific hepatomegaly and liver dysfunction are also common in sickle cell disease, thought to be related to centrilobular congestion. Chronic hepatitis C, related to multiple infections, is also a problem. Gallstones (pigmented type) are ubiquitous in sickle cell disease, and may be present in patients as young as 3 years.

- Pregnancy is a unique problem in sickle cell disease, with an increased rate of both maternal and fetal deaths. There is certainly an increased risk of pregnancy-induced hypertension (preeclampsia), but there is also an increased incidence of intrauterine growth retardation, intrauterine fetal demise, and prematurity.

- There are seven classic sickle cell nephropathies: gross hematuria, papillary necrosis, nephrotic syndrome, renal infarction, isosthenuria, pyelonephritis, and renal medullary carcinoma. The risk of the latter is also increased in sickle cell trait and SC.

- Priapism has been reported in up to 40% of males with sickle cell disease.

- Ocular complications (proliferative retinopathy) occurs with greater frequency in SC disease and sickle cell-β^+-thalassemia than in SS.

- Osteonecrosis is a common complication and may affect the vertebrae, hands, feet, and femoral and humeral heads.

□ Sickle cell trait (SA)

- SA is usually asymptomatic. Those affected may manifest mild isosthenuria, are at risk for splenic infarcts at high altitudes, and have a risk for renal medullary carcinoma.

- The peripheral blood smear shows no sickle cells.

- The electrophoresis shows **35% to 45% HbS,** <1% HbF, 1% to 3% HbA2, and 50% to 55% HbA. The roughly 60:40 ratio of A:S is due to a greater affinity of α chains for β^A chains over β S chains.

- As with all individuals with HbS, the metabisulfite and dithionate tests are positive.

□ S-α -thalassemia

- When α-thalassemia is coinherited with sickle cell trait, there is a **decreased** percentage of hemoglobin S.

- The degree to which HbS is decreased is relative to the number of α-globin genes deleted. In single gene alpha gene deletion (-α/$\alpha\alpha$), there is about 30-35% Hb S. In two α gene deletions (—/$\alpha\alpha$ or -α/-α) there is 25-30% Hb S.

□ S-β-thalassemia

- When, β-thalassemia is coinherited with HbS, there is an **increased** proportion of HbS (S usually >50%).

- Disease manifestations can be quite severe, depending upon the type of β-thalassemia defect.

□ SC disease

- Double heterozygosity for HbS and HbC results in about 50% HbS and clinical manifestations intermediate in severity between SS and SA.

- SC red cells have an average lifespan of 27 days (compared with 17 days for SS and 120 days for normal red cells).

- The various SS-associated complications are about half as frequent in SC, but avascular necrosis of bone and proliferative retinopathy are equally common or more common in SC.

- The peripheral smear is remarkable for mild sickling and abundant target cells.

■ HbA2' (hemoglobin A2 prime)

□ HbA2' is a clinically insignificant δ-chain variant that occurs in 1-2% of African Americans.

□ When heterozygotes for this variant undergo gel electrophoresis, A2' is barely detectable. This may lead to underestimation of the A2 and therefore underdiagnosis of β-thalassemia trait.

Diseases of Red Blood Cells>Hemobglobin Disorders

□ In looking for an elevated A2 as part of excluding β thal trait HbA2 and HbA2' levels must be added.

□ A2' is easily detectable by HPLC, in which it produces a minor peak in the S area.

■ HbC (β6glu→lys)

□ Hemoglobin C trait (heterozygous AC) has about 40 - 50% of hemoglobin in the in C band (HbA2 + HbC). C trait is generally asymptomatic, but the peripheral smear has scattered **target cells.**

□ Hemoglobin C disease (homozygous CC) manifests 90% HbC, 7% HbF, 3% HbA2, 0% HbA.

□ There is mild hemolytic anemia, splenomegaly, and numerous **target cells.** Hexagonal or rod-shaped **crystals** may be found in the red cells, especially after splenectomy.

■ HbE (β26glu→lys)

□ Hemoglobin E is common in Southeast Asia.

□ The CBC shows *thalassemic indices* and the peripheral smear numerous target cells.

■ HbD & G

□ Those with HbD or G are clinically normal

□ On cellulose acetate there is a band that runs with HbS and runs with HbA on citrate.

□ Often D & G can be distinguished because HbD is a β-chain defect, while HbG is an α chain defect; thus, HbG may produce two HbA2 bands (one normal, the other abnormal) separated by a distance equal to that separating HbA from HbG.

■ Hb$_{Lepore}$

□ Common near the Mediterranean, especially Italy.

□ Suspect Hb$_{Lepore}$ whenever less than 30% (usually around 15%) hemoglobin S is present on the electrophoresis. Actual HbS is rarely present in this quantity, unless aggressively transfused.

□ Hb$_{Lepore}$ is the result of a fusion between δ and β genes.

□ Hb$_{Lepore}$ runs with HbS on cellulose acetate but is inefficiently produced so that it only comprises 8 - 15% of total Hb.

□ HbF may be as high as 20%.

■ Hb Constant Spring (CS)

□ Hb CS is another cause of thalassemic indices.

□ Hb CS results from a mutation in the α gene stop codon, producing an *abnormally long transcript* that is unstable. The α^{cs} gene is thus inefficient, producing *thalassemia.*

□ In the heterozygote, the hemoglobins produced are: α-β (HbA), α^{cs}-β (HbCS), α-δ (HbA2), α^{cs}-δ (four bands are seen in the adult on cellulose acetate electrophoresis). In the newborn, α-γ (HbF), and α^{cs}-γ are also seen.

■ High oxygen affinity hemoglobins

□ A group of hemoglobins with left-shifted oxygen dissociation curves.

□ Examples include Hb$_{Chesapeake}$ and Hb$_{Denver}$.

□ Most of these cannot be resolved on either gel electrophoresis or HPLC, but the clue to their diagnosis is the common finding of *erythrocytosis* on the CBC.

□ The HbO$_2$ dissociation curve (P$_{50}$) is diagnostic.

■ Unstable hemoglobins

□ A group of hemoglobins that are associated with characteristic peripheral smear findings of *Heinz bodies and bite cells.*

□ Oxidative stresses may precipitate hemolytic crisis.

□ Screening for unstable hemoglobins is carried out by incubating lysed red cells with 17% isopropanol which causes precipitation of unstable hemoglobins.

Diseases of Red Blood Cells>Hemobglobin Disorders

□ Examples include Hbs Hasharon, Koln, & Zurich, but only Hb Hammersmith is associated with severe hemolysis.

- Methemoglobin (Hi, hemiglobin)

  □ Methemoglobin (Hi) is the form of hemoglobin in which iron is in the oxidized ferric (Fe^{+++}) state instead of the usual ferrous (Fe^{++}), often resulting from oxidation of hemoglobin. Hi is incapable of combining with oxygen.

  □ Under normal circumstances, there is a small degree of hemoglobin oxidation, and up to 1.5% of total Hb is normally Hi. The small amount of Hi that normally forms is reduced in the erythrocyte by the NADH-dependent methemoglobin reductase system. Cyanosis results when Hi reaches 10% of total Hb or around 1.5 g/dL. In such cases, the blood is grossly chocolate brown.

  □ The co-oximeter is capable of measuring methemoglobin directly. Recall that both pulse oximetry and arterial blood gas analyzers, however, estimate oxygen saturation by emitting a red light (wavelength of 660 nm) absorbed mainly by reduced hemoglobin and an infrared light (wavelength of 940 nm) absorbed by oxyhemoglobin. Since methemoglobin absorbs equally at both of these wavelengths, it is essentially undetectable by these modalities; in fact, increasing levels of methemoglobin result in regression of the measured oxygen saturation towards 85%. This is a form of oxygen saturation gap (see Chapter 1).

    - Hereditary methemoglobinemia can result from either deficiency in the reductase system or abnormal hemoglobins (HbM) upon which this enzyme cannot act.

    - Hb M is actually a group of hemoglobins that, due to various amino acid substitutions, prefer the ferric (methemoglobin) state, which binds oxygen poorly.

    - Cyanosis appears at 6 months of age, unless there is M fetal hemoglobin in which case cyanosis abates at about 6 months.

    - Most M hemoglobins run with A on routine gels.

□ Acquired methemoglobinemia results from exposure to drugs or chemicals that increase the formation of Hi, common examples being nitrites, quinones, phenacetin, and sulfonamides. Hi has a very high affinity for cyanide, so part of the treatment for cyanide toxicity involves administration of nitrites to generate Hi which will chelate cyanide.

□ Treatment for methemoglobinemia is methylene blue, which reduces Hi to Hb.

- Sulfhemoglobin (SHb)

  □ SHb ss formed when hemoglobin is oxidized in the presence of sulfur. If further oxidized, SHb precipitates to form Heinz bodies. SHb cannot transport oxygen.

  □ Unlike Hi, SHb cannot be reduced to Hb.

  □ Normally, SHb is less than 1% of total Hb. Cyanosis manifests at around 3% to 4% or 0.5 g/dL.

  □ Sulfhemoglobin may increase after exposure to sulfonamides and in the presence of *C. perfringens* bacteremia (enterogenous cyanosis).

- Carboxyhemoglobin (HbCO) (see Chapter 1).

Thalassemia

- General features

  □ Thalassemia refers to a quantitative abnormality of structurally normal globin chain synthesis. This is distinguished from hemoglobinopathy, which refers to the production of a structurally abnormal globin chain.

  □ Thalassemia is most prevalent in the Mediterranean, Africa and Southeast Asia, paralleling the prevalence of malaria.

  □ The α genes are located on chromosome 16, and β genes are located on chromosome 11p15.5.

    - There is one copy of the β gene on each chromosome 11, for a total of two productive genes in normal cells. The β-globin (*HBB*) gene is regulated by an upstream (5') promoter sequence and an

T4.7
Alpha Thalassemia Syndromes

Syndrome	Genotype	CBC	Electrophoresis
normal	αα/αα	normal	normal
silent carrier	−α/αα	normal	normal
α-thal trait	−α/−α or −−/αα	thalassemic	normal
HbH disease	−−/−α or −−/α^{CS}α	thalassemic Heinz bodies	fast-migrating Hb H, Hb H = β_4 tetramers.
Hb Bart disease (hydrops fetalis)	−−/−−	hypochromia nRBCs	fast-migrating Hb Barts. Hb Barts = γ_4 tetramers.

upstream regulatory gene known as the locus control region (LCR). Nearby (within the *HBB* gene cluster) are the genes for the delta globin chain, gamma globin chains, and a *pseudo-HBB* gene. There are a large number of possible abnormal alleles at the *HBB* gene locus (more than 200). The *vast majority of these consist of point mutations*. The type of large deletions that underlie α-thalassemia are rarely seen. Based upon their impact on β-globin chain production, these alleles can be categorized as β° alleles (result in complete absence of β-chain production—usually the result of nonsense or frameshift mutations), β+ alleles (diminished β-chain production—resulting from mutations in the promoter sequence, LCR, or 5' untranslated region), silent alleles (almost no impact on chain production—due to mutation of the promoter's CACCC box or the 5' untranslated region), or complex alleles (fusion δ-β- and γ-δ-β- chains resulting from deletion of noncoding intervening segments of the *HBB* gene cluster). β+ mediterranean tends to be more severe than in β+ american (seen in American blacks). Due to the large number of possible mutations, β-thalassemia lends itself to targeted mutation analysis. That is, within any given ethnic group, particular molecular defects will be more or less common. Using the appropriate primers for amplification or dot-blot analysis, one can screen for the most commonly expected alleles. Failing this, direct sequence analysis can be undertaken.

- There are two copies of the alpha genes on each chromosome 16, for a total of 4 α chain-producing gene loci in each normal cell. α thalassemia syndromes *usually result from a large structural deletion* within the translated portion of the gene, but occasionally result from a point mutation in the untranslated region (eg, Hb Constant spring). One potential genotype, α thal 2 (α+ thal) refers to a genotype in which chromosome 16 has one normal and one deleted alpha gene (-α/). This is the most common genotype in African Americans with thalassemia. Another genotype, α thal 1 (α° thal) refers to a genotype in which chromosome 16 has two deleted α genes (−−/). This is prevalent in Asians.

  □ Reduced synthesis of either α−or β−chains results in decreased total hemoglobin production, leading to hypochromasia and microcytosis.

  □ Continued synthesis of normal amounts of the unaffected chain leads to its relative abundance and precipitation of these chains in the red cell, reducing the cell's lifespan. Thus, in α−thalassemia, β_4 and γ_4 tetramers form, while in β−thalassemia, α_4 tetramers form.

- Clinical features

  □ CBC findings typical of thalassemia ('thalassemic indices') include an elevated RBC count (>5.5 × 10^{12} in men, >5.0 × 10^{12} in women), low MCV (65 to 75 fL in α−thalassemia, 55 to 65 fL in β−thalassemia), low hematocrit, and normal to slightly increased RDW. An MCV/RBC count ratio <13 favors thalassemia, while a ratio >15 favors iron deficiency.

  □ Peripheral smear findings include microcytic hypochromic anemia with occasional target cells (more in β−thalassemia than α−thalassemia), and basophilic stippling.

  □ When somebody is doubly heterozygous for β−thalassemia and an abnormal β−chain, this results in an *increased* percentage of the abnormal β−chain; eg, in S-β−thalassemia, there is >50% HbS with 1-15% Hb F. α thal leads to *decreased* percentage of abnormal beta chains; eg, in S-α−thalassemia there is 30-35%

HbS with one α gene deletion, and 25%-30% HbS with 2 α gene deletions.

□ α thalassemia syndromes **T4.7**

□ α thalassemia is most common in those of sub-Saharan African and southeast Asian descent. The α thal 1 gene is prevalent only in Asians, and it is they who are at risk for the very severe kinds of α thalassemia (hemoglobin Bart and hemoglobin H diseases). The α thal 2 gene is most prevalent in blacks.

□ Persons with single gene deletion α-thalassemia (silent carrier) are entirely asymptomatic, have normal CBC, and normal electrophoresis. Though they are of interest clinically for genetic counseling, the lab is of little use in identifying these individuals.

□ Persons with α thalassemia trait (2 gene deletions) manifest a CBC with thalassemic indices and an electrophoresis with normal A and A2 bands. A2 is not increased. In the absence of iron deficiency, this can be interpreted as consistent with α-thalassemia trait. Unlike β-thalassemia, the manifestations of α-thalassemia are present at birth.

● Acquired hemoglobin H may be seen in erythroleukemia (FAB M6), myeloproliferative disorders, and myelodysplastic syndromes.

● β-thalassemia syndromes **T4.8**

● β-thalassemia is most common in Mediterranean populations, and manifestations do not become evident until 6 to 9 months of age.

● Beta thal minor typically results from inheritance of one abnormal β gene, either β^+ or β^0. On hemoglobin electrophoresis, one of several patterns is found. In the most common situation, one sees high HbA2 (over 2.5%, usually 4- 8%) and normal HbF. In the second most common situation, the electrophoresis may show normal A2 (because the patient is also iron deficient). This electrophoresis may be erroneously interpreted as consistent with alpha thalassemia. When the electrophoresis is done for a CBC with thalassemic indices, many labs perform parallel iron studies to exclude this possibility. If the results of these indicate iron deficiency and the percent A2 is normal, electrophoresis should be repeated following iron repletion.

● In δ-β thal (deletion of both the δ and β genes) there is a normal quantity of HbA2 and elevated HbF (5- 20%);

● In heterozygous Hb Lepore (fusion of δ and β) there is a normal quantity of HbA2, slightly elevated HbF, and a band in the S region comprising 6- 15% (Hb Lepore).

● Beta thal major results from inheritance of two abnormal genes such as $\beta^0\beta^0$, $\beta^{+med}\beta^{+med}$, or β^0, β^{+med}. Individuals are not anemic at birth but develop anemia within one year. The most common cause of death in childhood is infection. The hemoglobin electrophoresis shows increased HbF (50-95%), normal to elevated HbA2, and little to no HbA. Beta thal intermedia and major (Cooley

T4.8
Beta-Thalassemia Syndromes

Syndrome	Genotype
β-thalassemia minor	β / β^+
	β / β°
β-thalassemia major	β / β°
	β^+ / β^+
	β^+ / β°

T4.9
Warm Autoimmune Hemolytic Anemia (WAIHA) vs Cold Agglutinin Disease (CAD) vs Paroxysmal Cold Hemoglobinuria (PCH)

	WAIHA	CAD	PCH
Ig	IgG Anti-Broad Rh	IgM anti-I, i	IgG anti-P
DAT	IgG only (2/3) IgG/C3 (1/4)	C3	C3
Serum	All cells in panel react (AHG phase)	Most cells in panel react (IS/AHG phases)	Antibody panel-negative, biphasic hemolysin
Setting	Lymphoma, medications	*M. pneumoniae* (anti-I), infectious mono (anti-i), lymphoma	Young children with viral syndrome, syphilis

anemia) are distinguished by the *dependence of the latter on transfusions*. The HbF in this condition, as in most things other than HPFH (below) is present in a heterocellular distribution (some cells with and some cells without on the Kleihauer-Betke stain).

Hereditary persistence of fetal hemoglobin (HPFH) results from a delayed switch from gamma to beta or delta chains. This can result from deletion of the beta and delta genes. Hemoglobin F is present in a pancellular distribution. Combined sickle cell-HPFH is found in about 1 in 100 of those with homozygous HbSS. These individuals have a pancellular distribution of about 25% HbF and suffer from neither anemia nor vasoocclusive episodes. An adult hemoglobin electrophoresis with Hb S, F, and A2 has two possible causes: combined sickle cell-HPFH and combined sickle cell-β-thalassemia. These can be distinguished by the pancellular distribution in the former and heterocellular in the latter.

Extrinsic Red Cell Disorders

Warm autoimmune hemolytic anemia (WAIHA)

- WAIHA is usually mediated by a warm-reacting IgG antibody.

- The responsible antibody usually has broad reactivity with red cell antigens, especially *Rh antigens*. Uncommonly, the antibody has a narrow specificity; eg, for a specific Rh antigen, Kell, Kidd, etc.

- The DAT (Antiglobulin test, Coombs test) is the crucial test in diagnosing AIHA. It is positive in nearly all cases of WAIHA, usually with polyspecific and anti-IgG reagents, sometimes with both anti-IgG and anti-C3, and uncommonly with anti-C3 reagents only. Infrequently, the DAT may be falsely negative, due to very rapid intravascular destruction of erythrocytes or very low titer antibody. Furthermore, a small percentage of healthy people have a positive DAT.

- The antibody binds to antigens on the red cell surface. In most cases, the bound antibody acts as an opsonin that provokes red cell destruction by splenic macrophages (*extravascular hemolysis*). In this instance, some partially degraded red cells may escape the spleen and are seen in the peripheral smear as *spherocytes*. In other cases, the antibody activates complement and, depending upon a

range of factors, may either produce intravascular hemolysis (through the completion of the cascade through the formation of C5-9 membrane attack complex) or opsonization (cascade arrested at the coating of red cells with C3b). In a few cases, the antibody is incapable of leading to red cell destruction and only *coats the red cell*. In fact, 5-10% of hospitalized patients develop a red cell antibody, most due to a medication, and most inconsequential. The specific consequence of antibody binding depends upon several factors: the density of the target antigen on the red cell surface, the avidity of the antibody, the titer of the antibody, the thermal amplitude of the antibody, and the isotype (complement can be activated by IgA, IgM, IgG₁, and IgG₃; IgG tends to produce extravascular hemolysis in the spleen; IgM tends to produce extravascular hemolysis in the liver).

- Patients present with variable severity. Some have an abrupt onset and severe symptomatic anemia, while others have a chronic low-grade hemolysis perhaps detected only incidentally. While these patients have less severe manifestations, the bad news is that they are much more likely to have a serious underlying disease.

- WAIHA may be primary (idiopathic) or secondary (about 70% of cases). Secondary WAIHA occurs in hematolymphoid neoplasms (especially CLL/SLL), inherited autoimmunity (especially antibody deficiency—common variable immunodeficiency, IgA deficiency, Bruton agammaglobulinemia), collagen vascular disease, and thymoma. Stem cell transplantation has also been associated with WAIHA.

Cold autoagglutinins

- Cold agglutinins are IgM antibodies with specificity that is *most commonly anti-I*. Others include *anti-i, anti-H, anti-Pr,* and *anti-IH*.

- These may be pathologic or nonpathologic. The most important laboratory features in predicting pathogenicity are *titer and thermal range* (thermal amplitude).

  □ Nonpathologic cold agglutinins **react most strongly at 4°C**, but they have variably wide thermal amplitudes and may react at up to 22°C.

  □ They may react at or near room temperature, making such things as automated CBCs unreliable.

The only reliable CBC index in the presence of cold agglutinins is the hemoglobin.

◻ The **titer** of benign cold agglutinins is **usually <64** at 4°C. Most are IgM and can activate complement in vitro, thus reactions may be seen at the antiglobulin phase using polyspecific antisera. If monospecific reagents are used, the cells are agglutinated by anti-C3d but not anti-IgG.

■ Pathologic cold agglutinins

◻ Are reactive over a **broad thermal range, up to 32-37°C** and cause spontaneous autoagglutination in anticoagulated blood at room temperature.

◻ As with benign cold agglutinins, automated CBCs may be unreliable.

◻ The **titer** is **often >1000** when tested at 4°C.

◻ There are two clinical types: idiopathic and secondary. Idiopathic cold autoimmune hemolytic anemia (CAIHA) or cold agglutinin syndrome (CAS) is a chronic condition found predominantly in older individuals complaining of acrocyanosis and Reynaud phenomenon with a moderate hemolytic anemia. The responsible antibody is usually an IgM that is monoclonal. It may have anti-I, anti-i, anti-IH, anti-IH or anti-Pr specificity **T4.10**,

T4.11. The antibody causes agglutination in the extremities and fixing of complement, leading to eventual intravascular lysis. Secondary CAIHA is a transient condition often associated with infection. *M pneumoniae* infection is associated with an anti-I, and EBV-associated infectious mononucleosis is associated with anti-i.

■ As with warm autoantibodies, the task is to look beyond the cold-reacting antibody for *masked alloantibodies*. Options include a prewarmed screen or cross-match, using serum from a cold autoadsorption or

T4.10
Reagents for Identifying Cold Agglutinins

Cells	I antigen	i antigen	H antigen
Type O cord blood	–	+++	+++
Type O adult blood	+++	–	+++
Type A1 adult blood	++	–	–
Type A2 adult blood	++	–	+
Saliva	–	–	+

T4.11
Antibody Specificities in Cold Agglutinin Disease

O cord	O adult	A1 adult	A2 adult	Specificity	Notes
–	+++	+++	+++	I	While often benign, anti-I is the most common cause of CAIHA; sometimes associated with M. *pneumoniae*; enzymes enhance effect
+++	–	–	–	i	Sometimes associated with EBV infectious mononucleosis
+++	+++	–/+	+	H	Neutralized by saliva almost always benign
+/–	+++	+/–	+++	IH	Neutralized by saliva almost always benign
+++	+++	+++	+++	Pr	Rare; destroyed by enzymes. Do not confuse with anti-P

adsorption with rabbit erythrocyte stroma (REST), or serum pretreated with DTT or 2-ME (disrupt IgM sulfhydryl bonds).

Paroxysmal cold hemoglobinuria (PCH)

■ This is uncommon, most often seen in *children with viral illnesses* such as measles, mumps, chickenpox, and infectious mononucleosis. Its original description was in the setting of *syphilis.*

■ PCH presents with paroxysmal episodes of hemoglobinuria associated with cold exposure. Sudden fever, chills, abdominal and back pain, hemoglobinuria, and jaundice characterize acute attacks. The resultant anemia is usually severe (eg, Hgb <5). Occasionally the peripheral blood smear shows unique *intraneutrophilic hemophagocytosis.*

■ Treatment consists of keeping the patient warm and transfusing as necessary.

■ The responsible antibody is an IgG *biphasic hemolysin* with *anti-P* specificity (Donath-Landsteiner antibody

T4.12
Positive Donath-Landsteiner Test

Procedure	Vial 1	Vial 2
30 minutes	37°C	4°C
30 minutes	37°C	37°C
Results	no hemolysis	hemolysis

T4.13
Manifestations of Iron Deficiency

Blood	Microcytosis (↓ MCV) Hypochromia (↓ MCH) Anemia Anisocytosis (↑ RDW) Poikilocytosis (thin elliptocytes = pencil cells) Thrombocytosis
Marrow	↓ Iron stores Mild erythroid hyperplasia
Chemistries	↑ Zinc protoporphyrin (ZPP) ↓ Iron ↑ Total iron binding capacity (TIBC) ↓ Iron saturation ↓ Ferritin

T4.12). It is called a biphasic hemolysin due to its capacity to produce hemolysis only when incubated at two different temperatures *in vitro.*

■ Like CAIHA, the DAT is positive with polyspecific AHG, negative with anti-IgG, and positive with anti-C3. To confirm the diagnosis, the Donath-Landsteiner test is performed on 2 vials of blood at 2 different temperatures: 4° and 37°C. A positive test is obtained if only incubation of the patient's red cells at 4°C then 37°C leads to hemolysis.

Cryoglobulinemia

■ Cryoglobulins are immunoglobulins that precipitate reversibly at low temperatures.

■ To detect cryoglobulins, blood is drawn and kept at 37°C until clotted. It is centrifuged at 37°, and the remaining serum is stored at 4°C for at least 3 days. It is then centrifuged at 4°. Any precipitate that forms is a cryoprecipitate which can be subjected to electrophoresis for characterization.

■ Three types of cryoglobulins are recognized: type I and the mixed types, II & III. Type I cryoglobulins are monoclonal immunoglobulins found in association with multiple myeloma or Waldenstrom macroglobulinemia. Type II cryoglobulins are a mixture of a monoclonal IgM and a polyclonal IgG. The IgM has rheumatoid factor activity (anti-IgG). Type II is the most common type of cryoglobulin. Type III is a mixture of two polyclonal immunoglobulins.

■ Mixed cryoglobulinemia (types II & III) affects individuals with a variety of clinical conditions, including lymphoproliferative disorders, chronic infections, chronic liver diseases, and autoimmune diseases (especially SLE). It is most common in women in the 4th and 5th decades. In the past, about 30%-50% were associated with no underlying disorder (essential mixed cryoglobulinemia). With the advent of testing for hepatitis C virus, it was found that most of these had underlying hepatitis C virus infection. Currently, *HCV is the most common cause of mixed cryoglobulinemia.*

■ Clinically, cryoglobulinemia is a systemic immune complex disease characterized by a distinctive clinical syndrome of palpable purpura (leukocytoclastic vasculitis), arthralgias, hepatosplenomegaly, lymphadenopathy, anemia, sensorineural deficits, and glomerulonephritis. Most patients are variably hypocomplementemic, reflecting the immune complex nature of the disease.

- Renal involvement trails the onset of disease by 4-5 years, manifests as either nephrotic or nephritic syndrome, and is associated with severe hypocomplementemia. In renal biopsies, the most common finding is membranoproliferative glomerulonephritis (MPGN) type II. In some cases, usually when acute, the deposits produce the appearance of thrombotic microangiopathy. In all tissues, as in the kidney, the basic pathologic lesion is vasculitis. Electron microscopy demonstrates large subendothelial immune complex deposits with a fibrillary or tubular structure in a fingerprint-like pattern.

Iron deficiency anemia (T4.13)

- There is a temporal progression of the laboratory manifestations of iron deficiency. A decrease in the serum ferritin is the earliest event, followed by a decrease in the percent saturation of transferrin, decreased serum iron, and increased zinc protoporphyrin (ZPP). It is only after these stages that there is a decrease in the hemoglobin, followed by what is initially a normocytic, normochromic anemia. The MCV progressively drops, eventually below 80, and the red cells become progressively hypochromic and poikilocytotic.

4.14
Iron Studies in Anemia of Chronic Disease and Iron-Deficiency Anemia

	Serum Iron	TIBC	% sat	Ferritin
Iron deficiency	↓	↑	<10%	↓
Anemia of Chronic Disease	↓	↓	>15%	Normal - ↑

T4.15
Causes of Iron Deficiency

Infant	Decreased intake; increased use with inadequate intake (growth spurts)
Adult	Blood loss (eg, colon cancer, menses); decreased intake (strict vegetarianism); decreased absorption (celiac sprue, small bowel resection); increased use with poor intake (pregnancy, lactation)

- The quickest way to confirm the diagnosis of iron deficiency is the serum ferritin, usually under $10 \mu g/L$ in established iron deficiency. Ferritin is an acute-phase reactant, however, and may be nonspecifically elevated in hepatic insufficiency (impaired clearance).

- Adjunctive tests come into play in these instances is which the ferritin is considered questionable, especially the serum iron (low), total iron binding capacity (raised), and percent transferrin saturation (low). Serum soluble transferrin receptor is elevated whenever there is a relative lack of iron (iron deficiency and in erythroid hyperplasia such as hemolytic anemia, hemorrhage, or polycythemia). The zinc protoporphyrin (ZPP) and free erythrocyte protoporphyrin (FEP) are elevated in iron deficiency but also elevated in lead poisoning and anemia of chronic disease. The last resort is direct microscopic examination of marrow for iron stores.

- Most of the body's iron is in heme (hemoglobin, myoglobin, oxidative enzymes) and in storage (ferritin, hemosiderin). For example, 1 mL of whole blood contains 0.5 mg of iron (1 mL of packed RBCs contains 1 mg of iron).

- Iron is ingested and absorbed predominantly in the duodenum, transported in bloodstream by transferrin, and eventually stored as ferritin.

- Causes of iron deficiency (T4.15)

- Particularly in children, there appears to be a relationship between iron and lead levels.

  □ Children with elevated lead levels are more likely to have iron deficiency, even after controlling for socioeconomic status.

  □ It appears that lead ingestion inhibits the intestinal absorption of iron. Furthermore, iron deficiency may enhance intestinal absorption of any ingested lead.

Folate and vitamin B_{12}

- The active form of folate, tetrahydrofolate (THF), acts as a cofactor in methyl transfer reactions. An important methyl transfer reaction is the conversion of dUMP to dTMP for use in DNA synthesis. Folate deficiency leads to impaired DNA synthesis, which leads to impaired nuclear maturation.

Diseases of Red Blood Cells>Extrinsic Red Cell Disorders

- B_{12} is a cofactor for methyltransferase enzymes necessary for the conversion of the circulating form of folate (N^5-methyl folate) to the active form (THF). In B_{12} deficiency, methyl folate accumulates (the "methyl folate trap"). It is also a cofactor for methylmalonyl CoA mutase which converts methylmalonyl CoA to succinyl CoA. In B_{12} deficiency, methylmalonyl CoA accumulates.

- B_{12} is ingested in animal products (mostly), bound to R factor in stomach, released from R factor in duodenum by pancreatic enzymes, and bound to gastric-derived intrinsic factor (IF). IF-bound B_{12} is absorbed in the ileum, bound to transcobalamin I & II (90%) in enterocytes, and exported to the blood stream.

- Folate is ingested in green vegetables (mostly), absorbed in jejunum, and released from enterocytes as N^5-methyl folate. After transport in blood stream, it is converted in target cells to THF by the B_{12}-dependent methyltransferase.

- Causes of folate and vitamin B_{12} deficiency **T4.16**

- The findings in B_{12} and folate deficiency are similar.

  □ The blood smear shows the classic features of megaloblastic anemia: marked oval macrocytosis, hypersegmented neutrophils, and large platelets.

  □ Erythropoiesis becomes ineffective, resulting in a hypercellular marrow. Nuclear maturation arrest associated with essentially normal cytoplasmic maturation leads to the characteristic nuclear:cytoplasmic dyssynchrony. Many erythroblasts perish while still

in the marrow. Thus megaloblastic anemia is in part a hemolytic anemia, and is commonly associated with a very high LDH and a mild to moderate elevation in serum bilirubin. The red cells that do proceed to maturity are macrocytic, with the MCV in fully developed megaloblastic anemia exceeding 115 fL.

□ Folate deficiency does not cause the same neurologic defect that vitamin B_{12} deficiency causes. However, supplementation of folate in early pregnancy is known to reduce the incidence of neural tube defects. No clear mechanism for this effect has been established, but there appears to be an increased incidence of anti-folate antibodies in women whose pregnancy has this complication.

□ The diagnosis of folate deficiency can be confirmed by measuring the serum or red blood cell folate. However, there are several confounding factors in the use of these tests. One or several balanced meals can quickly normalize the serum folate, but the red blood cell folate is more stable over time. Vitamin

T4.17
Manifestations of Folate and Vitamin B_{12} Deficiency

Peripheral blood/CBC		Oval macrocytosis Hypersegmented neutrophils Pancytopenia (when severe) Anisopoikilocytosis (variable)
Bone marrow		Hypercellularity Megaloblastic changes Erythroid hyperplasia with left shift
Chemistry	Folate deficiency	↑ LDH and indirect bilirubin ↓ serum and RBC folate ↑ urinary FIGLU (formiminoglutamic acid)
	B_{12} deficiency	↑ LDH and indirect bilirubin ↓ serum B_{12} ↑ urinary methylmalonic acid ↓ RBC folate (2/3 of cases)

T4.18
Laboratory Distinction of Intravascular and Extravascular Hemolysis

Intravascular hemolysis	Extravascular hemolysis
schistocytes ↑LDH ↓ haptoglobin ↑ free Hb, ↑ urine Hb hemosiderinuria	microspherocytes ↑ LDH normal to ↓ haptoglobin ↑ indirect bilirubin ↑ urine & fecal urobilinogen

T4.16
Causes of Folate and Vitamin B_{12} Deficiency

	Folate deficiency	B_{12} deficiency
Diet	Common (alcoholics)	Rare (strict vegetarians)
Malabsorption	Sprue	Pernicious anemia, post-gastrectomy, pancreatic insufficiency, Crohn disease, *D. latum* infestation
Increased requirements	Pregnancy, increased RBC destruction	Pregnancy, increased RBC destruction
Drugs	Methotrexate (MTX)	Dilantin
Inherited	none	Transcobalamin II deficiency

Diseases of Red Blood Cells>Extrinsic Red Cell Disorders

T4.19
Nonhemorrhagic causes of Acute Severe Anemia

Acute Intravascular Hemolysis	Acute Exacerbation of Chronic Hemolysis
Microangiopathic hemolytic anemia	Aplastic crisis (Parvovirus B19)
Mechanical hemolysis (eg, heart valve)	Splenic sequestration crisis
Toxins (eg, venoms)	Hyperhemolytic crisis
Infections (eg, malaria, *Clostridium*)	
Oxidant stress (especially in G6PD deficiency)	
Hemolytic transfusion reaction (ABO incompatibility)	
Paroxysmal nocturnal hemoglobinuria	
Paroxysmal cold hemoglobinuria	

B_{12} deficiency can produce a falsely low RBC folate, but it does not affect the serum folate.

□ Serum B_{12} levels are often low in patients with HIV infection, but true B_{12} deficiency is very uncommon in this situation. The mechanism for this is unclear.

□ B_{12} deficiency may be difficult to diagnose in patients with leukocytosis, especially in myeloproliferative diseases, since these conditions produce a falsely elevated B_{12} level.

□ If B_{12} deficiency is diagnosed, identifying its cause is the next step in the evaluation. The Schilling test is designed for this purpose. The patient is given a parenteral dose of unlabeled B_{12} followed by an oral

T4.20
Morphologic Findings in Red Cells

Finding	Definition	Associated conditions
Basophilic stippling	Small blue dots in red cells, due to clusters of ribosomes.	Hemolytic anemias, lead poisoning, thalassemia
Pappenheimer bodies	Larger, more irregular, and grayer than basophilic stippling, due to iron-containing mitochondria	Asplenia, sideroblastic anemia
Heinz bodies Bite cells	Heinz bodies: gray-black round inclusions, seen only with supravital stains (crystal violet). Bite cells: sharp bite-like defects in red cells where a Heinz body has been removed in the spleen. Both are due to denatured hemoglobin	Oxidative injury: G6PD deficiency or unstable hemoglobins
Howell-Jolly bodies Cabot rings	Howell-Jolly body: dot-like dark purple inclusion. Cabot ring: ring-shaped dark purple inclusion. Both represent a residual nuclear fragment	Asplenia
Target cells	Red cells with a dark circle within the central area of pallor, reflecting redundant membrane	Thalassemia, hemoglobin C, liver disease
Schistocytes	Fragmented red blood cells, taking shapes such as helmet-shaped cells, due to mechanical red cell fragmentation.	Microangiopathic hemolytic anemias (MHA): DIC, TTP, HUS, HELLP. Mechanical heart valves.
Dacrocytes (teardrop cells)	Teardrop or pear-shaped erythrocytes	Can be seen in relatively benign conditions (thalassemia, megaloblastic anemia), often seen in myelophthisis
Echinocytes (burr cells)	Red blood cells that have circumferential undulations or spiny projections with pointed tips	Uremia, gastric cancer, pyruvate kinase deficiency
Acanthocytes (spur cells)	Red blood cells that have circumferential blunt and spiny projections with bulbous tips	Liver disease, abetalipoproteinemia, Mcleod phenotype
Spherocytes	Red cells without central pallor due to decreased red cell membrane	Immune hemolytic anemia, hereditary spherocytosis
Elliptocytes	Red cells twice as long as they are wide	Iron deficiency, hereditary elliptocytosis
Stomatocytes	Red cells whose area of central pallor is elongated in a mouth-like shape	Alcohol, Dilantin, Rh null phenotype (absence of Rh antigens), hereditary stomatocytosis

dose of radiolabeled vitamin B_{12}. The purpose of the unlabeled dose is to fully saturate the body with B_{12} so that the radiolabeled dose will be quickly excreted in the urine. A 24-hour urine sample is then collected. A low level of urinary radioactivity confirms B_{12} malabsorption, but it does not identify the specific gastrointestinal defect. The second part of the Schilling test is then undertaken. The patient is given another oral dose of radiolabeled B_{12} in addition to oral intrinsic factor. Patients with pernicious anemia will demonstrate enhanced absorption (increased urinary radioactivity) in this second part of the test.

Anemia of chronic disease (ACD)

■ Systemic inflammation alters marrow iron utilization through several mechanisms. Furthermore, it appears to suppress erythropoietin secretion and red cell sensitivity to erythropoietin. This combination of factors leads to a mild, refractory, hyporegenerative anemia that is usually normocytic and normochromic, but is microcytic in up to a third of cases. *ACD is the most common cause of anemia in hospitalized patients* in the United States. The vast majority of cases are due to rheumatoid arthritis, collagen vascular disease (eg, lupus), chronic infection (eg, osteomyelitis, bronchiectasis), or malignancy.

■ The laboratory diagnosis of ACD depends upon demonstrating a hypoproliferative (low reticulocyte count) and normocytic or microcytic anemia in the presence of characteristic iron studies. The iron studies should document increased iron stores (normal to high serum ferritin or increased stainable iron in a bone marrow biopsy) and a low serum iron, low transferrin, and low total iron-binding capacity.

■ While a normal or elevated ferritin level distinguishes ACD from iron deficiency; ferritin must be interpreted in light of its positive acute phase response. While a low ferritin is essentially diagnostic of iron deficiency, a normal ferritin does not entirely exclude it. In confusing situations, the soluble serum transferrin receptor assay may be helpful. This analyte is increased in iron deficiency anemia and usually normal in ACD.

Approach to the Diagnosis of Anemia

The reticulocyte count is an essential piece of information. Anemia due to a production defect is associated with a normal reticulocyte count (hyporegenerative anemia).

Anemia accompanied by reticulocytosis (hyperregenerative anemia) suggests either hemolysis or hemorrhage. An exception is a partially treated production defect, such as in the early treatment of iron, folate, or B_{12} deficiency. Another exception is the rare autoimmune hemolysis that targets not only mature erythrocytes but also maturing marrow erythroid precursors. Hemorrhage is usually clinically apparent; however, significant blood loss into the retroperitoneum or pelvis may go unnoticed. In neonates, intracranial hemorrhage of sufficient quantity to cause anemia may occur. Both hemolytic and blood-loss anemia may eventually lead to depletion of iron, folate, or B_{12} and present as a production defect. Paroxysmal nocturnal hemoglobinuria (PNH) is a hemolytic anemia that may transform to aplastic anemia.

Hemolysis may occur within the blood stream (intravascular hemolysis) or within the reticuloendothelial system (extravascular hemolysis). Intravascular hemolysis is caused by microangiopathic hemolytic anemia (DIC, HUS, TTP, HELLP), complement fixation on the red cell surface (eg, ABO incompatibility, PNH, PCH), mechanical heart valves, snake envenomation, and certain infectious agents (malaria, babesiosis, *Clostridium*). Most other forms of hemolysis are extravascular. Good screening tests for hemolysis are the serum LDH (↑), haptoglobin (↓), and bilirubin (↑). Note that most of these tests, particularly bilirubin and LDH, will be abnormal in conditions associated with intramedullary hemolysis, such as vitamin B_{12} deficiency. In determining the cause of hemolysis, the differential diagnosis hinges first on whether the hemolysis is intra- or extravascular. T4.18

Anemia due to blood loss is seen most often as a result of surgery, trauma, or gastrointestinal pathology. Most often, hemorrhage is quite obviously present, but occasionally, it is either internal (large retroperitoneal or pelvic hemorrhages) or occurs in the pre-hospital setting (where its volume cannot be estimated). While acute blood loss is usually associated with symptoms, chronic slow blood loss is generally well tolerated and usually presents late, as iron deficiency anemia. Note also that acute blood loss is not the only form of anemia that can present abruptly. Causes other than hemorrhage that may present as rapid-onset severe anemia include intravascular hemolysis and acute exacerbations of a chronic compensated hemolytic anemia such as sickle cell disease.

Diseases of Red Blood Cells>Approach to the Diagnosis of Anemia

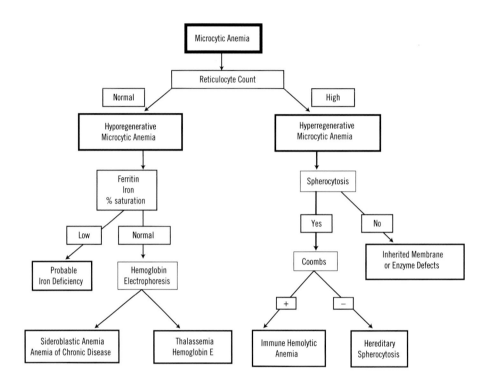

F4.5 Microcytic Anemia Algorithm

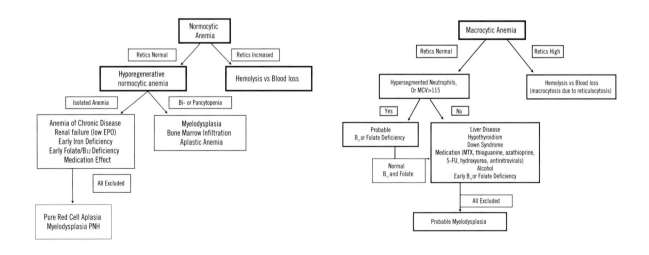

F4.6 Normocytic Anemia Algorithm   F4.7 Macrocytic Anemia Algorithm

4: Hematopathology

Diseases of Red Blood Cells>Approach to the Diagnosis of Anemia; Erythrocytosis I Nonneoplastic White Blood Cell Disorders>Functional and Morphologic Abnormalities

Beyond acute hemolysis and blood loss, the differential diagnosis is somewhat more complicated. Perhaps the best way to approach the diagnosis is according to red cell size (microcytic, normocytic, and macrocytic). The blood smear may display helpful morphologic findings. **T4.20**

- Microcytic anemia (MCV <80 fL) **F4.5**

- Normocytic anemia (MCV 80 to 100 fL) **F4.6**

- Macrocytic anemia (MCV >100 fL) **F4.7**

Erythrocytosis (T4.21 , p 276)

- The primary considerations are myeloproliferative disorders (CML, PV), reactive erythrocytosis, and spurious erythrocytosis due to dehydration (Gaisbock syndrome). Excluding the latter two through clinical history and serum erythropoi (EPO) measurements, a myeloproliferative disease (MPD) is suspected. The causes of reactive erythrocytosis are: hypoxia, high oxygen-affinity hemoglobins, and certain EPO-secreting neoplasms (renal cell carcinoma, cerebellar hemangioblastoma, uterine leiomyomas, and hepatocellular carcinoma). A transient neonatal polycythemia may be seen in infants of diabeteic mothers (IDM) and Down syndrome. Clues to MPD include basophilia, thrombocytosis, and splenomegaly.

Nonneoplastic White Blood Cell Disorders

Functional and Morphologic Abnormalities (see Chapter 6)

Quantitative abnormalities

- Neutrophilia

  □ Reactive neutrophilia usually does not exceed 30 × 10^3/μL, and is often accompanied by toxic granulation, Döhle bodies, and cytoplasmic vacuoles. While immature cells may be present (a left shift), these are mainly bands and some metamyelocytes. Myelocytes and promyelocytes are very uncommon, and there should be no blasts. Reactive neutrophilia is most commonly due to infection. Other causes include medications (epinephrine, corticosteroids), trauma, burns, systemic inflammation (collagen vascular diseases, gout), seizure, exercise, post-splenectomy, leuko-

cyte adhesion defect, and pregnancy. In children, juvenile rheumatoid arthritis (JRA) is a consideration.

  □ One expects reactive neutrophilia to resolve either spontaneously or following treatment. When neutrophilia is persistent or unassociated with an identifiable cause, the main concern is a myeloproliferative disorder (MPD). Features favoring MPD include basophilia, lack of 'toxic' morphology, and a 'myelocyte bulge' (myelocytes are present, often outnumbering metamyelocytes). The LAP score is decreased in CML, but it is increased in reactive neutrophilia and non-CML forms of MPD. Lastly, GM-CSF causes a marked leukocytosis with prominent toxic granulation, nRBCs, and abnormal nuclear segmentation.

  □ A type of reactive neutrophilia in which toxic changes are regularly absent is that associated with the Hantavirus pulmonary syndrome (HPS). During the HPS prodrome, thrombocytopenia is the only dependable finding. Once pulmonary edema is established, however, there is a highly reproducible pentad of findings: thrombocytopenia, left-shifted neutrophilia, *lack* of significant toxic granulation, increased hemoglobin concentration (hemoconcentration), and >10% of lymphocytes having immunoblastic morphology. In fact, having 4 of these 5 has a high sensitivity and specificity for HPS.

- Lymphocytosis

  □ Causes of reactive lymphocytosis include viral infection (EBV, CMV, HIV, etc), toxoplasmosis, and medications. Reactive lymphocytic proliferations in blood and bone marrow are composed principally of T lymphocytes, and these take the form of so-called atypical lymphocytes (ATLs) which have the appearance of enlarged lymphocytes with moderate to abundant cytoplasm, often granulated.

  □ An exception is the *syndrome of persistent polyclonal B lymphocytosis,* presents usually affects young adult females who smoke. It presents as a mild absolute increase in small lymphocytes with indented to bilobed nuclei and abundant pale-staining cytoplasm. There is a polyclonal IgM hypergammaglobulinemia, and there are no cytopenias. The vast majority of patients are HLA-DR7+.

□ Reactive lymphocytosis in children sometimes takes the form of small mature lymphocytes with clefted nuclei (Reider cells), classically associated with pertussis, in which the lymphocyte count can be quite high.

□ In adults, one may find ATLs in association with a transient infection or other immune stimulation. However, the absolute number of lymphocytes is usually not increased. An absolute lymphocytosis in an adult is reason for suspicion. A neoplastic disorder becomes more likely with higher lymphocyte counts, irregular nuclear contours, cytopenias, persistent lymphadenopathy, and increasing age. Chronic lymphocytic leukemia (CLL) is the most common neoplastic consideration.

■ Monocytosis

□ Monocytosis is a frequent reactive finding, but persistent monocytosis, if not otherwise explained, may represent chronic myelomonocytic leukemia (CMML).

□ Causes of reactive monocytosis include collagen vascular diseases, chronic infection (clasically listeria or tuberculosis), malignancy, and neutropenia (a compensatory response).

□ A monocytic neoplasm is suggested by the presence of promonocytes and/or splenomegaly.

□ Serum lysozyme is usually elevated in monocytic proliferations, but it is not useful to distinguish reactive from neoplastic conditions. It *is* useful to clarify that a neoplastic process (eg AML) has monocytic differentiation.

□ An additional caveat is that some automated counters may misclassify hairy cells, blasts, or immature hypogranular neutrophils as monocytes.

■ Eosinophilia

□ Eosinophilia is almost always a reaction, most commonly related to allergy. Worldwide, the most common cause is helminthic infections. Other causes of reactive eosinophilia include collagen vascular disease, malignancy (T-cell lymphoma/leukemia,

Hodgkin lymphoma, and colonic carcinoma), inflammatory bowel disease, and GM-CSF.

□ Of the cytokines, *interleukin-5 (IL-5) is the most specific for the eosinophil lineage* and is responsible for selective differentiation of eosinophils and release of eosinophils from bone marrow.

□ Several named syndromes are associated with eosinophilia and eosinophilic infiltration of specific organs: eosinophilic cellulitis (Well syndrome), eosinophilic pneumonia (Löeffler syndrome), eosinophilic fasciitis (Shulman syndrome), and eosinophilic vasculitis (Churg-Strauss syndrome).

□ After excluding the enormous list of causes of reactive eosinophilia, one may consider a myeloproliferative disorder or hypereosinophilic syndrome (HES). There are very few morphologic clues to help distinguish reactive from neoplastic eosinophilia, but if eosinophils are morphologically abnormal (trilobate, monolobate) and/or there is splenomegaly, the likelihood of a neoplastic eosinophilic proliferation is increased.

■ Blasts

□ The normal number of blasts in the peripheral blood is zero. Blasts are rarely a component of reactive leukocytosis or chronic clonal myeloid disorders.

□ When blasts are found, it is important to determine their lineage. *Truly reliable morphologic determinants of lineage are few and possibly limited only to Auer rods. Cytochemical and immunophenotypic studies are necessary for proper classification in nearly all cases.*

□ When myeloblasts are present, the criteria for the diagnosis of AML must be applied—in peripheral blood >20% blasts is required—if peripheral blood criteria are not met, then bone marrow examination is necessary. M3 AML (APML) must be recognized and distinguished from non-M3 AMLs. The decisive test for M3 is detection of the t(15;17) translocation, but this takes time. A less definitive though more rapid approach is often necessary, taking account of a combination of features: characteristic morphology, extensively positive cytochemical staining for MPO, and the combined CD34-/CD13+/CD33+/HLA-DR- immunophenotype.

☐ If the blasts are lymphoid, the possibilities include Burkitt, precursor-B-ALL, and precursor-T-ALL, which immunophenotype can quickly resolve.

☐ Chromosomal (conventional cytogenetic and/or molecular) studies should be initiated, but these results are seldom available sufficiently early in the evaluation.

■ Neutropenia (agranulocytosis) **T4.22**

☐ The most common cause of neutropenia is medication—antibiotics (penicillins, chloramphenicol), anti-thyroidals (methimazole, propylthiouracil, carbimazole), anticonvulsants (valproate, carbamazepine), procainamide, and NSAIDs. Agranulocytosis is a serious potential complication of antithyroid drugs (carbimazole, methimazole and propylthiouracil). This effect is not dose-dependent, and its incidence is somewhere between 0.05 and 0.5% of all users. In most patients, agranulocytosis occurs within the first 3 months of treatment. This often presents with pharyngitis, and patients are specifically instructed to seek attention if they develop sore throat, fever, an oral ulcer, or other symptoms of infection (pneumonia, UTI). Minor depressions in the neutrophil count, not requiring medical attention, are much more common than true neutropenia. At present, there is not consensus regarding a routine interval of leukocyte counts, and, following an initial baseline count, additional counts are performed only when signs of infection are present. Sulphasalazine, for which the incidence of agranulocytosis is similar, should be similarly monitored.

☐ Causes of increased neutrophil destruction include autoimmunity, splenomegaly, medications, or infection.

● Infections that cause neutropenia include typhoid fever, brucellosis, tularemia, rickettsial infection, and, particularly in neonates and the elderly, overwhelming sepsis of any bacterial cause.

● Autoimmune neutropenia takes 2 forms: (i) in adults, usually associated with lupus or rheumatoid arthritis (the triad of RA, splenomegaly and

neutropenia is Felty syndrome); (ii) in infants and children with no underlying disease.

☐ Decreased production, when isolated to neutrophils, may be due to medications, large granular lymphocytic leukemia, and the constitutional neutropenias.

● The constitutional neutropenias include cyclic/congenital (*ELA2*-related) neutropenia, Kostmann syndrome, Schwachman-Diamond syndrome, (not to be confused with Blackfann-Diamond syndrome which is similar but affects erythrocytes), Chediak-Higashi, Fanconi anemia, dyskeratosis congenita, benign familial neutropenias, glycogen storage disease type Ib, WHIM syndrome (myelokathexis), reticular dysgenesis, and Wiskott-Aldrich syndrome.

● Cyclic neutropenia and congenital neutropenia (*ELA2*-related neutropenias) present with recurrent fever, cervical lymphadenopathy, oral ulcers, gingivitis, sinusitis, and pharyngitis. The more severe form of the disease (congenital neutropenia) may present in the neonatal period with omphalitis, followed in infancy by infectious complications such as pneumonia, intractable diarrhea, and abscesses. The later development of acute myelogenous leukemia (AML) afflicts a significant minority. In the milder form (cyclic neutropenia), there are intervals of fever, often accompanied by one or more foci of inflammation—such as oral ulcers, pharyngitis, sinusitis, perianal ulceration, or colonic ulceration—during which neutropenia can be found. A compensatory monocytosis characterizes both conditions. In bone marrow examination, one finds maturation arrest at the promyelocyte stage. Maturation arrest is intermittent in cyclic neutropenia, but even in intercritical periods, the neutrophil count rarely exceeds 2000/μL. Mutations in the *ELA2* gene (19p13—encoding neutrophil elastase) are responsible for both conditions.

☐ In neutropenia, the peripheral smear often shows compensatory monocytosis.

4: Hematopathology

Nonneoplastic White Blood Cell Disorders>Functional and Morphologic Abnormalities; Nonneoplastic Lymph Node Proliferations

- Lymphopenia

  □ Isolated lymphopenia is uncommon but may be seen in systemic lupus erythematosis, HIV infection, severe acute respiratory syndrome (SARS), anti-CD20 (rituxan) therapy, steroid therapy, and certain congenital immunodeficiencies (Bruton, SCID, DiGeorge, CVI).

  □ Flow cytometry for lymphocyte subsets can be helpful.

- Monocytopenia

  □ Consider hairy cell leukemia or steroid therapy.

  □ In patients undergoing chemotherapy, monocytopenia heralds the onset of neutropenia.

Nonneoplastic Lymph Node Proliferations

The follicular pattern—reactive follicular hyperplasia (RFH)—displays an increase in the size of lymphoid follicles, usually due to an expansion of the germinal center. The reactive follicle has a mantle zone that is intact, at least partially if not completely, and is polarized towards the capsule. Polarization is manifested as a greater thickness of the mantle zone towards the capsule (or towards the crypt in the case of tonsils and towards the serosa in the case of intestine); in fact, the mantle is usually attenuated or absent in the direction of the node's center. Furthermore, the germinal zone itself is polarized, with a darker staining small lymphoid zone externally, and lighter staining transformed lymphocyte zone centrally. In contrast to follicular lymphoma, the germinal centers usually remain separate and vary in size

(but they may coalesce in some cases). The germinal centers contain numerous mitoses and tingible-body macrophages. Staining with bcl-2 is weak or absent within the germinal center (but strong in the surrounding mantle), while PCNA (Ki-67, proliferating cell nuclear antigen) is strongly expressed. In follicular lymphoma, follicles are often 'naked' (mantles are obliterated) and confluent. Mitoses are rare, as are tingible-body macrophages. Staining with bcl-2 is strong in the follicle, and PCNA is weak. The causes of a follicular pattern of hyperplasia includes:

- Nonspecific reactive follicular hyperplasia (etiology unknown) is the most common scenario.

- Some viruses are associated with a pattern of RFH. HIV infection produces a profound variety called florid follicular hyperplasia. This progresses through stages that parallel the clinical stages of disease. In early infection, the robust florid follicular hyperplasia is seen, with giant germinal centers that are often confluent, lose their mantles, and take on all sorts of abnormal shapes, including dumbbell shapes, geographic germinal centers, and clovers. This stage has many follicles demonstrating follicular lysis. This progresses to follicular involution, characterized by regressively transformed germinal centers that resemble hyaline-vascular Castleman disease, and finally, it progresses to lymphocyte depletion.

- Rheumatoid arthritis and Sjögren syndrome produce reactive follicular hyperplasia, frequently with interfollicular plasmacytosis.

- Syphilis, like rheumatoid lymphadenitis, produces reactive follicular hyperplasia with interfollicular plasma-

---

T4.21
Polycythemia Vera (PV) vs Secondary Erythrocytosis

Parameter	PV	Secondary
RBC mass	↑	↑
PaO$_2$	Normal	Normal to ↓
Leukocytes & basophils	↑	Normal
LAP score	↑	Normal
Serum B$_{12}$	↑	Normal
EPO	↓	↑
Serum iron / stainable iron	↓	Normal
Platelet aggregation studies	Abnormal	Normal

T4.22
Constitutional (Congenital) Neutropenias

Isolated Neutropenia	With Other Cytopenias
Kostmann syndrome	Shwachman-Diamond
Cyclic neutropenia	Dyskeratosis congenita
Glycogen storage dz type 1b	Congenital amegakaryocytic thrombocytopenia
WHIM syndrome	
Chediak-Higashi	Fanconi anemia
Reticular dysgenesis	Common variable immunodeficiency

cytosis. It also causes capsular and trabecular thickening (due to chronicity) and capsular infiltration by plasma cells.

- Castleman disease

  □ The hyaline vascular type, which is by far the most common, is usually localized to the mediastinum and does not have systemic manifestations. The germinal centers are atretic rather than hyperplastic and characterized by one or two central hyalinized blood vessels. Often the mantle is hyperplastic in an onion-ring fashion.

  □ The less common plasma cell variant may be multi-centric and may be associated with systemic manifes-tations such as the POEMS syndrome. The histologic pattern resembles rheumatoid lymphadenitis, with interfollicular plasmacytosis and either hyperplastic or regressed germinal centers. Some cases of plasma cell Castleman are caused by human herpes virus 8 (HHV8) infection, and a significant number of these cases arise in human immunodeficiency virus-1 (HIV-1) infection. HHV8-associated cases show blurring of the germinal center-mantle boundary (so-called regressive dissolution of the germinal center), atypical plasma cells (which may be clonal), and an increased number of immunoblasts.

The interfollicular pattern is characterized by expan-sion of the interfollicular (paracortical) zones. Lymphoid follicles are usually small. The interfollicular area may show a variety of cells, including small lympho-cytes, transformed lymphocytes, immunoblasts, and plasma cells. The differential diagnosis includes:

- Viral infections such as infectious mononucleosis, CMV, postvaccinial lymphadenitis

- Hypersensitivity reactions (eg, dilantin)

- Kimura disease is endemic in Asia and predominantly affects young men. This presents most commonly as a soft tissue mass of the head and neck with cervical lymphadenopathy, peripheral eosinophilia and increased IgE. Recurrences are common, but overall prognosis is excellent. The lymph nodes are characterized by florid follicular hyperplasia having increased vascularity and proteinaceous deposits, paracortical eosinophilia, increased prominence of postcapillary venules, and interfollicular viral-type immunoblasts. This entity is distinct from angi-

olymphoid hyperplasia with eosinophilia (AL&E) which does not appear to have any racial predilection, affects women more often than men, has skin rather than soft tissue lesions, and lacks lymphadenopathy, eosinophilia, and hyperimmunoglobulin E.

The sinus pattern is characterized by sinuses that are dilated and most often filled with histiocytes. The dif-ferential diagnosis includes

- Sinus histiocytosis, a nonspecific reaction to numerous lymph node stimuli.

- Sinus histiocytosis with massive lymphadenopathy (Rosai-Dorfman disease) presents most commonly with bilateral cervical lymphadenopathy. However, it has been reported in multiple extranodal sites including quite often the brain. The histopathologic characteristics include markedly distended sinuses filled with foamy histiocytes having *emperipolesis* (internalized cells not being digested—not true hemophagocytosis). The surrounding infiltrate is rich in *plasma cells*. The disease is usually self-limited and very rarely fatal. The histiocytes in this disorder express S100, CD11b, CD14, lysozyme, and HLA-DR, as would be expected. Unexpectedly, they have also been found to express CD31.

- Lymphangiogram effect is a classic cause of a sinus expansion pattern in lymph nodes. This change was found in intraabdominal nodes in association with lymphangiogram performed in the staging of Hodgkin lymphoma, a procedure that is not performed much any more. A very similar change is now seen in pelvic nodes following lower extremity joint replacement surgery, particularly when prostheses contain cobalt-chromium alloy and titanium. Affected nodes are found most often as part of a prostatectomy specimen and show sinus expanded by abundant large histiocytes. These foamy histiocytes contain particles (that may mimic internal-ized cells by light microscopy).

- Whipple disease affects predominantly *males (10:1)*. It is characterized by infiltration of multiple organs by foamy histiocytes, usually without much of a lymphoid reac-tion. Intestinal infiltration (with malabsorption), joint infiltration (causing arthralgias), CNS involvement, cardiac valve infiltration, and hepatosplenomegaly are common. In lymph nodes, the sinuses are dilated by foamy histiocytes containing PAS+, diastase-resistant, AFB− bacilli (*Tropheryma whippelii*).

277

- Hemophagocytic syndrome is characterized by histiocytes with internalized degenerated and partially digested lymphoid cells. It is associated with EBV and certain types of lymphoma.

- Dermatopathic lymphadenitis is found in patients with benign and malignant skin disorders and characterized by paracortical expansion by histiocytes containing faint pigment. In mycosis fungoides, this is an ominous sign.

Granulomatous lymphadenitis

- Suppurative granulomata characterize cat-scratch disease, lymphogranuloma venereum (LGV), and tularemia. Cat-scratch disease is caused by *Bartonella henselae,* transmitted by the scratch of a kitten. A Warthin-Starry stain is recommended in these cases but is rarely fruitful. While cat-scratch disease most often affects axillary and cervical nodes, an identical histologic picture may be seen in inguinal lymph nodes infected by lymphogranuloma venereum.

- Necrotizing granulomata without suppuration are seen in mycobacterial infection, brucellosis, fungal infection, and yersinial infection. In the thorax and mediastinum, these are often due to *M. tuberculosis, H. capsulatum,* and *C. immitis.* In cervical nodes, *M. scrofulaceum* causes a mat of caseating granulomatous lymph nodes. In immunocompetent patients, atypical mycobacteria such as *M. avium-intracellulare* (MAI) or *M. kansasii* also can cause a necrotizing granulomatous lymphadenitis; whereas well-formed granulomas may not form in immunocompromised hosts. Yersinial infection may cause this pattern in intraabdominal nodes, ileal Peyer patches, or the appendix.

- Rounded, nonnecrotizing granulomas are characteristic of sarcoidosis but may be caused by foreign material and atypical mycobacteria.

- Ill-formed granulomas *impinging on germinal centers* are seen in toxoplasmosis, most commonly affecting posterior cervical lymph nodes. The typical histologic triad includes reactive follicular hyperplasia; multiple small aggregates of epithelioid histiocytes often encroaching upon germinal centers; and monocytoid B-cell hyperplasia.

- Ill-defined sheets of histiocytes with karyorrhexis is characteristic of Kikuchi-Fujimoto disease (histiocytic necrotizing lymphadenitis), a benign self-limiting disease presenting as isolated cervical lymphadenopathy and fever in young women. Some feel this is a forme-fruste of systemic lupus erythematosis, and the histologic findings are the same as in lupus. *Neutrophils are absent* from the infiltrate.

  □ Kikuchi-Fujimoto disease is found worldwide, but is most common in people of Japanese or other Asian origin. Affected patients most often are adults younger than 40 years, with a male:female ratio of 1:4.

  □ Adenopathy presents abruptly, is tender, cervical, unilateral, and associated with fever. About ¼ have a peripheral lymphocytosis, and as many have a mild neutropenia.

  □ The histologic findings include necrotic areas within the paracortex having abundant karyorrhectic debris, histiocytes, plasmacytoid monocytes, and a mixture of lymphocytes, including immunoblasts that are predominantly CD8+ T cells. Neutrophils are absent, and plasma cells are scarce.

  □ The histologic differential diagnosis includes lupus, necrotic lymphoma, herpes lymphadenitis, and Kawasaki disease-associated lymphadenitis. Numerous plasma cells are considered a clue to lupus-associated lymphadenitis.

  □ Lymphadenopathy typically resolves within 4 months.

The diffuse pattern of nodal expansion, easy to confuse with lymphoma, is produced by several viruses, particularly Epstein-Barr virus (EBV). The affected areas are effaced by a proliferation of T lymphocytes, plasma cells, and immunoblasts that may be very atypical. The process can histologically mimic Hodgkin lymphoma or large cell lymphoma, and the clinical history is very important. Similar histologic findings may occur in CMV, HSV, measles, or post-vaccinia lymphadenitis. In CMV, typical inclusions may be seen. In HSV, focal necrosis is characteristic, and the typical inclusions may be seen. In measles, giant Warthin-Finkledy immunoblasts are typically present.

Nonlymphoid constituents

- Benign salivary, Müllerian, and breast epithelial rests may be present in lymph nodes in the appropriate locations.

4: Hematopathology

Nonneoplastic White Blood Cell Disorders>Nonneoplastic Lymph Node Proliferations I Neoplastic Hematopathology>
B-Cell Neoplasms

Benign salivary epithelial inclusions are common in para-salivary lymph nodes and are felt to be the precursors of Warthin tumors. Müllerian inclusions give rise to nodal endosalpingiosis. Benign breast epithelia are present in some axillary lymph nodes. Controversy exists as to whether lateral neck lymph nodes may sometimes contain benign thyroid follicles. Many consider this evidence of thyroid follicular carcinoma.

- Fatty infiltration is very common in lymph nodes, particularly those in the pelvis. Vascular transformation of lymph node sinuses (VTLNS) is an occasional finding, seen most commonly in intraabdominal lymph nodes. The vascular transformation is thought to result from obstruction. It must be distinguished from Kaposi sarcoma and bacillary angiomatosis. Other stromal proliferations include leiomyomas, palisaded myofibroblastoma, inflammatory pseudotumor, and mycobacterial spindle cell tumors.

Neoplastic Hematopathology

B-Cell Neoplasms

Small lymphocytic lymphoma/chronic lymphocytic leukemia (SLL/CLL)

- SLL presents as diffuse nodal effacement by predominantly small, mature-appearing lymphocytes. The lymphocytes have a *rounded nuclear contour* with *coarsely clumped chromatin* and scant cytoplasm. Mitoses are relatively low in number, higher numbers suggesting mantle cell lymphoma. Occasionally, the nuclear contours are irregular or clefted (resembling typical mantle cell or follicular lymphoma), and smaller populations of prolymphocytes and paraimmunoblasts may be present. Some cases have a plasmacytoid cytomorphology (distinguished from lymphoplasmacytic lymphoma by the expression of CD5 and CD23). Rarely, there may be Reed-Sternberg-like cells. Within the diffuse growth of an SLL, there are often so-called *proliferation centers,* notable at low magnification as a pale nodule and at high magnification for a large proportion of prolymphocytes and paraimmunoblasts. The peripheral blood is nearly always involved (CLL) at the time of presentation.

- CLL presents as a lymphocytosis, with numerous smudged cells (an EDTA artifact not seen on heparin smears). The count is high (>6000/µL) but usually not extremely high (usually <30,000/µL). As in the lymph node, the neoplastic cells are predominantly small, mature-appearing lymphocytes with scant cytoplasm, rounded nuclear contours, and *a coarsely clumped chromatin (block-like, checkerboard-like, cracked earth-like).* Prolymphocytes, characterized by an increased volume of cytoplasm, open chromatin, and central prominent nucleoli, comprise 10% or less of the population (11-55% prolymphocytes defines CLL/PLL).

- The bone marrow is very commonly involved at presentation. Involvement takes one of three patterns: nodular, interstitial, or diffuse. The diffuse pattern is associated with a worse prognosis, while the nodular pattern indicates a better prognosis. Infiltrates resembling B-CLL/SLL can be found in HCV-positive patients.

- Immunophenotype **F4.8**

  □ Positive for: CD19, CD20+ (dim), CD22, CD5, CD23, sIg (dim), CD43, CD79, CD11c.

  □ Negative for: FMC-7, CD10, bcl-1, bcl-6.

  □ As in the majority of neoplastic B lymphocytes, bcl-2 is expressed.

  □ CD38 and/or ZAP-70 expression is present in a subset of cases and implies an unfavorable prognosis.

  □ An increase in polyclonal lymphocytes coexpressing CD5/19 is sometimes seen in autoimmune disorders, *especially rheumatoid arthritis (RA), in HCV,* and *post-bone marrow transplant.*

- It was previously thought, as a result of access only to traditional cytogenetic techniques, that fewer than half of cases had chromosomal aberrations and that the most common of these was trisomy 12. This was biased by the fact that a trisomy is relatively easy to observe. It is now known, through the combined application of conventional cytogenetics and FISH, that only 20% of cases have a normal karyotype. The most common chromosomal anomaly is deletion of 13q14 (> half of cases). Other frequent findings are trisomy 12 (15-20%), del(11q), del(14q), and del(17p).

- SLL/CLL typically affects elderly patients, men more commonly than women. As is typical of low-grade lymphomas, it usually presents with *generalized involvement*—generalized adenopathy, splenomegaly, and bone marrow involvement. In contrast, high-grade lymphomas tend to be localized at presentation. Cytopenias are unusual and more likely represent autoimmune phenomena than marrow replacement. Hypogamma-globulinemia is common (about 50%). A small minority display hypergammaglobulinemia. An M protein is occasionally present.

■ The most common transformation is prolymphocytic, heralded immunophenotypically by stronger expression of CD22, sIg, and CD20, weaker CD5 and CD23. CLL/PLL is present when prolymphocytes comprise 11-55% of the neoplastic cells. Richter syndrome, the transformation to large cell lymphoma, occurs in 3-15% of cases.

■ Factors that affect prognosis

  □ CLL is generally an indolent disease, with most cases arising in old age and most affected patients dying of other things. Treatment is usually withheld.

Some cases, however, are rapidly progressive, and there is much interest in finding markers that can predict aggressive disease so that therapy can be appropriately initiated.

□ Stage may be assessed by one of several systems

  ● *The Rai staging system was initially proposed as a 5-tiered system and subsequently revised to 3 tiers: low-risk (original Rai stage 0), intermediate-risk (stages I and II), and high-risk (stages III and IV).*

  ● *The Binet staging system classifies non-cytopenic patients as stage A or B, depending upon the number of lymph node areas involved, and patients with anemia or thrombocytopenia as stage C. The 'lymph node areas' include cervical nodes, axillary nodes, inguinal nodes (each side counting as one), liver, and spleen.* **T4.23**

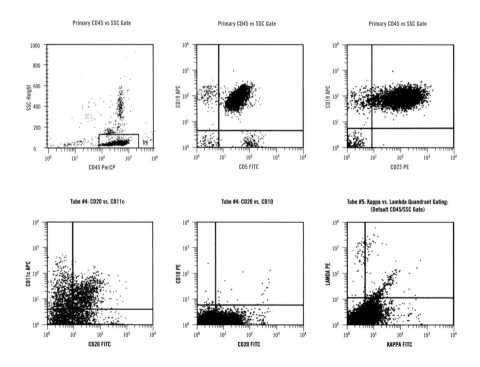

F4.8 Flow cytometry in a case of CLL. The primary CD45 vs side-scatter (SSC) gate selects the lymphocyte population (red axis). The cells co-express CD5, CD19, and CD23 (tube 2). Tube 4 demonstrates the weak to moderate expression of CD11c and dim CD20 that is typical of CLL. The cells express monotypic κ light chains dimly.

▫ B symptoms (fever, weight loss, and night sweats) are thought to correlate with shortened survival.

▫ Lymphocyte morphology, count, and rate of doubling may correlate with prognosis. Atypical morphology (irregularly contoured or clefted nuclei, for example), peripheral lymphocyte doubling time of ≤ 1 year, and higher initial lymphocyte count (especially >30,000) tend to correlate with worsened survival.

▫ The pattern of marrow infiltration may be nodular, interstitial, or diffuse. The nodular and interstitial patterns are correlated with a better prognosis, while the diffuse pattern correlates with a worse prognosis.

▫ The stereotypical immunophenotype of CLL/SLL includes expression of CD19, CD5, and CD23 with dim surface immunoglobulin (sIg) expression, dim CD20 expression, and weak to absent CD38. Atypical immunophenotypic features, including bright CD20, bright sIg, and CD38 expression, have been correlated with atypical morphology, an unmutated IgVH gene (see below), and a worsened prognosis. Lastly, the Z-chain-associated protein (ZAP)-70, a tyrosine kinase normally associated with the T-cell receptor (TCR) Z chain, is present in a subset of CLL cases. ZAP-70 expression, like CD38, correlates with an unmutated IgVH gene.

▫ More than 80% of CLL/SLLs have at least one structural chromosomal abnormality. A relatively stable clinical course is seen in those cases with del(13q) as the sole abnormality. The shortest survival has been noted in those with 11q and 17p deletions.

▫ The mutation status of immunoglobulin heavy chain gene variable region (IgVH) may be a pivotal prognostic factor. Somatic hypermutation of this gene is a physiologic feature of postgerminal center B cells ('memory' B cells) and is seen in about half of CLL cases; thus, it appears that there may be two types of CLL, one arising from pregerminal center B cells (no IgVH mutations), and one from postgerminal center cells (hypermutated IgVH). *IgVH hypermutation is associated with prolonged survival, and IgVH nonmutation is associated with poor survival.* Mutation analysis is not widely available, however, and CD38 and/or ZAP-70 (both tending to be positive in nonmutated cases) may serve as surrogate markers. For a designation of CD38+, at least 30% of neoplastic cells should express CD38.

Mantle cell lymphoma (MCL)

■ The neoplastic cell is a small to medium-sized lymphocyte with an *irregular nuclear contour and a small delicate nucleolus.* These proliferate in a diffuse to 'vaguely nodular' pattern. Typically there are admixed histiocytes in sheets and aggregates. Unlike SLL/CLL, there is typically not a peripheral blood lymphocytosis; however, it happens often enough that the leukemic phase of MCL must be excluded whenever a diagnosis of CLL is entertained. Furthermore, there is a subset of MCLs with a penchant for peripheral blood involvement; these tend to have cytogenetic aberrations involving chromosomes 17, 21, and 8 (in addition to the requisite t(11;14)).

■ A blastoid (blastic MCL) variant is occasionally observed, in which several varieties of high-grade lymphoma may enter into the differential. Lymphoblastic lymphoma/leukemia can be distinguished by its lack of bcl-1, lack of CD5, and expression of CD99 and tdt.

T4.23
CLL Staging

Original Rai stages	Modified Rai stages	Survival	Binet stages	Survival
0. lymphocytosis (>5000/mL)	Low risk	>13 years	A. <3 lymphoid areas	15 years
I. with lymphadenopathy II. with hepatosplenomegaly	Intermediate risk	8 years	B. >3 lymphoid areas	5 years
III. with anemia (<11 g/dL) IV. with thrombocytopenia (<100,000/mL)	High risk	2 years	C. Anemia (<11 g/dL) or thrombocytopenia (<100,000/mL)	3 years

Neoplastic Hematopathology>B-Cell Neoplasms

■ Immunophenotype **(F4.9)**

  □ Positive: CD19, CD20 (bright), CD22, FMC-7, CD5, sIg (bright), CD43, bcl-1 (cyclin D1, prad 1)

  □ Negative: CD23, CD11c

  □ More likely to be λ-restricted than κ-restricted

■ Its characteristic cytogenetic finding is t(11;14), which places the J_H region of the IgH (14q32) gene in proximity to the *CCND1* (11q13) gene, resulting in amplification.

  □ Most MCLs have more than just this molecular anomaly, most commonly of chromosome 13.

  □ Note that B cells with translocations involving IgH —especially involving bcl-2 and c-myc—can be found in a small percentage of normal adults. It is felt that these translocations may be necessary but insufficient in isolation to produce a B-cell neoplasm.

  □ Cyclin D1 (prad-1, bcl-1), the product of the *CCND1* gene, is a protein that appears to stimulate entrance into the G1-phase of the cell cycle.

  □ The rate at which t(11;14)/*BCL1* rearrangements are found in MCL is variable depending upon the methodology employed. About 50% of rearrangements involves a single breakpoint area, referred to as the major translocation cluster (MTC) region. This region is actually quite a bit away from the *BCL1* gene, producing gene amplification in some long-distance mechanism. Thus, Southern blot (SBA) using a single MTC region probe, or PCR, using flanking primers to this region, will detect only about half of rearrangements. The use of multiple probes or multiplex primers can raise this detection rate to about 70%. FISH assays, however, can detect nearly 100% of rearrangements and are therefore the clear choice for finding t(11;14)/*BCL1–IgH* fusions in MCL.

■ MCL's deceptively low-grade appearance belies its *aggressive clinical course*. MCL occurs mainly in adults and is likely to be generalized at the time of diagnosis. MCL is

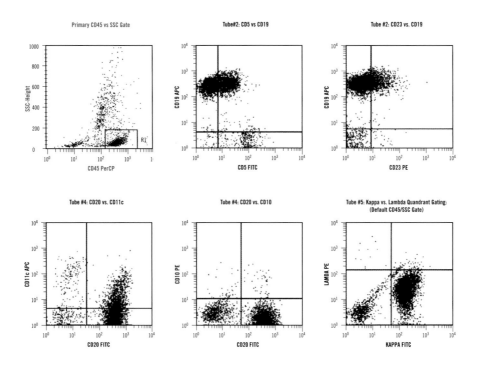

F4.9 Flow cytometry in a case of MCL. Tube 2 shows CD19 and CD5 co-expression, with CD23 being negative. Importantly, tube 4 shows the bright expression of CD20, and tube 5 shows bright expression of monotypic κ light chains.

more aggressive than other small lymphoid neoplasms, with a median survival of 3-4 years.

Follicular lymphoma (FL)

- Affected lymph nodes are effaced by back-to-back follicles having attenuated mantles, no tangible body macrophages, and diminished mitoses. The follicles are populated by two cell types in varying proportions: the small cleaved cell (centrocyte) and large noncleaved cell (centroblast).

- Grading is based on the proportion of large noncleaved cells (centroblasts).

  □ Grade I: 0-5 per 40× field or <25% of all neoplastic cells

  □ Grade II: 5-15 per 40× field or 25% to 50% of all neoplastic cells

  □ Grade III: >15 per 40× field or >50% of all neoplastic cells

- Immunophenotype (F4.10)

  □ Positive: CD19, CD20, FMC-7, CD22, CD10, sIg (bright), bcl-2, bcl-6

  □ Negative: CD5, CD43, CD11c

  □ The expression of CD23, CD19, CD10, bcl-6, and bcl-2 is variable. Many cases of FL are dim or variable for CD19. Many cases, particularly with ascending grade, are negative for CD10, bcl-6, and/or bcl-2.

  □ Bcl-6 expression is common in reactive germinal centers. Most FLs display strong nuclear expression, and bcl-6 is expressed by Burkitt lymphoma and many diffuse large B-cell lymphomas (DLBCLs).

  □ CD10 is expressed in early B-cell maturation then again in reactive germinal centers. Most FLs display cytoplasmic CD10 as do Burkitt lymphomas and many DLBCLs.

  □ Bcl-2 expression is not unique to FL. It is commonly expressed in various neoplastic B and T cells, so it must always be interpreted in context.

- In virtually all cases, the t(14;18)(p32;q21) translocation forms the basis for FL.

  □ This translocation juxtaposes the *BCL2* gene on chromosome 18 with the J region of the immunoglobulin heavy-chain gene (JH) on chromosome 14, with a resulting over-expression of the bcl-2 protein. Most of the t(14;18) translocations occur within a 150 base pair region (the major breakpoint region—MBR) that is amenable to amplification with PCR or probing with FISH.

  □ The gene product of *BCL2* is an antiapoptotic molecule capable of aborting the normal process of programmed cell death.

  □ The t(14;18) abnormality is the most common translocation encountered in B-lineage lymphoma. This anomaly is also found in a significant minority of diffuse large B-cell lymphomas (DLBCL) and in 90% of follicular lymphomas. It is rarely found in other B-cell lymphomas. Occasionally, a 5' region of *BCL2*, the variant cluster region (VCR) is rearranged in CLL/SLL. Among DLBCLs, the presence of the t(14;18) rearrangement has been associated with a 'germinal center' phenotype. It is felt that this subset of DLBCL has a relatively favorable prognosis.

  □ Note that while *BCL2* gene rearrangement is nearly always associated with overexpression of bcl-2 protein, the converse is not true. Many B-cell neoplasms display overexpression of bcl-2, and most of these do not have structural *BCL2* gene rearrangments. These other neoplasms appear to have dysregulated *BCL2* loci on other bases.

- Like all low-grade lymphomas, FL arises mainly in adults and tends to be generalized at the time of diagnosis, with a high rate of bone marrow involvement. When found in the marrow, it is usually in the form of *focal paratrabecular aggregates*. Only FL and TCRBCL are commonly found in this form. Bone marrow discordant morphology is a common finding—usually in the form of high-grade morphology in the lymph node with low-grade morphology in the marrow. This form of discordance implies a slightly better prognosis as compared to patients with concordant (high grade/high grade) findings.

- FL has a median survival of 8 to 10 years. Most eventually progress (transform) to high-grade FLs or DLBCL.

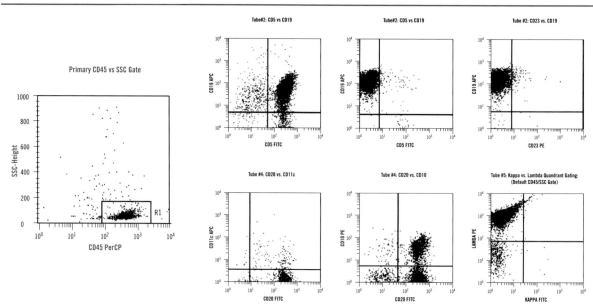

F4.10 Flow cytometry in a case of FL. Note the coexpression of CD38 and CD10, with very strong λ light chain expression. CD5, CD23, and CD11c are negative. Some cases of FL show dim or variable CD19 expression, and some may be entirely negative for CD10.

Factors known to correlate with progression include age, stage, bone marrow involvement, B symptoms, performance status, serum lactate dehydrogenase levels, and anemia. It appears that bcl-6 and CD10 expression favorably impact prognosis.

Marginal zone lymphoma (MZL)

■ Marginal zone B cell lymphomas may present as:

□ Nodal marginal zone B-cell lymphoma presents histologically as a proliferation of monocytoid B cells in a diffuse, sinusoidal or interfollicular pattern, usually with follicular permeation (colonization). Plasma cells with intranuclear Dutcher bodies can often be found.

□ Extranodal marginal zone B cell lymphoma of mucosa-associated lymphoid tissue (MALT lymphoma) presents as a mixture of small round lymphocytes with abundant pale cytoplasm and indented nuclei (monocytoid B cells), plasma cells (some of which can be found to contain Dutcher bodies), and lymphoepithelial lesions. Of note, the plasma cells in the infiltrate are monoclonal. Reactive lymphoid follicles with germinal centers may be seen.

□ Splenic marginal zone lymphoma presents as white pulp colonization. The leukemic phase of splenic

MZL is synonymous with splenic lymphoma with villous lymphocytes (SLVL). The leukemic cells morphologically resemble HCL, except that a *distinct nucleolus* is usually present in SLVL.

■ Immunophenotype

□ Positive: CD19, CD20, FMC-7, sIg

□ Plasma cells within infiltrate contain monoclonal cytoplasmic light chains

□ Negative: CD5, CD23, CD10, CD11c

□ Sometimes (<30%) CD43+, most often in the case of MALT lymphoma

■ Molecular: extranodal marginal zone (MALT) lymphomas demonstrate a t(11;18) or t(1;14). The t(11;18) translocation is associated with rearrangement of the *API2* and *MALT1* genes. *API2–MALT1* translocation tumors have largely been identified in the stomach and lung. The t(1;14) translocation results in a *MALT1–IgH* gene fusion. *MALT1–IgH* translocation tumors have been found largely in ocular, parotid, and cutaneous sites.

■ A monoclonal gammopathy is present in 30-50% of cases.

Hairy cell leukemia (HCL)

- HCL affects mainly the spleen, peripheral blood, marrow, and liver. It is very uncommon in lymph nodes.

- The diagnosis of hairy cell leukemia in the peripheral blood may be challenging. It may mimic aplastic anemia in its initial presentation. While the peripheral blood is nearly always involved, the cells are usually present in low numbers. Even when the cells are noted, the differential diagnosis is broad. Mild to moderate pancytopenia is common, with a disproportionate neutropenia and *monocytopenia*. In fact, some consider the diagnosis of HCL extremely unlikely without monocytopenia. Note, however, that many automated analyzers will mistake hairy cells for monocytes. In peripheral blood smears and cytologic preparations, the neoplastic cells have a classic cytologic appearance:

  - The hairy cell is larger than a mature lymphocyte, and its nucleus is about twice the size of a mature lymphocyte nucleus. The cell size tends to be remarkably uniform—lacking are the admixed larger 'transformed' cells seen so often in other low-grade lymphoid neoplasms.

  - The nuclei, however, do vary in outline—they may be round, oval, reniform, or bilobed. In tissue, they may even be spindled. In most cases, the largest number of cells have nuclei that are oval. The nuclear outline tends to be sharp and smooth. The chromatin is highly characteristic—usually desribed as 'ground glass' due to its even dispersal. The nucleolus is usually indistinct, but occasionally a single nucleolus is evident.

  - While hairy projections are the feature that gives HCL its name: it is neither a consistent nor a unique feature. The cytoplasmic margin may have hairy projections, and when they are present, they tend to be circumferential. More commonly, the cytoplasmic margin is indistinct and frayed, as though there is not a distinct cytoplasmic membrane. The cytoplasm is pale, textured, and flocculent.

- The morphologic features may be closely mimicked.

  - Splenic lymphoma with villous lymphocytes (SLVL) represents the leukemic phase of splenic marginal zone lymphoma (MZL). The cells of SLVL, like those of HCL, have moderate to abundant cytoplasm and may have cytoplasmic projections; however, these tend to be more polar, and the flocculent quality of HCL cytoplasm is lacking. The chromatin in SLVL lacks the dispersed ground-glass quality of HCL, being more clumped, and the nucleolus is typically more prominent in SLVL. In histologic sections, MZL can mimic HCL closely.

  - Prolymphocytic leukemia (PLL)

  - Mastocytosis may produce a cytologic and histologic appearance similar to HCL in many respects. The nuclei tend to be oval to reniform, there is dispersed chromatin, and there is abundant cytoplasm. Furthermore, both may be associated with fibrosis in tissue, and an infiltrate of mast cells is common in hairy cell infiltrates. The finding of granular cytoplasm and numerous admixed eosinophils are important clues to the diagnosis of mastocytosis.

  - In some cases, even AML (particularly M3 and M5) may enter the differential diagnosis.

- Bone marrow demonstrates features typical of hairy cell infiltration elsewhere: sheets of typical hairy cells, reticulin fibrosis, blood lakes, and a smattering of mast cells. While blood lakes are not as prominent as elsewhere (especially the spleen), there are often numerous extravascated red cells. The reticulin fibrosis is responsible for the typically inaspirable (dry tap) quality of the marrow. The hairy cells are exceedingly fragile, and aspirate smears often display numerous stripped nuclei. The bone marrow biopsy shows aggregates of hairy cells in addition to subtle but widespread interstitial infiltration. When present in aggregates, the abundant cytoplasm of the hairy cells results in an evenly spaced fried-egg appearance. When present only interstitially, the infiltrates may be very difficult to distinguish from hematopoietic elements. Occasionally the marrow is extremely hypocellular and the hairy cells so subtle as to tempt a diagnosis of aplastic anemia. The surrounding marrow is notable for erythroid predominance (due to relatively suppressed granulopoiesis). There is apparent reticulin fibrosis in many cases (due mainly to deposition of fibronectin).

- In the spleen HCL infiltrates the red pulp. Formation of blood lakes is highly characteristic.

- While the liver is frequently involved in HCL, this is not commonly seen as a surgical pathology specimen. The hairy cells infiltrate the hepatic sinusoids extensively. Angiomatoid foci have been described, which appear to represent the hepatic version of a blood lake.

- The lymph nodes of the splenic hilum and some regional intraabdominal nodes may be involved. The infiltrate in these instances tends to be sinusoidal.

- The cells ultrastructurally display ribosome-lamellar complexes.

- The cells contain tartrate-resistant acid phosphatase (TRAP). Other proliferations that may demonstrate weak to moderate TRAP positivity include PLL, Waldenstrom macroglobulinemia, mast cell disease, and Gaucher cells.

- The typical immunophenotype is **F4.11**

  □ Positive: CD19, CD20, CD22, sIg, CD11c, CD25, CD103, DBA.44, cyclin D1. Many also CD2+.

  □ Negative: CD5, CD43, CD23, CD10

  □ In the plot of CD45 vs side scatter, there is often a dual population, the HCL having strong CD45 and moderate side-angle light scatter, and appearing in the usual location for monocytes. In fact, in some automated leukocyte differentials, hairy cells may be counted erroneously as monocytes, thus masking monocytopenia.

  □ About 10% are CD10+, and these cases do not appear to differ clinically.

  □ While CD11c is commonly expressed in CLL and SLVL, expression is typically brighter in HCL.

  □ CD25 is also commonly expressed in CLL, but again, expression is much brighter in HCL.

  □ CD103 is the most specific of the hairy cell antigens, but there have been reports of expression in cases of SLVL.

  □ DBA.44 is also expressed in a majority of SLVL and a significant minority of follicular lymphoma, mantle cell lymphoma, and diffuse large B-cell lymphoma.

  □ Cyclin D1 shows dim to moderate nuclear staining in HCL.

- There are no signature molecular findings, and cytogenetic studies are often difficult in HCL due to low cellularity and low proliferative rate. Noted abnormalities include duplications of a region in 14q, t(14;18), and abnormalities of a region of chromosome 5. The finding of bcl-1 over-expression, in many cases of HCL, does not appear to be associated with structural rearrangements of the bcl-1 locus (11q13).

- HCL accounts for about 2% of all leukemias. It affects older males (over 50; 4:1 male:female ratio) who present with splenomegaly and pancytopenia (especially monocytopenia and neutropenia). Lymphadenopathy is not usually a feature.

Prolymphocytic leukemia (PLL)

- PLL mainly involves peripheral blood and bone marrow. The neoplasm is very uncommon and rarely involves lymph node. When it does, it must be distinguished from MZL and, in some cases, from blastoid MCL. By criteria, the neoplasm is composed of >55% prolymphocytes, defined as having a prominent nucleolus and a moderate quantity of slightly eccentric cytoplasm. Neoplasms having 11- 55% prolymphocytes are defined as CLL/PLL.

- PLL arises de novo with far greater frequency than it evolves from CLL. At presentation, the white count is usually quite high, >100,000/ÌL, and there is diffuse marrow effacement. While capable of mimicking HCL in marrow biopsies PLL usually displays distinct nucleoli.

- Immunophenotype

  □ The immunophenotype differs from SLL/CLL with no expression of CD5, strong CD11c, bright sIg, bright CD20, CD22, and FMC-7.

- Molecular findings include alterations of 14q32 (often in the form of t(11;14)) in about 20% of cases.

Lymphoplasmacytic lymphoma (LPL) / Waldenström macroglobulinemia

- LPL has morphologic resemblance to SLL/CLL, but contains at least a small population of cells with plasmacytoid differentiation. Fully developed plasma cells and Dutcher bodies can usually be found.

- An IgM monoclonal spike is usually detectable.

- Immunophenotype

    □ Positive: CD19, CD20, CD38, SIg, cIg

    □ CD5 is sometimes expressed, as is CD43

    □ Negative: CD10, CD23

- A recently described t(9;14)(p13;q32), involving the pax-5 gene, appears to be a reproducible finding.

Diffuse large B-cell lymphoma (DLBCL)

- This category includes several previously separate entities, including centroblastic, immunoblastic, and T-cell rich B-cell lymphomas (TCRBCL). In addition, any B-cell neoplasm with morphologic anaplasia, even when CD30 is expressed, is included in the category of DLBCL.

- There is diffuse effacement of the lymph node by predominantly large cells (larger than a macrophage or endothelial nucleus). In many cases, the large cells are "centroblastic," with vesicular nuclei having one or more nucleoli and basophilic cytoplasm. Some cases have immunoblastic cytology, with prominent single nucleoli. Others resemble anaplastic large cell lymphoma, and currently such cases, even if CD30+, are classified as DLBCL. Lastly, some take the form of T-cell rich B-cell lymphoma, in which the large neoplastic cells are obscured by abundant CD8+ T cells.

- Immunophenotype

    □ Positive: CD19, CD20, CD22, CD45

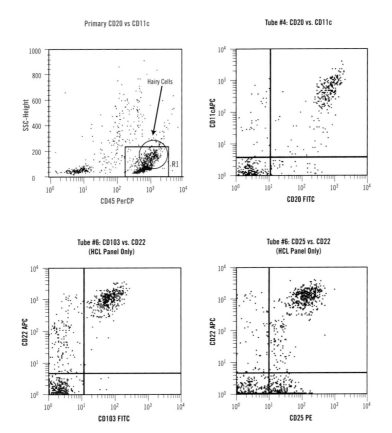

F4.11 Flow cytometry in a case of HCL. Note the strongly CD45+ population with increase side scatter in the gating plot. Note also the very strong expression of CD11c (in contrast to the relatively dim expression in CLL). CD25 and CD103 are additional signature markers.

□ Usually positive: bcl-2

□ Variable: CD10, CD5, bcl-6

- Molecular: bcl-2 or bcl-6 rearrangements in 20-30%. The *BCL6* gene is located on chromosome 3(q27), and it rearranges with a wide variety of partners. A common rearrangement involving *BCL6* is t(3;14)(q27;q32), joining *BCL6* with the IgH locus. Bcl-6 protein is over-expressed in FL, a large number of DLBCL, and Burkitt lymphoma/leukemia, but structural *BCL6* rearrangments are found in only 10% of FL and 30% of DLBCL. The subset of FL with *BCL6* rearrangement appears to represent a higher grade subtype. Unlike bcl-2, bcl-6 protein is normally expressed in germinal center B lymphocytes.

- DLBCL presents as a rapidly enlarging lymph node or extranodal (most often gastrointestinal) site. Unlike the low-grade lymphomas, they tend to be localized at the time of presentation. Bone marrow involvement at the time of diagnosis is uncommon; however, TCRBCL has a particular inclination to involve the marrow (>60%), especially in a paratrabecular fashion.

- Primary CNS lymphoma most often takes the form of DLBCL. Only rare examples of other lymphomas (T, low-grade B, and Hodgkin lymphoma) have been reported.

  □ Among immunocompetent patients, the peak age is about 60, while among AIDS patients, the median age is about 35.

  □ Most cases arise supratentorially, within the frontal, temporal, or parietal lobes. Usually they arise as a solitary lesion with radiographic features that mimic glioblastoma multiforme (GBM), including a tendency to extend across the midline.

  □ Histologically, the neoplastic cells are typically found in perivascular cuffs and express pan-B-cell antigens.

Burkitt lymphoma/leukemia

- Three clinicopathologic types of Burkitt lymphoma are recognized:

  □ African (endemic) Burkitt often presents as a jaw mass and is strongly associated with EBV.

  □ Western (sporadic) Burkitt often presents in intra-abdominal locations, particularly the ileocecal valve, and is not strongly associated with EBV.

  □ Immunodeficiency-associated Burkitt (so-called Burkitt-like lymphoma) most often presents nodally.

- In tissue, there is diffuse infiltration by monomorphic, cells with a distinct rim of basophilic cytoplasm and medium-sized (about the size of a tissue macrophage nucleus), round nuclei having 2 to 5 nucleoli. Numerous tingible-body macrophages are scattered throughout, and there is a high mitotic rate, imparting the classic starry sky appearance. In peripheral blood or tissue imprints, the cells have characteristic deep blue cytoplasm (Wright stains) with lipid-containing vacuoles.

- Immunophenotype

  □ Positive: CD19, CD20, CD22, CD10, bcl-6, sIg, c-myc

  □ Negative: CD5, CD23, TdT, CD34

  □ PCNA (Ki67) is + in >99% of cells by IHC

  □ Immunophenotyping can aid in the distinction from DLBCL. Burkitt is supported by c-myc expression, lack of bcl-2, and a Ki-67 score of >99.

- Molecular rearrangements involving the *C-MYC* gene of chromosome 8—t(8;14), t(2;8), or t(8;22)—are nearly always identified. Most commonly, the *C-MYC* gene is translocated to the IgH locus as a result of t(8;14); however, in many cases it is rearranged with Igλ (2p12) or IgK (22q11). The result of these translocations is *c-myc* protein over-expression. *C-myc* and its partner protein—called Max—combine to activate a number of genes involved in driving the cell into the cell cycle.

- The marrow is involved in 20-30% of cases.

Mediastinal (sclerosing) large cell lymphoma

- This is a sclerotic process that diffusely infiltrates mediastinal structures. The neoplastic cells, which are sometimes obscured by the bands of sclerosis, are large centroblast-like B cells. Often, the histologic differential diagnosis will initially include NS Hodgkin and sclerosing mediastinitis.

- Immunophenotype

  □ Positive: CD45, CD19, CD20, CD79a, CD30 (usually)

  □ Negative: CD10, CD5

- Mediastinal large cell lymphoma affects a broad age range, classically presenting in a young adult female (male:female ratio is about 1:2). Usually, the disease remains confined to the mediastinum.

Intravascular large B-cell lymphoma

- This lesion has in the past been referred to as angioendotheliomatosis, angiotropic lymphoma, and intravascular lymphomatosis.

- Symptoms are related to small-vessel obstruction by large neoplastic B cells.

Primary effusion lymphoma (PEL) is a lymphoma of immunosuppressed individuals, particularly those infected with HIV, that is associated with HHV-8 (the same virus that has been implicated in Kaposi sarcoma and multicentric Castleman disease). Like KS, PEL is disproportionately a disease of homosexual males with HIV. The patients present with effusions (pleural, pericardial, peritoneal) having large atypical B lymphocytes with cytoplasmic vacuolization. Cases of PEL have now been reported with primary soft tissue and lymph node presentations. The immunophenotype is distinctly unusual: the cells are negative for typical B-cell, T-cell, and myeloid antigens (CD20, CD79, CD19, CD10, CD3, CD5, CD13, CD14, CD33). While the cells are usually CD45+, some are not. Often, but not always, positive are CD30, CD38, CD138, and EMA. Southern blot analysis often shows clonal rearrangement of Ig heavy and light chain genes. HHV-8 can be displayed in all cases by immunohistochemistry or molecular studies.

Lymphomatoid granulomatosis (LG) is a lymphoma in which neoplastic cells destructively invade vessel walls in a pattern resembling primary vasculitis. The neoplastic B cells are often admixed with much greater numbers of reactive T cells, plasma cells, and histiocytes. Granulomas are actually very uncommon. It most consistently affects the lungs, where it presents as one or several tumors, but may involve the upper aerodigestive

tract, brain, kidneys, and liver. There is an association with EBV and immunodeficiency. This should be distinguished from nasal-type T/NK-cell angiocentric lymphoma.

Posttransplant lymphoproliferative disorder (PTLD)

- EBV has been implicated in most cases. There is a spectrum of B lymphoproliferative lesions, including reactive plasmacytosis, infectious mononucleosis-like proliferations, polymorphous (lymphocytes, immunoblasts, plasma cells) proliferations, and monomorphous PTLD. Most monomorphous PTLDs take the form of a conventional high-grade B-cell lymphoma.

- A smaller number of T-cell lymphomas and Hodgkin lymphomas occur in this setting.

Acute Lymphoblastic Leukemia and Lymphoma

Precursor B and T neoplasms (B-acute lymphoblastic leukemia/lymphoma and T-acute lymphoblastic leukemia/lymphoma)

- B-lineage neoplasms represent about 80% of acute lymphoblastic leukemia, but only about 20% of lymphoblastic lymphomas.

- T-lineage ALL represents about 20% of acute lymphoblastic leukemia, and about 80% of lymphoblastic lymphomas. T-ALL typically presents as an anterior mediastinal mass and may be associated with hypercalcemia.

- Morphologically, B- and T-ALLs present in tissue or peripheral blood as a monotonous proliferation of undifferentiated blasts. Initially, the morphologic differential includes undifferentiated varieties of AML (M0, M1, M2). In the tissue, T-ALL is sometimes associated with an infiltrate of eosinophils. In the leukemic phase, the FAB classification recognized three types of ALL, based on blast appearance: L1, L2 and L3.

  □ The L1 morphology predominates in childhood ALL. L1 blasts are characterized by homogeneity, a very high N:C ratio, scant cytoplasm, and inconspicuous nucleoli. Particularly in poor preparations, these lymphoblasts can sometimes be confused with mature lymphocytes. L1 comprises 85% of childhood and 31% of adult ALL.

◻The L2 morphology is the most common type seen in adults. L2 blasts are heterogeneous, large blasts with irregular nuclear contours, moderate cytoplasm, and one or more prominent nucleoli. L2 comprises 14% of childhood and 60% of adult ALL.

◻L3 blasts are homogeneous and large, with deep-blue vacuolated cytoplasm and one or more prominent nucleoli. The leukemic cells **bear surface immunoglobulin and lack TdT**. L3 is morphologically and immunologically identical to Burkitt lymphoma/ leukemia.

■ Immunophenotypes

◻Precursor B-ALL

◻*Positive: CD34, CD99, CD19, HLA-DR, TdT (nuclear).*

◻*CD20 is variable but usually negative.*

◻*Negative: sIg*

◻*CD19 is the earliest B-lineage-specific antigen; lack of CD19 essentially excludes B-lineage ALL. However, CD19 expression is not uncommon in AML. Whereas CD19 is usually bright in B-lineage ALL, dim CD19*

is seen in the positive cases of AML, especially AML with t(8;21).

◻*30-50% express at least one myeloid antigen, usually CD13 or CD33, usually dimly.*

◻*ALL with t(1;19) has a characteristic blast immunophenotype, with CD19+, CD9+ and CD10+, but negative CD34 and CD20.*

◻*Burkitt (L3) leukemia/lymphoma differs in key ways (see separate discussion), particularly in its tendency to express CD20 and surface immunoglobulin (sIg) with a negative TdT.*

◻**Precursor T ALL**

◻*Positive: CD34, CD99, CD7, CD2, CD5, CD3 (cytoplasmic), TdT (nuclear)*

◻*Negative: HLA-DR*

◻ *CD4 & CD8 are often both positive or both negative.*

◻*A diagnosis of T-lineage ALL should rarely be made in the absence of CD7. Since CD7 expression is not uncommon in myeloid and B-lineage acute leukemias, a diagnosis of T-lineage ALL should generally be made*

T4.24

Immunophenotypes of Mature B-Cell Neoplasms

	CD19	CD20	CD79	CD5	CD23	FMC-7	CD11c	CD25	CD10	sIg
CLL	+++	+	-/+	+	+	-	+	-	-	+/-
PLL	+++	+++	+	-/+	-	+	-	-	-	+++
MCL	+++	+++	+	+	-	+	-	-	-	+++
FL	++/+/-	+++	+	-	-	+	-	-	+	+++
MZL-LP/ SLVL	+++	+++	+	-	-	+	+	-/+	-	+++
HCL	+++	+++	+	-	-	+	+++	++	-	+++

CLL = chronic lymphocytic leukemia, PLL = prolymphocytic leukemia, MCL= mantle cell lymphoma, FL= follicular lymphoma, MZL/SLVL=marginal zone lymphoma/splenic lymphoma with villous lymphocytes, HCL= hairy cell leukemia

4: Hematopathology

Neoplastic Hematopathology>Acute Lymphoblastic Leukemia and Lymphoma I Plasma Cell Neoplasms>Plasma Cell
Myeloma or Multiple Myeloma

*when HLA-DR is negative and other T-cell markers
are present, such as CD2, CD3 and CD5.*

- Molecular: more than 70% of ALLs have chromosomal
  abnormalities, numerical or structural.

  □ Among these, so-called high hyperdiploidy (>52
  chromosomes) is associated with a favorable prognosis. Also favorable is the t(12;21)/TEL–AML1
  rearrangement.

  □ The most common structural abnormality is
  t(9;22)(q34;q11), the BCR/ABL translocation, present in 5% of childhood ALL and 20% of adult ALL,
  and distinctly unfavorable. At the cytogenetic level,
  the t(9;22) of ALL appears identical to that of CML.
  However, at the molecular level, the translocations
  differ. The major breakpoint (*M-bcr*) rearrangement
  results in a chimeric protein of 210kD and is common in CML. The minor breakpoint (*m-bcr*)
  rearrangement results in a chimeric protein of 190kD
  and is common in ALL. PCR and FISH are capable
  of distinguishing these rearrangements.

  □ Other findings with poor prognostic implications are
  t(1;19), 11q23/*MLL* rearrangements, and
  hypodiploidy (<40 chromosomes).

  □ t(4;11)(q21;q23) is seen in about 5% of cases and
  is associated with expression of CD15 and lack of
  CD10.

Acute leukemia with mixed immunophenotypes

- It is not at all uncommon for acute leukemias to express
  a mixture of lymphoid and myeloid antigens. In such
  cases, classification may be somewhat challenging, and
  one must consider the lineage-specificity of each positive marker as well as their strength of expression.
  Taking these into account (for which various scoring

systems have been devised), these leukemias can be classified as either (i) myeloid antigen positive ALL—
behaves like ALL, (ii) lymphoid antigen positive
AML—behaves like AML.

  □ While CD13 and CD33 are fairly specific for AML,
  CD117 is nearly 100% specific (the sensitivity of
  CD117 is only about 70-90%).

  □ Anomalous T-cell antigen expression—usually CD4,
  CD5, or CD7—is present in 20-40% of AMLs, and
  B-cell antigen expression—usually CD19—is pres-
  ent in 10-20% of cases.

  □ The lymphoid markers CD79a, CD10, CD2 and
  CD3 are virtually never present on pure AML.

- Mixed lineage acute leukemia is diagnosed rarely when
  there is non-committal morphology (M0, L1, L2),
  negative cytochemistries, and a roughly equal expression of myeloid and lymphoid antigens, both in
  number and intensity.

- Biphenotypic acute leukemia is also very rare and implies
  the presence of two distinct populations, one myeloid
  and one lymphoid.

Plasma Cell Neoplasms

Plasma Cell Myeloma or Multiple Myeloma (MM) (T4.26)

- A monoclonal immunoglobulin paraprotein is present in
  the vast majority of cases:

  □ The immunoglobulin heavy chain is most
  commonly IgG (55%), followed by IgA (22%),
  none—light chain only (18%), IgD (2%), biclonal
  (2%), IgE, and nonsecretory (1%). By convention,

4.25
Immunophenotypes in ALL

	TdT	HLA-DR	CD19	CD20	CD10	sIg	CD7
Precursor B	+	+	+	-/+	+	-	-
Burkitt	-	+	+	+	-/+	+	-
Precursor T	+	-	-	-	-	-	+

neoplasms producing IgM are considered non-myelomas (eg, LPL, SLL).

☐ The light chain is most commonly κ; interestingly, IgD myelomas are associated with λ in 90% of cases.

☐ Patients who appear to lack a paraprotein when routine SPEP is examined usually have a light chain- only myeloma (90%); others have IgD-producing myeloma (8%), or nonsecretory myeloma (2%). Most such patients will appear to have hypogammaglobulinemia.

■ Immunophenotype **F4.12**

☐ Neoplastic plasma cells do not usually express CD45 or B-cell antigens (CD19, CD20, CD21, CD22, sIg).

☐ Most neoplastic plasma cells express CD38, CD138, CD56, cytoplasmic κ or λ, and PCA-1. CD56 expression not only implies the neoplastic nature of a plasma cell population, but when present, it is suggestive of behavior that is more aggressive.

☐ 10-30% express myelomonocytic markers (CD117, CD13, CD33, CD11b, CD15)

☐ 10-50% express CALLA (CD10)

☐ Occasional expression of EMA and CD30

☐ Up to 10% may express moderately strong CD45 or CD20.

■ Incidence increases with age, and MM is twice as common in blacks as whites.

■ Primary (AL) amyloidosis develops in 20%, more commonly with λ light chains.

■ Molecular anomalies and prognosis

☐ The overall prognosis is relatively poor, with a mean survival of about 3-5 years.

☐ β_2 microglobulin is usually elevated. Higher levels correlate with poorer prognosis.

☐ A high plasma cell labeling index, which reflects the number of plasma cells in S-phase, correlates with poor prognosis.

☐ Stage correlates with prognosis.

☐ Chromosomal abnormalities are among the most important prognostic parameters in patients with myeloma. As plasma cells have been difficult to culture for cytogenetics, FISH studies are typically used to detect these anomalies. Over 80% of cases are found to have 4 or more chromosomal anomalies, the most common of which affect 13q14, 19p, 14q32, and 17p13.1. Chromosome 14q32 translocations (IgH translocations) appear to be common early events and are found in >70% of myeloma cases and 50% of MGUS cases. The t(11;14)(q13;q32) translocation is the most common translocation in multiple myeloma, present in about 20%, and affects the cyclin D1 locus. The breakpoint differs from that seen in MCL.

☐ Based upon FISH results, patients can be stratified into three distinct prognostic groups:

☐ *shortest survival median of about 24 months— t(4;14), t(14;16), or 17p13.1 deletion*

☐ *intermediate survival median of 42 months—13q14 deletions alone*

☐ *longest survival median of over 50 months— no anomalies or only the t(11;14)*

Plasma cell leukemia

■ Defined as >20% or >2.0×10^9/L plasma cells in the peripheral blood.

T4.26
Diagnostic Criteria for Multiple Myeloma

Major criteria	Minor criteria
>30% plasma cells in bone marrow Serum IgG >3.5 g/dL or IgA >2 g/dL Urine κ or λ light chain >1 g/24 hr Biopsy-proven plasmacytoma	10-30% plasma cells in bone marrow Monoclonal protein Suppression of other Ig classes Lytic bone lesions

Diagnosis requires 1 major criterion and 1 minor criterion or 3 minor criteria including the first 2.

Plasma Cell Neoplasms>Plasma Cell Myeloma or Multiple Myeloma

- Half present de novo, half develop in patients with established MM

- Presents abruptly and follows an aggressive course, with mean survival <1 year.

- High incidence of IgE paraprotein.

Solitary plasmacytoma

- A localized proliferation of plasma cells.

- Most have no detectable serum or urine monoclonal protein.

- Solitary plasmacytoma of bone

  □ Vertebrae > ribs > pelvis

  □ Most (75%) develop MM within 10 years.

- Solitary extramedullary plasmacytoma

  □ Nasal cavity, oropharynx or larynx

  □ Most do not develop MM.

Smoldering myeloma

- A disorder having many features of MM but following a stable course.

- Defined as marrow plasmacytosis of 10-30%, and no lytic bone lesions, renal failure, hypercalcemia, or anemia.

Indolent myeloma has the features of smoldering myeloma plus up to 3 lytic bone lesions.

Monoclonal gammopathy of unknown significance (MGUS)

- This term is applied to the very common scenario in which a patient is found to have a monoclonal gammopathy but lack criteria for the other plasma cell neoplasms defined above.

- MGUS is found in 3% of people over 70.

- 20 years after onset, about 1/3 have developed overt myeloma.

- Diagnostic criteria for MGUS

  □ Monoclonal gammopathy <3.5 g/dL

  □ <10% PCs in bone marrow

  □ Normal to high normal Ca^{2+}

  □ Normal renal function

  □ No lytic bone lesions

  □ Minimal to no Bence-Jones protein

  □ Normal β_2 microglobulin

  □ No amyloidosis

  □ No plasmacytoma

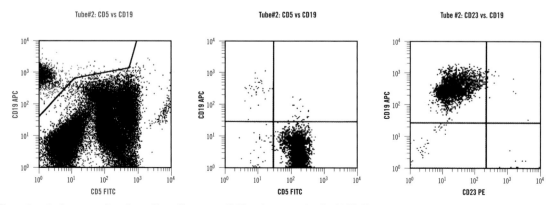

F4.12 Flow cytometry in a case of myeloma. The cells express CD56 and are negative for CD19. They are demonstrated to be clonal by cytoplasmic light chain restriction.

Osteosclerotic myeloma (POEMS syndrome)

- POEMS is an acronym for a very rare syndrome consisting of polyneuropathy, organomegaly, endocrinopathy, M-protein, and skin changes.

- Affected individuals usually have a solitary intra-osseous plasmacytoma with associated thickening of bony trabecula (osteosclerotic myeloma).

- There appears to be a greater-than-chance association between POEMS syndrome and the plasma cell variant of Castleman disease.

Heavy chain disease (Franklin disease)

- A lymphoproliferative disorder productive of heavy (H) chains only.

- The most common form is α heavy chain disease, seen in association with the immunoproliferative small intestine disease (IPSID, Mediterranean lymphoma).

- Less common are γ and μ heavy chain diseases.

T-Cell Neoplasms

Peripheral T-cell lymphoma (PTCL)

- The PTCLs are predominantly nodal-based neoplasms. Collectively, they represent the majority of T-cell lymphomas in the Western world.

- This is a group of lymphomas with wide-ranging morphology. Most often there is a diffuse proliferation of small and large cells, but small cells or large cells may predominate. The neoplastic lymphocytes are distinctive for their multilobated (cloverleaf) nuclei. Admixed eosinophils or histiocytes may be numerous. Architectural variants include an interfollicular (T-zone) variant and a Lennert-like (lymphoepithelioid/lymphohistiocytic) variant.

- Immunophenotype **F4.13**

  □ In the context of T-cell proliferations, immunophenotyping is frequently used to confirm T-lineage and to suggest clonality based upon immunophenotypic aberrancy; however, at this time it cannot be used to confirm clonality. Immunophenotypic aberrancy

may take several forms: an unnaturally large preponderance of T cells over B cells, of CD4 over CD8, of CD8 over CD4, the co-expression of CD4 and CD8, the lack of both CD4 and CD8, the loss of CD5, or the loss of CD7.

  □ PTCL is CD4+ and CD8-. There is commonly loss of one or several pan-T-cell markers: CD2, CD3, CD5, or CD7

  □ CD25 is negative

- PTCL is not associated with HTLV-1

- There is no consistent structural chromosomal abnormality, but trisomy 3 is frequent in Lennert-like variants.

Adult T-cell leukemia/lymphoma (ATCL)

- This is a peripheral T-cell neoplasm caused by HTLV-1 which is endemic in Southwest Japan, Southeast United States, and the Caribbean. Patients present with lymphadenopathy, splenomegaly, and leukocytosis. Some patients manifest a skin rash, hypercalcemia (caused by elaboration of OAF [osteoclast activating factor]), and lytic bone lesions.

- The neoplastic lymphoid cells have pronounced nuclear irregularity, producing *cloverleaf* forms.

- Immunophenotype

  □ Positive: CD2, CD3, CD5, CD7-, CD4, and CD25

  □ Negative: CD7, CD8

Cutaneous T-cell lymphoma (CTCL), mycosis fungoides (MF) and Sézary syndrome

- CTCL is an entity not specifically recognized in the WHO classification, but has been taken to refer to any primary dermal T-cell malignancy, most often composed of CD4+ T lymphocytes.

- MF is a CTCL which may later involve lymph nodes. It is an epidermotropic malignancy of small cells having cerebriform nuclei and admixed larger cells with similar features.

- Sézary syndrome represents peripheralized (circulating) mycosis fungoides, characterized by circulating cerebriform T lymphocytes. The incidence of circulating malignant cells is highest for the generalized erythroderma presentation (90%), while usual-type localized MF has a very low incidence of peripheralization. Curiously, the peripheral blood involvement is not commonly accompanied by marrow involvement, and when present, marrow involvement may be extremely subtle.

- Lymph nodes are often enlarged in MF, but their histology is usually that of dermatopathic lymphadenopathy. Later, there may be colonization of nodes by malignant T cells, first in paracortical areas and progressing to diffuse lymph node effacement.

- Immunophenotype

  □ Positive: CD2, CD3, CD5, CD4

  □ Negative: CD7 may be lost, CD8, CD25

Angioimmunoblastic T-cell lymphoma (AITCL)

- In the past, the uncommon entities known as angioimmunoblastic lymphadenopathy (AIL) and immunoblastic lymphadenopathy (IBL) were known to give rise to T-cell neoplasms which became known as AIL-like IBL-like T-cell lymphomas. It is now thought that both AIL and IBL are clonal disorders from the start, with characteristic clinicopathologic features.

- AITCL affects older adults who present abruptly with symptoms including fever, night sweats, weight loss, and generalized lymphadenopathy. Often there is a Coombs+ autoimmune hemolytic anemia and polyclonal hypergammaglobulinemia.

- The affected lymph nodes manifest diffuse effacement with a characteristic prominence of arborizing post-capillary venules, deposition of PAS+ extracellular material, and absence of follicles/germinal centers. This lack of germinal centers is key to distinguishing neoplasm from reactive lymphadenopathies. The cytology presents a mixed population of immunoblasts, lymphocytes, plasma

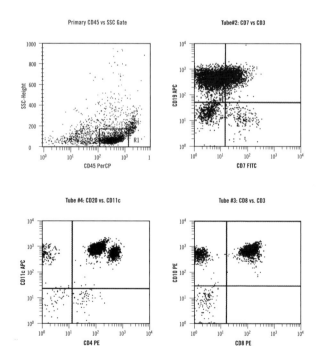

F4.13 In the context of T cell proliferations, a relative loss of CD7 (tube 2, above right) and co-expression of CD4/CD8 (tube 2/3, bottom) are examples of aberrancy

cells, and eosinophils. An increase in the numbers of CD21+ follicular dendritic cells is characteristic.

- Immunophenotype

    □ Positive: CD4 and most pan-T cell markers—CD2, CD3, CD5, CD7

    □ Negative: CD8, with loss of one or several pan-T cell markers—CD2, CD3, CD5, CD7

Anaplastic large cell lymphoma (ALCL)

- ALCL is a lymphoma of children and adults. It represents nearly half of childhood high grade lymphomas and about 5% of adult high-grade lymphomas.

- Most ALCLs have four things in common: nodal disease, anaplastic cytology, expression of CD30, and expression of Alk. There are many variations on this theme, however, including Alk– cases, leukemic presentations, and small cell variants.

    □ Most commonly, ALCL presents with lymphadenopathy, histologically displaying diffuse infiltration by large cells, many having pleomorphic nuclei containing one or more nucleoli, and a variable number of anaplastic cells (multinucleated forms, horseshoe-shaped, and Reed-Sternberg-like cells). The hallmark anaplastic cells tend to cluster near blood vessels. The neoplastic cells grow in a cohesive manner and often involve lymph node sinuses. In fact, the tumor is often initially mistaken for a carcinoma.

    □ Cases that are Alk+ and arise in children have the best prognosis overall (so long as there is not a leukemic component).

    □ Alk–ALCL is more aggressive than Alk+ ALCL and occurs in older individuals.

    □ In the leukemic cases, small cell cytology tends to predominate. The vast majority occur in children, express Alk, and the prognosis has been poor.

    □ In the small cell variant, the neoplastic cells are somewhat more uniform, and the process may be mistaken for a PTCL.

- Immunophenotype

    □ Usually positive: CD30 (usually membranous and Golgi staining), Alk (nucleus, cytoplasm, or both), clusterin (golgi), EMA, CD45, at least one T-cell antigen.

    □ Alk expression correlates with t(2;5) rearrangement.

    □ The Golgi pattern of staining for clusterin appears to be highly specific for ALCL.

    □ Negative: B-cell antigens, CD15, EBV antigens.

    □ Cases without demonstrable T antigens are called null cell type ALCL and have not been demonstrated to have any clinical differences with T-cell type ALCL. Note that anaplastic lymphomas that are CD30+ with B-cell antigen expression are classified as DLBCL.

- Molecular: the *t(2;5)(p23;q35)* rearrangement is present in > 95% of cases; clonal TCR rearrangement is present in about 90% of cases. The t(2;5) results in relocation of the *ALK* (anaplastic lymphoma kinase) gene on 2p23 to the *NPM* (nucleophosmin) gene on 5q35. Since the *ALK-NPM* rearrangement occurs regularly within the same intron, PCR has no difficulty detecting the fusion gene. Less common *ALK* rearrangements include t(1;2), t(2;3), and inv(2).

- *Alk positivity is the most important prognostic factor (favorable prognosis).*

Large granular lymphocytic leukemia (LGL)

- The large granular lymphocytes that, in healthy adults, circulate in low numbers are a mixture of T-cytotoxic and NK cells. This population expands in response to viral infection, rheumatoid arthritis, other autoimmune disorders, and splenectomy.

- LGL leukemia is a condition in which there is an unexplained sustained (>6 month) increase (>2 x 10^6/L) in LGLs. This condition has previously been called large granular lymphocytosis, T-CLL, T-γ lymphoproliferative disorder. In many cases, it is associated with neutropenia, a helpful finding when present. Most have splenomegaly. A small group experience aggressive disease that is often linked to morphologic blast-like immaturity of the cells.

■ Immunophenotype: there are 2 distinctive immunophenotypes

□ CD2+, CD3+, CD8+, CD16+, CD56−, CD7−, CD57+/− [Tc phenotype]. The distribution of CD5 in is characteristically bimodal.

□ CD2+, CD3−, CD8−/+, CD16+/−, CD56+/−, CD57+/− [NK phenotype]

Enteropathy-associated T-cell lymphoma

■ A high-grade T-cell lymphoma arising in patients with longstanding celiac sprue.

■ The development of lymphoma is often preceded by refractory sprue with mucosal ulceration (ulcerative jejunoileitis).

Hepatosplenic T-cell lymphoma

■ Splenic lymphomas account for perhaps 1% of NHLs, most being B-cell lymphomas.

■ Hepatosplenic γδ T-cell lymphoma is a well-recognized and distinct entity. It occurs in young males who present with constitutional ('B') symptoms, hepatosplenomegaly, cytopenias, and without lymphadenopathy.

■ Lymphomatous infiltrates are seen in the red pulp, and are composed of CD8+ cytotoxic T cells that express an γδ TCR, display isochrome 7q, and pursue an aggressive clinical course.

■ αβ T-cell lymphomas are very similar, except for a female predominance and wider age distribution.

■ In neither of these entities is peripheral blood or nodal involvement seen with any frequency.

Blastic NK-cell lymphoma

■ This is a neoplasm involving mainly the skin, with some cases also involving lymph nodes, peripheral blood, and bone marrow.

■ A lymphoblastic-appearing lymphoma with an NK immunophenotype expressing CD45, CD4, CD43, CD56, and the relatively unique antigen CD123 (shared only with so-called plasmacytoid dendritic cells).

■ They are nearly always negative for CD2, CD3, CD5, CD7, CD8, CD30, CD138, B-cell antigens, and myelomonocytic antigens.

■ TCR and Ig genes are usually germline. About ⅔ have cytogenetic anomalies, usually complex.

Extranodal (nasal) NK/T-cell lymphoma

■ Previously known as angiocentric T-cell lymphoma or polymorphic reticulosis, this entity is one of the causes of the syndrome known as lethal midline granuloma.

■ It is an EBV-associated vasculitis-like proliferation of neoplastic NK (CD3-, CD56+) or T (CD3+, CD56-) cells.

Subcutaneous panniculitic T-cell lymphoma

■ A T-cell lymphoma presenting as soft tissue masses and showing histologic involvement of the subcutaneous adipose tissue.

Hodgkin Lymphoma (HL)

Nodular lymphocyte predominant Hodgkin lymphoma (NLPHL)

■ Presents as lymph node effacement by a nodular or vaguely nodular proliferation of small lymphocytes and histiocytes. Classic Reed-Sternberg (RS) cells are very rare, and there is instead the characteristic L&H cell, a cell having abundant cytoplasm and a large vesicular convoluted (popcorn) nucleus.

■ Progressive transformation of germinal centers is thought to be a precursor lesion for NLP Hodgkin lymphoma.

■ Immunophenotype

□ The L&H cells are positive for CD45, CD20, bcl-6, EMA

□ They are negative for CD30 and CD15

□ Background lymphocytes are predominantly CD20+ B cells

• Classical hodgkin lymphoma (CHL)

- Morphologic types

  □ Nodular sclerosis (NS)

  - Effacement of lymph node in a pattern of nodules carved out by bands of sclerosis. Classic Reed-Sternberg and Hodgkins cells are present, but the characteristic and defining cell is the lacunar cell, a large cell with a round to convoluted vesicular nucleus and variably sized nucleoli. This lacune in which the cell is found is an artifact of formalin fixation not be seen with other fixatives such as B5. Mummified cells are also present. These large cells are scattered within a background of small mature lymphocytes, plasma cells, and eosinophils. Histiocytes, including well-formed epithelioid granulomas, are often present.

  - *NS is the most common type of HL in the Western world, commonly affecting young females. It has a tendency to involve the mediastinum more than other types of HL.*

  □ Mixed cellularity (MC)

  - *Diffuse effacement of lymph node by a mixture of mature lymphocytes, eosinophils, histiocytes, and plasma cells. Admixed are varying numbers of classic R-S cells and mononuclear Hodgkin cells.*

  - *MC is more common in underdeveloped parts of the world and in HIV-associated CHL.*

  □ Lymphocyte rich (LR)

  - *Morphologically similar to NLPHL, with the typical immunophenotype of classical HL.*

  □ Lymphocyte depleted (LD)

  - *Classic R-S cells and variants usually number >15/hpf. The background cells are markedly decreased compared to mixed cellularity type.*

  - *LD is more common in elderly patients and presents at a higher stage.*

- Immunophenotype

  □ The neoplastic (R-S) cells express CD15, CD30, fascin, EBV

  □ They are negative for CD45, CD20, EMA

  □ Background lymphocytes are *predominantly T-cells*

- HL demonstrates a bimodal peak in incidence. The first peak occurs between the ages of 15-35 and is predominated by the NS classical HL and NLPHL. The second peak occurs after age 50 and contains more cases of LD classical HL.

- HL presents with localized lymphadenopathy in the vast majority of patients. Disseminated disease is uncommon but may be seen in LD, MC, or HIV-associated HL. The cervical lymph nodes are most often affected. So-called "B" symptoms are present in some patients and include fever, night sweats, weight loss, and fatigue.

- The bone marrow is not frequently involved in HL. The incidence is highest for LD (50%) and HIV-associated HL (60%), lowest for LP (<1%) and about 10% overall. Marrow involvement usually takes the form of very focal collections of lymphocytes, histiocytes, plasma cells, and Reed-Sternberg cells, usually with a degree of fibrosis. Finding a Reed-Sternberg cell is mandatory for the diagnosis of bone marrow involvement. In the uninvolved marrows of patients with HL, hypercellularity, lymphoid aggregates, and epithelioid granulomas are not uncommon.

- HL is known for its habit of spreading via contiguous lymphatic sites. A tendency for noncontiguous spread is often manifested by LD classical HL, however.

- Mediastinal HL is nearly always of the NS type. Abdominal HL is more frequently MC.

Myeloid Neoplasms

Myelodysplastic syndromes (MDS) (T4.27)

- This group of diseases have in common: cytopenias, dyspoietic morphology, and a propensity for the development of acute leukemia. Each results from a clonal disorder of hematopoietic stem cells. The clinical presentation is reflective of progressive cytopenias—fatigue, infection, bleeding. Splenomegaly is usually absent.

Plasma Cell Neoplasms>Myeloid Neoplasms

■ Most cases arise de novo. Secondary MDS follows such things as chemotherapy (usually with alkylating agents), radiation exposure, benzene exposure, or Fanconi anemia.

■ Morphology

☐ The marrow is ordinarily hypercellular, and blasts are by definition less than 20%.

☐ Dyspoiesis is recognized within the granulocytic series as aberrant granulation and abnormal nuclear segmentation.

☐ Dyspoietic erythroids show basophilic stippling, circulating nRBCs, macrocytosis, megaloblastoid changes (nuclear:cytoplasmic maturation dyssyn-chrony), nuclear lobulation, internuclear bridging, multinuclearity, and karyorrhexis. Additional features may include ringed sideroblasts, cytoplasmic PAS positivity, and cytoplasmic vacuolization. A ringed sideroblast is defined in the WHO as a erythroid precursor with at least ten siderosomes that surround at least ⅓ of the nucleus. Acquired sideroblastic anemia is due to alcohol, INH, Pyrazinamide, lead, benzene.

☐ Dyspoietic megakaryocytes show hypogranulation, micromegakaryocytes, "pawn ball"(multinucleated) nuclei, and hypolobated nuclei.

☐ Note: In marrow aspirates from normal subjects, one can find scattered dyspoietic cells, ordinarily representing <5% any cell line, and there is a tendency for

T4.27
Myelodysplastic Syndromes

Type	Peripheral blood	Bone marrow
Refractory anemia (RA)	Anemia No blasts	Dysplastic erythroids <5% blasts <15% ringed sideroblasts
Refractory anemia with ringed sideroblasts (RARS)	Anemia Dimorphic red cell population Pappenheimer bodies No blasts	Dysplastic erythroids <5% blasts >15% ringed sideroblasts
Refractory cytopenia with multilineage dysplasia (RCMLD)	Bi- or pancytopenia <1% blasts No Auer rods	<5% blasts No Auer rods Dysplasia in >10% of >1 cell line <15% ringed sideroblasts
Refractory cytopenia with multilineage dysplasia with ringed sideroblasts (RCMLD-RS)	Bi- or pancytopenia <1% blasts No Auer rods	<5% blasts No Auer rods Dysplasia in >10% of >1 cell line > >15% ringed sideroblasts
Refractory anemia with excess blasts (RAEB)	Bi- or pancytopenia <5% blasts, no Auer rods—RAEB-1 5-19% blasts or Auer rods—RAEB-2	5-9% blasts, no Auer rods—RAEB-1 10-19% blasts or Auer rods—RAEB-2 Dysplasia
MDS with del(5q)—5q− syndrome	Anemia, normal to increased platelets <5% blasts No Auer rods	Hypolobated megakaryocytes <5% blasts No Auer rods Isolated 5q- karyotype
MDS, unclassified	Cytopenia <1% blasts No Auer rods	Dysplasia in one cell line <5% blasts No Auer rods

these findings to increase if the specimen is not immediately processed. Mild degrees of dysplasia and hypercellularity are particularly common in B_{12} and folate deficiencies.

□ Clusters of very immature cells located away from bony trabeculae or vessels are known as *abnormal localization of immature precursors (ALIP)*. This finding suggests an increased likelihood of leukemic evolution.

■ Cytogenetic abnormalities are present in about 30-40% of low-grade cases (RA, RARS) and 70-80% of higher grade cases. The most common (25%) karyotype is one with complex abnormalities (two or more clonal abnormalities), and this is associated with a poor prognosis. Second (15%) is isolated monosomy 7 or 7q–. Third (10%) is isolated 5q–, which is associated with a good prognosis.

■ Immunophenotyping has recently shown promise in evaluating the marrow for dysplasia. Certain reproducible patterns of abnormal antigenic maturation are demonstrable in these marrows. Among experienced observers, the sensitivity and specificity of this modality may be >90%, greatly exceeding that of morphology or cytogenetics alone.

■ Prognosis depends on four main variables: type of MDS, percentage of blasts, cytogenetics, and the number of depressed cell lines. With regard to type, RA and RARS are the most stable. Favorable cytogenetics include loss of Y, del(5q), and del(20q). Otherwise the overall rate of progression to acute leukemia is ~10% for RA and RARS, 45% for RAEB.

The overlapping myelodysplastic / myeloproliferative disorders (MD/MPD)

■ The MD/MPD category includes disparate entities united by the coexistence, *at presentation*, of dyspoiesis and *increased* production of mature cells. Hence these disorders have features of both MDS and MPD.

■ Chronic myelomonocytic leukemia (CMML)

□ CMML presents as persistent absolute monocytosis ($>1 \times 10^6$/mL) in peripheral blood, with marrow dysplasia, fewer than 20% blasts, and absence of a Philadelphia chromosome. The sum of blasts and promonocytes compose <20% of the marrow.

□ There may be hepatosplenomegaly, and there is often anemia and thrombocytopenia. Despite the requisite monocytosis, about half of CMMLs present with a normal or low white count, due to offsetting neutropenia. The monocyte morphology is not overtly abnormal.

□ When the spleen is enlarged, a leukemic infiltrate of monocytes is found. When (rarely) lymph nodes are enlarged, they are found to have an infiltrate of so-called plasmacytoid monocytes having an unusual immunophenotype (CD14+, CD68+, CD56+, CD4+, CD2+, and CD5+).

□ Some have clonal cytogenetic anomalies, but none that are specific for this entity.

□ CMML with eosinophilia ($>1.5 \times 10^9$/L) represents a distinct subset in which abnormalities of the TEL gene on chromosome 5 are common, often in the form of t(5;12). In CMML with eosinophilia, there may be significant tissue infiltration and damage.

■ Atypical chronic myelogenous leukemia (aCML)

□ Neutrophilia composed of a spectrum of forms (mature neutrophils, metamyelocytes, myelocytes, and promyelocytes), marrow dysplasia, fewer than 20% blasts, and absence of a Philadelphia chromosome.

□ Most have clonal cytogenetic anomalies, but none are specific.

■ Juvenile chronic myelomonocytic leukemia (JMML)

□ This is a disorder that usually affects children and presents with monocytosis and/or granulocytosis, hepatosplenomegaly, and constitutional symptoms. There is often anemia and thrombocytopenia, increased HgbF, and clonal chromosomal abnormalities (especially monosomy 7).

□ In vitro spontaneous formation of granulocyte-macrophage colonies that are hypersensitive to GM-CSF is confirmatory.

□ Nearly 10% of patients have neurofibromatosis type 1 (NF-1).

□ There must be fewer than 20% blasts and no Philadelphia chromosome.

Myeloproliferative disorders (MPDs) are the non-dysplastic proliferation of marrow (erythrocytic, granulocytic, megakaryocytic) elements, resulting in increased production of mature cells. MPD is nearly always associated with splenomegaly at presentation. All have a tendency to progress to eventual marrow failure and/or acute leukemia.

■ Chronic myelogenous leukemia (CML)

□ The Philadelphia chromosome involves a reciprocal translocation of chromosomes 9 and 22—t(9;22)(q34;q11)—in which the ABL locus at the 9q34 is translocated to the BCR locus at 22q11, producing a chimeric BCR-ABL product with enhanced tyrosine kinase activity. This is the defining feature of CML.

□ While this characteristic anomaly has been known for some time to be omnipresent in CML, the other MPDs have lacked such a marker. In fact, the absence of a Philadelphia chromosome is usually required before making the diagnosis of another MPD. Recently, a marker known as JAK-2 has been identified in the majority of non-CML MPDs (see below). JAK-2 is not seen in CML.

□ Without bone marrow transplant, most patients will progress, usually within 5 years, through an accelerated phase to an eventual blast phase. As with all MPDs, splenomegaly is common in CML. Of the MPDs, CML has the highest rate of progression to acute leukemia (95%), usually within 3-7 years. All others are around 10%. In addition, CML affects the youngest patients (average 35-50). Common to all MPDs is a platelet aggregation defect characterized by impaired aggregation in the presence of epinephrine. CML is a cause of *elevated B$_{12}$ levels*.

□ The initial *chronic phase* presents with leukocytosis due to increased neutrophils in all stages of maturation, a myelocyte "bulge," basophilia, eosinophilia, and thrombocytosis. Blasts are rare (<1%). At this stage there is the distinctively *low* leukocyte alkaline

phosphatase (LAP) score. In the marrow there is hypercellularity with an increased M:E ratio, a myelocyte "bulge," increased megakaryocytes, and reticulin fibrosis. One can easily find scattered histiocytes—gray-green crystal containing, Gaucher-like, and sea-blue histiocytes—that are merely indicative of increased cell turnover and nonspecific. One does not find a significant degree of dyspoiesis; however, dysgranulopoiesis in CML has a strong association with chromosome 17p abnormalities and may herald an accelerated phase.

□ The *accelerated phase* is marked by the emergence of one or more of the following: progressive basophilia (>20%), thrombocytopenia (<100 × 10^9/L), thrombocytosis (>1000 × 10^9/L), or leukocytosis, clonal cytogenetic progression (Ph plus +8, i(17q), +19, another Ph, etc), or increasing blasts (>10% but less than 20%). The LAP score tends to rise.

□ The *blast phase* is marked by one of the following: >20% blasts in blood or marrow, a tissue infiltrate of blasts (chloroma), or a prominent focal accumulation of blasts in the marrow biopsy. In the blast phase, 70% are of the AML type, and 30% are ALL (usually pre-B) type. Most patients in blast crisis have additional cytogenetic abnormalities, most commonly duplication of the Philadelphia chromosome, +8, or i17q.

■ Polycythemia vera (PV) **(T4.28)**

□ Presents at a mean age of 60, most commonly with manifestations—such as hypertension, thrombosis, pruritus, erythromelalgia, or headache—of a polycythemia.

□ PV must be distinguished from relative polycythemia, secondary polycythemia, and CML. Relative polycythemia is seen in the setting of stress or dehydration and has been called Gaisbock syndrome. Secondary polycythemia is associated with low PaO$_2$ states (such as smoking and living at high altitudes), abnormal hemoglobin variants, and certain neoplasms (renal cell carcinoma, cerebellar hemangioblastoma) in which there is elevated erythropoietin.

□ The erythrocytosis is usually normocytic, but may become microcytic and hypochromic.

T4.28
Criteria for Polycythemia Vera:
A1+A2+Any Other A Criterion or A1+A2+Any Two B Criteria

A1	Increased RBC mass or Hgb>18.5 g/dL (men), >16.5 g/dL (women)
A2	Erythrocytosis is primary—no familial erythrocytosis, hypoxemia (PaO_2<92%), high-affinity hemoglobin variant, truncated erythropoietin (EPO) receptor, or tumor that is producing EPO
A3	Splenomegaly
A4	Clonal cytogenetic abnormality other than Philadelphia chromosome
A5	Endogenous erythroid colony formation in vitro
B1	Thrombocytosis >400 x10^6/µL
B2	WBC>12 x10^6/µL
B3	Panmyelosis on bone marrow biopsy
B4	Low serum EPO

▫ Neutrophilia and basophilia are common, and sometimes there is thrombocytosis.

▫ The initial proliferative phase is marked by marrow hypercellularity, panmyelosis, and usually a low M:E ratio. Megakaryocyte hyperplasia is often quite prominent and may distract from the erythroid hyperplasia. Stainable iron is characteristically decreased or absent.

▫ The spent phase (post-polycythemic myelofibrosis with myeloid metaplasia—PPMM) is heralded by a peripheral myelophthisic pattern, marrow reticulin fibrosis, and extramedullary hematopoiesis.

▫ The cause of death is *most commonly thrombosis* (31%), followed by acute leukemia (19%). Myeloproliferative disorders, particularly PV, are *the most common cause of the Budd-Chiari syndrome.* PV alone accounts for 10-40% of cases. Endogenous erythroid colony formation may be seen in >80% of patients thought to have idiopathic Budd-Chiari syndrome.

▫ Red blood cell mass is measured using isotope dilution, in which a sample of patient red cells is labeled with a radioactive isotope and reinfused. The red cell mass can then be calculated from the degree of dilution of the labeled red cells. This direct measurement

of the red cell mass distinguishes reduced plasma volume from a true absolute erythrocytosis.

▫ In testing for endogenous erythroid colony formation, patient marrow is cultured. In PV, one can observe the spontaneous formation of erythroid colonies (without addition of erythropoietin). In healthy patients or those with secondary erythrocytosis, erythroid colony formation requires exogenous erythropoietin.

▫ **The JAK-2 (janus kinase 2)** mutation has now been identified in >80% of PV cases and >40% of ET and MMM. The JAK-2 mutation is a valine to phenylalanine substitution at codon 617 (Val617Phe) that appears to confer cytokine-independent growth to cells bearing it.

■ Essential thrombocythemia (ET) **(T4.29)**

▫ This is the least common MPD, possibly because its diagnosis is made only after the others have been excluded.

▫ ET has a bimodal incidence, with a peak at age 30 and again at age 60, and has a female preponderance.

▫ It has the longest survival of the MPDs, with the lowest likelihood (5%) of transformation to acute leukemia. Less than half of patients have splenomegaly.

▫ It presents most commonly as an isolated thrombocytosis, but some patients present with thrombosis or mucosal hemorrhages. Aside from variable size, the platelets are not morphologically noteworthy, red

T4.29
Criteria for Essential Thrombocthemia

Platelets >600×106/µL and megakaryocytic hyperplasia
No evidence of PV—normal red cell mass or Hgb < 18.5 g/dL (men), <16.5 g/dl (women); stainable iron in marrow, normal ferritin, or normal MCV
No evidence of CML—no Philadelphia chromosome or BCR/ABL
No evidence of MMM—neither collagen nor reticulin fibrosis present
No evidence of MDS—neither dysgranulopoiesis nor micromegakaryocytes; no del5q, t(3;3), or inv(3)
No evidence of reactive thrombocytosis

cell and white cell indices are typically normal, and there is not a significant suggestion of myelophthisis.

◻ The bone marrow shows an increase in mature-appearing, large, hyperlobated megakaryocytes which are clustered, paratrabecular, and display marked emperipolesis. ET must be distinguished from reactive thrombocytoposis that occurs in iron deficiency, chronic inflammation, asplenia, and other hematolymphoid malignancies (such as CML).

■ Myelofibrosis with myeloid metaplasia (MMM)/ agnogenic myeloid metaplasia (AMM) / chronic idiopathic myelofibrosis (CIMF)

◻ IMF is seen in older adults, usually between the ages of 60-70. About 30-40% present with unexplained splenomegaly or hepatosplenomegaly.

◻ The cellular (prefibrotic) phase is somewhat difficult to correctly classify. It presents with anemia, mild leukocytosis, and mild thrombocytosis. There may be occasional dacrocytes and nRBCs. The marrow at this stage shows predominantly hypercellularity with an increase in megakaryocytes that are both morphologically abnormal—aberrantly lobulated with clumped, hyperchromatic, and inky chromatin—and abnormally situated—in clusters found adjacent to sinuses and trabecula.

◻ In the fibrotic phase, where most patients present, the peripheral smear has a leukoerythroblastic pattern, with dacrocytosis and anisocytosis. The bone marrow is often inaspirable. Characteristic bone marrow findings include reticulin and/or collagen fibrosis, intrasinusoidal hematopoiesis, and increased numbers of abnormal and clustered megakaryocytes.

■ Chronic eosinophilic leukemia (CEL) / hypereosinophilic syndrome (HES).

◻ CEL and HES are characterized by peripheral eosinophilia (>1.5×10^9/L), often with evidence of tissue infiltration and damage, when no cause of secondary eosinophilia can be established.

◻ When evidence of clonality can be found, such as a cytogenetic abnormality or increased blasts (but not >20%), CEL is diagnosed.

◻ Lacking this, the diagnosis is HES.

◻ Causes of secondary eosinophilia include allergic reactions, parasitic infestations, collagen vascular disease, T cell lymphomas, Hodgkin lymphoma, mastocytosis, and other myeloproliferative disorders (CML, etc).

◻ The eosinophils may be hypogranular, in which case histochemical staining for cyanide-resistant myeloperoxidase (eosinophils are positive) can be helpful.

■ Chronic neutrophilic leukemia (CNL)

◻ CNL is characterized by marked neutrophilia (>25×10^9/L) which, unlike CML, is composed almost entirely of mature neutrophils and bands. Clearly, the diagnosis rests on excluding reactive neutrophilia and other MPDs, MDSs, and MD/MPDs.

◻ An absence of the Philadelphia chromosome is required. There are cases morphologically indistinguishable from CNL that have a variant of the Philadelphia chromosome productive of a variant bcr/abl protein, p230—such cases should be classified as CML.

Acute myeloid leukemia (AML) (T4.30)

■ AML is a disease predominantly of adults. It is very uncommon in childhood, but it represents a large proportion of neonatal/infantile acute leukemias.

■ While AML ordinarily presents with a very high WBC count due to circulating blasts, it may present with peripheral cytopenias, or as a soft tissue or visceral mass (so-called chloroma or extramedullary myeloid cell tumor).

■ The diagnosis of AML is principally established on the basis of a blast percentage >20% of all marrow nucleated cells. In some cases, the diagnosis can be made below this threshold, such as in acute erythroleukemia, or when certain cytogenetic abnormalities are detected (eg, t(8;21)). Additionally, in acute promyelocytic leukemia (APML) and acute monocytic leukemia, promyelocytes and promonocytes respectively are counted as blasts. Marrow percentages are to be based upon a 500-cell count, and peripheral blood percentages based upon a 200-cell count.

Plasma Cell Neoplasms>Myeloid Neoplasms

T4.30
AML Subtype Cytochemistry

Type	PAS	SBB	MPO	CAE	NSE	Auer rods
M0	–	–	–	–	–	rare
M1	–	+	+		50%	rare
M2	–	+	+	+	–	50%
M3	–	+	+	+	–	95%
M4	–	+	+	+	+	64%
M5	–	–	–		+	0%
M6	+	+	+	–	–	50%
M7	+	–	–		+/–	0%

- Immunophenotype—general features

  □ Most express CD13, CD33, HLA-DR, and CD45

  □ APML is negative for HLA-DR

  □ CD34 is present frequently, but this depends on the degree of maturation

  □ AML is usually negative for lymphoid markers, but up to 20% are positive for CD7

- AML is classified (WHO) into four main groups: AML with recurrent genetic abnormalities; AML with multilineage dysplasia; AML, therapy related; and AML, NOS.

  □ The first group recognizes the tendency of certain genetic abnormalities to relate directly to clinical behavior. For example AML with t(8;21), inv(16), or t(16;16) tends to affect younger adults and to respond well to chemotherapy.

  □ The next two groups are marked by affinity for older adults and chemoresistance.

  □ The last group represents a miscellany of *de novo* AMLs that loosely recapitulate the FAB (French-American-British) classification.

  - AML with recurrent cytogenetic abnormalities

- AML with t(8;21)(q22;q22)

- About 10% of AMLs will be found to contain this translocation, which results in the transposition of the AML1 and ETO genes. The AML1 gene encodes the α chain of core binding factor (CBFα). Interestingly, the CBFβ gene is involved in AML with inv(16) or t(16;16). This translocation may be found by conventional cytogenetics, or with greater sensitivity by FISH or PCR.

- The blasts are characterized by pronounced azurophilic granularity, sometimes having large (pseudo-Chediak-Higashi) granules, and Auer rods. Such blasts would otherwise be characterized as M2 (AML with maturation).

- The blasts express CD34, CD13, CD33, HLA-DR, many express CD19, and some express CD15. Since CD34 is a marker of immaturity, and CD15 is acquired late in development, their co-expression is anomalous and suggestive of t(8;21) AML. CD19 expression by AML is also suggestive of this translocation. CD56 is also often expressed, indicating a worse prognosis.

- Tends to affect younger adults and to be relatively chemosensitive.

  □ AML with inv(16)(p13q22) or t(16;16)(p13;q22)

- These structural abnormalities result in the apposition of the MYH11 (myosin) and CBFβ genes. This may be found by conventional cytogenetics, or with greater sensitivity by FISH or PCR.

- The resulting leukemia shows myelomonocytic differentiation with a prominent component of morphologically abnormal eosinophils. The eosinophils have granules that are abnormally large, some of them basophilic, and α naphthyl acetate esterase-positive (granules are usually negative in normal eosinophils and in the eosinophils of other types of AML). This increase in eosinophils is something noted in the marrow, but it is not commonly seen in the peripheral blood.

- The designation M4Eo (AMML Eo) was given to this morphology in the FAB.

- The blasts express CD13, CD33, CD14, CD64, CD11b, HLA-DR, lysozyme, and often express CD2.

- Tends to affect younger adults and to be relatively chemosensitive.

☐ AML with t(15;17)(q22;q21)

- This is the FAB subtype AML M3 (acute promyelocytic leukemia—APML) that is important to recognize due to its tendency to present in DIC and its responsiveness to all trans-retinoic acid (ATRA).

- The leukemic cells are abnormal promyelocytes that have kidney-shaped or bi-lobed nuclei, with cytoplasm varying from intensely granulated and replete with Auer rods to hypogranulated (microgranular variant). The microgranular variant may resemble acute monocytic leukemia. The MPO reaction is quite strong in both variants, being weak or negative in monoblasts.

- The Auer rods in APML differ ultrastructurally from Auer rods found in other settings.

- The typical variant often presents with very few leukemic cells in the peripheral blood; whereas in microgranular APML, the count is usually quite high.

- By flow cytometry **F4.14,** the neoplastic cells express CD33 strongly, express CD13 in a range of strength, and express CD15 weakly. They are negative for HLA-DR and CD34.

- CD34 expression is one of the features of so-called variant M3 (M3v). Additional features include more common expression of HLA-DR and CD2.

- The chromosomal abnormality results in juxtaposition of the retinoic acid receptor (RAR·) gene and the PML gene. Several variant translocations involving RAR· have been documented, usually resulting in morphologic APML that is relatively not as sensitive to ATRA. These include t(11;17) and t(5;17). In addition, there are three major breakpoints—bcr1 (located within intron 6), bcr2 (exon 6), and bcr3 (intron 3)—that lead to the production of three different transcripts—long, variable, and short. This last transcript (short, bcr3) more commonly has the features of variant M3 (M3v), with shorter survival and relative insensitivity to ATRA.

☐ AML with anomalies of 11q23 (MLL)

- This subtype is common in children and young adults, particularly those who have undergone therapy with topoisomerase II inhibitors.

- The leukemic cells usually show monoblastic (M4-M5) differentiation, with expression of CD4, CD14, CD64, CD11b, and lysozyme. CD34 is usually negative.

- Structural abnormalities of 11q23, which contains the MLL gene, is a finding in about 5% of ALLs and a similar percentage of AMLs. However, not all anomalies of 11q23 involve the MLL gene. Cytogenetics has limited sensitivity for 11q23 rearrangements; furthermore, cytogenetics cannot distinguish 11q23 rearrangements with and without MLL abnormalities. FISH is significantly more sensitive and is capable of making the MLL distinction. The most common rearrangements are t(9;11)(p21;q23), producing an MLL/AF9 gene fusion, and t(4;11), producing the MLL/AF4 gene fusion and common in infants.

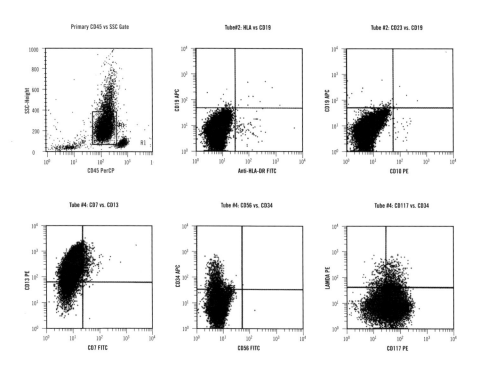

F4.14 Flow cytometry in a case of APML. The lack of HLA-DR expression is very important in this immunophenotype.

- AML with multilineage dysplasia affects mainly the elderly, often follows a period of MDS, but may arise de novo. By definition, there are >20% blasts, and dysplasia within >50% of the cells in at least 2 cell lines. They may present with any variety of immunophenotype, but are typically CD34, CD13, and CD33+. Their cytogenetics are typically quite complex, reflecting an evolving myelodysplastic substrate. Their prognosis is relatively poor.

- AML and MDS, therapy-related. In addition to the above-described topoisomerase II-related AML with MLL anomalies, alkylating agent-related AML and MDS are also recognized. They have an average latency of 5 years following treatment, and the incidence is dose-dependent. A period of MDS usually precedes the development of AML. The response to treatment is poor.

- AML not otherwise categorized

    • AML, minimally differentiated (FAB M0).

- The WHO criteria for M0 are: >20% of all marrow nucleated cells are blasts, but the blasts have agranular cytoplasm which lacks cytochemical evidence of myeloid differentiation. The myeloid differentiation, therfore, is demonstrable only by immunophenotyping (or ultrastructural cytochemical reactions—rarely available). Fewer than 3% of blasts stain positively with SBB, MPO, and NSE. The distinction from lymphoblasts is difficult on morphology alone.

- By flow cytometry, the blasts exhibit myeloid markers (CD13, CD33, CD117), CD34, and HLA-DR. Myeloid antigens indicative of greater degrees of maturation (CD14, CD15, CD11b) are negative. Lymphoid antigens are usually negative or of low intensity. TdT is positive in up to 30% of cases.

- M0 has a very poor prognosis.

- ☐ AML without maturation (FAB M1)
  - By WHO criteria, greater than 20% of all marrow nucleated cells are blasts, and greater than 90% of these are cells which have not matured beyond the myeloblast stage. The cells may display obvious granulation or Auer rods, but often do not. At least 3% of the blasts stain with MPO, CAE, or SBB.
  - The cells usually express CD34, CD13, CD33, HLA-DR, and CD117.
  - Prognosis is poor.
- ☐ AML with maturation (FAB M2)
  - In M2, greater than 20% of all marrow nucleated cells are blasts, with myeloblasts representing less than 89% of cells; that is, promyelocytes and other maturing forms make up 10% or more. Monocytic cells are less than 20% of nonerythroid cells (or else M4/M5 must be considered). Cytoplasmic granulation and Auer rods are frequent.
  - Neoplasms with this morphology may turn out to have the t(8;21) translocation, requiring reclassification as such.
  - In this variety of AML, CD34 may be present or absent, but the cells are usually positive for HLA-DR, CD13, CD33, CD117, and CD15.
  - Abnormalities of chromosome 12p may be present and are associated with increased basophils.
  - AML with maturation is frequently responsive to therapy.
- ☐ Acute myelomonocytic leukemia (FAB M4)
  - The criteria for M4 are: greater than 20% of all marrow nucleated cells are blasts, and the nonerythroid cells are composed of at least 20% monocytic and at least 20% neutrophilic precursors.
  - The immunophenotype is typically myelomonocytic: CD13, CD33, CD4, CD14, CD64, CC11b positive. A smaller population of cells may be CD34+.
  - M4 is frequently responsive to therapy.
- ☐ Acute monocytic/monoblastic leukemia (FAB M5)
  - In M5, >20% of all marrow nucleated cells are blasts, and >80% of nonerythroid cells are monocyte lineage (monoblasts, promonocytes, and monocytes).

- Monoblast nuclei are round and contain lacy chromatin, and nucleoli. Monoblasts have abundant cytoplasm that is usually basophilic, and may show pseudopod formation. Promonocytes have infolded or lobated nuclei, with nucleoli. Their cytoplasm is lighter blue-gray, and it may display granules and/or vacuoles.
- M5a (WHO acute monoblastic leukemia) exists when greater than 80% of the monocytic cells are monoblasts, while M5b (WHO acute monocytic leukemia) has fewer than 80% monoblasts.
- Prominence of promonocytes, with their lobated nuclei, may lead to confusion with the microgranular variant of acute promyelocytic leukemia. The distinction is easily made with cytochemistry, flow, and/or cytogenetics.
- Flow cytometry shows expression of HLA-DR, monocytic markers (CD4, CD14, CD64, CD11b, lysozyme), variable myeloid markers (CD13, CD33, CD117), and a usually negative CD34.
- The translocation t(8;16) is sometimes present, and this is associated with the presence of hemophagocytosis by the neoplastic cells.
- M5 is apt to affect younger individuals and often manifests bleeding disorders and some degree of soft tissue infiltration, notably gingival enlargement and CNS infiltration.
- The course is variable but the prognosis is relatively poor.

- ☐ Acute erythroid leukemia (FAB M6, diGuglielmo syndrome).
  - The criterion for M6 are: greater than 50% of all marrow nucleated cells are erythroid precursors. The WHO recognizes the more common erythroleukemia subtype, in which >20% of nonerythroids are myeloblasts, and a pure erythroid leukemia subtype.
  - Pure erythroid leukemia (true erythroleukemia, acute erythremic myelosis) includes extremely rare cases in which the neoplastic cells are immature erythroids without an excess of myeloblasts.

- Significantly more common is the type in which there are excess myeloblasts. Peripheral anemia, not erythrocytosis, is the rule, often with numerous circulating nRBCs. In the marrow, both the erythroid precursors and the myeloids are dysplastic and megaloblastoid. Erythroid cytoplasm may contain vacuoles and display globular PAS positivity (like ALL blasts are prone to do).

- The differential diagnosis includes, in addition to other acute leukemias, B12 and folate deficiency, in which the dysplastic features are not quite as pronounced. Note also that cases with >50% erythroids but <20% myeloblasts may be classified as MDS (RAEB).

- The neoplastic cells variably express CD34, HLA-DR, CD13, CD33, and CD117. They usually express glycophorin (CD235a).

- M6 responds poorly to treatment and has a poor prognosis.

  □ Acute megakaryoblastic leukemia (FAB M7)

- The criteria for M7 are: greater than 50% of blasts are demonstrably megakaryocytic either by the platelet peroxidase (PPO) technique (electron microscopy with staining for peroxidase), or by immunophenotyping (CD41 or CD61).

- There is an association with mediastinal germ cell tumors, with both neoplasms demonstrating i(12p).

- Note also that the AMLs and transient myeloproliferative disorders (TMD) that are associated with Down syndrome most often take the form of an M7 AML.

- Leukemia in Down syndrome (DS, trisomy 21). Acute leukemia in children with DS is somewhat evenly divided between acute lymphoblastic leukemia/lymphoma (ALL) and acute myeloblastic leukemia (AML). There is a many-fold increased risk of both.

  □ ALL in DS is in most ways similar to ALL in normal children, except for a reported increased sensitivity to methotrexate (MTX) and overall favorable prognosis.

□ AML in DS is peculiar in that it has the immunophenotypic and morphologic features of M7 (megakaryoblastic) AML. This subtype is unusual overall and exceedingly rare in children. DS-associated AML is highly sensitive to chemotherapy. AML in Down syndrome typically arises in young children (1-5 years of age); whereas, transient myeloproliferative disorder in Down syndrome arises in the first week or two of life.

□ Transient myeloproliferative disorder (transient leukemia). About 10% of neonates with Down syndrome (or trisomy 21 mosaicism) may manifest a transient myeloproliferative disorder (TMD). This nearly always arises in the first week of life (ranging from 30 weeks gestation to 6 months of age) with a very high white count and hepatosplenomegaly. It is somewhat difficult to distinguish from congenital acute leukemia, but when the baby has the obvious stigmata of DS, it is best to err on the side of TMD and withhold treatment. However, in many cases the child is either a trisomy 21 mosaic or, in some cases, the trisomy 21 anomaly is confined to the clone itself. Thus, in children with apparent congenital acute leukemia, a crucial first step in the evaluation, regardless of the child's morphology, is cytogenetics. The white count is initially quite high, and the blasts type as megakaryoblastic or mixed megakaryoblasts-erythroblasts. The blasts are characteristically negative for CD11b and CD13, in contrast to AML in DS which expresses CD11b and CD13. Some develop hepatic fibrosis, attributed to megakaryoblast infiltration of the liver. In others, complete clinicopathologic resolution, without therapy, is the rule. Nonetheless, about 30% go on to develop true AML, mostly of the M7 type. It has recently been reported that somatic (acquired, not germline) mutations in the *GATA-1* gene are present in the blasts of both TMD and DS-associated AML.

- Congenital acute leukemia, in contrast to other childhood acute leukemias, is most commonly (about 65%) an AML. About 25% of congenital acute leukemia is ALL, and most of the remaining are mixed. It is arbitrarily defined as an acute leukemia presenting before the age of 4 weeks and must be distinguished from a leukemoid reaction (sepsis, hemolytic disease of the newborn) and TMD. While the vast majority of congenital AML falls into the M4/M5 category, TMD usually has an M7 phenotype and, of course, trisomy 21. A significant minority (about 10%) of congenital acute leukemias have abnormalities of 11q23 (MLL).

Mastocytosis

This term encompasses a group of disorders ranging from the solitary cutaneous mastocytoma to mast cell leukemia. Types of cutaneous mastocytosis include solitary mastocytoma, diffuse erythrodermic mastocytosis, telangiectasia macularis eruptiva perstans (TMEP), and urticaria pigmentosa (UP). UP is the most common form and is characterized by oval or round red-brown macules. Urtication upon stroking is characteristic of these lesions and is called the Darier sign.

Useful laboratory tests include the serum tryptase level, urine N-methylhistamine (NMH), and urine prostaglandin D_2 (PGD2). Histamine levels are elevated but nonspecific, as hypereosinophilic states can also raise histamine.

The immunophenotype of nonneoplastic mast cells

- Mast cells are consistently positive for LCA, CD11c, CD33, CD43, CD117, and FcÂRI.

- They are consistently negative for CD25 and CD34, in addition to the plasma cell marker CD138, the monocyte markers CD14 and CD15, and the lymphoid markers CD2, CD3, CD5, CD19, and CD20.

Systemic mastocytosis

- In the bone marrow, mastocytosis appears as spindled or round cell infiltrates, usually with fibrosis and a smattering of eosinophils.

- Thus, the differential includes a wide range of entities—spindle cell infiltrates such as AILT; fibrotic processes such as MPD, HL, and HCL; round cell processes such as PLL and HCL.

- The neoplastic mast cell infiltrates are positive for CD117 (c-kit) and CD25. Expression of CD25 correlates with the presence of c-kit mutations and is indicative of malignancy. In addition, neoplastic mast cells appear to aberrantly express CD2.

Hematopathology Take Home Points

Peripheral blood manifestations of infectious disease

- Bacterial infection is reflected mostly within neutrophils. So-called toxic changes within neutrophils include pronounced primary (toxic) granulation, Döhle bodies, and cytoplasmic vacuolization. Vacuolization tends to suggest particularly severe infection. None of these findings is specific for bacterial infection, and Döhle bodies may be seen in normal pregnancy. Howell-Jolly body-like inclusions are sometimes seen within neutrophils in AIDS.

- Viral infection is usually reflected in lymphocytes. The classic atypical lymphocyte types, including Downey I-III lymphocytes, are typically associated with viral infection; however, these may be seen in collagen vascular disease and drug reactions. Plasmacytoid lymphocytes are suggestive of viral hepatitis. In Hantavirus infection, there is a characteristic pattern of findings, including thrombocytopenia, left-shifted neutrophilia without toxic granulation, hemoconcentration, and >10% immunoblastic lymphocytes.

- Infectious agents may be directly visualized in peripheral blood in a limited number of conditions.

  □ Intracellular bacteria are sometimes encountered in the peripheral blood. Only intracellular bacteria should be considered significant; otherwise, a stain contaminant is likely. This finding is uncommon and indicates overwhelming infection.

  □ In relapsing fever, *Borrelia recurrentis* can be found in the peripheral blood. *B. burgdorferi* cannot be found in the peripheral blood. The organisms can only be found during febrile episodes, they are fairly few in number, and extracellular. They are loosely coiled spirochetes, measuring about 40 μm in length with 3-10 coils.

  □ Human granulocytic and human monocytic Ehrlichiosis. The sensitivity of peripheral blood examination is much higher in HGE than HME. Nonspecific peripheral blood findings may include leukopenia and thrombocytopenia.

☐ Intracellular *Histoplasma capsulatum* may be seen in the peripheral blood, particularly in immunocompromised hosts.

☐ *Malaria and babesia* (see Chapter 3)

☐ Trypanosomiasis (see Chapter 3)

☐ In *filariasis* due to *Wuchereria bancrofti, Brugia malayi,* and *Loa Loa,* the organisms may be detectable in the blood. *W bancrofti* and *B malayi* are nocturnal, and *Loa Loa* is diurnal.

Hypocellular or acellular marrow may be due to paroxysmal nocturnal hemoglobinuria (PNH), myeloablative chemo/radiotherapy, hairy cell leukemia (HCL), hypoplastic myelodysplasia (MDS), hypoplastic acute myeloid leukemia (AML), and aplastic anemia. Causes of aplastic anemia include medications (chloramphenicol, anticonvulsants), toxins (benzene, radiation), HCV, and Fanconi anemia. Hypocellular AML, is not a specific subtype of AML nor is hypoplastic MDS a specific subtype of MDS; they are morphologic presentations. Hypoplastic AML is said to be present when the overall marrow cellularity is <20% but >20% of those cells are myeloblasts. In aplastic anemia, the cellularity tends to be much lower than hypoplastic AML, and the cells present are largely small mature lymphocytes. Immunohistochemical staining for CD34 can be extremely helpful to differentiate hypocellular AML from hypocellular MDS.

Hypercellular marrow may be seen in myeloproliferative diseases (MPD), myelodysplastic syndromes (MDS), leukemia, lymphoma, B_{12}/folate deficiency, peripheral blood cell loss/destruction, and GM-CSF therapy.

Lymphocytosis is defined according to age. In normal adults, lymphocytes comprise fewer than 20% of marrow nucleated cells, while in children, they may be up to 50%. Often, lymphocytes in pediatric marrows have immature features, with nuclear immaturity, TdT, and CD34 expression, and are called hematogones. Hematogones are present as very inconspicuous interstitially dispersed individual cells and *do not form aggregates*. With increasing age, there is a tendency for the formation of benign lymphoid aggregates in the marrow. Features of benign lymphoid aggregates include: perivascular, small size, circumscription, varied or uniform (small lymphs) composition, with or without ger-

minal centers, and, probably of greatest importance, T>B. Failure to meet the morphologic expectations of benign lymphoid aggregates—when aggregates are poorly-circumscribed, large, numerous, or cytologically atypical—raises the possibility of lymphomatous involvement. When this suspicion is present, immunophenotyping can be helpful. Any lymphoid aggregate composed largely or exclusively of B cells is strongly suggestive of lymphoma.

Osteoblasts and osteoclasts are not regularly seen in adult marrows and when present are usually pathologic, indicating bone destruction/repair. In children, they may be normal and numerous. An osteoblast is a mononuclear cell with an eccentric nucleus and can sometimes be confused with a plasma cell; however, the osteoblast nucleus lacks the clockface chromatin of a plasma cell, and the osteoblast hoff (Golgi zone), instead of being directly applied to the nucleus as the plasma cell hoff is, is separated from the nucleus by a certain quantity of normal cytoplasm. The osteoclast, a multinucleated cell, is distinguished from the megakaryocyte by having numerous distinct round nuclei rather than a single multilobate nucleus.

Serous fat atrophy (gelatinous transformation) is a term referring to a change in the marrow in which the adipocytes acquire a pale eosinophilic to amphophilic staining quality (serous atrophy), hematopoietic cellularity is decreased, and there is a myxohyaline (gelatinous) substance deposited between adipocytes. Patients with this finding have a wide range of underlying disorders—united perhaps by chronicity, debilitation, and malnutrition—including advanced malignancy, chronic infection, malabsorption, or primary malnutrition (eg, anorexia nervosa).

The postchemotherapy marrow often poses a dilemna: hematogones vs persistent acute leukemia (or minimal residual disease). Morphologic remission, usually defined as less <5% blasts, does not exclude the presence of residual leukemic cells. Below this level is what is called minimal residual disease, which may be detectable only by polymerase chain reaction or multiparameter flow cytometry. PCR is not always applicable to a particular leukemia but is particularly effective in Philadelphia chromosome-positive cases. With regard to flow cytometry, leukemias often display a characteristic immunophenotypic 'fingerprint'—an aberrancy of antigen coexpression, intensity, etc—that can be exploited to detect low numbers of residual cells. In the case of AML, examples include the anomalous expression of lymphoid antigens (CD2, CD5, CD7, CD19), or the co-expression of dyssynchronous antigens (CD34 with CD15; or CD34 with CD56). In T-ALL, the characteristic T lymphoblast or immature thymocyte immunophenotype would be very distinctive and unusual in normal marrow. In the case of B-ALL, however, the situation is more complicated. A small population of benign immature B cells (hematogones) is normally present in the marrow. Hematogones are usually few in number, but in pediatric marrows and in postchemotherapy or post-bone marrow transplant marrows, may be sufficiently increased to present a problem. Hematogones proceed through a maturation sequence, with early hematogones that are CD19+/CD10+/CD20- and later hematogones that are CD19+/CD10-/CD20+. This immunophenotypic maturational spread is the hallmark of hematogones. Furthermore, while young hematogones express TdT, the overall ratio of TdT- to TdT+ cells is greater than 1 in benign hematogone proliferations. If immunohistochemistry is applied to bone marrow biopsies using either CD34 or TdT, positive cells should not be present in clusters of >5 cells. Of course, when applicable, PCR is the more sensitive modality. The level of residual disease that is prognostically significant has yet to be settled.

Emperipolesis refers to the finding in normal marrows of megakaryocytes which have internalized other cells such as granulocytic precursors, erythroid precursors, and lymphocytes. This is to be distinguished from hemophagocytosis in which histiocytes engulf and destroy bone marrow cells. In true hemophagocytosis, the internalized cells are visibly degenerated; whereas in emperipolesis, they appear morphologically normal.

Sometimes a marrow biopsy shows extensive replacement by an apparently fibrous or spindled process. This differential includes myeloproliferative diseases (particularly ET and MMM), acute myelogenous leukemia (M7 or acute myelofibrosis), hairy cell leukemia (HCL), mastocytosis, Hodgkin lymphoma, T-cell lymphoma (AILT), metastasis with desmoplasia, or fibrosis due to prior bone marrow harvesting/biopsy.

Fever of unknown origin (FUO) in adults is defined as a temperature higher than 38.3°C (100.9°F) that lasts for more than 3 weeks with no obvious source despite appropriate investigation. The differential diagnosis is quite extensive, including infectious, neoplastic, autoimmune, and medication-related etiologies. Even in recent series, infection continues to be the most common identifiable cause of FUO. Lymphoma is the most common noninfectious cause. In published series, on average, 20-30% of cases remain undiagnosed after exhaustive evaluation. A bone marrow biopsy is often performed in these evaluations, particularly after non-invasive modalities have failed. The yield of bone marrow biopsy in immunocompetent individuals is low (in the range of 5-15%), but it is higher in HIV-infection (15-40%). The marrow should be cultured and examined for evidence of lymphoma, granulomatous disease, or stainable organisms.

Marrow histiocytes and granulomas. A mild increase in scattered histiocytes in the marrow accompanies high cell turnover states (often seen in MDS and MPD, for example). Sea-blue histiocytes have abundant cytoplasm that has a pale blue color on Wright-stained preparations. These are seen in myeloproliferative diseases, especially CML, and such storage diseases as Niemann-Pick. Histiocytes may be few or numerous in the hemophagocytic syndrome. Diffuse histiocytosis in marrow is seen in storage diseases, some infections, histiocytic neoplasms (malignant histiocytosis), and hemophagocytic syndrome. Note: Langerhans histiocytosis and Rosai-Dorfman disease (SHML) rarely involve the marrow. Leishmaniasis due to *L. donovani* or *L. braziliensis* is an example of an infection that may be identified in this setting. The organisms are visible in H&E or Wright-Giemsa stains as multiple tiny 2-5 μm intrahistiocytic amastigotes—oval structures with a nucleus adjacent to the distinct transverse bar-like kinetoplast.

Hemophagocytic syndrome (HPS, **T4.31**) is usually a disorder of nonneoplastic histiocytes, but a mild degree of hemophagocytosis has been observed in malignant histiocytosis. HPS can occur as a rare primary idiopathic syndrome but more commonly is secondary to a neoplastic (T-cell lymphoma), infectious (EBV), or autoimmune process. Clinically, HPS manifests as fever, hepatic dysfunction, hepatosplenomegaly, and low peripheral blood cell counts.

When granulomas are found in the marrow, as in other sites, the differential diagnosis depends on the nature of the granuloma. Lipogranulomas are common in bone marrow and are not usually associated with disease. Epithelioid granulomas should be considered pathologic,

311

however, and there are several variations. The cohesive aggregate of epithelioid histiocytes without central necrosis is a common finding. This type of granuloma is nonspecific, but the differential diagnosis includes sarcoidosis, a number of infections (fungi, rickettsiae, leishmania, brucellosis, leprosy), Hodgkin lymphoma, and drug reactions. A caseating granuloma is strongly suggestive of infection, particularly due to mycobacteria or fungi. So-called fibrin ring granulomas are typical of Q fever, but not diagnostic.

Extranodal lymphomas

- The most common location for extranodal lymphomas is the GI tract. The most common location within the GI tract is the stomach. Most of the extranodal lymphomas in the GI tract are low-grade. Several distinctive types exist

- B-cell lymphoma of the mucosa-associated lymphoid tissue (**MALT**) [Marginal zone B-cell lymphoma, Extranodal]. This lymphoma arises in the stomach in association with *H. pylori* infection. Immunohistochemically and morphologically, the gastric MALT lymphoma is identical to marginal zone lymphoma.

- Lymphomatous polyposis arises in the ileocecal region as several polypoid tumors composed of attenuated mucosa overlying aggregates of *mantle cell lymphoma.*

- Enteropathy-associated T-cell lymphoma (EATCL) is a high-grade T-cell lymphoma that arises in the small bowel in association with longstanding celiac sprue.

- Mediterranean lymphoma is an IgA-secreting lymphoplasmacytic lymphoma arising in the small bowel in association with longstanding helminthic infestation.

T4.31

Hemophagocytic Syndrome (HPS) vs Malignant Histiocytosis (MH)

Parameter	HPS	MH
Fever	+	+
Cytopenias	+	+
Hemophagocytosis	Florid	Inconspicuous
Nuclear atypia	–	+/+++
Clonal molecular rearrangements	–	+

Bibliography

Ahmed S. Diagnostic Yield of Bone Marrow Examination in Fever of Unknown Origin. *Am J Med* 2003; 115(7): 591-592.

Akasaka T, Ueda C, Kurata M, et al. Nonimmunoglobulin (non-Ig)/*BCL6* Gene Fusion In Diffuse Large B-Cell Lymphoma Results In Worse Prognosis Than Ig/*BCL6*. *Blood* 2000; 96: 2907-2909.

Albinger-Hegyi A, Hochreutener B, Abdou M-T, et al. High Frequency of t(14;18)-Translocation Breakpoints Outside Of Major Breakpoint And Minor Cluster Regions In Follicular Lymphomas: Improved Polymerase Chain Reaction Protocols For Their Detection. *Am J Pathol* 2002; 160: 823-832.

Amin HM, Medeiros LJ, Manning JT, Jones D. Dissolution of the Lymphoid Follicle Is a Feature of the HHV8+ Variant of Plasma Cell Castleman's Disease. *Am J Surg Pathol* 2003 Jan;27(1):91-100.

Ataga KI. Hypercoagulability In Sickle Cell Disease: A Curious Paradox. Am J Med 2003; 115(9): 721-728.

Baens M, Maes B, Steyls A, et al. The Product of the t(11;18), an API2–MLT fusion, Marks Nearly Half Of Gastric MALT Type Lymphomas Without Large Cell Proliferation. *Am J Pathol* 2000; 156: 1433-1439.

Bain BJ. The Bone Marrow Aspirate of Healthy Subjects. *British Journal of Haematology* 1996; 94: 206-209.

Bajwa RPS, Skinner R, Windebank KP, Reid MM. Demographic Study of Leukaemia Presenting Within the First 3 Months of Life in the Northern Health Region o f England. J Clin Pathol 2004; 57: 186-188.

Baxter EJ, Scott LM, Campbell PJ, East C, Fourouclas N, Swanton S, Vassiliou GS, Bench AJ, Boyd EM, Curtin N, Scott MA, Erber WN, Green AR; Cancer Genome Project.Acquired mutation of the tyrosine kinase JAK2 in human myeloproliferative disorders. *Lancet* 2005; 365:1054-1061.

Bene MC, Castoldi G, Knapp W. Proposals for the Immunological Classification of Acute Leukemias. *Leukemia* 1995; 9: 1783-1786.

Berliner N, Horwitz M, Loughran TP. Congenital and Acquired Neutropenia. *Hematology* 2004; 63-79.

Beutler E, Waalen J. The definition of anemia: what is the lower limit of normal of the blood hemoglobin concentration? *Blood* 2006; 107:1747-1750.

Bilalovic N, Blystad AK, Golouh R, Nesland JM, Selak I, Trinh D, Torlakovic E. Expression of bcl-6 and CD10 Protein is Associated with Longer Overall Survival and Time to Treatment Failure in Follicular Lymphoma. *Am J Clin Pathol* 2004; 121: 34-42.

Binet JL, Auguier A, Dighiero G, Chastang C, Piguet H, Goasguen J, et al. A New Prognostic Classification of CLL Derived From a Multivariate Survival Analysis. *Cancer* 1981;48:198-206.

Bilalovic N, Blystad AK, Golouh R, Nesland JM, Selak I, Trinh D, Torlakovic E. Expression of bcl-6 and CD10 Protein Is Associated With Longer Overall Survival and Time to Treatment Failure in Follicular Lymphoma. *Am J Clin Pathol* 2004;121:34-42.

Bohm J. Gelatinous Transformation of the Bone Marrow: The Spectrum of Underlying Diseases. *Am J Surg Pathol* 2000; 24(1): 56-65.

Bibliography

Bosch X, Guilabert A, Miquel R, Campo E. Enigmatic Kikuchi-Fujimoto Disease: A Comprehensive Review. *Am J Clin Pathol* 2004;122:141-152.

Bresters D, Reus ACW, Veerman AJP, VanWering ER, Does-Van Den Berg A, Kaspers GJL. Congenital Leukaemia: The Dutch Experience and Review of the Literature. *Brit J Haematol* 2002; 117: 513-524.

Campo E. Genetic and Molecular Genetic Studies in the Diagnosis of B-Cell Lymphomas I: Mantle Cell Lymphoma, Follicular Lymphoma, and Burkitt's Lymphoma. *Human Pathology* 2003; 34(4): 330-335.

Caraway NP, Stewart J. Primary Effusion Lymphoma. *Pathology Case Reviews* 2006; 11:78-84.

Cataldo KA; Jalal SM; Law ME; Ansell SM; Inwards DJ; Fine M; Arber DA; Pulford KA; Strickler JG. Detection of t(2;5) in anaplastic large cell lymphoma: Comparison of immunohistochemical studies, FISH, and RT-PCR in paraffin-embedded tissue. *Am J Surg Pathol* 1999;23:1386-1392.

Carella M, Stewart G, Ajetunmobi JF, et al. Genomewide Search for Dehydrated Hereditary Stomatocytosis (Hereditary Xerocytosis): Mapping of Locus to Chromosome 16 (16q23-qter). *Am J Hum Genet* 1998;63:810-816.

Chan WC, Hans CP, Kadin ME. Genetic and Molecular Genetic Studies in the Diagnosis of T-Cell Malignancies. *Human Pathology* 2003; 34(4): 314-321.

Chen Y, Tallman MS, Goolsby C, Peterson L. Immunophenotypic Variations in Hairy Cell Leukemia. *Am J Clin Pathol* 2006; 125:251-259.

Chng WJ, Lai HC, Earnest A, Kuperan P. Haematological Parameters in Severe Acute Respiratory Syndrome. *Clin Lab Haem* 2005; 27:15-20.

Clark BE, Thein SL. Molecular Diagnosis of Haemoglobin Disorders. *Clin Lab Haem* 2004; 26: 159-176.

Cook JR, Shekhter-Levin S, Swerdlow SH. Utility of Routine Classical Cytogenetic Studies in the Evaluation of Suspected Lymphomas: Results of 279 Consecutive Lymph Node/Extranodal Tissue Biopsies. *Am J Clin Pathol* 2004;121:826-835.

Cooper DS, Goldminz D, Levin AA, Ladenson PW, Daniels GH, Molitch ME, Ridgway EC. Agranulocytosis Associated With Antithyroid Drug: Effects of Patient Age and Drug Dose. *Ann Intern Med* 1983; 98: 26-29.

Cournoyer D, Toffelmire EB, Wells GA, Barber DL, Barrett BJ, Delage R, Forrest DL, Gagnon RF, Harvey EA, Laneuville P, Patterson BJ, Poon M, Posen GA, Messner HA. Anti-Erythropoietin Antibody-Mediated Pure Red Cell Aplasia after Treatment with Recombinant Erythropoietin Products: Recommendations for Minimization of Risk. *J Am Soc Nephrol* 2004; 15: 2728–2734.

Cox MC, Panetta P, Lo-Coco F, Del Poeta G, Venditti A, Maurillo L, Del Principe MI, Mauriello A, Anemona L, Bruno A, Mazzone C, Palombo P, Amadori S. Chromosomal Aberration of the 11q23 Locus in Acute Leukemia and Frequency of MLL Gene Translocation Results in 378 Adult Patients. *Am J Clin Pathol* 2004;122:298-306.

Bibliography

Crespo M, Bosch F, Villamor N, Bellosillo B, Colomer D, Rozman M, et al. ZAP-70 Expression as a Surrogate for Immunoglobulin-Variable-Region Mutations in CLL. *N Engl J Med* 2003;348: 1764-1775.

Cushing T, Clericuzio CL, Wilson CS, Taub JW, Ge Y, Reichard KK, Winter SS. Risk For Leukemia In Infants Without Down Syndrome Who Have Transient Myeloproliferative Disorder. J *Pediatr* 2006;148:687-689.

DeKleijn E, Vandenbroucke JP, van der Meer JWM. Fever Of Unknown Origin (FUO): A Prospective Multicenter Study Of 167 Patients With FUO, Using Fixed Epidemiologic Entry Criteria. *Medicine* 1997; 76: 392-400.

Delaunay J. The Hereditary Stomatocytoses: Genetic Disorders of the Red Cell Membrane Permeability to Monovalent Cations. *Semin Hematol* 2004;41:165-172.

Delgado J, Matutes E, Morilla AM, Morilla RM, Owusu-Ankomah KA, Rafiz-Mohammed F, delGiudice I, Catovsky D. Diagnostic Significance of CD20 and FMC7 Expression in B-Cell Disorders. *Am J Clin Pathol* 2003; 120: 754-759.

Dickinson JD, Smith LM, Sanger WG, Zhou G, Townley P, Lynch JC, Pavletic ZS, Bierman PJ, Joshi SS. Unique Gene Expression and Clinical Characteristics are Associated with the 11q23 Deletion in Chronic Lymphocytic Leukaemia. *Brit J Haematol* 2005; 128:460-471.

Dohner H, Stilgenbauer S, Benner A, Leupolt E, Krober A, Bullinger L, et al. Genomic Aberrations and Survival in CLL. N *Engl J Med* 2000; 343: 1910-1916.

Du MQ, Liu H, Diss TC, Ye H, Hamoudi RA, Dupin N, Meignin V, Oksenhendler E, Boshoff C, Isaacson PG. Kaposi Sarcoma-Associated Herpesvirus Infects Monotypic (IgM lambda) but Polyclonal Naive B cells in Castleman Disease and Associated Lymphoproliferative Disorders. *Blood* 2001;97:2130-2136.

Einerson RR, Kurtin PJ, Dayharsh GA, Kimlinger TK, Remstein ED. FISH Is Superior to PCR in Detecting t(14;18)(q32;q21)–IgH/bcl-2 in Follicular Lymphoma Using Paraffin-Embedded Tissue Samples. *Am J Clin Pathol* 2005;124: 421-429.

Elliot MA, Tefferi A. Thrombosis and Haemorrhage in Polycythemia Vera and Essential Thrombocythaemia. *Brit J Haematol* 2004; 128:275-290.

Emile C, Danon F, Fermand JP, Clauvel JP. Castleman Disease in POEMS Syndrome With Eevated Interleukin-6. *Cancer* 1993;71(3):874.

Escribano L, Montero ACG, Nunez R, Orfao A. Flow Cytometric Analysis of Normaland Neoplastic Mast Cells: Role in Diagnosis and Follow-Up of Mast Cell Disease. *Immunol Allergy Clin N A*m 2006; 26: 535-547.

Eshoa C, Perkins S, Kampalath B, Shidham V, Juckett M, Chang CC. Decreased CD10 Expression in Grade III and in Interfollicular Infiltrates of Follicular Lymphoma. *Am J Clin Pathol* 2001; 115: 862-867.

Bibliography

Facon T; Avet-Loiseau H; Guillerm G; Moreau P; Geneviève F; Zandecki M; Laï JL; Leleu X; Jouet JP; Bauters F; Harousseau JL; Bataille R; Mary JY. Intergroupe Francophone du Myélome. Chromosome 13 abnormalities identified by FISH analysis and serum beta2-microglobulin roduce a powerful myeloma staging system for patients receiving high-dose therapy. *Blood* 2001;97:1566-1571.

Fais F, Ghiotto F, Hashimoto S, Sellars B, Valetto A, Allen SL, et al. CLL B-cells Express Restricted Sets of Mutated and Unmutated Antigen Receptors. *J Clin Invest* 1998;102:1515-1525.

Fohlem-Walter A, Jacob C, Lecompte T, Lesesve JF. Laboratory Identification of Cryoglobulinemia from Automated Blood Cell Counts, Fresh Blood Samples, and Blood Films. *Am J Clin Pathol* 2002; 117: 606-614.

Foucar K. Bone Marrow Pathology, 2nd ed. (Chicago: American Society of Clinical Pathology, 2001), Chapters 7-18.

Frost M, Newell J, Lones MA, Tripp SR, Cairo MS, Perkins SL. Comparative Immunohistochemical Analysis of Pediatric Burkitt Lymphoma and Diffuse Large B-Cell Lymphoma. *Am J Clin Pathol* 2004;121:1-9.

Garcia DP, Rooney MT, Ahmad E, Davis BH. Diagnostic Usefulness of CD23 and FMC-7 Antigen Expression Patterns in B-Cell Lymphoma Classification. *Am J Clin Pathol.* 2001; 115: 258-265.

Gascoyne RD; Aoun P; Wu D; Chhanabhai M; Skinnider BF; Greiner TC; Morris SW; Connors JM; Vose JM; Viswanatha DS; Coldman A; Weisenburger DD Prognostic significance of anaplastic lymphoma kinase (ALK) protein expression in adults with analplastic large cell lymphoma. *Blood* 1999;93:3913-3921.

Hagland U, Juliusson G, Stellan B, *et al.* Hairy Cell Leukemia is Characterized by Clonal Chromosome Abnormalities Clustered to Specific Regions. *Blood* 1994; 83: 2637-2645.

Hasserman RP, Howard J, Wood A, Henry K, Bain B. Acute Erythremic Myelosis (True Erythroleukemia): A Variant of AML FAB-M6. *J Clin Pathol* 2001; 54:205-209.

Hoyer JD. Leukocyte Differential. *Mayo Clin Proc* 1993; 68: 1027-1028.

Huang L, Abruzzo LV, Valbuena JR, Medeiros LJ, Lin P. Acute Myeloid Leukemia Associated with Variant t(8;21) Detected by Conventional Cytogenetic and Molecular Studies: A Report of Four Cases and Review of the Literature. *Am J Clin Pathol* 2006; 125:267-272.

Ibrahim S, Keating M, Do KA, O'Brien S, Huh YO, Jilani I, et al. CD38 Expression as an Important Prognostic Factor in B-Cell CLL. *Blood* 2001;98:181-186.

Illoh OC. Current Applications of Flow Cytometry in the Diagnosis of Primary Immunodeficiency Diseases. *Arch Pathol Lab Med.* 2004; 128: 23-31.

Ioachim, Ratech. Ioachim's *Lymph Node Pathology,* 3rd ed. (Philadelphia: Lipincott Williams & Wilkons, 2002).

International Agranulocytosis and Aplastic Anaemia Study. Risk of Agranulocytosis and Aplastic Anaemia in Relation to Use of Antithyroid Drugs. *BMJ* 1988; 297: 2651-2665.

Jaffe, Harris, Stein, Vardiman Eds., *Tumours of Haematopoietic and Lymphoid Tissues* (Lyon: International Agency for Research on Cancer, 2001).

Jamal S, Picker LJ, Aquino DB, McKenna RW, Dawson DB, Kroft SH. Immunophenotypic Analysis of Peripheral T-Cell Neoplasms. *Am J Clin Pathol* 2001; 116: 512-526.

Jasionowski TM, Hartung L, Greenwood JH, Perkins SL, Bahler DW. Analysis of CD10+ Hairy Cell Leukemia. *Am J Clin Pathol* 2003; 120: 228-235.

Bibliography

Joutovsky A, Hadzi-Nesic J, Nardi MA. HPLC Retention Time as a Diagnostic Tool for Hemoglobin Variants and Hemoglobinopathies: A Study of 60,000 Samples in a Clinical Diagnostic Laboratory. *Clinical Chemistry* 2004; 50(10): 1736-1747.

Kadin ME. Genetic and Molecular Genetic Studies in the Diagnosis of T-Cell Malignancies. *Human Pathology* 2003; 34(4): 322-329.

Keren DF, McCoy JP, Carey JL Eds., *Flow Cytometry in Clinical Diagnosis 4th Ed* (Chicago: American Society of Clinical Pathology, 2007)

Kiss TL, Ali MAM, Livine M, Lafferty JD. An Algorithm to Aid in the Investigation of Thalassemia Trait in Multicultural Populations. *Arch Pathol Lab Med.* 2000; 124: 1320-1323.

Koster F, Foucar K, Hjelle B, Scott A, Chong YY, Larson R, McCabe M. Rapid Presumptive Diagnosis of Hantavirus Cardiopulmonary Syndrome by Peripheral Blood Smear Review. *Am J Clin Pathol* 200;116(5): 665-672

Kralovics R, Passamonti F, Buser AS, Teo S, Tiedt R, Passweg JR, Tichelli A, Cazzola M, Skoda RC. Gain-of-Function Mutation of JAK2 in Myeloproliferative Disorders. *N Engl J Med* 2005;352:1779-1790.

Kussick SJ, Fromm JR, Rossini A, Li Y, Chang A, Norwood TH, Wood BL. Four-Color Flow Cytometry Shows Strong Concordance With Bone Marrow Morphology and Cytogenetics in the Evaluation for Myelodysplasia. *Am J Clin Pathol* 2005;124: 170-181.

Kussick SJ, Wood BL. Four-Color Flow Cytometry Identifies Virtually all Cytogenetically Abnormal Bone Marrow Samples in the Workup of Non-CML Myeloproliferative Disorders. *Am J Clin Pathol* 2003; 120: 854-865.

Kyle RA, Therneau TM, Rajkumar SV, Jr, Offord, Larson DR, Plevak MF, Melton LJ III.A Long-Term Study of Prognosis in Monoclonal Gammopathy of Undetermined Significance. *NEJM.* 2002; 246: 564-569.

Kyle RA, Gertz MA, Witzig TE, Lust JA, Lacy MQ, Dispenzieri A, Fonseca R, Rajkumar SV, Offord JR, Larson DR, Plevak ME, Therneau TM, Greipp PR. Review of 1027 Patients with Newly Diagnosed Multiple Myeloma. *Mayo Clin Proc* 2003; 78: 21-33.

Lesesve J, Salignac S, Alla F, Defente M, Benbih M, Bordigoni P, Lecompte T. Comparative Evaluation of Schistocyte Counting by an Automated Method and by Microscopic Determination. *Am J Clin Pathol* 2004;121:739-745.

Levine RL, Loriaux M, Huntly BJP, Loh ML, Beran M, Stoffregen E, Berger R, Clark JJ, Willis SG, Nguyen KT, Flores NJ, Estey E, Gattermann N, Armstrong S, Look AT, Griffin JD, Bernard OA, Heinrich MC, Gilliland DG, Druker B, Deininger MWN. The JAK2V617F Activating Mutation Occurs in Chronic Myelomonocytic Leukemia and Acute Myeloid Leukemia, but not in Acute Lymphoblastic Leukemia or Chronic Lymphocytic Leukemia. *Blood,* 2005; 106(10): 3377-3379.

Lin P, Hao S, Medeiros LJ, Estey EH, Pierce SA, Wang X, Glassman AB, Bueso-Ramos C, Huh YO. Expression of CD2 in Acute Promyelocytic Leukemia Correlates With Short Form of PML-RAR· Transcripts and Poorer Prognosis. *Am J Clin Pathol* 2004;121:1-9.

Lin P, Owens R, Tricot G, Wilson CS. Flow Cytometric Immunophenotypic Analysis of 306 Cases of Multiple Myeloma. *Am J Clin Pathol* 2004;121:482-488.

Liu H; Ye H; Ruskone-Fourmestraux A; De Jong D; Pileri S; Thiede C; Lavergne A; Boot H; Caletti G; Wündisch T; Molina T; Taal BG; Elena S; Thomas T; Zinzani PL; Neubauer A; Stolte M; Hamoudi RA; Dogan A; Isaacson PG; Du MQ. t(11;18) is a marker for all stage gastric MALT lymphomas that will not respond to H. pylori eradication. *Gastroenterology* 2002;1286-1294.

Bibliography

Mackay IR, Rosen FS. The Immune System: Second of Two Parts. *NEJM*. 2000; 343: 108-117.

Mackay IR, Rosen FS. The Immune System: First of Two Parts. *NEJM*. 2000; 343: 37-49.

Macon WR, Levy NB, Kurtin PJ, Slhany KE, Elkhalifa MY, Casey TT, Craig FE, Vnencak-Jones CL, Gulley ML, Park JP, Cousar JB. Hepatosplenic ·, T-Cell Lymphomas: A Report of 14 Cases and Comparison with Hepatosplenic Á‰ T-Cell Lymphomas. *Am J Surg Pathol* 2001; 25(3): 285-296.

Mauro FR, DeRossi G, Burgio VL, Caruso R, Giannarelli D, Monarca B, et al. Prognostic Value of Bone Marrow Histology in CLL: A Study of 335 Untreated Cases From a Single Institution. *Haematologica* 1994;79:334-341.

Means RT Jr, Allen J, Sears DA, Schuster SJ. Serum Soluble Transferrin Receptor and the Prediction of Marrow Aspirate Iron Results in a Heterogeneous Group of Patients. *Clin Lab Haem* 1999; 21:161-167.

Miranda RN, Briggs RC, Kinney MC, et al. Immunohistochemical Detection of Cyclin D1 Using Optimized Conditions is Highly Specific for Mantle Cell Lymphoma and Hairy Cell Leukemia. *Mod Pathol* 2000;13:1308-1314.

MW Morris, FR Davey. Basic Examination of Blood. *Clinical Diagnosis and Management by Laboratory Methods,* 19th ed. (Philadelphia: W.B. Saunders Company, 1996).

Nascimento AF, Pinkus JL, Pinkus GS. Clusterin, a Marker for Anaplastic Large Cell Lymphoma: Immunohistochemical Profile in Hematopoietic and Nonhematopoietic Malignant Neoplasms. Am J Clin Pathol 2004;121:709-717

Natkunam Y, Rouse RV. Utility of Paraffin Section Immunohistochemistry for C-kit (CD117) in the Differential Diagnosis of Systemic Mast Cell Disease Involving the Bone Marrow. *Am J Surg Pathol* 2000; 24(1): 81-91.

Needleman H. Lead Poisoning. *Annu Rev Med* 2004; 55: 209-222.

Ng A, Taylor GM, Wynn RF, Eden OB. Effects of Topoisomerase 2 Inhibitors on the MLL Gene in Children Receiving Chemotherapy: A Prospective Study. *Leukemia* 2005; 19: 253-259.

Ng SB, Lai KW, Murugaya S, Lee KM, Loong SLE, Fook-Chong S, Tao M, Sng I. Nasal-type Extranodal Natural Killer/T-cell Lymphomas: A Clinicopathologic and Genotypic Study of 42 Cases in Singapore. *Mod Pathol* 2004; 17:1097-1107.

O'Brien LA, James, Othman M, et al. Founder von Willebrand factor haplotype associated with type 1 vonWillebrand disease. *Blood* 2003;102:549-557.

O'Connell FP, Pinkus JL, Pinkus GS. CD138 (Syndecan-1), a Plasma Cell Marker: Immunohistochemical Profile in Hematopoietic and Nonhematopoietic Neoplasms. *AJCP* 2004; 121: 254-263.

Ogawa M. Differentiation and Proliferation of Hematopoietic Stem Cells. *Blood*. 1993; 81: 2844-2853.

Onciu M, Schlette E, Medeiros LJ, Abruzzo LV, Keating M, Lai R. Cytogenetic Findings in Mantle Cell Lymphoma: Cases With a High Level of Peripheral Blood Involvement Have a Distinct Pattern of Abnormalities. *Am J Clin Pathol* 2001; 116: 886-892.

Onciu M, Behm FG, Raimondi SC, Moore S, Harwood EL, Pui CH, Sandlund JT. Alk-Positive Anaplastic Large Cell Lymphoma with Leukemic Peripheral Blood Involvement is a Clinicopathologic Entity With an Unfavorable Prognosis: Report of Three Cases and Review of the Literature. *Am J Clin Pathol* 2003; 120: 617-625.

Orchard JA, Ibbotson RE, Davis Z, Wiestner A, Rosenwald A, Thomas PW, et al. ZAP-70Expression and Prognosis in CLL. *Lancet* 2004;363:105-111.

Pagliuca A, Mufti GJ, Janossa-Tahernia M, Eridani S, Westwood NB, Thumpston J, Sawyer B, Sturgess R, Williams R. In Vitro Colony Culture and Chromosomal Studie s in Hepatic and Portal Vein Thrombosis: Possible Evidence of an Occult Myeloproliferative State. *Quarterly Journal of Medicine* 1990; 76(281):981-989.

Bibliography

Petrella T, Bagot M, Willemze R, Beylot-Barry M, Vergier B, Delaunay M, Meijer CJLM, Courville P, Joly P, Grange F, DeMuret A, Machet L, Dompmartin A, Bosq J, Durlach A, Bernard P, Dalac S, Dechelotte P, D'Incan M, Wechsler J, Teitell MA. Blastic NK-Cell Lymphomas (Agranular CD4+, CD56+ Hematodermic Neoplasms) *Am J Clin Pathol* 2005; 123: 662-675.

Prassouli A, Papadakis V, Tsakris A, Stefanaki K, Garoufi A, Haidas S, Dracou C. Classic Transient Erythroblastopenia of Childhood with Human Parvovirus B19 Genome Detection in the Blood and Bone Marrow. *J Pediatr Hemaol Oncol* 2005; 27(6): 333-336.

Rai KR, Wasil T, Iqbal U, Driscoll N, Patel D, Janson D, Mehrotra M. Clinical Staging and Prognostic Markers in Chronic Lymphocytic Leukemia. *Hematol Oncol Clin N Am* 2004; 18: 795– 805.

Rai KR, Sawitsky A, Cronkite EP, Chanana AD, Levy RN, Pasternak BS. Clinical Staging of Chronic Lymphocytic Leukemia. *Blood* 1975; 46:219-234.

Rao SP, Miller ST, Cohen BJ. Transient Aplastic Crisis in Patients with Sickle Cell Disease. *Am J Dis Child* 1992; 146:1328.

Raimondi SC; Chang MN; Ravindranath Y; Behm FG; Gresik MV; Steuber CP; Weinstein HJ; Carroll AJ. Chromosomal abnormalities in 478 children with acute myelod leukemia: Clinical characteristics and treatment outcome in a cooperative Pediatric Oncology Group study-POG 8821. *Blood* 1999;94:3707-3716.

Rajmkumar SV, Kyle RA, Therneau TM, Melton LJ III, Bradwell AR, Clark RJ, Larson DR, Plevak MF, Dispenzieri A, Katzmann JA. Serum Free Light Chain Ratio is an Independent Risk Factor for Progression in Monoclonal Gammopathy of Undetermined Significance. *Blood* 2005; 106: 812-817.

Ray S, Craig FE, Swerdlow SH. Abnormal Patterns of Antigenic Expression in Follicular Lymphoma: A Flow Cytometric Study. *Am J Clin Pathol* 2005;124: 576-583.

Rimsza LM, Larson RS, Winter SS, Foucar K, Chong YY, Garner KW, Leith CP. Benign Hematogone-Rich Lymphoid Proliferations can be Distinguished from B-Lineage Acute Lymphoblastic Leukemia by Integration of Morphology, Immunophenotype, Adhesion Molecule Expression, and Architectural Features. *Am J Clin Pathol* 2000; 114: 66-75.

Robbins BA, Ellison DJ, Spinosa JC, et al. Diagnostic Application of Two-Color Flow Cytometry in 161 Cases of Hairy Cell Leukemia. *Blood* 1993;82:1277-1287.

Ross JS, Ginsburg GS. The Integration of Molecular Diagnostics with Therapeutics. *Am J Clin Pathol.* 2003; 119: 26-36.

Rothenberg ME. Eosinophilia. *N Engl J Med* 1998; 338: 1592-1600.

Schlette E, Fu K, Medeiros LJ. CD23 Expression in Mantle Cell Lymphoma: Clinicopathologic Features of 18 Cases. *Am J Clin Pathol* 2003; 120: 760-766.

Sen F, Lai R, Albitar M. Chronic Lymphocytic Leukemia With t(14;18) and Trisomy 12: Report of 2 Cases and Review of the Literature. *Arch Pathol Lab Med* 2002;126:1543–1546.

Setty S, Khalil Z, Schori P, Azar M, Ferrieri P. Babesiosis: Two Atypical Cases from Minnesota and a Review. *Am J Clin Pathol* 2003; 120: 554-559.

Shastri KA, Logue GL. Autoimmune Neutropenia. *Blood* 1993; 81(8): 1984-1995.

Sibanda EN, Stanczuk G. Lymph Node Pathology in Zimbabwe: A Review of 2194 Specimens. *Q J Med* 1993; 86: 811-817.

Slone SP, Fleming DR, Buchino JJ. Sinus Histiocytosis with Massive Lymphadenopathy and Langerhans Cell Histiocytosis Express the Cellular Adhesion Molecule CD31. *Arch Pathol Lab Med* 2003;127(3):341-344.

Sotlar K, Horny HP, Simonitsch I, Krokowski M, Aichberger KJ, Mayerhofer M, Printz D, Fritsch G, Valent P. CD25 Indicates the Neoplastic Phenotype of Mast Cells. *Am J Surg Pathol* 2004; 28(10): 1319-1326.

Bibliography

Staudt LM. Molecular Diagnosis of the Hematologic Cancers. *NEJM*. 2003; 348:1777-1785.

Tajiri J, Noguchi S, Murakami T, Murakami N. Antithyroid Drug-Induced Agranulocytosis: The Usefulness of Routine White Blood Cell Count Monitoring. *Arch Intern Med* 1990; 150: 621-624.

Tefferi A. Anemia in Adults: A Contemporary Approach to Diagnosis. *Mayo Clin Proc.* 2003;78:1274-1280.

Thalhammer-Scherrer R, Mitterbauer G, Simonitsch I, Jaeger U, Lechner K, Schneider B, Fonatsch C, Schwarzinger I. The Immunophenotype of 325 Adult Acute Leukemias. *Am J Clin Pathol* 2002; 117: 380-389.

Thomas C, Thomas L. Biochemical Markers and Hematologic Indices in the Diagnosis of Functional Iron Deficiency *Clinical Chemistry* 2002; 48(7): 1066-1076.

Timura€ao€lua A, Erkan Ç, Erbasan F. The Importance of Platelet Indexes in Discriminating between ß-Thalassemia Trait and Iron Deficiency Anemia. Acta *Haematol* 2004;111:235–236.

Tischkowitz M, Dokal I. Fanconi Anemia and Leukemia—Clinical and Molecular Aspects. *British Journal of Haematology* 2004; 126: 176-191.

Trueworthy R, Shuster J, Look T, et al. Ploidy of lymphoblasts is the strongest predictor of treatment outcome in B progenitor cell ALL of childhood: A Pediatric Oncology Group study. *J Clin Oncol* 1992;10:606–613.

Tworek JA, Singleton TP, Schnitzer B, Hsi ED, Ross CW. Flow Cytometric and Immunohistochemical Analysis of Small Lymphocytic Lymphoma, Mantle Cell Lymphoma, and Plasmacytoid Small Lymphocytic Lymphoma. *Am J Clin Pathol.* 1998; 110: 582-589.

Valla D, Casadevall N, Lacombe C, Varet B, Goldwasser E, Franco D, Maillard JN, Pariente EA, Leporrier M, Rueff B. Primary Myeloproliferative Disorder and Hepatic Vein Thrombosis: A Prospective Study of Erythroid Colony Formation In Vitro in 20 Patients With Budd-Chiari Syndrome. *Annals of Internal Medicine* 1985; 103(3): 329-334.

Van Kirk R, Sandhaus LM, Hoyer JD. The Detection and Diagnosis of Hemoglobin A2'by High-Performance Liquid Chromatography. *Am J Clin Pathol* 2005;123: 657-661.

Vyasa P, Crispino JD. Molecular insights into Down syndrome-associated leukemia. *Curr Opin Pediatr* 2007; 19:9–14.

Wang LJ, Glasser L. Spurious Dyserythropoiesis. *Am J Clin Pathol* 2002; 117: 57-59.

Ward PCJ. Modern Approaches to the Investigation of Vitamin B_{12} Deficiency. *Clin Lab Med* 2002; 22: 435–445.

Went PT, Zimpfer A, Pehrs AC, et al. High Speci ficity of Combined TRAP and DBA.44 Expression for Hairy Cell Leukemia. *Am J Surg Pathol* 2005;29:474-478.

Willis MS, McKenna RW, Peterson LC, Coad JE, Kroft SH. Low Blast Count Myeloid Disorders with Auer Rods: A Clinicopathologic Analysis of 9 Cases. *Am J Clin Pathol* 2005;124:191-198.

Wolf AW, Jimenez E, Lozoff B. Effects Of Iron Therapy on Infant Blood Lead Levels. *J Pediatr* 2003;143:789-795.

Wu M, Anderson AE, Kahn LB. A report of Intracranial Rosai-Dorfman Disease with Literature Review. *Ann Diagn Pathol* 2001; 5(2):96-102.

Xu Y, Dolan MM, Nguyen PL. Diagnostic Significance of Detecting Dysgranulopoiesis in Chronic Myeloid Leukemia. *Am J Clin Pathol* 2003; 120: 778-784.

Chapter 5

Coagulation and Thrombosis

Normal Hemostasis

Normal Hemostasis Occurs in 3 Steps

Vasoconstriction is the initial reaction to a vascular injury. This is mediated by vascular smooth muscle in response to local cytokines. There are vascular diseases that can result in bleeding (eg, Osler-Weber-Rendu) and thrombosis which clinically tend to resemble bleeding due to platelet defects. Vascular causes of abnormal bleeding are not discussed in detail here.

Platelet aggregation is the second step, mediated by platelets in response to circulating and fixed agonists.

Fibrin formation is the final step, mediated by the coagulation cascade.

Normal Platelet Function

Normal platelet survival time is 7-10 days.

Mean platelet volume (MPV) tends to vary inversely with the platelet count.

Platelets are anucleate structures consisting of a cytoskeleton and granules. Platelet α granules contain fibrinogen, platelet-derived growth factor (PDGF), von Willebrand factor (vWF), P-selectin, and platelet factor 4 (PF4)—all large proteins. Platelet dense granules contain adenosine diphosphate (ADP), adenosine triphosphate (ATP), serotonin (5-HT), and calcium—all small molecules.

Platelets bear a limited number of cell-surface antigens

- The GP (glycoprotein) Ib/V/IX complex (CD42): the *receptor for vWF.*

- The GP IIb/IIIa complex: the *receptor for fibrinogen.* The platelet antigen known as PL^A is associated with GP IIIa. PL^A has two alleles, PL^{A1} and PL^{A2}. Platelet antigens bak^a and bak^b are associated with GP IIb. CD41 = GP IIb/IIIa, CD61 = GP IIIa.

- GP Ia/IIa complex: collagen receptor. Br^a/ Br^b.

- GP Ic/IIa complex: fibronectin receptor.

- The red cell antigens ABO, P, I, i, & Le (no Rh antigens).

- Class I MHC antigens.

- Passively adsorbed IgG and coagulation factors.

Primary hemostasis, referring to the platelet phase of hemostasis, consists of three steps: adhesion, degranulation (the release reaction), and aggregation.

- Adhesion (attachment to a surface) is mediated by GPIb, which acts as a receptor for vWF, and GPIa-IIa, acting as a receptor for collagen. VWF and collagen are exposed on the subendothelial basement membrane. The receptor GPIb is activated by shear forces *in vivo* and by ristocetin *in vitro.*

- Degranulation (release reaction) refers to the release of α and dense granules and the synthesis and release of thromboxane A_2 (TXA_2). This process is stimulated by any one of the platelet agonists: epinephrine, ADP, thrombin, platelet activating factor (PAF), collagen, or TXA_2.

- Aggregation (attachment to other platelets) is mediated by GPIIb/IIIa and fibrinogen. The latter is free in the extracellular space and can crosslink two platelets together via their respective GPIIb/IIIa receptors.

Normal Coagulation (F5.1)

For purposes of understanding and testing the coagulation cascade, the distinction of three phases has significant relevance. These are the extrinsic pathway, intrinsic pathway, and common pathway.

The only factor unique to the extrinsic pathway is FVII. The extrinsic pathway is initiated when tissue injury leads to the release of tissue factor (aka, factor III). Activated factor VII (FVIIa), cleaves factor X to factor Xa. Factor VIIa is capable of activating factor IX to IXa, so *in vivo* activation of VII can propel the intrinsic pathway; furthermore, this is felt to be a major mechanism by which the administration of FVIIa exerts its therapeutic effect.

Intrinsic pathway factors include FXII, FXI, FIX, FVIII, prekallikrein, and HMWK (plus calcium and phospholipids). Like the extrinsic pathway, the endpoint is conversion of factor X to factor Xa. The intrinsic pathway is initiated by the proximity of prekallikrein, HMWK, FXII and FXI to one another and to a negatively charged surface (the contact phase). This results in conversion of prekallikrein to kallikrein, which in turn activates FXII to FXIIa. Factor XIIa can then activate more prekallikrein to kallikrein, establishing a cycle. The ultimate activation of FX is carried out by the so-called tenase complex (Calcium, FVIIIa, FIXa) on the surface of platelets. Platelets, when activated, express an abundance of phosphatidylserine (PS) and phosphatidylinositol (PI) on their surfaces, facilitating attachment of the tenase complex. Factor Xa is capable of activating VII to VIIa, thus providing a link with the intrinsic pathway.

The common pathway, while conceptually distinct, is required by the intrinsic and extrinsic pathways to produce a clot. Thus, while it is possible to separately test the pathways by mental subtraction, they are not truly isolatable *in vivo or in vitro*. Common pathway constituents include FX, FII, and fibrinogen. It begins at

the convergence in the intrinsic and extrinsic pathways, with the activation of FX to FXa. Xa converts FII (prothrombin) to FIIa (thrombin), and thrombin converts fibrinogen (I) to fibrin (Ia). The so-called prothrombinase complex, like the tenase complex, forms on the surfaces of platelets, anchored by PS and PI, and consists of Va and Xa. Fibrinogen is composed of pairs of three polypeptides: A-α, B-β, γ. A and B are referred to as fibrinopeptides (FpA and FpB). **T5.1**

Control of Coagulation

The control of the thrombin concentration can be viewed as the dynamic part of this process (fibrin degradation being the other major part). At nearly every step of the intrinsic and extrinsic pathways, there are feedback loops that are activated, usually leading to the rapid degradation of the step's product. A major mechanism in the extrinsic pathway is the inhibition

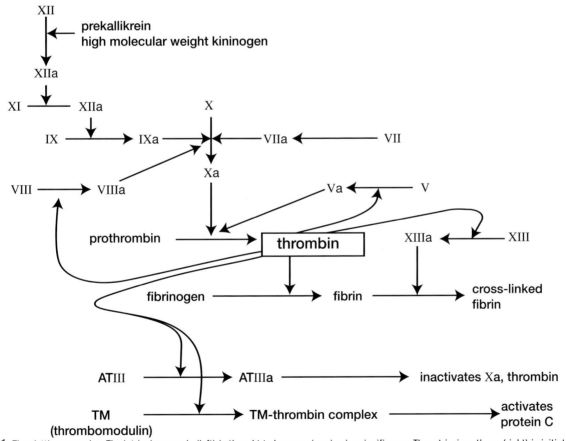

F5.1 The clotting cascades. The intrinsic cascade (left) is thought to have a minor in vivo significance. The extrinsic pathway (right) is initiated upon vascular injury, which leads to exposure of tissue factor (TF, factor III). There is thought to be a biologically significant interrelation of the extrinsic and intrinsic pathway, mediated by FVIIa crossing over and activating FIX.

Normal Hemostasis>Control of Coagulation

of the tissue factor-FVIIa-FXa complex by a protein known by several names: lipoprotein-associated coagulation inhibitor (LACI)/extrinsic pathway inhibitor (EPI)/tissue factor pathway inhibitor (TFPI)/anticonvertin. Furthermore, the activation of thrombin is directly controlled through the action of numerous factors: Antithrombin, α_2-macroglobulin, heparin cofactor II, and α_1-antitrypsin. Antithrombin inactivates not only thrombin but also FIXa, FXa, FXIa and FXIIa. Antithrombin can be further stimulated by heparin, forming the basis for heparin therapy. Lastly, thrombin combines with thrombomodulin on endothelial cell surfaces forming a thrombin-TM complex that converts protein C to activated protein C (APC). APC in turn inactivates FVa and FVIIIa, with protein S as its cofactor.

T5.1
Coagulation Factors

Factor	Other Names	Vitamin K Dependent	Where Produced	Half-Life (Hours)	% Activity Required for Normal Coagulation
I	Fibrinogen	−	Liver	100-150	30
II	Prothrombin	+	Liver	50-80	30
V		−	Liver	24	10-20
VII		+	Liver	6	10-20
VIII	Antihemophilic factor	−	Liver (Kuppfer cells)	12	30
IX	Christmas factor	+	Liver	24	30
X	Stuart-Prower factor	+	Liver	25-60	10-20
XI		−	Liver	40-80	10-20
XII	Hagemann factor	−	Liver	50-70	<5
XIII	Fibrin stabilizing factor	−	Liver	150	<5
vWF	von Willebrand factor	−	Endothelial cells Megakaryocytes	24	30
Prekallikrein	Fletcher factor	−	Liver	35	<5
High molecular weight kininogen (HMWK)	Fitzgerald factor	−	Liver	150	<5

Others are FIV (calcium) and FIII (tissue factor); activated factor V (Va) is sometimes called FVI (accelerin)

Plasmin is the primary agent of fibrin degradation, formed from plasminogen which is structurally incorporated into the fibrin clot. Tissue plasminogen activator (tPA) converts plasminogen to plasmin, and tPA is released from vascular endothelial cells following injury; thus the mechanisms for fibrin degradation and fibrin formation are set into motion simultaneously. Exposure to fibrin activates tPA. Plasmin itself is controlled by rapid degradation by α2-antiplasmin as wells as inhibition by several agents: plasminogen activator inhibitors (PAI-1 and PAI-2).

Laboratory Evaluation of Hemostasis

Laboratory Evaluation of Platelets

The bleeding time

- The bleeding time was proposed as an *in vivo* assessment of platelet function at a time when there were no other available tests of platelet function. However, the bleeding time test actually is of limited use. The bleeding time is not a useful test for predicting the risk of bleeding during surgery. The only current indication for the bleeding time is to screen for qualitative platelet disorders and von Willebrand disease. The bleeding time is expected to be prolonged in von Willebrand disease, other inherited platelet disorders, uremia, aspirin ingestion, or low platelet counts (<100,000/μL). It is currently the position of both the College of American Pathologists and the American Society for Clinical Pathology that the bleeding time is not effective as a screening test in patients without a history of excessive bleeding, including patients who have recently taken aspirin or NSAIDs.

- In the so-called Ivy bleeding time, a blood pressure cuff is placed around the arm and inflated to 40 mm Hg. Two standard incisions are made on the volar surface of the forearm. The cuts are blotted every 30 seconds until bleeding stops. The times for the two incisions are averaged. A normal adult falls between 1½ and 9½ minutes. The Duke bleeding time is based upon an incision in the earlobe or fingertip. In the Mielke bleeding time, a template is used to standardize the incision depth and length. Despite extensive attempts at standardization, however, the bleeding time test has not achieved acceptable sensitivity, specificity, or precision.

PFA-100 is an instrument that may be used for platelet disorder screening. It utilizes an artificial vessel, and under standardized flow conditions measures the time required for anticoagulated blood to occlude a standard aperture. Results are reported in terms of closure times (CT). Like the bleeding time, the CT is affected by both platelet count and platelet function.

Platelet aggregometry (platelet function tests)

- Standard pre-analytic conditions must be maintained for reliable platelet aggregometry. Generally, the assay should be scheduled in advance so that there is not a significant delay in testing. Patients should not have taken aspirin or NSAIDs for >7 days. Tubes should be kept at room temperature (cold causes platelet activation), and the test should be performed within 2 hours.

- Platelet aggregometry is performed on a sample of platelet-rich plasma (the result of slow-centrifugation of whole blood). The sample is stirred continuously within a cuvette while being exposed to various agonists, in response to which the initially turbid mixture clears as aggregation takes place. Light transmission through the sample increases as aggregation takes place. Normally there is no significant spontaneous aggregation. The normal adult displays >60% platelet aggregation in response to platelet agonists: ADP, epinephrine, arachidonate, collagen, and ristocetin. Normal newborns tend to have decreased aggregation as compared to adults.

- A graph is generated with time on the x-axis and transmittance on the y-axis. When transmittance is plotted against time, aggregation produces stereotypical curves.

  □ A biphasic curve is normally seen with low-dose ADP and epinephrine, resulting from a primary and secondary wave of aggregation, the latter due to platelet degranulation.

  □ A monophasic curve (primary aggregation only) is seen with high-dose ADP, collagen and ristocetin.

  □ The response to ristocetin is normally seen with ristocetin concentration exceeding 1.2 mg/mL. There is normally little to no response to ristocetin < 0.8 mg/mL.

☐ The response to collagen normally follows a short lag.

☐ The release of platelet dense granules, reflected in the secondary wave, can be monitored during aggregation by assaying secreted ATP using the firefly luminescence assay.

■ Abnormal aggregometry

☐ The most common cause of abnormal aggregometry is a medication. The typical result of aspirin and aspirin-like agents is decreased aggregation with arachidonate.

☐ Poor response to all agents (ADP, epinephrine, arachidonate, collagen) except ristocetin is typical of Glanzmann thombasthenia (rare).

☐ An absent secondary phase (with epinephrine and ADP) is seen in with storage pool defects and aspirin.

☐ A poor response to epinephrine is seen in myeloproliferative diseases

☐ Response to everything but risotocetin (**F5.2**) is the hallmark of von Willebrand disease. This pattern is also seen in Bernard-Soullier syndrome.

Clot retraction is a normal component of the physiologic formation of a thrombus and the beginning of wound healing. The normally functioning GPIIb-IIIa receptor is needed for proper clot retraction. Platelets from patients with Glanzmann thrombasthenia demonstrate diminished clot retraction. The *in vitro* clot retraction test was traditionally used to detect Glanzmann thrombasthenia. The blood is kept at 37° C and observed at intervals for clot retraction. Normal adults should produce clot retraction within 4 hours. When the clot retracts, it pulls away from the walls of the tube, often resulting in the extrusion of a few red blood cells and a quantity of plasma. The test is not used very much anymore.

The platelet count is performed by automated counters using impedance counting or light scatter technology. The platelet count must be within normal limits in order to interpret all of the above tests.

Platelet flow cytometry

■ Since flow cytometry is capable of detecting cell surface expression, it can be adapted to the diagnosis of most of the inherited platelet defects, particularly those in which a platelet surface receptor is quantitatively decreased. Furthermore, since platelet activation is associated with predictable changes in the expression of membrane constituents, functional defects can also be assessed.

■ Currently, antibodies are available for a variety of platelet markers, including GPIIb-IIIa, CD62 (a component of the platelet α granule that is externalized if these are properly secreted), CD63 (lysosomal granule membrane protein), and the particular conformation of fibrinogen assumed only within the GPIIb-IIIa receptor.

Laboratory Evaluation of Coagulation

Activated clotting time (ACT)

■ The ACT is a point-of-care test that can be used to monitor high-dose heparin therapy, particularly at ranges where the aPTT is immeasurable (>150 seconds). This has utility in bypass surgery as well as in other instances when an immediate result is desired (dialysis, etc). If time permits, an anti-Xa assay is a favorable alternative to the ACT. The ACT is performed on whole blood. Blood is collected into a tube that contains an intrinsic pathway activator (kaolin, glass, etc) and an analyzer measures the clotting time.

■ In a normal adult, the ACT runs about 70 to 180 seconds. In high dose heparin therapy, a time of >400 seconds is often sought.

■ The ACT is less precise than the aPTT, and, since it is performed on whole blood, a number of noncoagulation factors (platelet count, hematocrit, etc) influences it.

Activated partial thromboplastin time (aPTT)

■ Phospholipid, a contact activator of FXII (silica, kaolin, etc), and excess calcium are added to citrated plasma. The time to clot formation is the PTT.

■ The aPTT can be used to screen for factor deficiency.

Normal Hemostasis>Laboratory Evaluation of Coagulation

□ Prolongation of the PTT is caused by deficiencies of factors XII, XI, IX, VIII (intrinsic pathway constituents), X, V, II, or fibrinogen (common pathway) or by an inhibitor.

□ Prolongation of both the PT and PTT is caused by deficiencies of factors X, V, II, or fibrinogen (the common pathway) or an inhibitor.

□ A factor generally must be below 30% to cause a prolonged PTT. With multiple factor deficiencies, higher levels may shorten the PTT. The PTT is more sensitive to deficiencies in intrinsic pathway factors than common pathway factors.

□ An elevated FVIII level is capable of shortening the PTT.

■ The PTT is used to monitor heparin therapy (unfractionated heparin) **T5.2**. With very high doses of heparin, as used in cardiac bypass surgery, the aPTT is unmeasurable (often reported as >150 seconds). In this circumstance, the ACT is often used. The aPTT may also be used to monitor hirudin or argatroban. Xa assays are used to monitor therapy with low molecular weight heparins and to monitor unfractionated heparin in circumstances where the PTT is unreliable.

□ The therapeutic PTT range for heparin is generally that which corresponds to anti-Xa level of 0.3-0.7 U/mL.

□ In some patients, heparin fails to prolong the PTT (heparin resistance). Often this is due to an acute phase response (combined effect of increased FVIII and binding of heparin by acute phase reactants) or antithrombin deficiency.

■ Determining the cause of a prolonged aPTT **T5.3**

□ The first step is to exclude the effect of heparin through the use of a heparin neutralization procedure.

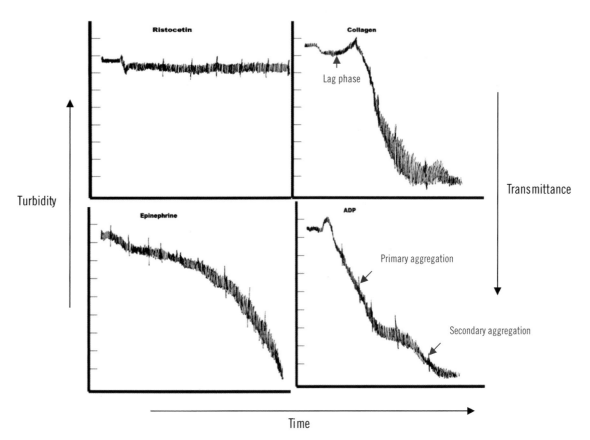

F5.2 Platelet aggregometry in a patient with von Willebrand disease.

T5.2
Sources of Error in the aPTT Monitoring of Anticoagulation

The aPTT may overestimate the degree of anticoagulation (be inappropriately prolonged)	The aPTT may underestimate the degree of anticoagulation (be inappropriately shortened)
Antiphospholipid syndrome Liver disease Inherited factor deficiencies DIC	Post-thrombosis acute phase reaction Pregnancy ATIII deficiency Renal disease (acquired ATIII deficiency) Congenitally high factor VIII
Check	**Check**
Lupus anticoagulant factor levels D-dimer	ATIII levels FVIII levels

□ If heparin neutralization does not correct the aPTT, then a mixing study (see below) is performed.

□ *If a mixing study fails to correct the aPTT, then an inhibitor is suspected (lupus anticoagulant, anti-factor VIII antibody).*

□ *If a mixing study corrects the aPTT, then a factor deficiency is suspected. Specific assays for factors activities (XII, XI, IX, VIII) can be performed. If these are* normal, consider common factor assays and/or a test for lupus anticoagulant (weak inhibitors sometimes correct in a 1:1 mix).

□ Mixing studies may be performed to help determine the cause of prolonged clotting times (PT, PTT, or TT) and to screen for inhibitors.

□ The patient's plasma is mixed with normal plasma, in 1:1 proportions, and the abnormal test (eg PTT) is repeated, both immediately and after a 1-2 hour incubation.

T5.3
Causes of a Prolonged PTT

Etiology	Protime	Additional tests
Deficiencies of FXII, XI, IX, VIII, pre-kallikrein, HMWK	Normal	Specific factor assays
Deficiencies of FX, V, II	Prolonged	Specific factor assays
Lupus anticoagulant	Normal or prolonged (PTT>PT)	LAC assay
Anti-FVIII antibody	Normal	Anti-FVIII antibody assay
Heparin	Usually normal (PTT>PT)	Heparin neutralization procedure
Hirudin	Prolonged	History
DIC	Prolonged (PT>PTT)	D-dimer
Liver disease	Prolonged (PT>PTT)	History, LFTs
Vitamin K deficiency / coumadin	Prolonged (PT>PTT)	Assays for II, VII, IX, X show selective decrease

□ A 1:1 mix results in at least 50% activity of all clotting factors. Correction of the clotting time is the expected result if the prolongation is due to any factor deficiency. Anything less than complete correction to within the normal range suggests an inhibitor.

□ Some inhibitors show a correction in the immediate aPTT, but prolongation of the incubated aPTT. This is particularly a feature of antibodies against specific factors (eg, anti-FVIII antibody).

□ A 4:1 (4 parts patient plasma to 1 part normal plasma) mix has been advocated for the detection of weak inhibitors. Some inhibitors, especially weak ones, will correct with a 1:1 mix and may be missed. When a percent correction was calculated in one study, a percent correction cutoff of 50% in a 4:1 mix had a 100% sensitivity and 88% specificity for inhibitor. The sensitivity and specificity both approached 100% if a 10% cutoff is applied after incubation for 1 hour. For the 1:1 mix, the results were poor with any cutoff, with cutoffs of <58% indicating inhibitor, and >70% indicating deficiency.

$$\% \text{ correction} = \frac{(\text{Patient clotting time} - \text{Mix clotting time})}{(\text{Patient clotting time} - \text{Normal clotting time})}$$

□ In the past, mixing with various blood products was useful in determining the identity of a missing factor. For example, aged plasma lacks factors II, V, VIII, XIII. When a prolonged clotting test corrects with aged plasma, the prolongation cannot be due to any of these factors. Adsorbed plasma lacks factors II, VII, IX, X. Serum lacks fibrinogen and factors II, V, VIII, XIII.

□ For all clot-based assays, including the aPTT, plasma should be separated from cells as soon as possible. This is particularly true when the PTT is being used for heparin monitoring, since platelets begin to release platelet factor 4 (PF4) which can artifactually shorten the PTT. The plasma should be kept cool until testing is completed (to minimize loss of coagulation factors). If testing will be delayed > 4 hours, the specimen should be frozen.

□ The normal neonate has a PTT up to 55 seconds. This shortens to the adult range by 6 months of age.

Activated protein C resistance (APCR) screening assay

■ Activated protein C (APC) exerts its anticoagulant properties through the degradation of activated factors V and VIII. APC cleaves FVa and FVIIIa at specific arginine residues, but the factor V Leiden mutation results in substitution of glutamine for arginine at one of the cleavage sites, leading to a form of FV that is resistant to APC degradation.

■ In the clot-based APCR assay, the patient's plasma is first diluted 1:5 with reagent FV-deficient plasma. Then the PTT is measured under two separate conditions: first, with no added protein C; second, after the addition of activated protein C. In normal adults, the ratio of the second PTT to the first PTT (sensitivity ratio) should be >2:1.

■ If the sensitivity ratio is <2, then APCR is suggested. The sensitivity of this assay, of course, depends on the cut-off used.

■ Note that normal neonates have protein C resistance due to low endogenous protein C levels. A modification of this technique, using an initial 1:11 dilution, has been recommended for neonates and infants under 6 months.

■ The presence of a lupus anticoagulant can affect the reliability of this assay and is one of the indications for a DNA-based assay.

Anti-cardiolipin antibody (ACA)—IgG, IgA, & IgM.

■ In order to diagnose the antiphospholipid syndrome (see below), one must demonstrate either anti-cardiolipin (ACA) antibody or lupus anticoagulant (LAC). ACA tests are usually ELISA-based, and LAC tests are clot-based.

■ About 80% of patients with the antiphospholipid syndrome have ACA.

■ ACA should be tested in a β_2 glycoprotein I (β_2-GPI)-dependent manner. Many anti-cardiolipin antibodies are directed against cardiolipin bound to β_2-glycoprotein I, and while other ACAs and ACA assays exist, it is the β_2-GPI-linked antigen that appears to be clinically significant. Non-β_2-GPI-linked ACAs are of doubtful clinical significance at this time.

□ Syphilis, Q fever, and HIV infection can produce a false-positive ACA test (usually an IgM ACA). Furthermore, the anti-cardiolipin antibody may produce a false-positive syphilis test (RPR).

Anti-Xa assay (heparin antifactor Xa assay)

■ The anti-Xa assay can be used to monitor either unfractionated or low molecular weight heparin (LMWH). It is the test of choice for monitoring low molecular weight heparins and danaparoid. It is a useful alternative to the aPTT for monitoring unfractionated heparin, particularly in patients having abnormal baseline coagulation studies due to LAC, FXII deficiency, etc.

■ Blood should be drawn 4 hours after a dose of LMWH; 6 hours after danaparoid.

■ In the chromogenic assay, the patient's plasma is added to a known amount of factor Xa with excess antithrombin. Heparin (or danaparoid) in the patient's plasma stimulates anti-thrombin to inhibit factor Xa. The quantity of residual factor Xa is measured with a chromogenic substrate which Xa cleaves to produce a colored compound that is detected by a spectropho-tometer. The residual Xa is subtracted from the initial Xa to determine the anticoagulant concentration (expressed in antifactor Xa units/mL). Thus, when there has been no heparin administered, the antifactor Xa should be zero. The higher the heparin (or dana-paroid), the higher the antifactor Xa.

■ Unlike unfractionated heparin, LMWH and dana-paroid do not require strict monitoring in most patients. Monitoring may be required in renal failure, pregnancy, extremes of weight, and in children (particularly neonates).

Antithrombin (AT, previously antithrombin III)

■ 100% activity is by definition normal, but any level above 60% is essentially normal. In neonates, antithrombin levels are much lower (>40% is normal), increasing to adult values within 6 months. In adults, heparin will lead to decreased AT, but rarely <70%. Over the age of 6 months, an AT level <60%, even in heparinized patients, is abnormal. Acquired AT defi-ciency is more common in clinical practice than inher-ited deficiency and is seen in nephrotic syndrome, L-asparaginase therapy, liver failure, acute thrombosis, and DIC.

■ There are two varieties of AT assays: functional and antigenic. Of the two, the functional assay yields more clinically useful information. If the result is abnormal, one may elect to perform an antigenic assay to distin-guish types I and II inherited AT deficiency. Functional assays are usually chromogenic and based upon the antithrombin's ability to inhibit thrombin and Xa. These are performed by adding patient plasma to heparin, a known quantity of either thrombin or Xa, and a chromogenic substrate. Any uninhibited thrombin (or Xa) will convert the substrate to a colored product that can be measured spectrophoto-metrically. The quantity of product is inversely propor-tional to the antithrombin activity.

Bethesda assay (factor VIII inhibitor assay, anti-FVIII antibody assay)

■ While FVIII is the most common factor to which anti-bodies arise; this assay can be adapted to any factor (anti-FV, anti-FIX, etc).

■ Anti-FVIII antibodies (FVIII inhibitors) have the following properties:

□ In coagulation screening assays, they behave as inhibitors; that is, they prolong the aPTT and fail to correct in a 1:1 mix

□ While the immediate aPTT following a 1:1 mix may correct, the aPTT performed after 1-hour incubation will be prolonged.

□ If factor assays are performed, FVIII will appear decreased. If serial dilutions are performed, each dilution will show progressively *more* FVIII activity.

□ In contrast to the most common inhibitor, the lupus anticoagulant, patients with factor inhibitors tend to have severe bleeding.

■ The Bethesda assay is performed by first making several dilutions of the patient's plasma with citrated saline. Each dilution is then mixed 1:1 with normal plasma and incubated for 1-2 hours. Factor VIII activity assays are then performed on each dilution. The dilution at which the FVIII activity is 50% represents the inhibitor titer. The result is expressed in Bethesda units (if the 1:160 dilution results in 50% factor activity, then the result is 160 Bethesda units).

Normal Hemostasis>Laboratory Evaluation of Coagulation

- Since one of the major therapeutic options in patients with anti-FVIII antibodies is the use of porcine FVIII, it can be helpful to know whether the patient's antibody will cross-react with the porcine product. Porcine factor VIII can be substituted for normal plasma in the above-described assay to make this determination.

Clot stability test (urea solubility test, factor XIII deficiency screen)

- When fibrinogen is converted into fibrin monomers, these associate through the formation of relatively weak noncovalent hydrogen bonds. It is the function of factor XIII to generate covalent bonds between fibrin monomers, thus stabilizing the clot.

- This test looks at the ability of an *in vitro* clot to withstand degradation by 5M urea. In patients with >1%-2% FXIII activity, the clot should be stable for >24 hours; thus, this test is mainly for detecting homozyotes.

- The test is only valid if fibrinogen is qualitatively and quantitatively normal. This test will not detect heterozygotes

- Abnormal results should be confirmed by quantitative FXIII activity.

D-dimer and fibrin-degradation products (FDPs)

- D-dimer is a type of fibrin-degradation product (FDP) or fibrin split product (FSP). D-dimer is formed only by plasmin-mediated degradation of fibrin. It is not formed in the plasmin-mediated degradation of fibrinogen (which produces fibrinogen degradation products). Thus, the presence of D-dimer indicates that fibrin has been formed and then degraded. Assays for FDPs are a little less specific, because they detect fibrin degradation products, fibrinogen degradation products, and D-dimer.

- D-dimers and FDP can be positive with DIC, thrombosis, or significant bleeding. They may also be elevated in cirrhotic patients who, due to difficulty in clearance of these products, may have persistent low-level chronic DIC. Patients with certain tumors, particularly mucin-secreting adenocarcinomas, may have elevated D-dimer and FDP.

- A normal D-dimer largely (90%) excludes an ongoing *in vivo* thrombosis. Sensitive varieties of the d-dimer assay can be used to exclude deep venous thrombosis and pulmonary embolism. D-dimer assays are most useful in patients with a low probability, based upon clinical parameters, of acute thromboembolic disease, as evidence against PE. A positive D-dimer is relatively nonspecific in this setting, but some would consider this an indication for further radiographic testing to exclude PE.

- Assays

  □ Latex agglutination assays are available for FDPs and D-dimers. Patient plasma is mixed with latex particles that are coated with anti-FDP or anti-D-dimer antibodies. If these are present, the latex particles will agglutinate as visible particles. Positive specimens can be serially diluted to provide a semi-quantitative FDP or D-dimer titer. Automated versions of this assay, capable of providing quantitative results, are also available.

  □ ELISA assays are available which can provide quantitative FDP or D-dimer measurements.

Factor assays (II, V, VII, VIII, IX, X, XI, XII)

- Specific factors can be assayed directly.

  □ The patient's plasma is mixed with reagent plasma having a known factor deficiency.

  □ The resulting PT or PTT of this mixture can be compared to a standard curve, generated by plotting known factor levels against clotting times. Factor VIII, IX, XI, and XII assays are PTT-based. Factor II, VII, and X assays are PT-based. Factor V can be either.

  □ Serial dilutions are usually performed. An inhibitor is suggested if serial dilutions result in an apparent increase in factor activity.

  □ Chromogenic assays and antigenic assays are available for some factors (II, VII, VIII, IX, X).

- Factor assays are usually performed when a screening assay (PT, PTT, TT) is prolonged and mixing studies indicate a deficiency (full correction in a 1:1 mix). The specific factors assayed depend upon the screening test.

  □ Prolonged PTT, normal PT: factors XII, XI, IX, VII.

  □ Normal PTT, prolonged PT: factor VII

  □ *In addition, consider common pathway constituents (I, II, X, V), since the PTT is insensitive to mild-moderate common factor deficiencies. Thus, these can sometimes produce a prolonged PT with normal PTT.*

  □ *Also, since coumadin is a common cause of a prolonged PT with normal PTT, it is often helpful to simultaneously assay other vitamin K-dependent factors (II, VII, IX, X).*

  □ Prolonged PT and PTT: factors I, II, X, V (common pathway). Consider performing additional factors, as multiple factor deficiencies can produce this pattern.

- In clinical practice, isolated inherited factor deficiencies are less common than multiple acquired factor deficiencies (eg, DIC, liver disease, coumadin, etc). Even when an apparent isolated factor deficiency is found, one must consider an acquired inhibitor (eg, anti-factor VIII antibody) **T5.4**.

- The plasma should be separated as soon as possible, preferably within 2 hours. Plasma that cannot be tested within 4 hours should be frozen.

- Results are expressed as percent activity. Normal plasma, by definition, contains 100% activity (1 U/mL) for each factor; however, in actuality results for normal adults usually fall between 60% to 150%.

- With the exception of FVIII, all factors are relatively low in neonates, reaching adult levels by 6 months of age.

Fibrinogen activity

- There are several assays for fibrinogen activity. The most common assays (the Clauss assay and the Ellis assay) are very similar to the thrombin time (see below). In the Clauss assay, the patient's plasma is diluted before the addition of excess thrombin. The lower the fibrinogen, the longer the clotting time. When compared to a standard curve, the fibrinogen activity can be determined.

T 5.4
Multiple Factor Deficiencies

Condition	Prolonged clotting times	Comment
DIC	PT and PTT	All factors decreased
Coumadin / vitamin K deficiency	PT >> PTT	Decreased FII, VII, IX, X; FVII is earliest deficiency
Liver disease	PT >> PTT	Most factors decreased, often normal FVII, XI, XII
Heparin	PT << PTT	Inhibits factors II, X, IX, XI, XII
Hirudin	PT and PTT	
Lupus anticoagulants (LAC)	PT << PTT	Inhibits assays that are phospholipid dependent. Nearly all levels appear decreased. Activities increase with serial dilution.
Degraded specimen (eg, delayed transport)	PT and PTT, sometimes PT < PTT	Loss of labile factors V and VIII
Nephrotic syndrome	PT < PTT	Loss of factor XI and XII (loss of ATIII shifts balance in favor of thrombosis, however)
Amyloidosis	PT and PTT, sometimes PT > PTT	Chelates FX

- In addition to specific fibrinogen assays, dys- and afibrinogenemia result in prolonged PT and PTT. The thrombin time and Reptilase time are prolonged as well.

Lupus anticoagulant (LAC) assays

- In order to diagnose the antiphospholipid syndrome (see below), one must demonstrate either anti-cardiolipin (ACA) antibody or lupus anticoagulant (LAC), on two separate occasions (8-12 weeks apart).

- Lupus anticoagulant tests are clot-based assays, based upon the observation that LACs can prolong phospholipid-dependent clotting times. In order to diagnose an LAC, one must demonstrate both:

  □ Prolongation of a phospholipid-dependent clotting time, and

  □ Correction of the clotting time with excess phospholipid.

- Either the activated partial thromboplastin time (aPTT) or the dilute Russell viper venom time (DRVVT) may be used for this purpose.

- In patients receiving oral anticoagulation, the plasma should be mixed with normal plasma (to correct factor deficiencies) before testing.

Plasminogen activator inhibitor type 1 (PAI-1) activity

- Decreased PAI-1 is a cause of abnormal bleeding, usually coagulation-type.

- Increased PAI-1is a cause of abnormal thrombosis, usually arterial-type.

- In the patient with recent abnormal thrombosis, it is best to wait 2 weeks or more before testing, as PAI-1 is a highly reactive acute-phase reactant. Tests of PAI-1 activity are best performed parallel with a C-reactive protein as a 'control' for this possibility.

- PAI-1 shows moderate diurnal variation, with levels highest in the morning and lowest in the evening. Standardization is best achieved by drawing samples between 0800-0900 (and certainly not outside 0700-1000). This will be compared with normal ranges based on 0800-0900 samples.

- Plasminogen activator inhibitor type 1 (PAI-1) antigen essentially parallels activity, and all the caveats regarding PAI-1 activity apply.

Protein C activity

- This is the preferred test for protein C deficiency.

- The patient should be off anticoagulants for >1 week and >1 month post-thrombosis.

- Blood drawn prior to initiation of anticoagulant therapy can be useful if the activity is within the normal range, but low levels in this setting should be confirmed at a later time.

- Protein C antigen essentially parallels protein C activity; however, there are types of protein C deficiency characterized by functional defects in quantitatively adequate protein C antigen. Some have used the protein C activity in conjunction with the protein C antigen to subclassify patients into quantitative (type I) and qualitative (type II) protein C deficiencies, but this is of little clinical significance.

Protein S activity

- This is the preferred test for protein S deficiency.

- Protein S activity (and antigen) normally decrease substantially in pregnancy. Normal ranges for protein S activity in pregnancy are as follows:
  1st trimester—50%-100%; 2nd trimester—25%-75%; 3rd trimester—20%-50%.

- Protein S antigen essentially parallels protein S activity, but as in the case of protein C there are types of congenital activity deficiency with low protein S antigen (quantitative or type I protein S deficiency) and types with normal protein S antigen (functional or type II protein S deficiency). Again, it is of no clinical importance to distinguish the two. Protein S circulates bound to C4b with a small proportion of free protein S. The free moiety is the ideal measurement, but total can also be assayed. In pregnancy, the normal ranges are:
  1st trimester—60%-100%; 2nd trimester—50%-130%; 3rd trimester—40%-90%.

Prothrombin variant (prothrombin 20210) test is a DNA-based test to determine whether the patient is harboring the abnormal allele 20210A or is homozygous for the normal allele 20210G. The variant allele is present in up to 20% of Dutch-ancestried patients with thrombosis.

Prothrombin fragment 1+2 (PF 1+2). A product of prothrombin activation, PF 1+2 is an excellent marker for incipient or ongoing *in vivo* thrombosis.

Prothrombin time (PT)

- A source of tissue factor and phospholipid (thromboplastin) is added to citrated plasma with excess calcium. The time to clot formation is the PT.

- Prolongation of the PT is caused by deficiencies of factors VII as well as common factor deficiencies (X, V, II, or fibrinogen) and inhibitors.

- While it seems intuitive that a common pathway factor deficiency should prolong the PT and PTT equally, in fact the PT is more sensitive to common pathway factor deficiencies than is the PTT. Thus, these deficiencies are sometimes associated with a prolonged PT and normal PTT.

- The PT is used to monitor warfarin (coumadin) therapy.

- Variations among thromboplastins result in differing sensitivity to coumadin and can result in differing PT results for the same level of anticoagulation. For this reason, the international sensitivity index (ISI) and international normalized ratio (INR) were invented. The manufacturer provides the ISI, based on comparisons between their thromboplastin and an international reference thromboplastin. A laboratory should calibrate/confirm the ISI locally through the use of a reference plasma and seek to use higher sensitivity reagents (low ISI reagents). When you use this manufacturer's thromboplastin in your lab to determine a PT, the INR is calculated as follows:

$$INR = (PT_{measured}/PT_{mean})^{ISI}$$

- Note that the INR is meant to reduce interlaboratory variation that results from differing thromboplastin sensitivities to coumadin. The INR is mainly valid as a standardizing calculation in *coumadinized* patients with PTs in the low range. In other clinical scenarios, the INR does not seek to nor does it succeed in reducing interlaboratory variation.

- Chromogenic factor X assays are useful for monitoring warfarin in the presence of a lupus anticoagulant, hirudin, or argatroban. In these circumstances, the INR can overestimate the amount of coumadinization, leading to inappropriate dosing. The chromogenic assay for factor X is not affected by these agents. The laboratory must establish a curve that correlates factor X levels with INRs.

Thrombin time (TT)

- Thrombin is added to patient plasma. The time to clot formation is the thrombin time.

- Prolongation of the TT is caused by deficiency of fibrinogen, defective fibrinogen (dysfibrinogenemia), or an inhibitor such as heparin, hirudin, argatroban, or fibrin degradation products (FDPs). In dysfibrinogenemia, both the thrombin time and reptilase time are prolonged (whereas inhibitors such as heparin do not affect the reptilase time).

- A prolongation of both the TT and reptilase time may also be caused by amyloidosis.

- The thrombin time can be used to determine that heparin is present in a specimen, as a cause of a prolonged PTT. The TT is exquisitely sensitive to the presence of heparin, and the other main cause of prolongation, dysfibrinogenemia, is very rare. If the TT is prolonged, the presence of heparin can be confirmed by either the reptilase time or a mixing study. The reptilase time, a test of the same portion of the coagulation cascade *that is unaffected by heparin,* is normal in the presence of heparin. Alternatively the plasma can be mixed 1:1 with normal plasma. A 1:1 mix will fail to correct in the presence of heparin, but it will correct with dysfibrinogenemia. Note that these results can also be obtained with hirudin, argatroban, or FDPs. More commonly, a heparin neutralization procedure is used for this purpose.

- Distinguishing dysfibrinogenemia from hypofibrinogenemia is difficult but of some clinical importance. In this regard, it is important to remember that an abnormal molecular form of fibrinogen (dysfibrinogenemia) is a bit of an inhibitor and will therefore show only partial correction in mixing studies; whereas hypofibrinogenemia will typically correct entirely.

Tissue plasminogen activator (TPA) activity

- Like PAI-1, tPA undergoes diurnal variation and is best measured at 0800-0900. Unlike PAI-1 tPA is lowest in the morning and highest in the evening.

- Decreased tPA is associated with an enhanced risk of thrombosis.

- Elevated tPA is seen when there is ongoing thrombosis.

Von Willebrand factor (vWF) assays

- The assays for vWF include:

  □ Ristocetin cofactor assay (vWF activity assay) is a version of a platelet aggregation study in which patient plasma is added to formalin-fixed normal platelets in the presence of ristocetin. Under these circumstances, the plasma of a normal person will cause platelet agglutination. Plasma deficient in vWF will cause decreased aggregation.

  □ The low-dose ristocetin cofactor assay is used to detect type 2B vWD. In this test, patient plasma is added to the patient's own platelets in the presence of a low dose of ristocetin. Type 2B vWD patients show pronounced aggregation (hyperaggregation) under these conditions.

  □ Platelet-type vWD also shows increased aggregation in this assay, due to a mutation on platelet GPIb which increases its affinity for vWF. In contrast, other types of vWD may show decreased ristocetin-induced platelet aggregation due to decreased vWF quantity and/or function. Further specialized coagulation testing can be performed to distinguish type 2B from platelet-type vWD.

  □ Von Willebrand factor antigen (vWF:Ag) assay is usually based upon an ELISA format. An older assay is the so-called Laurell rocket immunoelectrophoresis.

□ Factor VIII assay is an indirect test of vWF. Since FVIII is bound to vWF in blood, adequate vWF must be present in order for FVIII levels to be maintained. The PTT is often prolonged in vWD, but is often normal as well.

□ Von Willebrand factor multimer analysis is performed by gel electrophoresis. Recall that vWF in blood exists in an array of sizes—monomers, dimers, and various multimers. When plasma is subjected to electrophoresis on a gel, vWF multimers separate according to size. Labeled anti-vWF antibody is added to permit visualization. The multimer patterns permit subclassification of vWD (see below).

□ The bleeding time is often prolonged in vWD.

- Normal vWF activity depends upon the patient's blood type. Mean vWF levels are lowest for blood type O (75%), slightly higher for A (100%), and highest for B and AB (120%). Newborns vWF activity is *higher* than adult values, normalizing by about 6 months of age. In general, a vWF activity >70% is considered normal, <40% is definitely abnormal. Results falling between 40%-70% are suspicious but require further evaluation.

- Patients who are strongly suspected of having vWD should undergo repeat testing if their initial results are normal. The features of vWD vary over time, and patients often display transient normal values. Furthermore, both vWF and factor VIII become elevated during acute phase reactions, pregnancy, and estrogen use. Newborns tend to have high vWF activity, and the disease may not be detectable until 1 year of age.

- In female carriers of the hemophilia A gene, ratio of factor VIII to vWF ratio is about 1:2 (0.5). The ratio in noncarriers and vWD is 1:1.

Causes of Excessive Bleeding (Hemophilia)

Clinically, most bleeding disorders present as either platelet-type bleeding or coagulation-type bleeding **T5.5**.

- Platelet-type bleeding may be due to thrombocytopenia, defective platelets, von Willebrand factor, or defective vasculature (eg, hereditary hemorrhagic telangiectasia/Osler-Weber-Rendu). The most

T5.5
Clinical Manifestations of Bleeding Disorders

Findings	Coagulation-Type Bleeding Disorders	Platelet-Type Bleeding Disorders
Petechiae	Rare	Common
Hemarthroses	Common	Rare
Deep hematomas	Common	Rare
Delayed bleeding	Common	Rare
Mucosal bleeding	Rare	Common
Sex	Males	Females

common congenital cause of platelet-type bleeding is von Willebrand disease, but acquired defects outnumber congenital ones and include: alcohol, aspirin, penicillin, uremia, DIC, and myeloproliferative disorders (which have a complex set of platelet abnormalities detectable on platelet aggregation assays).

■ Coagulation-type bleeding is usually due to a coagulation factor disorder.

Some clues to the diagnosis of bleeding in infants can be gleaned from the family history. Of course, male infants are at higher risk for the X-linked disorders (hemophilia A and hemophilia B). A negative family history does not exclude hemophilia, as about 30% are the result of new mutations. Onset of bleeding after one to several weeks of life suggests the possibility of vitamin K deficiency. Prenatal exposure to phenytoin or phenobarbital may lead to vitamin K deficiency. Upper extremity defects may suggest the thrombocytopenia-absent radii (TAR) syndrome. Beyond these clues, the approach is as for adults. Laboratory testing must be interpreted in the light of an immature neonatal coagulation system, in which only factors VIII, fibrinogen, and vWF can be expected to have normal adult values. For all other values, repeat testing at around 6 months of age may be necessary.

Platelet Disorders (T5.6)

Bernard-Soulier syndrome (BSS) is due to decreased platelet GPIb/V/IX complex. This manifests with thrombocytopenia and giant platelets. In aggregometry studies, the platelets aggregate with all agonists except ristocetin (resembling the pattern of vWD). Unlike vWD, the peripheral smear contains large platelets.

Platelet storage pool disorders include abnormalities of dense granules (Hermansky-Pudlak, Chédiak-Higashi, Wiskott-Aldrich) and abnormalities of α granules (grey platelet syndrome). In the dense granule disorders, only first wave aggregation is seen with all agents. Dense granule secretion, as quantified by ATP secretion using chemiluminescence, is markedly diminished. The absence of dense granules can be confirmed by electron microscopy.

■ Both Hermansky-Pudlak and Chédiak-Higashi manifest oculocutaneous albinism. In Hermansky-Pudlak, the macrophages contain ceroid-like inclusions, while in Chédiak-Higashi, granulocytes and platelets contain giant inclusion granules.

□ Particularly common in Puerto Rico.

□ Epistaxis occurs frequently, particularly in childhood.

□ Platelet counts are usually normal, though the bleeding time is often prolonged.

□ Ultrastructural examination of platelets shows the complete absence of dense granules. Recall that dense granules (essentially neurosecretory granules) store small molecules such as ADP, ATP, and serotonin and mediate the second wave of platelet aggregation.

□ As would be expected, platelet aggregation studies are notable for blunted secondary aggregation.

□ The genes associated with Hermansky-Pudlak syndrome include: HPS1, HPS3, HPS4, HPS5, HPS6, AP3B1, and DTNBP1. HPS1 is found at 10q23. In those of Puerto Rican ancestry, nearly all cases are caused by a single duplication in HPS1, and targeted mutation analysis is available for this defect. Among those of non-Puerto Rican descent, mutations are more variable or yet uncharacterized, and testing is not clinically available.

□ Pulmonary fibrosis and granulomatous colitis complicated by bleeding have been reported in a significant minority of affected persons. Biopsies in affected tissues show ceroid-like material within macrophages (eg, alveolar macrophages).

■ Wiskott-Aldrich presents with the triad of thrombocytopenia, eczema, and immunodeficiency. The platelets are small.

In α granule disorders (grey platelet syndrome), aggregation is blunted with all agents except ADP. The lack of platelet α granules imparts a uniform pale-grey tinctorial quality on Wright-stained blood films. Platelets fail to express CD62 following stimulation by high-dose thrombin, and ELISA shows abnormally low PF4. Thrombocytopenia is common.

Glanzmann thrombasthenia is an autosomal recessive disease due to deficient GPIIb/IIIa complex. Platelets lack the PL^{A1} antigen. The peripheral smear shows a normal number of normally sized, dispersed platelets. In aggregometry studies, the platelets fail to aggregate with all agonists but ristocetin. Clot retraction is poor or absent **T5.6**.

Von Willebrand disease (vWD) is the most common inherited bleeding diathesis, present in up to 1% of the population. Since von Willebrand factor (vWF) participates in both the coagulation system (by maintaining high levels of factor VIII) and the formation of platelet thrombi, vWD results in a combined platelet and coagulation defect.

■ The incidence of vWD varies from 1/100 in Italy to 1/100,000 in Great Britain. vWF has two main functions: it assists in platelet aggregation, and it binds factor VIII in plasma, protecting it from inactivation and clearance. The clinical manifestations of von Willebrand disease reflect this dual role, with a combination of platelet-type and coagulation-type bleeding.

■ The ABO blood type is an example of a genetic modifier in the case of VWD. Normal individuals with blood group O have slightly low vWF levels—about 75% of normal. Thus, for a given genotype, affected individuals with the O blood type will be relatively more severely affected, and those with A, B, or AB will be less severely affected. However, the incidence of vWD is no different among the blood types.

■ Von Willebrand factor (vWF) physiology

□ vWF mediates platelet adhesion by binding GPIb.

□ vWF is synthesized in endothelial cells and megakaryocytes.

□ vWF is stored in Weibel-Palade bodies of endothelium and α granules of megakaryocytes.

□ vWF is released by these cells as a large multimer and broken down in serum by a protease. Thus, it circulates in variably sized multimers, most commonly dimers.

□ vWF is sometimes called factor VIII-related antigen (FVIIIR:Ag). It complexes with FVIII in the circulation.

□ vWF activity is referred to as ristocetin cofactor activity.

T5.6
Summary of Platelet Disorders

Phase	Mediators	Inherited Defects	Acquired Defects
Adhesion	GPIb & vWF	Bernard-Soulier syndrome von Willebrand disease	Paraproteinemia
Release reaction	Granules & agonists	Platelet release defect Storage pool disesae	Aspirin
Aggregation	GPIIb/IIIa & fibrinogen	Glanzmann dysfibrinogenemia	Dysfibrinogenemia

Causes of Excessive Bleeding (Hemophilia)>Platelet Disorders

□ vWF levels fluctuate. There is significant day-to-day variation, and levels increase with age. VWF increases with exercise, stress, and pregnancy.

□ Levels of vWF are lowest in blood type O individuals; however, there is no greater incidence of vWD in any particular blood type. A distinct vWF normal range for blood type O persons should be established by the laboratory. In one study, the mean vWF in each blood type were: O—75%, A—105%, B—117%, and AB—123%.

■ There are 4 main types of vWD and a type of pseudo-vWD. Type I vWD is a quantitative defect, while the type II variants are qualitative (functional) defects. Often the quantity of vWF is also reduced, however.

□ Type I vWD is a quantitative defect. It is the most common type and results in a mild bleeding disorder. Type I usually has normal PT and platelet count, with a prolonged PTT and bleeding time, and decreased FVIII, vWF:Ag and vWF activity. The multimer pattern shows a normal distribution, globally dim in comparison with normal adults. However, these parameters vary, and in fact the diagnosis of type I vWD can be challenging, requiring repeated testing over extended periods of time. Despite being responsible for 70%-80% of VWD

cases, there has been remarkably little progress in characterizing the underlying molecular defect in type I VWD. This may reflect the possibility that loci outside the VWF gene—perhaps those involved in biosynthesis or transport—are responsible. A Canadian study found a single dominant mutation—Tyr1584Cys—in about 15% of type 1 families.

□ Type IIa (10%-15% of vWD cases) is a moderately severe bleeding disorder. Multimer analysis shows absence of high weight multimers. The PT, fibrinogen, and TT are normal, while the PTT may be slightly prolonged. The FVIII and vWF antigen are normal to decreased. The ristocetin cofactor is decreased (<50%). Thus, there may be *discordance* between the markedly decreased ristocetin cofactor assay and normal to mildly decreased FVIII and vWF:Ag.

□ Like IIa, type IIb shows decreased high molecular weight multimers; however, IIb is unique in two important respects: there is *enhanced* ristocetin-induced platelet aggregation; and there is profound thrombocytopenia and bleeding upon exposure to DDAVP. Do not give DDAVP to type IIb vWD. Type IIb results from spontaneous binding of VWF to platelets. Most cases are due to a 'gain of function' point mutation in the GP1b-binding domain.

T5.7
von Willebrand Disease Types

Type	FVIII	VWF:Ag	Ristocetin-Induced Platelet Aggregation	Multimeric Analysis
I	↓	↓ - Nl	↓	Normally distributed but slightly decreased
IIa	Nl - ↓	Nl - ↓	↓↓	Decreased high molecular weight
IIb	Nl - ↓	Nl - ↓	↑	Decreased high molecular weight
III	↓↓	↓↓	↓↓	Globally decreased

Type IIb VWD must be distinguished from platelet-type VWD, which is due to mutations in the gene that encodes the platelet GP1b receptor. In both cases, the enhanced binding is selective for high molecular weight multimers and results in clearance of both platelets and high molecular weight multimers from the blood. Thus, thrombocytopenia and decreased high molecular weight multimers are characteristic laboratory features in both disorders. In most other laboratory assays, it mimics type IIa.

□ Type IIM is extremely rare. The basic defect prevents binding of vWF to GPIb. Multimer analysis appears entirely normal.

□ Type IIN (Normandy) vWD is also quite rare. A defect in vWD reduces its ability to bind FVIII. Multimer analysis is normal, RIPA is normal, and vWF antigen is normal. However, FVIII levels are quite low, causing easy confusion with hemophilia A. The autosomal dominant pattern of inheritance is key to making this distinction.

□ Type III is a severe disorder with virtually no vWF. FVIII is low, vWF antigen and activity are low, and multimers are quite faint across the size spectrum. Type III must be considered in kindreds in whom apparent hemophilia follows an autosomal recessive rather than X-linked inheritance.

□ Pseudo- or platelet-type vWD mimics some of the laboratory findings of type IIb. It is caused by an abnormality in platelet GPIb, leading to increased avidity for vWF. It can be distinguished by the observation that in pseudo-vWD, the platelets aggregate if exposed to cryoprecipitate, while in IIb they do not.

□ Type Vicenza von Willebrand disease is believed to be due to increased clearance of von Willebrand factor (vWF) from the blood. This variant is characterized by discrepant plasma (low) and platelet (normal) vWF and unusually large vWF multimers.

■ The laboratory diagnosis of vWD begins with a panel of tests: ristocetin cofactor (vWF activity), vWF antigen, and FVIII activity. It is often helpful to include an indicator of acute inflammation, such as the CRP or fibrinogen. In some cases, a pregnancy test is important. Based upon the results of the initial panel, additional testing may include multimer analysis.

□ Normal vWF activity, vWF antigen, and FVIII— largely (though not entirely) excludes vWD. Patients with vWD may test as normal in the first year of life, in acute phase reactions, pregnancy, and exogenous estrogen use. Furthermore, if the diagnosis is strongly suspected, the tests should be repeated at a separate time.

□ If all tests are reduced mildly and proportionately, this is most consistent with type I vWD (if all tests are reduced profoundly, this is suggestive of type 3 vWD).

□ When the vWD activity is reduced out of proportion to the vWF antigen and FVIII, this is most consistent with a variant of type II vWD. Multimer analysis and low-dose ristocetin aggregation are necessary to further elucidate these findings.

□ When FVIII is reduced out of proportion to vWF, consider hemophilia A, female hemophilia A carrier, specimen degradation (FVIII is labile) or type IIN wVD.

■ It is still uncertain which laboratory test is best to follow the course of vWD severity and the efficacy of treatment. In surgical and acute bleed settings, factor VIII activity is considered the best monitoring test. FVIII levels should be monitored every 12 hours during these circumstances, both to ensure therapeutic effect and to prevent supranormal (>200%) FVIII levels which may lead to thrombosis.

■ Treatment of type I is DDAVP or cryoprecipitate. DDAVP (desmopressin, 1-deamino-8-d-arginine vasopressin) is a synthetic derivative of antidiuretic hormone (ADH). Administration of desmopressin transiently increases factor VIII and vWF levels. Desmopressin must be given parenterally (usually by intravenous infusion in acute settings, but also available for subcutaneous injections and nasal inhalation). The effect of a single dose lasts for 8 to 10 hours. DDAVP is contraindicated in Type IIb. The adverse effects of desmopressin include, in addition to the generally mild tachycardia, headache, and facial flushing, an important tachyphylaxis effect (the need for stronger dosing over time). While desmopressin is effective in patients with type 1 von Willebrand disease, it is usually not useful in type 2 and 3 disease (type 2A patients experience an increase in the dysfunctional vWF they were already making, in 2B patients it is contraindicated, and type 3 patients can't mount a significant secretory response). Thus, in most non-type 1 patients, administration of vWF is preferable. Fresh-frozen plasma contains both factor VIII and von Willebrand factor, but large amounts are needed to attain hemostatic concentrations (20-25 mL/kg). Ten bags of cryoprecipitate, which also contains both factors, provide roughly equal clinical efficacy. Commercial concentrates (eg, Humate-P) contains vWF and factor VIII and have the advantage of being virus inactivated. Purified factor VIII products should not be used. Alloantibodies against vWF develop in 10%-15% of patients with type 3 disease who undergo multiple transfusions.

■ An acquired form of von Willebrand disease occurs rarely. It has been associated with lymphoproliferative disorders, autoimmune disease, essential thrombocythemia, and aortic stenosis.

Acquired platelet defects are the most commonly encountered platelet disorders

■ Aspirin and NSAIDs

□ These agents cause platelet impairment by inhibiting cyclooxygenase type 1 (COX-1), a key enzyme involved in the production of thromboxane A_2 (TXA_2). TXA_2 exerts autocrine platelet stimulation, leading to dense granule release and the secondary wave of aggregation. The inhibitory effect of aspirin persists for the lifetime of the platelet (10 days), since it actually acetylates the enzyme; while the effect of other NSAIDs is reversible.

□ This effect is detectable in the laboratory in the aggregometry responses of platelets to the so-called weak agonists: epinephrine, ADP, arachidonate, low-dose collagen, and low-dose thrombin. These are considered 'weak agonists' because, by themselves, they are capable of producing only the first, reversible, wave of aggregation; they depend upon

TXA_2 to generate secondary-wave, irreversible, aggregation. The lag phase in collagen-induced aggregation is often prolonged, and there is complete failure to aggregate in response to arachidonate. This combination of findings is collectively called the aspirin-like effect.

□ The storage pool defect induced by aspirin can be distinguished from inherited storage pool defects by studying platelet secretion in response to high-dose thrombin (normal in aspirin-like effect). High-dose thrombin (and high-dose collagen) are capable of producing complete aggregation without TXA_2.

□ COX-2, an enzyme present in endothelial cells, is involved in the production of prostacyclin, a platelet inhibitor. COX-2 is relatively resistant to the effect of aspirin, however. Furthermore, since endothelial cells have nuclei, they are able to replace COX-2; whereas, platelets cannot replace COX-1; the balance, therefore, is shifted in favor of platelet inhibition.

□ Aspirin often, but inconsistently, prolongs the bleeding time.

■ Ticlopidine and Clopidogrel cause blunted platelet aggregation, particularly in response to ADP. These agents (the thienopyridines) exert their effect through inhibition of ADP-mediated platelet activation.

■ Inhibitors of GPIIb-IIIa ($\alpha_{IIb}\beta_3$ antagonists) are used clinically to prevent thrombosis. These include Abciximab (ReoPro), Eptifibatide (Integrilin), and Tirofiban (Aggrastat). Platelet aggregation resembles that seen in Glanzmann thrombasthenia—impaired aggregation to all agonists, except Ristocetin.

■ In myeloproliferative disorders (MPD), particularly polycythemia vera and essential thrombocythemia, thrombosis (and sometimes bleeding) is an extremely common cause of morbidity and mortality. These complications occur even with normal platelet counts, due presumably to clonal defects in the megakaryocytes and platelets. The bleeding time is prolonged in only a small number of patients and predicts neither bleeding nor thrombosis. Very high platelet counts (>1.5 million) have been associated with an acquired von Willebrand disease. The most common finding in platelet aggregometry is decreased aggregation and secretion in response to epinephrine, ADP, and/or collagen.

- Uremia impairs platelet function to a variable extent. It is capable of prolonging the bleeding time and altering platelet aggregation *in vitro*; however, the clinical effects appear to be milder than the *in vitro* effects. Dialysis seems to improve platelet function in this scenario, as does DDAVP and estrogen therapy.

- Cardiopulmonary bypass circuits cause both thrombocytopenia and platelet dysfunction. A prolonged bleeding time is a common finding in this circumstance, in addition to abnormal aggregometry (particularly with ristocetin). There appears to be depletion of dense granules and α granules.

- Paraproteinemia is a common cause of platelet dysfunction. This is particularly common in the immunoglobulin classes capable of forming multimers—IgA and IgM—but, due to its higher incidence, is seen commonly in IgG paraproteinemia. This is thought to be due to platelet 'coating' with immunoglobulin, and the effect is noted to be proportional to the paraprotein concentration.

Thrombocytopenia

- The particular differential diagnosis depends on age of onset.

  □ In childhood, ITP is the most common cause.

  □ In neonates, the common causes are bone marrow suppression due to infection (toxoplasmosis, rubella, CMV), neonatal alloimmune thrombocytopenia (NAIT), maternal ITP (passive transfer of antibodies), and chromosomal anomalies (trisomy 18, trisomy 13, trisomy 21, Turner syndrome). Inherited thrombocytopenia should be considered most strongly when the presentation is early (1st year of life) or when chronic or recurrent. Note that milder disorders may be noted only much later, either at the time of menarche, trauma, or surgery, or on a routine CBC. A poor response to steroids but good response to transfused platelets is consistent with an inherited syndrome. Since many of the inherited syndromes have recognizable changes in platelet morphology, examination of the peripheral blood

smear should be carried out in all cases of newly recognized thrombocytopenia, particularly in search of giant platelets (megathrombocytes), very small platelets (microthrombocytes), abnormal platelet granules, and Döhle bodies.

□ In adults, thrombocytopenia is caused most commonly by ITP, a drug, or hypersplenism. The most common drugs implicated in thrombocytopenia are antibiotics, alcohol, anti-arrhythmics, thiazides, and heparin. Hypersplenism that results in significant thrombocytopenia is most often secondary to liver disease. ITP is then left as a usual diagnosis of exclusion. Other causes of thrombocytopenia include systemic lupus or other autoimmune disease (secondary ITP), antiphospholipid syndrome, B-cell malignancies, HIV infection, HCV infection, and *H. pylori* infection. Particularly in older individuals or those who do not respond to treatment, a bone marrow biopsy may be undertaken to exclude MDS. Thrombotic thrombocytopenic purpura (TTP) is an uncommon cause of thrombocytopenia but one always worth considering, particularly because platelet transfusion is absolutely contraindicated. Lastly, while not a cause of bleeding, the heparin-induced thrombocytopenia (HIT) syndrome must always be considered in new-onset thrombocytopenia.

- It is important to review the peripheral smear, first to exclude platelet satellitosis and platelet clumping. Platelet clumping is an EDTA-related artifact that can be ameliorated by a re-draw in sodium citrate. Second, observe the size of the platelets. Large and variably sized platelets (with the exception of the rare Bernard-Soulier syndrome or May-Hegglin anomaly) indicate increased marrow production (eg, ITP). Third, look for schistocytes. When thrombocytopenia is associated with abundant schistocytes, a microangiopathic hemolytic anemia (DIC, TTP, HUS, HELLP) should be considered. Usually clotting times are normal in TTP/HUS and prolonged in DIC/HELLP.

- A marrow biopsy may disclose underlying marrow pathology responsible for decreased platelet production (eg, myelodysplasia). A marrow showing numerous and focally clustered morphologically normal megakaryocytes would support peripheral destruction (eg, ITP).

■ *Immune thrombocytopenic purpura (ITP)*

□ The antigenic target in ITP varies, and may be GPIIb, GPIIIa, GPIb, or GPV.

□ Definitive diagnosis, though not usually pursued, can be made by flow cytometry or ELISA to demonstrate increased platelet surface immunoglobulin. Most often, ITP is a clinical diagnosis of exclusion that, in the most straightforward cases, is made in an otherwise healthy individual who presents with isolated thrombocytopenia, an otherwise unremarkable peripheral smear, and no other obvious causes of thrombocytopenia.

□ A substantial response to immunomodulatory treatment is the best diagnostic test for ITP, and >80% of ITP patients will respond to initial therapy, usually consisting of methylprednisolone with or without intravenous immunoglobulin (IVIG). Failure to respond suggests either an incorrect diagnosis or refractory ITP.

□ Approximately 10% of patients with ITP have refractory disease, meaning that a platelet count of 30,000 cannot be achieved with initial therapy. Another 5% or so can be maintained about 30K only with chronic treatment.

□ Splenectomy is considered for those who are refractory to medical treatment. Splenectomy is often an effective treatment for ITP, with 2/3 of patients achieving a sustained complete response. Some patients either fail to respond to splenectomy or suffer relapses after an initial response. No pre-operative factor has been found to correlate with the likelihood of response, although younger age has been associated with response in some studies. In postsplenectomy patients who still require treatment, anti-CD20 antibodies may be used. The mortality rate for open splenectomy is around 1%, with 0.2% mortality from laparoscopic splenectomy. Alternatives to splenectomy, including corticosteroids and other immunosuppressives, also carry significant risks.

■ *Neonatal alloimmune thrombocytopenia (NATP)* is usually caused by anti-PL^{A1} antibodies. 98% of the US population have platelets that are PL^{A1} positive. 80% of NATP cases occur due to sensitization of a PL^{A1} negative mother by the PL^{A1} positive fetal platelets. Nearly half of cases affect the *first pregnancy,* unlike hemolytic disease of the newborn. Affected neonates should be transfused with maternal platelets.

■ *Posttransfusion purpura (PTP),* like NATP, is caused by an *antibody response* in PL^{A1} *negative individuals to* PL^{A1} *positive platelets.* It classically presents as severe thrombocytopenia in a female recipient of cellular blood products, approximately 7-10 days following transfusion. Often there is a history of prior pregnancy or transfusion. For unknown reasons, the recipient's own platelets are destroyed in addition to the antigen-positive platelets, causing profound thrombocytopenia. Usually platelet counts recover within several weeks.

■ *Heparin-induced thrombocytopenia (HIT)*

□ Type I HIT, in which the platelet count drops to around 100,000 but does not decrease beyond 50% of baseline, arises in about 5% of heparinized patients. This can occur as early as day 1 of heparinization and does not appear to be immune mediated. Type I HIT is not a contraindication to future heparin use and only rarely produces hemorrhage or thrombosis.

□ In Type II HIT, the platelet count becomes very low (often <50,000, <50% of baseline), and thrombosis is an enormous risk. Like TTP (discussed next) this entity is included here not as a cause of bleeding but as an important consideration in thrombocytopenia.

□ Arterial thromboses outnumber venous, and bleeding is not usually a problem. Arterial thrombosis often involves the extremities (5%-10%), stroke (3%-5%), or myocardial infarction (3%-5%). Venous thrombosis manifests as lower-limb deep-vein thrombosis (50%), pulmonary embolism (25%), upper limb deep-vein thrombosis (10%), or adrenal hemorrhagic necrosis. Microvascular thrombosis may occur, particularly in patients treated with coumadin, and it is for this reason that coumadin is relatively contraindicated. Erythematous plaques or skin necrosis may form at the site of subcutaneous heparin injections.

Causes of Excessive Bleeding (Hemophilia)>Platelet Disorders

□ The typical onset of type II HIT is 5-10 days following the start of heparinization. Rapid-onset HIT may be seen in those previously exposed to heparin. The HIT syndrome can occur after cessation of heparin therapy, for up to 3 weeks; thus, patients may suffer a thrombotic event after discharge from a hospitalization during which they were exposed to heparin. This delayed-onset HIT is often quite severe. Furthermore, re-exposure to heparin while anti-PF4 antibodies are still present (within up to 124 days) may produce a rapid onset of HIT syndrome. However, once anti-PF4 antibodies disappear, there does not appear to be an anamnestic response.

□ Type II arises in about 1% of heparinized patients. There is a slightly decreased risk in patients treated only with LMWH, but the risk is present whenever patients are exposed to the heparin antigen, no matter how little (heparin-coated [hep-locked] intravenous catheters are an under-recognized stimulant). Risk factors for HIT include use of unfractionated heparin (10-40× risk compared to LMW heparin), longer duration of heparin (5-10× risk after 10-14 days compared to less than 4 days), surgery (3-5× risk as compared to medical patients), and female gender (2× risk).

□ The differential diagnosis of HIT includes other entities that may cause thrombocytopenia in a heparinized patient, including pulmonary embolus and sepsis. *Anti-PF4 antibodies are not diagnostic of HIT*, and they may be seen in nonthrombocytopenic heparinized patients. Most patients with HIT have mild or moderate thrombocytopenia, and platelet count nadirs less than $20 \times 10^9/L$ should raise suspicion for another etiology. Greater than 90% have at least a 50% drop in platelet count, but the platelet count nadir does not necessarily fall below normal.

□ Type II HIT is mediated by antibodies against platelet factor 4 (PF4). If HIT is suspected, an assay should be initiated. If the platelet count falls below 50% of baseline, or if an arterial thrombosis occurs, heparin should be discontinued. Management consists of discontinuing all forms of heparin and using instead recombinant hirudin, lepirudin, argatroban, or other agent with no cross-reactivity with the HIT antibodies. While low molecular weight heparins rarely induce HIT, they should be avoided in the midst of HIT, because they will cross react with anti-PF4 antibodies. Warfarin should be avoided because of the risk of microvascular thrombosis. Platelet transfusions are contraindicated.

□ The laboratory confirmation of type II HIT can involve one of three lab tests

- The serotonin release assay (SRA) is the gold standard test but not generally available.

- The heparin-induced platelet aggregation assay (HIPA) essentially involves a platelet aggregation study in which heparin is added as the 'agonist.' Enhanced aggregation with heparin is abnormal. This test is considered to be around 95% specific but its sensitivity ranges from 30%-80%.

- The anti-PF$_4$ antibody test by ELISA is reported to be around 90% sensitive and 95% specific. Once antibodies are formed, they are detectable (by ELISA) for a median duration of 85 days (up to 124 days) and functionally active (by SRA) for a median of 50 days (up to 64 days).

■ Thrombotic thrombocytopenia purpura (TTP) and hemolytic uremic syndrome (HUS)

□ TTP is a syndrome resulting from the widespread formation of microvascular platelet thrombi, particularly affecting the central nervous system, kidneys, gastrointestinal tract, and other organs. It presents with a classic pentad: thrombocytopenia, microangiopathic hemolytic anemia, neurologic abnormalities, renal abnormalities, and fever. Platelets usually number less than 20,000 /μL, and schistocytes are numerous in the peripheral smear. The serum LDH is very high, a feature that is used to follow the disease course and therapy.

□ HUS is another syndrome of microvascular platelet thrombi, with effects that are limited to the renal circulation. While there may be little etiologic commonality between HUS and TTP, they share the feature of thrombotic microangiopathy and there is some clinical overlap between the two syndromes.

□ TTP is usually idiopathic, and, if survived, an isolated event. In some cases of idiopathic TTP, there are recurrent bouts. Familial (chronic relapsing) TTP has been reported, as have some cases associated with ticlopidine and pregnancy.

□ It has been known for some time that TTP is associated with abnormally large circulating multimers of von Willebrand factor (vWF). Recall that vWF is released into the circulation by endothelial cells and megakaryocytes as large multimers which are

343

the face of an unidentified factor VIII mutation, RFLP linkage analysis can be applied if family members of the affected relative from two generations are available and willing to give blood samples.

- FVIII is administered for (1) treating spontaneous bleeds or (2) prophylaxis in surgery. FVIII is a high molecular weight compound that, when administered intravascularly, remains largely in the intravascular compartment (100% recovery of dose). The half-life ($t_{\frac{1}{2}}$) is 12 hours. The dose of FVIII depends on the target activity desired and is repeated every 12 hours. Alternatively, DDAVP (desmopressin) can be used in mild hemophiliacs. Amicar (epsilon aminocaproic acid) is an inhibitor of fibrinolysis that can be used as an adjunct.

- Antibodies to FVIII develop in 10%-25% of patients who receive FVIII replacement therapy. Acquired factor VIII inhibitors (anti-factor VIII antibodies) arise most commonly in hemophiliacs exposed to exogenous factor VIII. However, some nonhemophiliacs spontaneously develop anti-FVIII antibodies. This latter scenario presents either in an elderly adult or a young pregnant female as a spontaneous deep muscle hematoma. 17% have an associated autoimmune disease, 12% have an associated malignancy, and 11% are post-partum. If factor levels are done, FVIII appears extremely low (<1%). Characteristically, the inhibitor displays time dependence: the 1:1 mix must be incubated for 2 hours to bring out the inhibition. Most such anti-FVIII antibodies are transient, disappearing within a few months.

Hemophilia B (Christmas disease)

- Hemophilia B is clinically indistinguishable from hemophilia A. It is an X-linked recessive congenital deficiency of FIX. The incidence is about 1 in 25,000 male births.

- Like hemophilia A, the PT and TT are normal, while the PTT is prolonged.

- The FIX gene is much smaller than the factor VIII gene, having 8 exons. It is found at Xq27, close to FVIII, but far enough away to assort independently. Factor IX is synthesized in hepatocytes and released as the inactive form (IX). It is converted to the active form (IXa) by factor VII, combines with its cofactor

(factor VIII), and activates X to Xa. Mild to moderate hemophilia B is most commonly caused by missense point mutations in the Factor IX gene. Severe hemophilia B is usually associated with a nonsense mutation, microdeletion, gross deletion, or frameshift mutation. As is the case with hemophilia A, mutations resulting in essentially no production of antigenic factor IX (nonsense mutations and gross deletions) are associated with the greatest likelihood of developing anti-factor IX antibodies. Since the laboratory diagnosis of hemophilia B is usually straightforward, up to 30% of affected persons may show a normal aPTT. For detection of these cases, detection of carrier females, and for prenatal diagnosis direct sequence analysis is clinically available.

- Factor IX replacement therapy differs from FVIII. There is only 30% dose recovery, and the t½ is 8 hours.

Hereditary deficiency of other coagulation factors

- With the exception of factors XII and XIII, the other congenital factor deficiencies (II, V, VII, X, XI) have several features in common. They display autosomal recessive inheritance. Heterozygotes have approximately 50% factor activity, while homozygotes have activity in the range of 1-5%. Heterozygotes are usually asymptomatic; however, FXI heterozygotes may have bleeding symptoms. Lastly, homozygotes tend to have somewhat milder disease than hemophilia A and B.

- Factor V deficiency is rare and often associated with a consanguineous pedigree. It is inherited as an autosomal recessive trait. The factor V gene is located at 1q21-25, and there is much homology with the factor VIII gene. Like factor VIII, the gene is quite large, and a variety of molecular defects have been described. (Of course, the most common mutation in the FV gene is that leading to FV-Leiden.) Factor V is synthesized in the liver (plasma factor V) and in megakaryocytes (platelet factor V, stored in α granules, molecularly identical to plasma factor V), is activated to Va by thrombin, and serves as a cofactor for Xa, which converts prothrombin to thrombin. Va is inactivated by activated protein C, which requires the cofactor protein S. Severe factor V deficiency manifests as typical hemophilia. The PT and PTT are prolonged, and the thrombin time is normal. The bleeding time may be prolonged, due to a lack of platelet factor V. Isolated hereditary factor V deficiency is overall less common than the sum of the other rare etiologies of factor V deficiency—combined deficiency of factors V and VIII, acquired factor V deficiency (liver disease, amyloidosis), disseminated intravascular coagulation, and anti-factor V antibody inhibitors. The latter may develop spontaneously or after the administration of bovine thrombin preparations (which contain factor V).

- Factor VII deficiency is very uncommon but is associated with a serious bleeding disorder. A unique feature of FVII deficiency is the complete lack of association between factor VII levels and bleeding severity. The factor VII gene is located on chromosome 13q. Factor VII is a vitamin K-dependent factor synthesized in the liver. Circulating VII is activated by tissue factor to VIIa which can catalyze the formation of additional VIIa and activate factors X and IX. Thus, it is capable of driving both the extrinsic and intrinsic pathways. Factor VII deficiency is essentially the only cause of an isolated prolongation of the PT. The PTT, TT, and bleeding times are usually normal. A factor VII assay will confirm the diagnosis. Clinical severity appears only weakly associated with genotype, suggesting other counterbalancing influences. In general, a complete absence of factor VII production is incompatible with life, and a severe bleeding phenotype is mainly seen in those who are homozygous for a mutation (rather than the more common scenario of compound heterozygosity) that results in factor VII activities under 1%-2%. However, there are many with activities in this range that have only mild disease or no disease. Acquired factor VII deficiency can be caused by liver disease, warfarin, and vitamin K deficiency. These can be distinguished in the laboratory by the concomitant deficiency in other vitamin K-dependent factors.

- Factor X deficiency is a rare autosomal recessive condition. Like factor VII, the factor X gene is located at 13q. Factor X is synthesized in the liver as a vitamin K-dependent factor. In the circulation, it is activated either by the factor VIIa or the factor IXa-VIIIa complex. Russell viper venom (RVV) also can activate factor X in vitro. Xa converts prothrombin to thrombin. A multitude of gene mutations have been described in cases of factor X deficiency. The PT, PTT, and DRVVT are prolonged, with a normal TT and bleeding time. Amyloidosis is essentially the only cause of an acquired deficiency isolated to factor X. Interestingly, in this setting, transfused factor X does not effectively raise factor X levels. Acquired factor X

deficiency in association with other factor deficiencies may be seen in liver disease, warfarin therapy, and vitamin K deficiency.

- Factor XI deficiency is an autosomal recessive condition that is unique in many respects when compared to other isolated coagulation factor deficiencies. While most of the conditions in this group are spread widely among geographic and ethnic groups, factor XI deficiency is found mainly in the Ashkenazim. In this population, the gene frequency may be as high as 5%-10%. In addition, unlike the long list of unique mutations that give rise to other inherited factor deficiencies, three main mutation types give rise to most cases of factor XI deficiency. Furthermore, genotype-phenotype correlations are not strong, and even very low factor XI levels may not result in a significant bleeding diathesis. Interestingly, deficiency in factor XII, the primary activator of factor XI, essentially never results in a bleeding diathesis.

- Factor XIII deficiency

  □ Factor XIII deficiency is rare. Inheritance is autosomal recessive, but while clinical abnormalities are most apparent in homozygotes, heterozygotes can have mild bleeding symptoms.

  □ FXIII deficiency is associated with essentially normal PT, PTT, and TT. There is a very mild bleeding disorder, especially producing a tendency for delayed bleeding. Delayed bleeding is a reflection of the role of FXIII. Although a normal fibrin clot can form initially, it is weak due to an absence of FXIII-mediated covalent cross-linking. Other symptoms include umbilical stump bleeding, frequent miscarriages, delayed wound healing and the formation of hypertrophic scars.

  □ Factor XIII consists of two catalytic A subunits and two noncatalytic B subunits, encoded on two separate chromosomes (6p and 1q). Most mutations causing factor XIII deficiency have so far been found in the A subunit.

  □ A factor XIII gene polymorphism (Val34Leu) is present in nearly half the population. It is believed to play a role in prevention of deep venous thrombosis. The polymorphism is found somewhat more commonly in patients with intracranial hemorrhage than in the general population.

Causes of Excessive Bleeding (Hemophilia)>Coagulation Defects

□ Acquired FXIII deficiency has been described in liver disease, DIC, inflammatory conditions (Crohn colitis, ulcerative colitis, Henoch-Schönlein purpura), and hematolymphoid neoplasms.

- Contact factor deficiency (factor XII, HMWK, or prekallikrein) cause marked prolongation of the aPTT without clinical bleeding (see Causes of Excessive Thrombosis [Thrombophilia]).

- Inherited combined factor deficiency

  □ While most single-factor deficiencies are due to mutations within the gene that encodes the factor, there are mutations that affect genes involved in intracellular transport or post-translational modification of clotting factors. These can cause inherited combined deficiency states.

  □ The most common inherited combined deficiency is the combined factor V and factor VIII deficiency. The combined deficiency of FV and FVIII displays low levels of coagulant activity and antigen of both factors. It appears that a gene on 18q—the *LMAN1* gene which encodes ERGIC-53—is responsible. ERGIC-53 is found within the rough endoplasmic reticulum and Golgi where it acts as a chaperone in the intracellular transport of factors V and VIII.

  □ Second most common is the combined deficiency of vitamin K–dependent factors. The syndrome of multiple deficiencies of vitamin K–dependent coagulation factors shows deficient factors II, VII, IX, X, and proteins C and S.

- Fibrinogen deficiency: afibrinogenemia, hypofibrinogenemia, and dysfibrinogenemia.

  □ A cluster of three genes on chromosome 4q—fibrinogen α (FGA), fibrinogen β (FGB), and fibrinogen γ (FGG)—encode the protein fibrinogen. The fibrinogen molecule is a dimer, with each half composed of three polypeptide chains—Aα, Bβ, and γ. Disease-causing mutations are most often found in the Aα locus. In the clotting cascade, fibrinogen is cleaved into fibrin by thrombin; fibrin then polymerizes noncovalently and finally is stabilized by covalent bonds mediated by factor XIIIa. In the formation of platelet thrombi, fibrinogen binds to platelet GPIIb/IIIa to mediate platelet aggregation.

□ Afibrinogenemia and hypofibrinogenemia (autosomal recessive) are due to mutations that severely truncate the protein, and inherited dysfibrinogenemia (autosomal dominant) is due to various missense mutations.

□ Congenital afibrinogenemia is associated with an immeasurably prolonged PT and PTT and a clinical bleeding disorder similar to moderate to severe hemophilia A. Hypofibrinogenemia may be congenital or acquired (DIC, hepatic failure, and L-asparaginase therapy). Bleeding occurs when fibrinogen falls below 50 mg/dL. Umbilical cord hemorrhage is often the first manifestation of inherited hypo- or afibrinogenemia, followed by a life-long bleeding diathesis. Some patients, whose basic defect is the hepatocellular secretion of fibrinogen, succumb instead to cirrhosis (in a manner similar to that operative in α1-antitrypsin deficiency).

□ Dysfibrinogenemia may be congenital or acquired (liver disease, biliary disease, hepatocellular carcinoma, and renal cell carcinoma). Clinically, it may be asymptomatic (50%-60%), cause bleeding (30%-40%) or cause thrombosis (10%-20%), depending upon the particular mutation.

□ Recurrent miscarriages are a feature of dysfibrinogenemia and FXIII deficiency.

Acquired factor deficiencies

- Factor X deficiency is seen in some patients with amyloidosis.

- Liver disease causes
  (a) decreased synthesis of most clotting factors, leading to clotting prolongation, particularly evident in the PT
  (b) hypo- and dysfibrinogenemia reflected in prolonged TT
  (c) poorly understood platelet functional abnormalities
  (d) chronic DIC due to impaired clearance of D-dimer

Causes of Excessive Bleeding (Hemophilia)>Coagulation Defects

- Vitamin K deficiency leads to impaired production of the *vitamin K-dependent factors II, VII, IX, X, protein C, and protein S.* Vitamin K is necessary for γ-carboxylation of these factors within their so-called Gla domains. Note that, of these, factor VII has the shortest half-life (2-5 hrs). Protein C (6-8 hrs) is a close second, and this, particularly in patients congenitally deficient in protein C, may lead to a transient thrombotic state often manifested by skin necrosis when treated with warfarin. Causes of vitamin K deficiency include

  □ Hemorrhagic disease of the newborn- typically presents at around 3 days of age and is due to vitamin K deficiency. It is prevented by prophylactic vitamin K administration at birth.

  □ Antibiotics—diminish intestinal flora which are the source of some of our vitamin K.

  □ Malabsorption/malnutrition

  □ Warfarin therapy

Disseminated intravascular coagulation (DIC)

- The formation of widespread microvascular thrombi is stimulated when there is a circulating substance capable of behaving like tissue factor. The fibrinolytic system responds by attempting to degrade the newly formed fibrin. The consumption of coagulation factors in numerous small clots leads to a bleeding diathesis, producing the seemingly paradoxical coexistence of excess bleeding and thrombosis.

- Causes of DIC include overwhelming infections (gram negative, usually), obstetric complications (abruption, amniotic fluid emboli), mucin-secreting adenocarcinomas, extensive trauma, prostatic surgery, and venomous snake bites.

- Laboratory tests useful to detect DIC are antithrombin (AT), fibrinopeptide A, D-dimer, prothrombin fragment 1+2 (PF 1+2), and the platelet count. The PT, PTT, and fibrinogen level are helpful if they are abnormal, but they are frequently normal or fast. D-dimer and PF1+2 are among the most sensitive tests for DIC (95% sensitive). AT and fibrinopeptide A are a close 3rd and 4th (85%).

- The first principle of DIC treatment is to eliminate, whenever possible, the cause identified as underlying. Often this is either not possible or not yet identified, and the treating physician must attempt to control the clotting process. Treatment may target thrombosis, the process that most affects morbidity and mortality, bleeding, or both. The complexity of vicissitudes facing the DIC patient has led to much controversy regarding treatment. Among a multitude of studies, the sole unequivocally beneficial measure in the management of DIC is the eradication of the underlying disorder. Most patients, except those suffering from DIC resulting from obstetric accidents or massive liver failure, will need some form of anticoagulant therapy, often administered in the form of subcutaneous low-dose heparin. Anticoagulant replacement therapy may be indicated if the patient does not respond. Intravenous unfractionated heparin is sometimes given, but aggravation of hemorrhage is a potential risk. The use of heparin is somewhat risky in fulminant DIC, DIC in the setting of central nervous system insults, DIC associated with fulminant hepatic failure, and DIC due to obstetric accidents. Antithrombin concentrates may be the optimal treatment for fulminant DIC. Further efforts may be directed at replenishing specific factor deficiencies. Generally, the safest components in patients with active, uncontrolled, DIC are washed packed red cells, platelet concentrates, and antithrombin concentrates. Components containing clotting factors or fibrinogen may be associated with enhanced thrombosis, but may be necessary when uncontrolled bleeding is the major feature. When fibrinogen is <100 mg/dL, FFP (15-20 mL/kg of body weight) or cryoprecipitate (1 U/10 kg of body weight) should be considered. In the instances in which bleeding continues, consider inhibition of the fibrinolytic system (ε-aminocaproic acid and tranexamic acid). These agents should be administered after heparin has been infused.

T5.9
DIC vs TTP

Assay	DIC	TTP
Fibrinopeptide A	Elevated	Normal
D-dimer	Elevated	Normal/elevated
Prothrombin 1+2	Elevated	Normal

Thrombocytosis

Reactive Thrombocytosis

Reactive thrombocytosis must be distinguished from a myeloproliferative disease (such as CML or ET). Clinical evaluation is initially centered upon identifying clues to a secondary thrombocytosis—elevated C-reactive protein, erythrocyte sedimentation rate, iron studies.

- Nearly all cases of childhood thrombocytosis are reactive, benign, and self-limited. In young infants, the likelihood of finding an underlying cause is low, but in older children, thrombocytosis is often an acute-phase reaction to an identifiable condition. In a Japanese study, the most common underlying condition was infection, followed by Kawasaki disease, and iron deficiency. In a smaller study from Ireland, infection was also the most common cause, followed by iron deficiency and malignancy (most commonly ALL).

- In adults, the causes of reactive thrombocytosis include systemic inflammation, malignancy, and splenectomy. Post-splenectomy thrombocytosis does not often exceed 600×10^9/L.

- Neither thrombosis nor hemorrhage is usually a risk in secondary thrombocytosis, even at very high counts.

Myeloproliferative disease

- It is difficult to give a particular number at which thrombocytosis definitely represents a myeloproliferative disorder. The likelihood of MPD is >90% at 2 million platelets per dL, >80% at 1 million, and >70% at 600,000.

- Patients with thrombocytosis due to a myeloproliferative disorder are at risk for thrombosis and bleeding and may require at least aspirin for prophylaxis.

Anticoagulation Therapy

Coumadin (Warfarin)

Coumadin inhibits post-translational modification of the vitamin K-dependent coagulation factors: II, VII, IX, and X (and C & S). It appears that the most important of these factors in anticoagulation therapy is prothrombin (factor II) whose half-life is about 96 hours.

The anticoagulant effect of coumadin can be altered by interference with absorption, metabolism, or inherent responsiveness to the warfarin effect. Cholestyramine and some antibiotics inhibit absorption, blunting the warfarin effect. Many agents, including metronidazole, TMP-SMT, cimetidine, and omeprazole, inhibit warfarin metabolism, thus enhancing its effect. Other agents, by way of upregulation of the cytochrome p450 system, stimulate metabolism and thereby reduce the warfarin effect: barbiturates, alcohol, etc.

Hereditary resistance to warfarin, requiring up to 20× higher doses for therapeutic effect, is present in some individuals and is due to a mutated warfarin receptor. In addition, there are individuals with mutations in factor IX that result in excessive warfarin-induced bleeding despite a minimally prolonged PT and INR. In response to coumadin, factor IX activity in this condition decreases to <3%, while other vitamin K–dependent factors remain >40%.

Dietary intake of vitamin K (leafy vegetables) can alter the warfarin effect.

The PT test is the most common method for monitoring coumadin therapy. The PT responds to reduction of three of the four vitamin K-dependent factors (II, VII, X). Note that during the first few days of warfarin therapy, the prolongation of the PT reflects mainly a reduction of factor VII and only later also reflects a reduction of factors X and II. A particular target INR, often of 2.0 to 3.0, has been made for most indications. Some types of mechanical prosthetic heart valves and certain patients with the antiphospholipid syndrome who may require a higher targeted INR.

Heparin should be given concurrently with warfarin initially. Heparin can be discontinued when the INR has been in the therapeutic range for two consecutive days. The concurrent use of heparin is necessary for two reasons: it provides immediate anticoagulation, and it prevents the creation of a transient hypercoagulable state in patients with underlying protein C deficiency.

Coumadin reversal may be needed for patients with supratherapeutic INRs and bleeding. The most conservative approach (often applied to patients with INRs < 9.0 who do not have significant bleeding) is to omit one or several doses and resume therapy at a lower dose when the INR is in the therapeutic range. In some

Causes of Excessive Bleeding (Hemophilia)>Coagulation Defects

- Vitamin K deficiency leads to impaired production of the *vitamin K-dependent factors II, VII, IX, X, protein C, and protein S.* Vitamin K is necessary for γ-carboxylation of these factors within their so-called Gla domains. Note that, of these, factor VII has the shortest half-life (2-5 hrs). Protein C (6-8 hrs) is a close second, and this, particularly in patients congenitally deficient in protein C, may lead to a transient thrombotic state often manifested by skin necrosis when treated with warfarin. Causes of vitamin K deficiency include

  □ Hemorrhagic disease of the newborn- typically presents at around 3 days of age and is due to vitamin K deficiency. It is prevented by prophylactic vitamin K administration at birth.

  □ Antibiotics—diminish intestinal flora which are the source of some of our vitamin K.

  □ Malabsorption/malnutrition

  □ Warfarin therapy

Disseminated intravascular coagulation (DIC)

- The formation of widespread microvascular thrombi is stimulated when there is a circulating substance capable of behaving like tissue factor. The fibrinolytic system responds by attempting to degrade the newly formed fibrin. The consumption of coagulation factors in numerous small clots leads to a bleeding diathesis, producing the seemingly paradoxical coexistence of excess bleeding and thrombosis.

- Causes of DIC include overwhelming infections (gram negative, usually), obstetric complications (abruption, amniotic fluid emboli), mucin-secreting adenocarcinomas, extensive trauma, prostatic surgery, and venomous snake bites.

- Laboratory tests useful to detect DIC are antithrombin (AT), fibrinopeptide A, D-dimer, prothrombin fragment 1+2 (PF 1+2), and the platelet count. The PT, PTT, and fibrinogen level are helpful if they are abnormal, but they are frequently normal or fast. D-dimer and PF1+2 are among the most sensitive tests for DIC (95% sensitive). AT and fibrinopeptide A are a close 3rd and 4th (85%).

- The first principle of DIC treatment is to eliminate, whenever possible, the cause identified as underlying. Often this is either not possible or not yet identified, and the treating physician must attempt to control the clotting process. Treatment may target thrombosis, the process that most affects morbidity and mortality, bleeding, or both. The complexity of vicissitudes facing the DIC patient has led to much controversy regarding treatment. Among a multitude of studies, the sole unequivocally beneficial measure in the management of DIC is the eradication of the underlying disorder. Most patients, except those suffering from DIC resulting from obstetric accidents or massive liver failure, will need some form of anticoagulant therapy, often administered in the form of subcutaneous low-dose heparin. Anticoagulant replacement therapy may be indicated if the patient does not respond. Intravenous unfractionated heparin is sometimes given, but aggravation of hemorrhage is a potential risk. The use of heparin is somewhat risky in fulminant DIC, DIC in the setting of central nervous system insults, DIC associated with fulminant hepatic failure, and DIC due to obstetric accidents. Antithrombin concentrates may be the optimal treatment for fulminant DIC. Further efforts may be directed at replenishing specific factor deficiencies. Generally, the safest components in patients with active, uncontrolled, DIC are washed packed red cells, platelet concentrates, and antithrombin concentrates. Components containing clotting factors or fibrinogen may be associated with enhanced thrombosis, but may be necessary when uncontrolled bleeding is the major feature. When fibrinogen is <100 mg/dL, FFP (15-20 mL/kg of body weight) or cryoprecipitate (1 U/10 kg of body weight) should be considered. In the instances in which bleeding continues, consider inhibition of the fibrinolytic system (ε-aminocaproic acid and tranexamic acid). These agents should be administered after heparin has been infused.

T5.9
DIC vs TTP

Assay	DIC	TTP
Fibrinopeptide A	Elevated	Normal
D-dimer	Elevated	Normal/elevated
Prothrombin 1+2	Elevated	Normal

5: Coagulation and Thrombosis

Causes of Excessive Bleeding (Hemophilia)>Coagulation Defects I Causes of Excessive Thrombosis
(Thrombophilia)>Specific Causes of Thrombophilia

Causes of Excessive Thrombosis (Thrombophilia)

All patients with a thromboembolic event under age 55 deserve an evaluation for an underlying nonanatomic cause. One should not be deterred by the presence of a clinical 'explanation' for the event (such as trauma or recent surgery), as more than half of individuals with an inherent thrombophilia experience their first event under such circumstances. Furthermore, elderly patients experiencing their first thrombotic event should be selectively considered for further evaluation as well. Hagemann himself, for whom factor XII is named, did not die of his massive PE until well into his golden years.

The differential diagnosis of thrombophilia depends on the type of thrombosis—arterial or venous. In *venous thrombosis,* the most common sites are the deep veins of the lower extremities and iliofemoral veins. Other uncommon but characteristic sites include the mesenteric veins, renal veins, retinal veins, cerebral veins, and hepatic vein (Budd-Chiari syndrome). *Arterial thrombosis* generally takes the form of MI in the young (<55, but often <35 year old) patient but can also manifest as thrombosis in carotid arteries, cerebral arteries, retinal arteries, subclavian or axillary artery, or mesenteric arteries.

Effective management, in addition to the specific measures discussed below, includes family studies to identify individuals at risk for thrombosis. Counseling for affected individuals is important, so that risk factors, such as obesity, oral contraceptive use, and immobility, can be avoided, and prophylactic use of anticoagulants can be started in appropriate clinical situations, such as pregnancy, immobilization, and surgery.

The optimal laboratory evaluation takes place >2 months following the acute episode and >14 days following cessation of (coumadin) anticoagulant therapy. Alternatively, blood drawn immediately before the institution of anticoagulant therapy may be useful. Specifically, assays for protein C and protein S are unreliable when anticoagulant therapy is ongoing. Note: the APCR assay can be run anytime.

Specific Causes of Thrombophilia

Activated protein C resistance (Factor V Leiden, APCR)

- In the normal course of events, activated protein C (APC) degrades activated factors V and VIII by proteolytic cleavage, thus inhibiting coagulation. APCR is an autosomal dominant inherited condition that is responsible for about 50% of the cases of hereditary thrombophilia. APC resistance is almost always due to heterozygosity for factor V Leiden and is the major heritable risk factor for thrombophilia. It is found in about 20%-50% of those under age 50 who present with a thromboembolic event, and the incidence in unselected Caucasians is about 2%-5%. The factor V Leiden allele appears to be quite infrequent in those of sub-Saharan African, Chinese, Japanese, or Native American descent. Heterozygotes for factor V Leiden manifest a 5- to 8-fold increased risk of thrombosis, and the risk increases dramatically for homozygotes and compound heterozygotes having factor V Leiden and protein C deficiency or antithrombin III deficiency.

T5.10

Thrombophilia: Differential Diagnosis by Type of Thrombosis

Arterial thrombosis: eg, MI		Venous thrombosis: eg, DVT	
Common	Antiphospholipid syndrome (ACA) Prothrombin mutation (20210) HIT syndrome	Common	APCR prothrombin mutation (20210) Antiphospholipid syndrome (ACA & LAC) Protein C deficiency Protein S deficiency ATIII deficiency
Uncommon	Elevated PAI-1 activity Hyperhomocysteinemia t-PA deficiency	Uncommon	Hyperhomocysteinemia Heparin cofactor II Factor XII deficiency
Also consider	Anomalous coronary arteries Vasculitis	Also consider	Immobilization Trauma Pregnancy

Causes of Excessive Thrombosis (Thrombophilia)>Specific Causes of Thrombophilia; Prothrombin Variant (Prothrombin G20210A Mutation)

- The factor V gene is found on 1q (near the antithrombin gene). APCR is due to a G to A point mutation at nucleotide 1691 in the factor V gene that results in a glutamine for arginine substitution at position 506 (FV R506Q) in the factor V protein. This change affects 1 of 3 APC cleavage domains. The result is a type of factor V (factor V Leiden) that is resistant to proteolytic cleavage by activated protein C (APC). Heterozygotes have a 5- to 10- fold increased risk of thrombosis.

- Laboratory tests include a screening clotting assay (phenotypic analysis) and confirmatory DNA-based assay (genotypic analysis).

  □ In the screening test, 2 aPTTs are performed, one with patient serum alone, and the other with patient serum in the presence of APC. The ratio of the clotting time with APC to the clotting time without APC (the resistance ratio) is normally >2. This test is unreliable in patients undergoing anticoagulation. The APCR screen otherwise correlates very well with the results of DNA testing. Discrepant results may be seen in compound heterozygotes having both the factor V Leiden mutation and a type I quantitative factor V deficiency, as well as in other rare scenarios. The overall sensitivity and specificity of this assay are around 85%. In a modification to this assay, plasma deficient only in factor V is added to the patient plasma (to control for any other factor deficiencies such as those due to warfarin therapy and to mitigate the effects of any lupus anticoagulants), and a heparin neutralizer is added (to control for any heparin). This modified APC resistance assay has sensitivity and specificity >95%.

  □ Clinically available molecular testing most often is in the form of RFLP analysis. The factor V Leiden mutation results in the loss of a restriction endonuclease recognition site, permitting discernment of the mutated allele from the normal allele. The sensitivity is about 100%.

  □ 58% of APC-resistant patients had an associated risk factor at their first thrombotic event, and one very important risk factor is estrogen: pregnancy and oral contraceptive use are associated with the first thrombotic episode in 35% and 30% of women, respectively.

Prothrombin Variant (Prothrombin G20210A Mutation)

- The prothrombin variant is an autosomal dominant condition that is the second most common cause of inherited thrombophilia, responsible for ~20% of cases. The mutation is present in around 1-2% of those with European ancenstry and about 0.5% of the black population. It is also interestingly present in up to 10% of those with the FV Leiden mutation.

- It is due to a point mutation in the prothrombin gene in which a guanine to adenine (G to A) substitution at nucleotide 20210 (within the 3' untranslated region) occurs. This mutation is believed to enhance prothrombin gene transcription and translation. Direct gene sequencing by PCR is clinically available to detect the prothrombin 20210 mutation in genomic DNA extracted from circulating leukocytes. In fact, methods are now available to detect both the prothrombin G20210A mutation and factor V Leiden in the same reaction.

- Carriers have *elevated* prothrombin levels.

- The laboratory diagnosis is made only by direct DNA-based detection of the nucleotide substitution, usually using a PCR-based method.

Antithrombin deficiency (antithrombin III deficiency)

- Antithrombin (AT), when activated by heparin or heparan, inhibits factors II, IXa, Xa, FXIa and FXIIa.

- AT deficiency is an autosomal dominant disorder characterized by recurrent venous thrombosis. These events may begin to appear in the mid to late teenage years. Heterozygotes have a 5- to 10-fold increased risk for venous thrombosis, and the homozygous state is considered incompatible with life. The age at onset of thrombosis is usually between 10-40 years. The prevalence of hereditary AT deficiency appears to be around 1 in 2000. It is estimated to cause around 3% of of unexplained venous thrombosis. Particular attention must be paid to AT-deficient individuals during pregnancy (the combined AT-lowering effect of pregnancy and the prothrombotic effect of pregnancy are a dangerous combination).

- Acquired AT deficiency is seen in nephrotic syndrome, L-asparaginase therapy, estrogen therapy, pregnancy, acute thrombosis, DIC, and colitis. AT levels may increase with coumadin therapy.

- AT deficiency may come to clinical attention by an apparent inability to achieve therapeutic responses to heparin therapy, as measured by the aPTT and Xa assay, and patients who are unresponsive to heparin should be tested for AT deficiency. Note that heparin therapy reduces the AT activity, but never below 70%. Patients whose activity is tested below 60% should be considered AT deficient. For AT-deficient individuals, infusions of antithrombin concentrate will permit therapeutic heparinization.

- With regard to laboratory diagnosis, an antithrombin activity <60%, even in heparinized patients, is abnormal. Heterozygotes generally have antithrombin levels between 40% to 70%. Also, note that about 70% of individuals with a recent DVT or PE have decreased levels of AT before the initiation of anticoagulant therapy, due to consumption of this factor. Estrogens may reduce antithrombin levels by about 15%.

- Over 100 disease-causing mutations have been identified in the antithrombin gene.

Protein C or Protein S deficiency

- Protein C is activated *in vivo* by thrombin-thrombomodulin complexes. Activated protein C (APC) proteolytically cleaves factors such as Va and VIIIa into the inactive forms Vi and VIIIi. Protein S is the cofactor for protein C.

- The incidence of each condition in the general population is about 1 in 200, and each is responsible for 1%-5% of thrombophilia. Both are autosomal dominant conditions in which heterozygotes have a 5 to 7-fold increased risk of thrombosis and are at risk for coumadin-induced skin necrosis. Homozygotes present as newborns with purpura fulminans, a rapidly fatal form of DIC that requires immediate treatment with anticoagulation and FFP.

- Acquired protein C deficiency may result from coumadin therapy, liver disease, and pregnancy.

- Coumadin (warfarin) may be used for long-term prophylaxis; however, it must be started at very low doses in conjunction with porcine heparin or LMW heparin to prevent skin and fat necrosis. Alternatively, long-term low-dose subcutaneous porcine mucosal heparin/LMW heparin may be used. Protein C concentrates have been developed for treatment in deficiency states.

- Both functional (coagulation based) and antigenic (immunologic) assays are available for proteins C and S. The deficiencies of protein C are classified as type I (quantitative) or type II (qualitative). Type I deficiency, in which both qualitative and quantitative results are low, is by far the most common. In type II deficiencies, there is a normal antigenic level of the protein but reduced activity, and detecting the relatively uncommon type II deficiency is the reason for the widespread recommendation that a functional assay be used for screening. Protein C activity levels in healthy adults range from 70%-140% and increase slightly with age. Protein C levels in heterozygous protein C deficiency usually fall below 55% but sometimes fall into an indeterminate zone between 55%-70%. In these patients, it may be helpful to document two low levels on separate occasions. Protein C activity levels in newborns are normally around 20%-40%.

- Normally about 60% of plasma protein S is bound to C4b-binding protein. Both free and total antigenic assays are available. Thus three types of protein S deficiency states can be identified: type I is a quantitative defect, type II is a qualitative defect (the functional activity of protein S is decreased, but the antigen levels are normal), and type III is characterized by decreased free protein S (but a normal total protein S antigen). Type I is by far the most common. There is more overlap between normal and abnormal ranges for protein S than protein C, so that repeat sampling on separate occasions is advised. Protein S in healthy newborns is about 15%-30% of normal. Levels of protein S are normally slightly lower in females than males, and an acquired form of protein S deficiency can occur during both pregnancy oral contraceptives use. Protein S is reduced in HIV infection. Unlike AT III, levels of both protein S and protein C tend to increase in nephrotic syndrome.

5: Coagulation and Thrombosis

Causes of Excessive Thrombosis (Thrombophilia)>Prothrombin Variant (Prothrombin G20210A Mutation); Elevated
Plasminogen Activator Inhibitor Type 1 (PAI-1) Activity, Congenital or Acquired

MTHFR gene mutation and hyperhomocysteinemia

- Homocysteine is an amino acid that is formed in the breakdown of proteins. It is normally not an end-product in itself, but rather is a temporary intermediary in the interconversion of methionine and cysteine, both of which can then go on to be used for other purposes. Whenever the utilization of methionine or cysteine is blocked, excess homocysteine may accumulate.

- A point of possible confusion is the relationship between homocystinuria and hyperhomocysteinemia. Homocystinuria is a manifestation of extreme *hyperhomocysteinemia* (>100 µmol/L) that leads to a syndrome characterized by overflow of homocysteine into the urine (homocystinuria), mental retardation, ectopia lentis, premature atherosclerosis, and thrombosis. This syndrome is most commonly due to homozygous cystathionine-β-synthase deficiency or homozygous methylenetetrahydrofolate reductase (MTHFR) deficiency and is extremely rare. Mild to moderate hyperhomocysteinemia (16-100 µmol/L) is not associated with a recognizable clinical syndrome, is quite common, and is the subject of this section.

- **Mild to moderate hyperhomocysteinemia** affects 5%-7% of the population and is considered an independent risk factor for both atherosclerosis and recurrent arteriovenous thromboembolism. Hyperhomocysteinemia is classified as mild (16-24 µmol/L), moderate (25-100 µmol/L), or severe (>100). It is usually diagnosed by measuring plasma levels of homocysteine using high-pressure liquid chromatography. Very mild defects can be amplified by demonstrating an abnormal increase in plasma homocysteine after an oral methionine load. Hyperhomocysteinemia is present in up to 40% of patients with premature atherosclerosis and about 15%-20% of those with thrombophilia. The most common inherited cause of hyperhomocysteinemia is the *MTHFR* gene mutation, followed by heterozygous cystathionine-β-synthase deficiency. Deficiency of folate, B6, and B12 are common acquired causes of hyperhomocysteinemia.

- Genetic testing for the Ala677Val (C677T) mutation in *MTHFR* is clinically available. The alanine to valine substitution at amino acid 677 results in thermolability of the *MTHFR* protein and loss of activity. This mutation results in the so-called T allele for the *MTHFR* gene, located at 1p36.3.

- Elderly patients, smokers, and patients with renal failure frequently have elevated plasma homocysteine concentrations in the absence of vitamin deficiencies.

- People who have elevated homocysteine levels due to the *MTHFR* mutation can often achieve normal homocysteine with folate and/or B6 supplementation.

Paroxysmal nocturnal hemoglobinuria (PNH)

- PNH is associated with thromboembolic events and, to a much lesser extent, bleeding. Despite this, when subjected to such measures of global platelet function as thromboelastography and aggregometry, a marked reduction of platelet reactivity is observed. This is compounded by the frequent development of thrombocytopenia. For these reasons, it is thought that the thrombotic tendency in PNH is based upon some alteration in the coagulation system.

Elevated Plasminogen Activator Inhibitor Type 1 (PAI-1) Activity, Congenital or Acquired

- Acquired deficiency of tissue plasminogen activator (t-PA) is associated with several conditions. Patients with unstable angina, acute myocardial infarction, and status post percutaneous transluminal coronary angiography (PTCA) may be deficient in t-PA activity; in post-PTCA patients, this is a risk factor for restenosis.

- Heparin cofactor II (HCII) is another inhibitor that, like AT, is activated by heparin. Thrombotic tendencies are associated with levels less than 60% HCII activity, but HC-II deficiency appears to be a rare cause of unexplained thrombosis (around 1%). HC-II activity has been studied in patients with nephrotic syndrome and found to remain normal, in contrast to AT activity, which is commonly decreased in nephrotic syndrome.

- Factor XII (Hagemann factor) deficiency produces a markedly prolonged PTT without clinical bleeding. The PTT is often >100 seconds, while the PT and TT are normal. When the 1:1 mix is performed, there is initial correction, followed by prolongation after a 10 minute incubation. The PTT can be corrected by exposure to glass. Often, there is an increased tendency for thrombosis but not much risk of bleeding.

Thrombocytosis

Reactive Thrombocytosis

Reactive thrombocytosis must be distinguished from a myeloproliferative disease (such as CML or ET). Clinical evaluation is initially centered upon identifying clues to a secondary thrombocytosis—elevated C-reactive protein, erythrocyte sedimentation rate, iron studies.

- Nearly all cases of childhood thrombocytosis are reactive, benign, and self-limited. In young infants, the likelihood of finding an underlying cause is low, but in older children, thrombocytosis is often an acute-phase reaction to an identifiable condition. In a Japanese study, the most common underlying condition was infection, followed by Kawasaki disease, and iron deficiency. In a smaller study from Ireland, infection was also the most common cause, followed by iron deficiency and malignancy (most commonly ALL).

- In adults, the causes of reactive thrombocytosis include systemic inflammation, malignancy, and splenectomy. Post-splenectomy thrombocytosis does not often exceed 600×10^9/L.

- Neither thrombosis nor hemorrhage is usually a risk in secondary thrombocytosis, even at very high counts.

Myeloproliferative disease

- It is difficult to give a particular number at which thrombocytosis definitely represents a myeloproliferative disorder. The likelihood of MPD is >90% at 2 million platelets per dL, >80% at 1 million, and >70% at 600,000.

- Patients with thrombocytosis due to a myeloproliferative disorder are at risk for thrombosis and bleeding and may require at least aspirin for prophylaxis.

Anticoagulation Therapy

Coumadin (Warfarin)

Coumadin inhibits post-translational modification of the vitamin K-dependent coagulation factors: II, VII, IX, and X (and C & S). It appears that the most important of these factors in anticoagulation therapy is prothrombin (factor II) whose half-life is about 96 hours.

The anticoagulant effect of coumadin can be altered by interference with absorption, metabolism, or inherent responsiveness to the warfarin effect. Cholestyramine and some antibiotics inhibit absorption, blunting the warfarin effect. Many agents, including metronidazole, TMP-SMT, cimetidine, and omeprazole, inhibit warfarin metabolism, thus enhancing its effect. Other agents, by way of upregulation of the cytochrome p450 system, stimulate metabolism and thereby reduce the warfarin effect: barbiturates, alcohol, etc.

Hereditary resistance to warfarin, requiring up to 20× higher doses for therapeutic effect, is present in some individuals and is due to a mutated warfarin receptor. In addition, there are individuals with mutations in factor IX that result in excessive warfarin-induced bleeding despite a minimally prolonged PT and INR. In response to coumadin, factor IX activity in this condition decreases to <3%, while other vitamin K–dependent factors remain >40%.

Dietary intake of vitamin K (leafy vegetables) can alter the warfarin effect.

The PT test is the most common method for monitoring coumadin therapy. The PT responds to reduction of three of the four vitamin K-dependent factors (II, VII, X). Note that during the first few days of warfarin therapy, the prolongation of the PT reflects mainly a reduction of factor VII and only later also reflects a reduction of factors X and II. A particular target INR, often of 2.0 to 3.0, has been made for most indications. Some types of mechanical prosthetic heart valves and certain patients with the antiphospholipid syndrome who may require a higher targeted INR.

Heparin should be given concurrently with warfarin initially. Heparin can be discontinued when the INR has been in the therapeutic range for two consecutive days. The concurrent use of heparin is necessary for two reasons: it provides immediate anticoagulation, and it prevents the creation of a transient hypercoagulable state in patients with underlying protein C deficiency.

Coumadin reversal may be needed for patients with supratherapeutic INRs and bleeding. The most conservative approach (often applied to patients with INRs < 9.0 who do not have significant bleeding) is to omit one or several doses and resume therapy at a lower dose when the INR is in the therapeutic range. In some

Anticoagulation Therapy>Coumadin (Warfarin) | Bibliography

patients this is supplemented with oral vitamin K, particularly if the patient is at increased risk for bleeding. For patients with very high INRs (>20) or with serious bleeding, discontinue warfarin therapy and administer vitamin K by slow IV infusion, supplemented with fresh plasma or prothrombin complex concentrate, depending on the urgency of the situation.

For planned invasive procedures, coumadin may be discontinued 4 days before surgery and placed on heparin. Heparin can be discontinued hours before surgery.

Adcock DM. Factor VIII Inhibitors in patients with hemophilia A. *Clin Hemostasis Rev* 2002; 16: 1.

Adcock DM, Fink L, Marlar RA. A laboratory approach to the evaluation of hereditary hypercoagulability. *Am J Clin Pathol* 1997; 108:434-449.

Ananyeva NM, Lacroix-Desmazes S, Hauser CAE, Shima M, Ovanesov MV, Khrenov AV, Saenko EL. Inhibitors in hemophilia A: mechanisms of inhibition, management and perspectives. *Blood Coagul Fibrinolysis* 2004; 15(2):109-124.

Andrew M, Paes B, Milner R, Johnston M, Mitchell L, Tollefsen DM, Powers P. development of the human coagulation system in the full-term infant. *Blood* 1987; 70: 165-172.

Ariëns RAS, Lai TS, Weisel JW, Greenberg CS, Grant PJ. Role of factor XIII in fibrin clot formation and effects of genetic polymorphisms. *Blood* 2002; 100: 743-754.

Bayston TA and Lane DA. Antithrombin: molecular basis of deficiency. *Thromb Haemost* 1997; 78(1):339-343.

Behrens WE. Mediterranean macrothrombocytopenia. *Blood* 1975; 46: 199-208.

Bernard GR, Vincent JL, Laterre PF. Efficacy and safety of recombinant human activated protein C for severe sepsis. *N Engl J Med* 2001; 344 699–709.

Blackall DP, Uhl L, Spitalnik SL. Cryoprecipitate-reduced plasma: rationale for use and efficacy in the treatment of thrombotic thrombocytopenic purpura. *Transfusion* 2001; 41: 840-844.

Casonato A, Pontara E, Sartorello F, Cattini MG, Gallinaro L, Bertomoro A, Rosato A, Padrini R, Pagnan A. Identifying type Vicenza von Willebrand disease. *J Lab Clin Med* 2006;147:96–102.

Catto AJ, Kohler HP, Coore J, et al. Association of a common polymorphism in the factor XIII gene with venous thrombosis. *Blood* 1999; 93(3):906-908.

Chang S, Tillema V, Scherr D. A Percentage correction formula for evaluation of mixing studies. *Am J Clin Pathol* 2002; 117: 62-73.

Bibliography

Laposata M, Green D, Van Cott EM et al. College of American Pathologists conference XXXI on laboratory monitoring of anticoagulant therapy: the clinical use and laboratory monitoring of low-molecular weight heparin, danaparoid, hirudin and related compounds, and argatroban. *Arch Pathol Lab Med* 1998; 122(9):799-807.

Lederer DJ, Kawut SM, Sonett JR, Vakiani E, Seward SL Jr, White JG, Wilt JS, Marboe CC, Gahl WA, Arcasoy SM. Successful bilateral lung transplantation for pulmonary fibrosis associated with the Hermansky-Pudlak syndrome. *J Heart Lung Transplant* 2005; 24:1697-1699.

LeGal G, Righini M, Roy P, Sanchez O, Aujesky D, Bounameaux H Perrier A. Prediction of pulmonary embolism in the emergency department: the revised Geneva score. *Ann Int Med* 2006; 144:165-171.

Lehman CM, Blaylock RC, Alexander DP, Rodgers GM. Discontinuation of the bleeding time test without detectable adverse clinical impact. *Clin Chem* 2001 47: 1204-1211.

Levi M, TenCate H. Disseminated intravascular coagulation. *New Engl J Med* 2002; 341: 586-592.

Levine JS, Branch DW, Rauch J. The antiphospholipid syndrome. *New Engl J Med* 2002; 346: 752-763.

Lind SE. The bleeding time does not predict surgical bleeding. *Blood* 1991;77:2547-2552.

Ma J, Hennekens CH, Ridker PM, et al. A prospective study of fibrinogen and risk of myocardial infarction in the physician's health survey. *J Am Coll Cardiol* 1999; 33(5):1347-1352.

Macy PA. Identification and clinical significance of platelet antibodies. *Clin Hemostasis Rev* 2003; 17: 5.

Mannucci PM, Duga S, Peyvandi F. Recessively inherited coagulation disorders. *Blood* 2004;104:1243-1252.

Mannucci PM. Treatment of von Willebrand's disease. *N Engl J Med* 2004; 351: 683-694.

Matsubara K, Fukaya T, Nigami H, Harigaya H, Hirata T, Nozaki H, Baba K. Age-dependent changes in the incidence and etiology of childhood thrombocytosis. *Acta Haematol* 2004;111:132–137.

McGlennen RC, Key NS. Clinical and laboratory management of the prothrombin G20210A mutation. *Arch Pathol Lab Med* 2002; 126: 1319-1324.

Meijers JC, Tekelenburg WLH, Bouma BN, et al. High levels of coagulation factor XI as a risk factor for venous thrombosis. *N Engl J Med* 2000; 342(10):696-701.

Michelson AD. Platelet function in the newborn. *Semin Thromb Hemost* 1998; 24(6):507-512.

Miller JL. Blood Platelets. *Clinical Diagnosis and Management by Laboratory Methods, 19th ed.* (Philadelphia: W.B. Saunders Company, 1996).

Miller JL. Blood Coagulation and Fibrinolysis. *Clinical Diagnosis and Management by Laboratory Methods, 19th ed.* (Philadelphia: W.B. Saunders Company, 1996).

Miller JL. Platelet-type von Willebrand's disease. *Thromb Haemost* 1996; 75(6):865-869.

Moake JL. Thrombotic microangiopathies. *New Engl J Med* 2002; 347: 589-600.

Moake JL. Thrombotic thrombocytopenia purpura and the hemolytic uremic syndrome. *Arch Pathol Lab Med* 2002; 126: 1430-1433.

Moeller A, Weippert-Kretschmer M, Prinz H, Kretschmer V. Influence of ABO blood groups on primary hemostasis. *Transfusion* 2001; 41: 56-60.

Moll S, Ortel TL. Monitoring warfarin therapy in patients with lupus anticoagulants. *Ann Intern Med* 1997; 127(3):177-185.

Nair S, Ghosh K, Kulkarni B, Shetty S, Mohanty D. Glanzmann's thrombasthenia: updated. *Platelets* 2002; 13: 387-393.

Neerman-Arbez M, de Moerloose P, Bridel C, Honsberger A, Schonborner A, Rossier C, Peerlinck K, Claeyssens S, Di Michele D, d'Oiron R, Dreyfus M, Laubriat-Bianchin M, Dieval J, Antonarakis SE, Morris MA. Mutations in the Fibrinogen Aα−gene account for the majority of cases of congenital afibrinogenemia. *Blood* 2000;96:149-152.

Norman KE, Cotter MJ, Stewart BJ. Combined anticoagulant and antiselectin treatments prevent lethal intravascular coagulation. *Blood* 2003;101: 921–928.

patients this is supplemented with oral vitamin K, particularly if the patient is at increased risk for bleeding. For patients with very high INRs (>20) or with serious bleeding, discontinue warfarin therapy and administer vitamin K by slow IV infusion, supplemented with fresh plasma or prothrombin complex concentrate, depending on the urgency of the situation.

For planned invasive procedures, coumadin may be discontinued 4 days before surgery and placed on heparin. Heparin can be discontinued hours before surgery.

Adcock DM. Factor VIII Inhibitors in patients with hemophilia A. *Clin Hemostasis Rev* 2002; 16: 1.

Adcock DM, Fink L, Marlar RA. A laboratory approach to the evaluation of hereditary hypercoagulability. *Am J Clin Pathol* 1997; 108:434-449.

Ananyeva NM, Lacroix-Desmazes S, Hauser CAE, Shima M, Ovanesov MV, Khrenov AV, Saenko EL. Inhibitors in hemophilia A: mechanisms of inhibition, management and perspectives. *Blood Coagul Fibrinolysis* 2004; 15(2):109-124.

Andrew M, Paes B, Milner R, Johnston M, Mitchell L, Tollefsen DM, Powers P. development of the human coagulation system in the full-term infant. *Blood* 1987; 70: 165-172.

Ariëns RAS, Lai TS, Weisel JW, Greenberg CS, Grant PJ. Role of factor XIII in fibrin clot formation and effects of genetic polymorphisms. *Blood* 2002; 100: 743-754.

Bayston TA and Lane DA. Antithrombin: molecular basis of deficiency. *Thromb Haemost* 1997; 78(1):339-343.

Behrens WE. Mediterranean macrothrombocytopenia. *Blood* 1975; 46: 199-208.

Bernard GR, Vincent JL, Laterre PF. Efficacy and safety of recombinant human activated protein C for severe sepsis. *N Engl J Med* 2001; 344 699–709.

Blackall DP, Uhl L, Spitalnik SL. Cryoprecipitate-reduced plasma: rationale for use and efficacy in the treatment of thrombotic thrombocytopenic purpura. *Transfusion* 2001; 41: 840-844.

Casonato A, Pontara E, Sartorello F, Cattini MG, Gallinaro L, Bertomoro A, Rosato A, Padrini R, Pagnan A. Identifying type Vicenza von Willebrand disease. *J Lab Clin Med* 2006;147:96–102.

Catto AJ, Kohler HP, Coore J, et al. Association of a common polymorphism in the factor XIII gene with venous thrombosis. *Blood* 1999; 93(3):906-908.

Chang S, Tillema V, Scherr D. A Percentage correction formula for evaluation of mixing studies. *Am J Clin Pathol* 2002; 117: 62-73.

Bibliography

Cines DB, Blanchette VS. Immune thrombocytopenic purpura. *NEW ENGL J MED* 2002; 346: 995-1008.

Cunningham MT, Brandt JT, Laposata M, Olson JD. Laboratory diagnosis of dysfibrinogenemia. *Arch Pathol Lab Med* 2002; 126(4): 499–505.

Danilenko-Dixon DR, Van Winter JT, Homburger HA. Clinical implications of antiphospholipid antibodies in obstetrics. *Mayo Clin Proc* 1996; 71: 1118-1120.

DeRossi SS and Glick MG. Bleeding time: an unreliable predictor of clinical hemostasis. *J Oral Maxillofac Surg* 1996; 54(9):1119-20.

De Stefano V, Martinelli I, Mannucci PM, Paciaroni K, Chiusolo P, Casorelli I, Rossi E, Leone G. The risk of recurrent deep venous thrombosis among heterozygous carriers of both factor V Leiden and the G20210A prothrombin mutation. *N Engl J Med* 2000; 342(3): 214-215.

De Moerloose P, Reber G, Perrier A, Perneger T, Bounameaux H. Prevalence of factor V Leiden and prothrombin G20210A mutations in unselected patients with venous thromboembolism. *Br J Haematol* 2000; 110(1): 125-129.

Drachman JG. Inherited Thrombocytopenia: When a low platelet count does not mean ITP. *Blood* 2004;103: 390-398.

Dumenco LL, Blair AJ, Sweeney JD. The results of diagnostic studies for thrombophilia in a large group of patients with a personal or family history of thrombosis. *Am J Clin Pathol* 1998; 110: 673-682.

Elliot MA, Tefferi A. Thrombosis and haemorrhage in polycythemia vera and essential thrombocythaemia. *Brit J Haematol* 2004; 128:275-290.

Emilia G, Longo G, Luppi M, Gandini G, Morselli M, Ferrara L, Amarri S, Cagossi K, Torelli G. *Helicobacter pylori* eradication can induce platelet recovery in idiopathic thrombocytopenic purpura. *Blood* 2001; 97: 812-814.

Fabris F, Ahmad S, Cella G, Jeske WP, Walenga JM, Fareed J. Pathophysiology of heparin-induced thrombocytopenia. *Arch Pathol Lab Med* 2000; 124: 1657-1666.

Franchini M, Manzato F. Update on the treatment of disseminated intravascular coagulation. *Hematology* 2004; 9(2): 81–85.

Francis CW. Plasminogen activator inhibitor-1 levels and polymorphisms. *Arch Pathol Lab Med* 2002; 126: 1401-1404.

Frost SD, Brotman DJ, Michota FA. Rational use of D-dimer measurement to exclude acute venous thromboembolic disease. *Mayo Clin Proc* 2003;78:1385-1391.

Furlan M, Robles R, Galbusera M, Remuzzi G, Kyrle PA, Brenner B, Krause M, Scharrer I, Aumann V, Mittler U, Solenthaler M, Lämmle B. von Willebrand factor-cleaving protease in thrombotic thrombocytopenic purpura and the hemolytic-uremic syndrome. *NEW ENGL J MED* 1998; 339:1578-1584

Garay SM, Gardella JE, Fazzini EP, Goldring RM. Hermansky-Pudlak syndrome: pulmonary manifestations of a ceroid storage disorder. *Am J Med* 1979; 66:737-747.

Gewirtz AS, Miller ML, and Keys TF. The clinical usefulness of the preoperative bleeding time. *Arch Pathol Lab Med* 1996; 120(4):353-356.

Gill JC, Endres-Brooks J, Bauer PJ, Marks WJ Jr, Montgomery RR. The effect of ABO blood group on the diagnosis of von Willebrand's disease. *Blood* 1987; 69(6):1691-1695.

Griffin JH, Evatt B, Wideman C, Fernandez JA. Anticoagulant protein C pathway defective in the majority of thrombophilic patients. *Blood* 1993; 82:1989-1994.

Grunewald M, Grunewald A, Schmid A, Schopflin C, Schauer S, Griesshammer M, Koksch M. The platelet function defect of paroxysmal nocturnal haemoglobinuria. *Platelets* 2004; 15(3): 145–154.

Hanley JP. Warfarin reversal. *J Clin Pathol* 2004; 57: 1132–1139.

Hassell K. The management of patients with heparin-induced thrombocytopenia who require anticoagulant therapy. *Chest* 2005; 127(2): 1S-8S

Bibliography

Heath KE, Campos-Barros A, Toren A, Rozenfeld-Granot G, Carlsson LE, Savige J, Denison JC, Gregory MC, White JG, Barker DF, Greinacher A, Epstein CJ, Glucksman MJ, Martignetti JA. Nonmuscle myosin heavy chain IIA mutations define a spectrum of autosomal dominant macrothrombocytopenias: May-Hegglin anomaly and Fechtner, Sebastian, Epstein, and Alport-like syndromes. *Am J Hum Genet* 2001; 69: 1033–1045.

Hirsh J, Dalen JE, Aiuleison DR, Foller U, Btissei H, Anftell J, Deykin D. Oral anticoagulants: mechanism of action, clinical effectiveness, and optimal therapeutic range. *Chest* 2001; 119: 8S-21S.

Hohlfeld P, Forestier F, Kaplan C, Tissot JD, Daffos F. Fetal Thrombocytopenia: a retrospective survey of 5,194 fetal blood samplings. *Blood* 1994; 84(6): 1851-1856.

Hosler GA, Cusumano AM, Hutchins GM. Thrombotic thrombocytopenic purpura and hemolytic uremic syndrome are distinct pathologic entities. *Arch Pathol Lab Med* 2003; 127: 834-839.

Hoyer LW. Hemophilia A. *N Engl J Med* 1994; 330(1):38-47.

Iacoviello L, Di Castelnuovo A, de Knijff P, et al. Polymorphisms in the coagulation factor VII gene and the risk of myocardial infarction. *N Engl J Med* 1998; 338(2):79-85.

Jensen R. The antiphospholipid antibody syndrome. *Clin Hemostasis Rev* 2001; 15.

Jorquera JI, Montoro JM, Fernandez MA. Modified test for activated protein C resistance. *Lancet* 1994; 344:1162-1163.

Kane WH and Davie EW. Blood coagulation factors V and VIII: structural and functional similarities and their relationship to hemorrhagic and thrombotic disorders. *Blood* 1988; 71(3):539-555.

Kapiotis S, Quehenberger P, Jilma B, Handler S, Pabinger-Fasching I, Mannhalter C, Speiser W. Improved characteristics of APC-resistance assay: Coatest APC resistance by predilution of samples with factor V deficient plasma. *Am J Clin Pathol* 1996; 106(5): 588-593.

Karpatkin S. Autoimmune Thrombocytopenias. *Autoimmunity* 2004; 34(4): 363-368.

Kankirawatana S, Berkow RL, Marques MB. A neonate with bleeding and multiple factor deficiencies. *Lab Med* 2006; 37(2): 95-97

Kelley MJ, Jawien W, Ortel TL, Korczak JF. Mutation of MYH9, encoding non-muscle myosin heavy chain A, in May-Hegglin anomaly. *Nature Genet* 2000; 26: 106-108.

Kelton JG, Warkentin TE. Diagnosis of heparin-induced thrombocytopenia. *Am J Clin Pathol* 1995; 104: 611-613.

Key NS, McGlennen RC. Hyperhomocysteinemia and thrombophilia. *Arch Pathol Lab Med* 2002; 126: 1367-1374.

Kitchens CS. The Contact System. *Arch Pathol Lab Med* 2002; 126: 1382-1386.

Kitchens CS, Alving BM, Kessler CM, eds. *Consultative Hemostasis and Thrombosis* (Philadelphia: WB Saunders Company, 2002).

Kohda K, Kuga T, Kogawa K, Kanisawa Y, Koike K, Kuroiwa G, Hirayama Y, Sato Y, Matsunaga T, Niitsu Y. Effect of *Helicobacter pylori* eradication on platelet recovery in Japanese patients with chronic idiopathic thrombocytopenic purpura and secondary autoimmune thrombocytopenic purpura. *Br J Haematol* 2002; 118: 584.

Kojouri K, Vesely SK, Terrell DR, George JN. Splenectomy for adult patients with idiopathic thrombocytopenic purpura: a systematic review to assess long-term platelet count responses, prediction of response, and surgical complications. *Blood* 2004; 104: 2623-2634.

Kottke-Marchant KK, Duncan A. Antithrombin deficiency: issues in laboratory diagnosis. *Arch Pathol Lab Med* 2002; 126: 1326-1336.

Kottke-Marchant KK, Corcoran G. The laboratory diagnosis of platelet disorders: an algorithmic approach. *Arch Pathol Lab Med* 2002; 126: 133-146.

Bibliography

Laposata M, Green D, Van Cott EM et al. College of American Pathologists conference XXXI on laboratory monitoring of anticoagulant therapy: the clinical use and laboratory monitoring of low-molecular weight heparin, danaparoid, hirudin and related compounds, and argatroban. *Arch Pathol Lab Med* 1998; 122(9):799-807.

Lederer DJ, Kawut SM, Sonett JR, Vakiani E, Seward SL Jr, White JG, Wilt JS, Marboe CC, Gahl WA, Arcasoy SM. Successful bilateral lung transplantation for pulmonary fibrosis associated with the Hermansky-Pudlak syndrome. *J Heart Lung Transplant* 2005; 24:1697-1699.

LeGal G, Righini M, Roy P, Sanchez O, Aujesky D, Bounameaux H Perrier A. Prediction of pulmonary embolism in the emergency department: the revised Geneva score. *Ann Int Med* 2006; 144:165-171.

Lehman CM, Blaylock RC, Alexander DP, Rodgers GM. Discontinuation of the bleeding time test without detectable adverse clinical impact. *Clin Chem* 2001 47: 1204-1211.

Levi M, TenCate H. Disseminated intravascular coagulation. *New Engl J Med* 2002; 341: 586-592.

Levine JS, Branch DW, Rauch J. The antiphospholipid syndrome. *New Engl J Med* 2002; 346: 752-763.

Lind SE. The bleeding time does not predict surgical bleeding. *Blood* 1991;77:2547-2552.

Ma J, Hennekens CH, Ridker PM, et al. A prospective study of fibrinogen and risk of myocardial infarction in the physician's health survey. *J Am Coll Cardiol* 1999; 33(5):1347-1352.

Macy PA. Identification and clinical significance of platelet antibodies. *Clin Hemostasis Rev* 2003; 17: 5.

Mannucci PM, Duga S, Peyvandi F. Recessively inherited coagulation disorders. *Blood* 2004;104:1243-1252.

Mannucci PM. Treatment of von Willebrand's disease. *N Engl J Med* 2004; 351: 683-694.

Matsubara K, Fukaya T, Nigami H, Harigaya H, Hirata T, Nozaki H, Baba K. Age-dependent changes in the incidence and etiology of childhood thrombocytosis. *Acta Haematol* 2004;111:132–137.

McGlennen RC, Key NS. Clinical and laboratory management of the prothrombin G20210A mutation. *Arch Pathol Lab Med* 2002; 126: 1319-1324.

Meijers JC, Tekelenburg WLH, Bouma BN, et al. High levels of coagulation factor XI as a risk factor for venous thrombosis. *N Engl J Med* 2000; 342(10):696-701.

Michelson AD. Platelet function in the newborn. *Semin Thromb Hemost* 1998; 24(6):507-512.

Miller JL. Blood Platelets. *Clinical Diagnosis and Management by Laboratory Methods, 19th ed.* (Philadelphia: W.B. Saunders Company, 1996).

Miller JL. Blood Coagulation and Fibrinolysis. *Clinical Diagnosis and Management by Laboratory Methods, 19th ed.* (Philadelphia: W.B. Saunders Company, 1996).

Miller JL. Platelet-type von Willebrand's disease. *Thromb Haemost* 1996; 75(6):865-869.

Moake JL. Thrombotic microangiopathies. *New Engl J Med* 2002; 347: 589-600.

Moake JL. Thrombotic thrombocytopenia purpura and the hemolytic uremic syndrome. *Arch Pathol Lab Med* 2002; 126: 1430-1433.

Moeller A, Weippert-Kretschmer M, Prinz H, Kretschmer V. Influence of ABO blood groups on primary hemostasis. *Transfusion* 2001; 41: 56-60.

Moll S, Ortel TL. Monitoring warfarin therapy in patients with lupus anticoagulants. *Ann Intern Med* 1997; 127(3):177-185.

Nair S, Ghosh K, Kulkarni B, Shetty S, Mohanty D. Glanzmann's thrombasthenia: updated. *Platelets* 2002; 13: 387-393.

Neerman-Arbez M, de Moerloose P, Bridel C, Honsberger A, Schonborner A, Rossier C, Peerlinck K, Claeyssens S, Di Michele D, d'Oiron R, Dreyfus M, Laubriat-Bianchin M, Dieval J, Antonarakis SE, Morris MA. Mutations in the Fibrinogen Aα–gene account for the majority of cases of congenital afibrinogenemia. *Blood* 2000;96:149-152.

Norman KE, Cotter MJ, Stewart BJ. Combined anticoagulant and antiselectin treatments prevent lethal intravascular coagulation. *Blood* 2003;101: 921–928.

Bibliography

Olson JD, Arkin CF, Brandt JT. College of American Pathologists conference XXXI on laboratory monitoring of anticoagulant therapy: laboratory monitoring of unfractionated heparin therapy. *Arch Pathol Lab Med* 1998; 122(9):782-798.

O'Shea J, Sherlock M, Philip R. Thrombocytosis in childhood [letter]. *Acta Haematol* 2005; 113: 212.

Passam FH, Krilis SA. Laboratory tests for the antiphospholipid syndrome: current concepts. *Pathology* 2004; 36(2): 129–138.

Portielje J, Westendorp R, Kluin-Nelemans H, Brand A. Morbidity and mortality in adults with idiopathic thrombocytopenic purpura. *Blood* 2001;97:2549-2554.

Press RD, Bauer KA, Kujovich JL, Heit JA. Clinical utility of factor V Leiden (R506Q) testing for the diagnosis and management of thromboembolic disorders. *Arch Pathol Lab Med* 2002; 126: 1304-1318.

Rao AK, Niewiarowski S, Guzzo J, et al. Antithrombin III levels during heparin therapy. *Thromb Res* 1981; 24:181-186.

Rees DC, Cox M, and Clegg JB. World distribution of factor V Leiden. *Lancet* 1995; 346: 1133-1134.

Ridker PM, Miletich JP, Hennekens CH, et al. Ethnic distribution of factor V Leiden in 4047 men and women. *JAMA* 1997; 277(16):1305-1307.

Rodgers RP and Levin J. A critical reappraisal of the bleeding time. *Semin Thromb Hemost* 1990, 16(1):1-20.

Roelse J, Koopman R, Büller H, Berends F, ten Cate JW, Mertens K, van Mourik JA. Association of idiopathic venous thromboembolism with single point-mutation at Arg506 of factor V. *Lancet* 1994; 343:1535-1539.

Rozman P. Platelet Antigens: The role of human platelet alloantigens (HPA) in blood transfusion and transplantation. *Transpl Immunol* 2002; 10: 165-181.

Ruggeri ZM, Pareti FI, Mannucci PM, Ciavarella N, Zimmerman TS. Heightened interaction between platelets and factor VIII/von Willebrand factor in a new subtype of von Willebrand's disease. *N Engl J Med* 1980; 302:1047-1051.

Schinella RA, Greco MA, Cobert BL, Denmark LW, Cox RP. Hermansky-Pudlak syndrome with granulomatous colitis. *Ann Intern Med* 1980; 92:20-23.

Seligsohn U, Lubetsky A. Genetic susceptibility to venous thrombosis. *NEW ENGL J MED* 2001; 344: 1222-1231.

Seri M, Cusano R, Gangarossa S, Caridi G, Bordo D, Lo Nigro C, Ghiggeri GM, Ravazzolo R, Savino M, Del Vecchio M, d'Apolito M, Iolascon A, Zelante LL, Savoia A, Balduini CL, Noris P, Magrini U, Belletti S, Heath KE, Babcock M, Glucksman MJ, Aliprandis E, Bizzaro N, Desnick RJ, Martignetti JA. Mutations in MYH9 result in the May-Hegglin anomaly, and Fechtner and Sebastian syndromes. *Nat Genet* 2000; 26(1):103-105.

Strobl FJ, Hoffman S, Huber S, et al. Activated protein C resistance assay performance: improvement by sample dilution with factor V-deficient plasma. *Arch Pathol Lab Med* 1998, 122(5):430-433.

Svensson PJ and Dahlbäck B. Resistance to activated protein C as a basis for venous thrombosis. *N Engl J Med* 1994; 330(8):517-522.

Tollefson DM. Heparin cofactor II deficiency. *Arch Pathol Lab Med* 2002; 126: 1394-1400.

Triplett DA. Antiphospholipid antibodies. *Arch Pathol Lab Med* 2002; 126: 1424-1433.

Tsai HM, Lian EC. Antibodies to von Willebrand factor-cleaving protease in acute thrombotic thrombocytopenic purpura. *New Engl J Med* 2002; 339:1585-1594.

Tollefson DM. Heparin cofactor II deficiency. *Arch Pathol Lab Med* 2002; 126: 1394-1400.

Van Cott EM, Laposata M, Prins MH. Laboratory evaluation of hypercoagulability with venous or arterial thrombosis. *Arch Pathol Lab Med* 2002; 126: 1281-1294.

Van Oerle R, van Pampus L, Tans G, et al. The clinical application of a new specific functional assay to detect the factor V (Leiden) mutation associated with activated protein C resistance. *Am J Clin Pathol* 1997; 107(5):521-526.

Bibliography

Vincentelli A, Susen S, LeTourneau T, Six I, Fabre O, Juthier F, Bauters A, Decoene C, Goudemand J, Prat A, Jude B. Acquired von Willebrand syndrome in aortic stenosis. *N Engl J Med* 2003; 349:343-349.

Warkentin TE. Platelet count monitoring and laboratory testing for heparin-induced thrombocytopenia. *Arch Pathol Lab Med* 2002; 126: 1415-1422.

Warkentin TE, Kelton JG. Temporal aspects of heparin-induced thrombocytopenia. *New Engl J Med* 2001; 344:1286-1292.

Warkentin TE. Heparin-induced thrombocytopenia. *Dis Mon* 2005; 51: 141-149.

Warkentin TE. New approaches to the diagnosis of heparin-induced thrombocytopenia. *Chest* 2005; 127(2): 35S-45S.

Warkentin TE, Kelton JG. Delayed onset heparin-induced thrombocytopenia and thrombosis. *Ann Intern Med* 2001;135:502-506.

Warren BL, Eid A, Singer P. High-dose antithrombin III in severe sepsis: a randomized controlled trial. *JAMA* 2001: 1869–1878..

Weiss EJ, Bray PF, Tayback M, Schulman SP, Kickler TS, Becker LC, Weiss JL, Gerstenblith G, Goldschmidt-Clermont PJ. The platelet glycoprotein IIIa polymorphism PLA2 : an inherited platelet risk factor for coronary thrombotic events. *N Engl J Med* 1996; 334:1090-1094.

Wildenberg SC, Fryer JP, Gardner JM, Oetting WS, Brilliant MH, King RA. Identification of a novel transcript produced by the gene responsible for the Hermansky-Pudlak syndrome in Puerto Rico. *J Invest Dermatol* 1998; 110:777-781.

Wilson DB, Gard KM. Evaluation of an automated, latex-enhanced turbidimetric D-dimer test (advanced D-dimer) and usefulness in the exclusion of acute thromboembolic disease. *Am J Clin Pathol* 2003; 120: 930-937.

Zehnder JL and Benson RC. Sensitivity and specificity of the APC resistance assay in detection of individuals with factor V leiden. *Am J Clin Pathol* 1996, 106(1):107-111.

Zotz RB, Winkelmann BR, Nauck M, Giers G, Maruhn-Debowski B, März W, Scharf RE. Polymorphism of platelet membrane glycoprotein IIIa: human platelet antigen 1b (HPA-1b/PLA2) is an inherited risk factor for premature myocardial infarction in coronary artery disease. *Throm Haemost* 1998; 79:731-735.

Chapter 6

Immunology and Autoimmunity

Immune System Components

Immune system cells begin with a pluripotential stem cell that gives rise to lymphoid and myeloid stem cells. The lymphoid stem cell differentiates into three cell types: T lymphocytes, B lymphocytes, and natural killer (NK) lymphocytes. The myeloid stem differentiates into histiocytes, monocytes, dendritic cells, mast cells, neutrophils, eosinophils, basophils, megakaryocytes and erythrocytes.

B Cells

B cells originate in the marrow and undergo a stepwise maturation there **T6.1**. During this process they undergo rearrangement of their immunoglobulin genes.

- A single immunoglobulin (Ig) molecule consists of 4 chains bound together by disulfide bonds: 2 heavy chains and 2 light chains.

  □ Light chains have two domains: 1 variable and 1 constant.

  □ Heavy chains have 4 to 5 domains: 1 variable and 3 to 4 constants. The terminal constant region may insert into the membrane of B cells or, if free in serum, is called the Fc portion. This Fc may bind to Fc receptors (FcR) on the surfaces of phagocytic cells. Mast cells bear an Fcε receptor that renders them capable of binding IgE.

  □ The variable regions of a light and heavy chain combine to form the antigen binding site (paratope). This recognizes a specific molecular structure (epitope) which is often a tiny part of a larger molecule or cell (the antigen, which may contain several epitopes).

- Genes for light chains are found on chromosomes 2 (κ) and 22 (γ). Genes for the heavy chains (γ, α, μ, δ, ε) are found on chromosome 14.

  □ During B-cell development, these genes are physically rearranged. This process begins when the variable regions for both the light and heavy chain genes rearrange. The final variable region gene is created when separate V and J (light chain) or V, D, and J (heavy chain) segments are brought together (rearranged) in a fashion that has tremendous built-in randomness.

  □ The rearranged variable region is then joined to a light chain or heavy chain constant region. The latter is always initially a μ heavy chain gene, resulting in a completed IgM protein with some particular epitope specificity. Mature B cells co-express surface IgM and IgD. The randomness that is built into rearrangement leads to a population of B cells with a nearly infinite variety of variable regions; ie, specificities for a nearly infinite variety of antigens. Any B cells capable of producing self-reactive Ig are destroyed.

T6.1
B- and T-Cell Maturation Sequences

B-cell stage	Definition	T-cell stage	Definition
Lymphoid stem cell	CD34+, TdT+, HLA-DR+	Lymphoid stem cell	CD34+, TdT+, HLA-DR+
Pro-B cell (Pre-pre-B cell)	CD34+, TdT+, HLA-DR+, CD19+, CD10+, Ig H chain rearranging	Prothymocytes	CD34+, TdT+, CD7+
Pre-B cell	CD34–, TdT–, HLA-DR+, CD19+, CD10+, CD20+, *Cytoplasmic* μ heavy chains+Ig L chain rearranging	Immature/Common thymocytes	CD34–, TdT+, CD1+, CD2+, cytoplasmic CD3+ (surface CD3–), CD5+, CD7+, CD4 and CD8+, TCR rearranged
B cell	All of the above plus surface Ig, CD21+, CD22+	Mature thymocyte	All of the above, except: TdT– and CD1–. Surface CD3 becoming +, CD4 or CD8+
Plasma cell	Loss of B cell markers (CD19–, CD20–) and cytoplasmic (not surface) Ig+.	Mature T cell	All of the above, except surface CD3+

□ Up to this point, the process proceeds without antigen stimulation. Subsequent differentiation of the IgM+/IgD+ mature B cells awaits stimulation by an antigen which is complementary to the antigen binding site (paratope) of the surface Ig. Once stimulated by antigen in the presence of T_h cells the mature B cells proliferate and each progeny B cell rearranges its DNA yet again, rejoining their pre-fabricated variable genes with a different heavy chain gene (isotype switch). During this isotype switch, additional variability is created, leading to a group of B cells having an array of epitope specificities very nearly approximating that of the parent B cell, some having greater and some lesser affinity for the initiating antigen.

■ Since any protein can be an epitope, the variable end of the antibody itself may act as one. An epitope formed by the variable end of an Ig molecule is referred to as an idiotope, and anti-idiotype antibodies may be formed against it.

■ There are 5 Ig classes, based on the heavy chain **isotype:** IgG, IgA, IgM, IgD, and IgE (listed in order of serum concentration). There are 4 subclasses of IgG: IgG1, IgG2, IgG3, IgG4. All classes of IgG behave similarly, except that IgG2 cannot cross the placenta and IgG4 cannot activate complement. There are 2 subclasses of IgA: IgA1, IgA2. Other details worth knowing are included in **T6.2**.

T Cells

■ Undergo stepwise maturation in the thymus. T lymphocytes outnumber B lymphocytes in blood and other tissue by a ratio of about 2:1. They are found in paracortical areas of lymph nodes and within periarteriolar lymphatic sheaths in the spleen.

■ Their T-cell receptor (TCR) genes ($\alpha, \beta, \gamma, \delta$) on chromosome 7 rearrange in a fashion similar to the immunoglobulins.

■ T-cells differentiate into several types that are separable on the basis of cell surface antigens. T-helper (T_h) cells are the pivotal cell in most immune responses and bear the antigen CD4. T-suppressor (T_s), and T-cytotoxic (T_c) cells bear the antigen CD8. The usual CD4:CD8 ratio is about 2:1.

■ T-cell receptors (TCR) are found on the surfaces of T cells.

□ TCRs are highly analogous to immunoglobulin, but unlike Ig can only respond to epitopes presented in conjunction with MHC/HLA molecules. CD4+ (T_h) cells must be presented antigen in conjunction with class II MHC molecules (they are said to be class II MHC-restricted), while CD8+ (T_c) cells must be presented antigen in conjunction with class I MHC molecules (class I-restricted).

□ Each TCR is composed of a pair of equally-sized chains. Each chain has variable and constant domains. There are two classes of TCR: TCR $\alpha\beta$ (composed of one α and one β chain) and TCR $\gamma\delta$.

□ Like immunoglobulin, TCRs get the variability in the variable domains from the randomness built into the rearrangement of the V, D, and J segments of the variable region gene. But there is an additional degree of variability created by the terminal deoxynucleotidyl transferase (TDT) enzyme which randomly adds nucleotides into the gene.

T6.2
Immune System Components

Ig Class	Form found in blood	Activates complement	Immunopathogenic reactions
IgG	Monomers (2 binding sites)	+ (classical)	Immune complex (type III)
IgA	Dimers (4 binding sites)	+ (alternate)	Immune complex, rarely
IgM	Pentamers (10 binding sites)	+ (classical)	Cytotoxic (type II)
IgD	Bound to B cells	–	None
IgE	Bound to mast cells	–	Immediate-type hypersensitivity/ Allergic (type I)

6: Immunology and Autoimmunity

Laboratory Tests of Immune Function>Testing T-Cell Function; Testing NK-Cell Function; Testing Neutrophil Function; Testing Complement | Immunodeficiency>B-Cell Defects

Testing T-Cell Function

■ A test of delayed-type hypersensitivity (DTH) is the usual screening test for T-cell function. A tuberculin skin test is the classic example of this phenomenon. Antigen is inoculated subcutaneously and the skin is observed for the development of a lesion, usually by 24 to 48 hours, indicative of T-cell activation.

■ Alternatively, a gross estimation of the number of circulating T cells is obtained from the blood total lymphocyte count, since most circulating lymphocytes are T cells.

■ By flow cytometry, the proportion of all lymphocyte subsets, including T-cell subsets can be determined. The total CD3+ count is the most accurate way to enumerate T cells. The ratio of CD4:CD8 cells is normally around 2:1. Deviation from this ratio, particularly a decrease, is found in T-cell immunodeficiency states.

■ Proliferation assays can be performed by exposing T cells to mitogen, such as phytohemagglutinin or concanavalin A. Proliferation is measured by the uptake of radioactive DNA precursors (tritiated thymidine).

Testing NK-Cell Function

■ By flow cytometry, NK cells (CD3–, CD16+, CD56+, CD57+) can easily be enumerated. Isolated NK-cell deficiency is rare. Severe herpes virus infections have been reported in this context.

■ NK-cell function can be assessed by chromium release assays.

Testing Neutrophil Function

■ An excellent screening test for neutrophils is simply the neutrophil count and peripheral smear, since most inherited defects in this arm of the immune system have readily identifiable numerical and/or morphologic findings.

■ In addition, one can specifically look at chemotaxis, phagocytosis, or oxidative burst functions with various assays. One such assay is the nitroblue tetrazolium (NBT) assay in which yellow NBT dye is added to neutrophils which are then stimulated.

  □ Cells capable of a normal oxidative burst will reduce the yellow NBT to a purple-blue formazan precipitate, and are said to be f+. Normal individuals will have nearly 100% f+ cells.

  □ An abnormal result, with perhaps <10% f+ cells, is expected in chronic granulomatous disease (CGD), in which deficiency of NADPH oxidase prevents the oxidative burst.

■ Myeloperoxidase staining can disclose myeloperoxidase deficiency, an autosomal recessive trait which produces at most mild immunodeficiency.

Testing Complement

■ The screening test for complement is the CH50. This test determines what percentage of immunoglobulin-coated sheep red cells are lysed by the patient's serum and is thus a gross evaluation of the classical complement pathway. Quantitative deficiencies of any of the complement components, C1-C9, will lead to a reduced CH50.

■ Assays for quantitation of specific complement components are clinically available as well. C3 levels are used to look at the alternative pathway. Decreased levels of C3 reflect either primary C3 deficiency or activation of the alternate complement pathway. Levels of C4 or C1q are typically used to look at the classical pathway.

Immunodeficiency

B-Cell Defects

■ Defective B-cell function is characterized by recurrent bacterial sinopulmonary infections (due to staphylococci, streptococci, and hemophilus) and recalcitrant intestinal infection with *G lamblia*. Opportunistic fungal and viral infections are not a particular problem. B cell defects often present at or after 6 months of age, due to persistence of maternal antibodies in the infant serum.

Bruton (X-linked) agammaglobulinemia

■ Patients present with recurrent pyogenic infections, affecting primarily males, starting around 6 months of age. Often this leads to eventual bronchiectasis.

■ They commonly undergo duodenal biopsies for evaluation of chronic diarrhea, often before the diagnosis of an immunodeficiency has been made. When reviewing such a biopsy, particularly in a child or young adult, one must look for organisms such as *Giardia;* however, it is also important to ensure that there are plasma cells in the lamina propria. The absence of plasma cells in the intestinal mucosa is distinctly abnormal and should prompt evaluation for a B-cell defect.

■ Serum IgG levels are markedly reduced as are circulating mature B cells. Pre-B cells are found in lymph nodes and bone marrow where they do not mature normally into B cells.

■ Lymph nodes lack germinal centers, and plasma cells are absent. Tonsils are rudimentary.

■ Such individuals have normal immunity against most viral and fungal pathogens; although, they show susceptibility to polio, hepatitis, and enteroviruses.

■ They also suffer from a high incidence of leukemia/lymphoma and autoimmune diseases.

■ The responsible gene on the X chromosome encodes a tyrosine kinase called Atk (agammaglobulinemia tyrosine kinase).

■ Common variable immunodeficiency (CVI) is characterized by low serum immunoglobulin (IgG, IgM, and IgA). Some also have a component of T-cell deficiency. The clinical severity and age of onset are somewhat variable; the typical onset is around the second or third decade. Most patients suffer from recurrent upper and lower respiratory tract infections (*Streptococcus pneumoniae, Haemophilus influenzae,* and *Mycoplasma*), intestinal bacterial overgrowth, and intestinal *Giardia lamblia* infection. The development of bronchiectasis is extremely common. A normal number of B cells are found in blood and tissue which lack the capacity to differentiate into plasma cells. Germinal centers are hyperplastic; the typical small bowel morphology includes pronounced reactive follicular lymphoid hyperplasia in the face of a distinctly low number of plasma cells.

■ Selective IgA deficiency is the most common inherited immunodeficiency disease, affecting around 1/700 of people. These patients suffer from recurrent respiratory and gastrointestinal bacterial infections, a high incidence of autoimmunity, and are at risk for anaphylaxis due to transfusion of IgA-containing blood products.

■ Job (hypergammaglobulinemia E) syndrome presents with abnormally high serum IgE, high levels of specific IgE anti-staphylococcal antibody, exquisite susceptibility to staphylococcal infection, eosinophilia and eczema. These appear to result from a defect in granulocyte chemotaxis.

T-Cell Defects

■ Defective T-cell function is characterized by susceptibility to chronic viral, fungal, and protozoal infections. T-cell disorders often engender a certain degree of B-cell dysfunction due to their role in orchestrating B-cell activities. They tend to present at an earlier age, often in the neonatal period.

■ DiGeorge syndrome/velocardiofacial syndrome is due to failure of the 3rd and 4th pharyngeal pouches to adequately develop. In addition to T-cell deficiency, such individuals have a hypoplastic thymus, hypoplastic parathyroids, anomalies of the great vessels, typical facies (hypertelorism, low set ears, mandibular hypoplasia), bifid uvula, and a higher than usual incidence of esophageal atresia. They have depleted paracortical areas in lymph nodes, and poorly developed peri-arteriolar lymphatic sheaths (PALS) in the spleen. Deletion of 22q11.2 is associated with DiGeorge syndrome, velocardiofacial syndrome (VCFS), Shprintzen syndrome, and occasionally isolated conotruncal cardiac defects, while deletions on 10p13p14 (DiGeorge syndrome II locus) have also been associated with the phenotypic features of DiGeorge syndrome (DiGeorge syndrome II). A dual-probe FISH assay for these loci is available for these loci, with a sensitivity of about 95%. Most will demonstrate a deletion of 22q11, with the deletion of 10p13p14 being rare. Di George syndrome does not display Mendelian inheritance and occurs sporadically. Some cases have been associated with in utero exposure to *accutane*. Affected individuals suffer from hypocalcemia (with neonatal tetany), increased susceptibility to opportunistic pathogens such as fungi, viruses, and *Pneumocystis carinii,* and increased risk of transfusion-associated graft-vs-host disease.

■ Severe combined immunodeficiency (SCID) is a syndrome characterized by decreased or absent T-cell function, low or undetectable immunoglobulin levels, and thymic dysplasia. It results in severe, life-threatening,

371

immunodeficiency that is only treatable by bone marrow transplantation. SCID has various genetic bases.

☐ Most (50%) are X-linked recessive and due to a defect in the IL-2 receptor.

☐ Many (40%) of the remaining cases are autosomal recessive and due to deficiency in the enzyme adenosine deaminase (ADA).

☐ Other forms include JAK3 deficiency, purine nucleoside phosphorylase (PNP) deficiency, CD3 deficiency, and RAG1/RAG2 deficiency.

■ Wiskott-Aldrich syndrome (WAS) is an X-linked disease characterized by the triad of eczema, thrombocytopenia, and immunodeficiency. The platelets are small and uniform. The immunodeficiency is due to defects in both the T cell and B cell arms of the immune system. It has also been noted that there is loss of the CD43 antigen on circulating leukocytes and platelets. Such individuals have increased susceptibility to infection by pneumococci and other encapsulated bacteria, *Pneumocystis carinii,* and herpes virus. In addition, they have a 12% incidence of fatal malignancies. The gene responsible for WAS, on the X chromosome, has also been associated with other forms of disease, including X-linked thrombocytopenia and X-linked congenital neutropenia. Wiskott-Aldrich syndrome protein (WASP) refers to the product of the *WAS* gene. WASP is found mainly within hematopoietic cells and appears to be responsible for the cytoskeletal malleability that is necessary for physiologic activities.

■ Ataxia-telangiectasia (Louis-Bar syndrome) is an autosomal recessive disease caused by mutations in the *ATM* gene, on 11q22.3, which encodes the ATM protein kinase (involved in DNA repair). It is characterized by cerebellar ataxia, oculocutaneous telangiectasia, recurrent sinopulmonary infections, and a high incidence of malignancies. On MRI, the cerebellum is frequently small. The immunodeficiency is a combined T-cell and B-cell defect. IgA is usually deficient, and there is impaired antibody response to pneumococcal vaccine. Affected individuals have very high serum AFP and CEA for unknown reasons. The lifetime risk for malignancy is 38%, and hematolymphoid malignancies account for most of these. An immunoblotting assay is available for the ATM protein in nuclear lysate, as well as assays for ATM kinase activity. There is a radiosensitivity assay that determines the survival of lymphoid cells following irradiation, and this is abnormal in >95% of affected individuals. Routine cytogenetics can detect the t(7;14) in about 10% of cases, but direct sequence analysis of the *ATM* gene is required for a definitive molecular diagnosis in most cases.

■ Chronic mucocutaneous candidiasis is a highly selective defect in T-cell immunity to candidal infection that leads to chronic, recalcitrant, mucocutaneous candidal infections. Affected individuals often have associated endocrinopathies.

■ Duncan disease (X-linked lymphoproliferative disease) typically presents as a fulminant and often fatal immune response to Epstein-Barr virus (EBV) infection. EBV infection induces a fulminant hemophagocytic syndrome, the development of a neoplastic B-cell proliferation, and/or fulminant hepatic failure, concomitant with an inverted CD4:CD8 ratio in the peripheral blood. Even before EBV infection occurs, affected individuals often have a common variable immunodeficiency-like immune system defect, especially manifesting hypogammaglobulinemia with or without decreased B-, T-, or NK-subsets. The median survival is about 10 years of age. The *SH2D1A* gene, found at Xq25, has been implicated in this disease. Direct sequence analysis is clinically available. Flow cytometry, to measure surface expression of SAP, can be applied for screening, but it is not confirmatory.

Neutrophil/Phagocytic Defects

■ Defects in phagocytosis lead to particular susceptibility to infections with staphylococci, *E coli, S pneumoniae, Pseudomonas aeruginosa,* and *C albicans.*

■ Chronic granulomatous disease (CGD) results from defective intracellular oxidative killing of ingested organisms, most commonly due to deficiency in the enzyme NADPH oxidase. It is characterized by chronic suppurative infections due to bacteria and fungi that are catalase positive, especially staphylococci, enterobacter, and aspergillus. Such individuals almost never have streptococcal infections. At the sites of infection, there is extensive granuloma formation. CGD has several genetic bases, the most common of which is an X-linked form. About 1/3 show autosomal recessive inheritance. The screening test is the nitroblue tetrazolium (NBT) test, in which phagocytic cells with normal oxidative function can convert the yellow dye to a blue product. Affected leukocytes are also deficient in C3b receptors. Red cells often bear the McLeod phenotype (absence of Kell antigen Kx).

- Chediak-Higashi syndrome is an autosomal recessive condition that presents as neutropenia, recurrent infection, thrombocytopenia, and oculocutaneous albinism. Granulocytes, lymphocytes, and monocytes show giant cytoplasmic granules, representing abnormally fused lysosomes. The basic abnormality is defective degranulation. In late stages, an accelerated phase may develop, characterized by lymphoma-like proliferations within viscera.

- Neutrophil chemotaxis defects (lazy leukocyte syndromes) include the previously mentioned hyper-IgE syndrome.

- Integrin deficiencies, due to deficiencies of the integrins LFA-1 or MAC-1, characteristically manifest as periodontitis and delayed cord separation.

- May-Hegglin anomaly is an autosomal dominant condition manifesting as Döhle-like bodies in granulocytes and monocytes, large platelets, and thrombocytopenia. The Döhle-like bodies can be abolished by addition of ribonuclease. About half of patients have an abnormal bleeding history, but bleeding complications have only been documented when the platelet count falls below 80,000. Platelet aggregation studies are usually normal, and there does not appear to be much of an immune defect.

- Alder-Reilly anomaly is another mainly morphologic finding. It is an autosomal dominant condition manifesting as large azurophilic granules resembling toxic granulation in all white blood cells. There is an association with mucopolysaccharidoses.

- Pelger-Huet anomaly is due to an autosomal dominant disorder with dysfunctional segmentation of neutrophils. Bilobed neutrophils are seen rather than normally segmented forms. In homozygotes, monolobated neutrophils (Stodtmeister cells) are seen. Functionally, the cells are normal.

- Jordan anomaly is characterized by vacuolization of leukocyte cytoplasm by fat vacuoles.

Complement Deficiencies

- Deficiency of classical pathway components (C1q, C2, C4) lead to autoimmune phenomena such as lupus.

- Deficiency of C2 and C3 lead to recurrent infections with gram-positive encapsulated organisms.

- Deficiency of membrane attack complex components or so-called terminal complement components (C5-C9) leads to recurrent serious systemic infections, especially due to *N meningitidis* and *N gonorrhea*.

- C1 esterase inhibitor (C1 Inh) deficiency is an autosomal dominant disorder also called *hereditary angioedema (HAE)*. Classic HAE displays a fairly characteristic temporal and spatial pattern of edema episodes. On average, women have a more severe disease than men, and patients with an early onset of symptoms have more severe disease than those with late onset. For most with HAE the pattern is as follows: a symptom-free infancy and early childhood period is followed by the onset of clinical symptoms, usually in late childhood or adolescence. After onset, the disease persists for the life of the patient, with critical and intercritical periods. With regard to the spatial pattern, swelling is seen most consistently in the skin (upper extremity > lower) and intestinal tract (abdominal pain episodes). Laryngeal edema, though classic and potentially lethal, is present in only about 1% of episodes but has a lifetime incidence of about 50%. Facial swelling is rare, and while there is swelling of the soft palate and uvula, it spares the tongue. Acute episodes are treated with androgenic agents. There are two forms: either C1 Inh is absent (type I) or C1 Inh is present but functionally defective (type II). A third type of HAE has been described that is not associated with C1-INH deficiency, and its underlying mechanism is unknown. Urinary histamine levels and serum C1 levels are elevated during attacks, while serum CH50, C4, and C2 are decreased. Between attacks, C4 is always low, while C2 levels are normal.

Autoimmunity

Notes on Immunofluorescence Testing

There are 2 main types of immunofluorescence tests for autoantibodies

- Direct immunofluorescence (DIF) involves incubating cryostat sections of patient tissue with fluorescein-labeled anti-human globulin (AHG). Positive DIF tests confirm the in vivo presence of *bound autoantibodies* in the patient's tissues. Examples include skin IF (for SLE, dermatitis herpetiformis, etc.), and renal IF (for glomerulonephritides).

- Indirect immunofluorescence (IIF) involves incubating patient serum with cells/tissue known to contain specific antigens, then adding fluorescein-labeled anti-human globulin (AHG). Positive IIF tests confirm the presence of *circulating autoantibodies.*

Screening for ANA using HEp-2 cells

- Incubate patient serum (diluted 1:40) with HEp-2 cells, add fluorescein-labeled anti-human globulin (AHG) and counterstain.

- Examine for presence and pattern of fluorescence.

  □ Homogenous (mitoses+) = dsDNA, ssDNA, histone

  □ Rim (mitoses+) = dsDNA

  □ Speckled (mitoses–) = Sm, RNP, Scl70, SS-B

  □ Nucleolar (mitoses–) = scleroderma

  □ Centromere (mitoses+ in centromeric pattern) = CREST

  □ Cytoplasmic = AMA, ASMA, etc

- Serially dilute all positives to determine titer

Screening for antibodies to cytoplasmic constituents

- Incubate patient serum (diluted 1:40) with cryostat sections of tissue 'sandwich' consisting of rat liver, kidney, and stomach (fundic mucosa & smooth muscle). Add fluorescein-labeled anti-human globulin (AHG). Add counterstain

- Examine for fluorescence

  □ AMA+ in gastric parietal cells, renal tubular cells, and hepatocytes

  □ ASMA+ in gastric smooth muscle and renal parenchymal arteries

  □ APA+ in gastric parietal cells

  □ Anti-LKM+ in cytoplasm of hepatocytes and renal tubular cells

- Titer all positives

Screening for ANCA

- Incubate patient serum with alcohol-fixed neutrophils

- Add fluorescein-labeled anti-human globulin (AHG)

- Add counterstain

- Examine for presence and type (cytoplasmic or perinuclear) fluorescence

- Run ANA screen on all positives

Anti-dsDNA

- Anti-dsDNA can be detected either by indirect immunofluorescence assay using the substrate *Crithidia luciliae* or by ELISA.

Detecting anti-thyroid antibodies

- Incubate serum with cryostat sections of thyroid. Add fluorescein-labeled AHG

- Examine

  □ Fluorescence that highlights follicular epithelial cell cytoplasm: anti-thyroid microsomal

  □ Fluorescence that highlights follicular contents: anti-thyroglobulin

Autoantibodies and Their Clinical Implication (T5.3)

Antinuclear antibodies (ANA)

- Traditionally, this and other autoantibody tests have been performed by indirect immunoflourescence, combining patient serum with test cells (commonly HEp-2 cells). Currently, EIA techniques are emerging that may supplant fluorescence-based ANA testing.

- The diagnosis of SLE requires the presence of numerous clinical and laboratory criteria, of which the ANA results can only satisfy a couple.

Autoimmunity>Autoantibodies and Their Clinical Implication

T5.3
Clinically Useful Serum Autoantibodies

Antibody	Clinical utility	
Anti-nuclear antibody (ANA)	This test is nonspecific. Individuals are more likely to be ANA positive with age, achieving a 50% incidence by age 80, but this is usually low titer.	
	Patterns of immunofluorescence	*Antibody specificity*
	Peripheral (rim)	anti-dsDNA
	Homogeneous	anti-histone, anti-dsDNA
	Speckled	anti-Smith, anti-RNP, anti-SS-A/SS-B
	Nucleolar	anti-nucleolar (scleroderma)
	Centromere	anti-centromere (CREST)
Anti-dsDNA	Also called anti-native DNA, has high specificity for SLE. The substrate, *Crithidia luciliae,* a flagellate with a giant mitochondrion that contains double stranded DNA concentrated in an area called the kinetoplast. Antibodies to ssDNA do not react with *C luciliae.*	
Anti-Jo1	Also called anti-tRNA synthetase. Implies high likelihood of developing interstitial lung disease in polymyositis/dermatomyositis.	
Anti-histone	High specificity for drug-induced systemic lupus. Associated drugs include hydralazine, procainamide, isoniazid, dilantin, aldomet, and penicillin.	
Extractable nuclear antigens	A number of antigens, the so-called extractable nuclear antigens (ENAs), are present in the extract of calf thymus. ENAs typically give a speckled pattern on fluorescent ANA testing. ENAs include Smith, Ribonucleoprotein (RNP), SS-A (Ro), and SS-B(La).	
Anti-Smith (Sm)	Virtually diagnostic of SLE	
Anti-RNP	Suggests mixed connective tissue disease (MCTD)	
Anti-nucleolar	Scleroderma	
Anti-SS-B/Anti SS-A	SS-A (Ro) is present in 70% of patients with Sjögren syndrome and 30% of patients with SLE. SS-B(La) is present in 50% of patients with Sjögren and 15% of patients with SLE. Anti–SS-A/SS-B are found in children with neonatal lupus. Patients who are ANA+, SS-A+ but SS-B– are very likely to have lupus nephritis.	
Anti-mitochondrial (AMA)	AMA is detected in 85% of patients with primary biliary cirrhosis (PBC). AMA is reactive with the cytoplasm of parietal cells of the stomach and renal tubular cells in the mouse stomach/kidney substrate.	
Anti-smooth muscle (ASMA)	Lupoid (autoimmune) hepatitis is characterized by titers of >1:80. ASMA are specifically directed at F-actin. ASMA are detected on the mouse stomach/kidney substrate where they are reactive with the muscle underlying the gastric mucosa.	
Anti-microsomal	High specificity (90%) and sensitivity (95%) for Hashimoto disease, although up to 50% of patients with Graves disease will have antibodies.	
Anti-endomysial antibody	Endomysin is present in the reticular investment of muscle fibers. Anti-endomysial antibodies are IgA antibodies. They are highly sensitive and specific for celiac sprue and dermatitis herpetiformis. Antibody titers respond to a gluten-free diet.	
Cold agglutinin	Cold agglutinins are IgM antibodies directed against I or i antigens on red cells. In infectious mono, they are anti-i antibodies. In cold-agglutinin disease, they are monoclonal IgM kappa antibodies. Mycoplasma pneumonia is associated with anti-I cold agglutinin. Titers are found in 50% of infected individuals, peaking at 14-21 days.	
Anti-centromere	High specificity for CREST variant of scleroderma	
Anti-GBM	Goodpasture syndrome; the epitope is the M2 subunit of type IV collagen	
Anti-IF	Polymyositis/dermatomyositis (IF = intermediate filament)	
Anti-Scl-70	Anti-Scl-70 antibody is an anti-topoisomerase Ig seen in 20% of patients with scleroderma.	
Anti-PM1	Overlap syndrome with overlapping features of scleroderma and dermatomyositis	
cANCA	High specificity for Wegener syndrome; cANCA is anti-proteinase 3 (PR3)	
Anti-thyroglobulin	Hashimoto disease	
Thyroid-stimulating antibody	Also called LATS, it is present in 90% of individuals with Graves disease.	

T5.3
Clinically Useful Serum Autoantibodies (Continued)

Rheumatoid factor (RF)	RFs are IgM antibodies directed against the Fc fragment of IgG. RF may be "falsely" positive in a multitude of conditions including SBE, syphilis, infectious mononucleosis, and many rheumatologic diseases.
Anti-parietal cell Ab (APCA)	80% sensitive for pernicious anemia, but only 70% specific. Presence of the APCA antibody does not correlate with B12 malabsorption. The APCA antibody is identified by its reaction with the gastric parietal cells but not renal epithelial cells in the mouse stomach/kidney substrate.
Anti-intrinsic factor Ab	50-75% sensitive for adult pernicious anemia, but 90% sensitive for pediatric pernicious anemia. There are two types: type I, blocking antibody, reacts only with unbound IF, and is extremely specific; type II, binding antibody, reacts with unbound and bound IF, and is both less specific and less sensitive than type I.
Cryoglobulin	Cryoglobulins may be present in Waldenström macroglobulinemia, myeloma, CLL, SLE, CAH, and viral infections.

- The ANA test has a sensitivity of around 99%. A negative ANA virtually excludes active SLE.

- For specificity, both the pretest probability and the titer are important. In randomly screened populations (**as for any test**), the specificity of ANA is lower than in populations with signs and symptoms of SLE.

  - A large number of individuals with no disease or with unrelated diseases have a positive ANA. Around 20% of normal individuals have an ANA titer of 1:40, while only about 5% of normals have a titer as high as 1:160.

  - When a cutoff titer of 1:40 is used, the specificity is around 80%. When 1:160 is used, the specificity is around 95%.

  - The number of false positives **increases with age.**

  - Conditions associated with a positive ANA include: other autoimmune diseases (Sjögren syndrome, scleroderma, rheumatoid arthritis), multiple sclerosis, infections, malignancies, and fibromyalgia.

- Once the ANA is found to be positive, additional testing can help confirm the diagnosis of SLE, particularly testing for anti-dsDNA, anti-Sm, and anti-phospholipid antibodies. Tests for the detection of anti-dsDNA include the Farr assay (RIA-based testing) and an indirect immunofluorescence assay using the substrate *Crithidia luciliae.*

- Frequency in SLE

  - dsDNA = 40%

  - Sm = 30%

  - RNP = 30%

  - SS-A (Ro) = 30%

  - SS-B (La) = 30%

  - Histone = 70%

- Anti-dsDNA & Anti-Sm antibodies are essentially restricted to SLE. Increases in anti-dsDNA Ab titers predict flares in SLE.

- High-titered Anti-RNP (>1:10,000) is characteristic of mixed connective tissue disease (MCTD), particularly if unaccompanied by other ANAs. Anti-RNP is commonly seen in SLE, but titers are usually modest.

- Anti-Ro & Anti-La with negative dsDNA & Sm is compatible with Sjögren Syndrome.

- Anti-Scl-70 (anti-topoisomerase 1) is seen exclusively in progressive systemic sclerosis (PSS)

- Anti-centromere Ab strongly suggests CREST syndrome and is occasionally seen in PSS and Raynaud syndrome.

- Drug-induced lupus develops mostly in 'slow acety-laters' who are taking hydralazine, procainamide, or isoniazid. This form of lupus is usually negative for dsDNA, Sm, and RNP but is characterized by ANA & anti-histone antibodies directed at H2 (H2A and H2B) histone proteins. Drug-induced lupus is a slightly different disease than usual-type lupus: having a very low incidence of serious visceral manifestations (especially low incidence of renal and CNS manifestations) and manifests primarily with rash, serositis, and arthritis.

Antibodies to cytoplasmic constituents

- Anti-mitochondrial antibodies are associated with primary biliary cirrhosis.

  □ Anti-mitochondrial antibodies are directed against a mitochondrial antigen from the inner mitochondrial membrane, called M2, which is thought to be dihydrolipoamide acetyltransferase, a component of the pyruvate dehydrogenase enzyme complex.

  □ Anti-M2 mitochondrial antibodies are found in about 90% of patients with primary biliary cirrhosis (PBC) and is highly (about 95%-99%) specific.

  □ M1 has been found in syphilis, M5 in collagen vascular diseases, M6 in isoniazid-induced hepatitis, and M7 in cardiomyopathy.

- Anti-parietal cell Abs are associated with pernicious anemia.

- Anti-smooth muscle Abs are associated with autoimmune hepatitis.

- Anti-endomyseal antibody is associated with celiac sprue.

- Anti-liver kidney microsomal antibody is associated with autoimmune hepatitis.

- Anti-thyroid microsomal and anti-thyroglobulin antibodies are identified in patients with Hashimoto disease.

Anti-neutrophil cytoplasmic antibodies (ANCAs)

- When patient sera is incubated with alcohol-fixed neutrophils (IIF), two major patterns of reactivity can be recognized. The first, recognized as a cytoplasmic granular pattern with perinuclear accentuation, is called cytoplasmic ANCA. The second, characterized by predominantly perinuclear immunofluorescence, is called perinuclear ANCA. All positive ANCA results are titered.

- Testing for ANAs is performed on all positives to exclude a false-positive ANCA due to the presence of ANAs.

- c-ANCA appears to have anti-proteinase 3 (PR3) specificity, while p-ANCA has predominantly anti-myeloperoxidase (MPO) activity.

- c-ANCA is positive in approximately 90% of Wegener granulomatosis, and its presence correlates with activity. It is highly (95% to 99%) specific for Wegener.

- c-ANCA titers can be used to monitor Wegener activity.

- P-ANCA is less specific than c-ANCA but still has clinical utility, since it is seen in a small number of disorders: microscopic polyangiitis (MPA), polyarteritis nodosum (PAN), primary sclerosing cholangitis (PSC) and ulcerative colitis (UC).

Other Markers of Autoimmune Diseases

The LE cell is a traditional marker of SLE. In tissue samples and body fluids, the LE (lupus erythematosis) cell is any phagocytic cell that has an engulfed denatured nucleus. The LE cell test is performed by agitating a test tube, thus damaging some nucleated cells whose liberated nuclei are then engulfed. A smear from this fluid is then examined for LE cells. The LE cell test is positive in 70% of cases of SLE.

Angiotensin converting enzyme (ACE)

- ACE is an enzyme found in high concentrations in pulmonary endothelium where it functions to convert angiontensin I to angiotensin II, the active form of the hormone.

- ACE is an extremely useful test in the evaluation of patients with suspected sarcoidosis, in which it is nearly always elevated when the disease is active. Inactive sarcoidosis is associated with normal levels of ACE.

- Other causes of elevated ACE are: primary biliary cirrhosis (PBC), Gaucher disease, and leprosy. All of these have in common the formation of granulomas; however, most other granulomatous diseases are not associated with an elevated ACE.

Autoimmune Diseases

Pathophysiology

- During fetal development, a process occurs in the thymus whereby self-reactive T and B cells are selectively destroyed (the acquisition of self-tolerance). Developing T and B cells undergo rearrangement of their TCR and Ig genes with such a huge degree of built-in randomness that a nearly infinite degree of variety of TCR/Ig genes result, leading to a proportionately high degree of variety of antigenic specificities. Thus, we are endowed with lymphocytes that can more or less recognize any antigen we may one day encounter. Exposure to that antigen in postnatal life leads to proliferation of clones whose TCR/Ig receptor most closely recognizes the antigen. During this proliferation, more variety arises during the process of isotype switching, leading to more clones with greater or lesser antigen specificity. In the fetal thymus, however, the entire array of self antigens are presented to developing lymphocytes (the role of Hassal corpuscles?), and those whose surface TCR or Ig has avidity for the expressed antigens are either removed from the population or rendered ineffective.

- Loss of self-tolerance is theoretically required in order for autoimmunity to develop. The way this happens is a bit of a mystery, but some theories have been proposed. One is the hapten theory, which holds that a foreign antigen closely presented in conjunction with a self-antigen may promote the proliferation of lymphocyte clones with sufficient avidity for the self-antigen alone that autoimmunity ensues. This may explain the association of certain autoimmune disorders with antecedent infection or drug exposure (drug-induced lupus; rheumatic fever).

- Major histocompatibility complex (MHC)/human leukocyte antigens (HLA) seem to play a role in autoimmunity. One reason may be that all foreign antigens are presented to lymphocytes on the surfaces of human cells in conjunction with HLA proteins. Thus, if the hapten mechanism is a reality, then it would follow that these proteins would be a major target for autoimmunity. And in fact there are strong associations with several diseases and particular HLA types.

  - HLA-DR3 with insulin-dependent diabetes mellitus (IDDM), systemic lupus erythematosus (SLE), Sjögren syndrome, myasthenia gravis, dermatitis herpetiformis (DH), celiac sprue, and Grave disease

  - HLA-DR4 with IDDM, rheumatoid arthritis (RA), pemphigus vulgaris

  - HLA-DR2 with multiple sclerosis (MS), narcolepsy; protective for IDDM

  - HLA-B27 with ankylosing spondylitis and other 'reactive' arthritides

- Autoimmune diseases are most prevalent in women of reproductive age. Exceptions worth noting are ankylosing spondylitis (males>>females) and Sjögren syndrome (postmenopausal females). Several diseases, most notably RA, are typically more severe when they affect males.

- Examples of exposures triggering autoimmunity

  - Coxsackie B virus infection is associated with the development of IDDM

  - HBV infection is associated with polyarteritis nodosum (PAN)

  - K pneumonia infection is associated with the onset of ankylosing spondylitis

  - The drug aldomet can lead to autoimmune hemolytic anemia (warm type)

  - Penicillamine is linked to systemic vasculitis

  - Procainamide, hydralazine, & isoniazid are associated with drug-induced SLE

Autoimmunity>Autoimmune Diseases

Classically defined hypersensitivity reactions are the basis of all autoimmune diseases, whether systemic or organ-confined.

- Type I hypersensitivity (immediate-type hypersensitivity)

  □ Mechanism: Antigen binding to IgE on the surfaces of mast cells (bound by the F_cR) leads to IgE crosslinking and resulting degranulation (histamine, heparin, serotonin, arachidonate)

  □ Examples: Anaphylaxis, urticaria, asthma, eczema

  □ *Anaphylactoid reactions result from mast cell degranulation **without** IgE intermediation (heat, cold, trauma)*

  □ *Hereditary angioedema (HAE) also has **nothing to do with IgE** and is due to deficiency of C1 esterase inhibitor (C1Inh).*

- Type II hypersensitivity (antibody-mediated cellular cytotoxicity)

  □ Mechanism: Ab binds to antigen and leads to complement activation and/or opsonization

  □ Examples: Goodpasture syndrome, myasthenia gravis, immune hemolysis, erythroblastosis fetalis

- Type III hypersensitivity (immune complex)

  □ Mechanism: Antibody binds to antigen and activates complement leading to deposition of immune complexes

  □ Examples: SLE, Henoch-Schönlein purpura (HSP), serum sickness, post-streptococcal glomerulonephritis (PSGN), membranous glomerulonephritis (MGN), arthrus rxn

- Type IV hypersensitivity (delayed-type hypersensitivity)

  □ Mechanism: T-cell reaction to antigen, usually with granuloma formation.

  □ Example: tuberculin skin test

Autoimmune disorders T5.4

- **Celiac sprue**

  □ Celiac sprue tends to cluster within families, and there is a strong association with HLA-DQ2 and HLA-DQ8. While the link is strong among relatives of affected individuals, it is far from autosomal; and while >90% of cases arise in HLA-DQ2/8, only about 1% of those with this HLA type have disease.

T5.4
Autoimmune Disorders

Disease	Antibodies	Detection	Manifestations	
Pemphigus vulgaris	Anti-desmosomal	DIF on cryostat sections of skin: chicken wire IgG in epidermis	Suprabasal vesiculation	Skin
Bullous pemphigoid (BP)	Anti-epithelial basement membrane/ anti-hemidesmosome	DIF on cryostat sections of skin: linear IgG along BM. In salt-split skin, reactivity in roof	Subepithelial vesiculation	Skin
Epidermolysis bullosa acquisita (EBA)	EBA Ag	DIF on cryostat sections of skin: linear IgG along BM. In salt-split skin, reactivity in floor	Subepithelial vesiculation	Skin
Dermatitis herpetiformis	Gluten	DIF on cryostat sections of skin: granular IgA, especially in tips of dermal papillae	Subepithelial vesiculation	Skin
Wegener syndrome	c-ANCA	IIF on ethanol-fixed neutrophils	Systemic vasculitis: lungs, nasopharynx, kidneys, etc Necrotizing GN	Vasculitis
Polyarteritis nodosum (PAN)	p-ANCA	IIF on ethanol-fixed neutrophils	Systemic vasculitis: mesenteric arteries, kidneys, sparing lung	Vasculitis
Microscopic polyarteritis (MPA)	p-ANCA	IIF on ethanol-fixed neutrophils	Systemic vasculitis: lungs, kidneys, mesentery, etc Necrotizing GN	Vasculitis

T5.4
Autoimmune Disorders (continued)

Disease	Antibodies	Detection	Manifestations	
Hashimoto disease	Anti-microsomal, Anti-thyroglobulin	IIF on cryostat sections of thyroid tissue; latex agglutination	Lymphocytic thyroid inflammation with associated hypothyroidism	Organ-confined
Graves disease	Anti-TSH (TSI/LATS)	Bioassay	Hyperthyroidism ± ophthalmopathy	
Atrophic gastritis (PA)	Anti-parietal cell Ab Anti-IF Ab	IIF on cryostat sections of rat stomach/liver/kidney	Dyspepsia, B_{12} deficiency, gastritis, gastric adenocarcinoma	
Ulcerative colitis	pANCA	IIF on ethanol-fixed neutrophils	Colitis, colonic adeno, primary sclerosing cholangitis	
Celiac sprue	Anti-gliadin; Anti-endomyseal Anti-transglutaminase	ELISA IIF on cryostat sections of rat stomach/liver/kidney.	Weight loss, iron deficiency, duodenitis, DH, lymphoma (EATCL)	
Autoimmune hepatitis	Anti-smooth muscle Ab	IIF on cryostat sections of rat stomach/liver/kidney	Chronic hepatitis, cirrhosis, hepatocellular carcinoma	
Primary biliary cirrhosis	Anti-mitochondrial Ab	IIF on cryostat sections of rat stomach/liver/kidney	Pruritus, ductopenia, biliary cirrhosis, eventual jaundice	
Insulin-dependent diabetes mellitus	Anti-islet cell Ab; Anti-glutamic acid decarboxylase (GAD) Anti-insulin receptor	IIF on cryostat sections of pancreas ELISA; Bioassay	Absolute insulin deficiency, metabolic d/o, acanthosis nigricans	
Autoimmune hemolytic anemia	Anti-Rh complex	Not routinely done	Anemia, reticulocytosis, +DAT	
Immune thrombocytopenic purpura	Anti-GPIIb, GPIIIa, GPIb, or GPV	Not routinely done	Thrombocytopenia, meg hyperplasia	
Myasthenia gravis	Anti-AChR	Bioassay, ELISA	Weakness, thymoma	
Systemic lupus erythematosus (SLE)	ANA, Anti-dsDNA, Anti-Sm, Anti-RNP, etc	IIF on *C lucilae* or HEp-2 cells ELISA	Systemic: malar & discoid lesions, photosens, oral ulcers, polyarthritis, serositis, GN, CNS, cytopenias	Systemic
Mixed connective tissue disease (MCTD)	ANA– Anti-RNP+	IIF on *C lucilae* or HEp-2 cells ELISA	Systemic: overlapping features of SLE, scleroderma, and/or PM/DM	
Drug-induced lupus	ANA, Anti-histone	IIF on *C lucilae* or HEp-2 cells ELISA	SLE with mild to no renal or CNS involvement	
Sjögren syndrome (SS)	ANA, Anti-SS-A (Ro), Anti-SS-B (La), Anti-nucleolar	IIF on *C lucilae* or HEp-2 cells ELISA	Sialadenitis (keratoconjunctivitis sicca & xerostomia), ILD, pancreatitis; lymphoma 1° or 2° (RA)	
Scleroderma (PSS)	ANA, anti-nucleolar, anti-Scl-70 (anti-topoisomerase I)	IIF on *C lucilae* or HEp-2 cells ELISA	Obliterative vasculopathy, dermal sclerosis, epidermal atrophy, tenosynovitis, esopha-geal sclerosis, ILD, pulmonary htn, telangi-ectasia, calcinosis, renal hypertension	
CREST	Anti-centromere	IIF on *C lucilae* or HEp-2 cells ELISA	Calcinosis, Raynaud syndrome, esophageal dysmotility, sclerodactyly, telangiectasis	
Polymyositis/Dermatomyositis	Anti-Jo1 (tRNA synthetase)	IIF on *C lucilae* or HEp-2 cells ELISA	Proximal motor weakness and pain, heliotrope rash, Göttren syndrome papules, ILD. Possible internal malignancy	
Rheumatoid arthritis	RF (IgM anti-IgG); Anti-keratin Ab (AKA); Anti-RA33; Anti-RA-associated nuclear antigen (RANA); ANA-negative	Latex agglutination	Arthritis (proliferative synovitis), rheumatoid nodules, systemic vasculitis, pleuritis, ILD, 2° Sjögren (RANA+ pts), Felty syndrome	
Seronegative spondyloarthropathies (AS, Reiter syndrome, Psoriatic arthritis)	RF– ANA– HLA-B27+		AS: Spondylitis, kyphosis, iridocylitis Reiter syndrome: post-infectious (*Shigella, Yersinia, Chlamydia*), Spondylitis, urethritis, conjunctivitis. Psoriatic: psoriasis, polyarthritis	

T5.5

Antibodies Associated With Diagnoses of Autoimmune Thyroid Disorders

Diagnosis	Anti-thyroglobulin Ab	Anti-microsomal Ab	LATS (TSI)
Hashimoto thyroiditis	60%-100%	80%	0
Other thyroiditis (de Quervain & lymphocytic)	30%-50%	50%	0
Graves disease	30%	60%-80%	100%
Carcinoma of thyroid	20%-50%	15%	0

☐ The disease may arise at any time after eating begins. Many cases present in the pediatric age group, but new diagnoses are frequently made in the elderly.

☐ Celiac sprue affects the intestine and extra-intestinal sites. Histologically, the duodenum is the site of greatest severity. In fully developed lesions, there is villus atrophy, but many of those affected have only an increase in intraepithelial lymphocytes without architectural changes. Furthermore, many with histologic findings have no symptoms. After prolonged inflammation, there is a risk of malnutrition (a common cause of idiopathic short stature and unexplained iron deficiency anemia) and developing a T-cell lymphoma (enteropathy-associated T-cell lymphoma). Extra-intestinal manifestations include arthritis and dermatitis herpetiformis.

☐ There is a strong association of sprue with diabetes mellitus, IgA deficiency, and cystic fibrosis.

☐ Serologic markers in celiac sprue include anti-gliadin antibodies, anti-endomyseal antibodies, and anti-transglutaminase antibodies. Due to a high incidence of IgA anti-transglutaminase antibodies in patients with chronic liver diseases (particularly among those with autoimmune liver diseases) the specificity of these antibodies for celiac sprue in the setting of chronic liver disease is low.

☐ Anti-transglutaminase antibodies, anti-endomysial antibodies and antigliadin antibodies vary with exposure to gluten, but none correlates with mucosal recovery in celiac sprue. Tests of mucosal absorption, such as the D-xylose absorption test, may be useful in this regard. Transthyretin (a rapidly responsive indicator of nutritional status) correlates very well with mucosal recovery.

■ **Anti-thyroid autoantibodies T5.5**

☐ Like most autoantibodies, these are detected by indirect immunofluorescence, applying fluorescent-labeled anti-human globulin after incubating patient serum with control tissue (normal human thyroid). Anti-microsomal antibodies (anti-thyroid peroxidase antibodies) are identified when the follicular epithelium is highlighted. Anti-thyroglobulin antibody is present when the colloid is highlighted. Long-acting thyroid-stimulating (LATS) antibodies are also called thyroid-stimulating immunoglobulin (TSI), and TSH receptor antibodies.

☐ Hashimoto thyroiditis is characterized by anti-microsomal and anti-thyroglobulin antibodies. LATS are not identified in Hashimoto. Graves disease is highly likely to have long-acting thyroid stimulating (LATS) antibodies which are capable of acting upon TSH receptors as agonists. In addition, it is important to know that a proportion have either anti-microsomal or anti-thyroglobulin antibodies and that these antibodies are not restricted to Hashimoto thyroiditis.

■ **Autoimmune (lymphoplasmacytic, sclerosing) pancreatitis**

☐ Presents as a sonolucent enlargement of the pancreas associated with segmental narrowing of the pancreatic duct, and obstructive jaundice; ie, the presentation of pancreatic adenocarcinoma. Preoperative distinction of these two lesions is, of course, desirable. Preoperative fine needle aspiration may display a lymphoplasmacytic infiltrate, reflective of the histopathologic process (dense lymphoplasmacytic infiltrate with fibrosis).

☐ Autoimmune pancreatitis is associated with elevation of serum IgG4 in most (>70%) cases. Lesions

381

with histologic similarity to autoimmune pancreatitis may occur in various organs such as the lungs, liver, spleen, and thyroid. In addition, idiopathic retroperitoneal fibrosis and sclerosing mediastinitis both share histologic similarities with these lesions.

◻Features common to autoimmune pancreatitis and these other similar lesions include: lymphoplasmacytic infiltration, densely hyaline interstitial fibrosis, atrophy of the background parenchyma, infiltration into adjacent soft tissue, marked periductal inilration with duct stenosis, vascular thrombosis, eosinophilic infiltration, and many (but not purely) IgG4-positive plasma cells by immunohistochemistry.

◻All of these lesions are associated with increased serum IgG4. In normal individuals, IgG4 is present in concentrations lower than any other IgG subclass, representing about 5% of total IgG.

■ **Autoimmune hepatitis, autoimmune cholangitis, and primary biliary cirrhosis**

◻**Autoimmune hepatitis** has a peak incidence in adolescence and young adulthood, especially in females. Laboratory findings include hypergammaglobulinemia (predominantly increased IgG levels) and a specific subset of autoantibodies: ANA, anti-smooth muscle antibody (SMA), anti-liver kidney microsome antibody (LKM1, an antibody against CYP 2D6), and in some cases anti-soluble liver antigen/liver pancreas (SLA/LP) antibody. ANA/ASMA and LKM1 tend to be found in different patients, rarely both positive in an individual patient. Affected persons present with acute hepatitis with nonspecific constitutional symptoms. In some cases there are associated extrahepatic autoimmune phenomena, especially ulcerative colitis, arthritis, immune thrombocytopenic purpura (ITP), autoimmune hemolytic anemia (AIHA), thyroiditis, and diabetes. Histologically, there is chronic hepatitis characterized by a lymphoplasmacytic portal infiltrate with characteristically brisk limiting plate necrosis. Bile ducts are largely spared.

◻**Primary biliary cirrhosis (PBC)** presents histopathologically as a lymphoplasmacytic infiltrate with direct bile duct infiltration and progressive bile duct destruction (chronic nonsuppurative destructive cholangitis). Anti-mitochondrial antibodies (AMA) are present in >95% of cases. PBC is also associated with elevated IgM levels.

◻**Autoimmune cholangitis** has histologic features similar to PBC but the AMA is negative. Instead, these patients test positive for antinuclear antibodies (ANA) and/or anti-smooth muscle autoantibodies (ASMA). Some have termed this condition AMA-negative PBC. IgG and IgM levels are just slightly elevated.

■ **Giant cell arteritis (GCA)**

◻**GCA** is characterized by the granulomatous involvement of large and medium-sized branches of the aorta with predilection for the extracranial branches of the carotid artery. Headache is the main presenting symptom, and is characteristically of sudden onset and temporal. Ischemic sequela include jaw claudication, loss of vision, and stroke, in particular in the vertebrobasilar territory. About 5-10% of patients with biopsy-proven GCA present without obvious vascular manifestations. These patients with subclinical (silent) GCA, may present with only polymyalgia rheumatica (PMR) or fever of unknown origin. The temporal artery biopsy remains the gold standard diagnostic modality for GCA, but numerous laboratory tests may be abnormal at the time of diagnosis.

◻Abnormal laboratory tests in GCA include an elevated erythrocyte sedimentation rate (ESR). An ESR greater than 50 mm/h is one of the 1990 American College of Rheumatology criteria for the classification of GCA, and it is elevated in 95%-100% of cases of GCA. Other acute phase reactants, particularly C-reactive protein (CRP) and the platelet count, are also elevated in GCA. A normochromic-normocytic anemia is common, and it appears that anemic patients are more likely to present as subclinical (silent) GCA and suffer fewer ischemic complications. Abnormal liver function tests, particularly alkaline phosphatase elevation and albumin depletion, have also been described in these patients.

■ **Inflammatory myopathies** typically present with proximal symmetrical muscle weakness, elevated serum creatine kinase, and characteristic EMG findings. Several distinct categories are recognized: isolated inflammatory myositis, connective tissue disease-associated myositis, malignancy-associated myositis, polymyositis (PM), dermatomyositis (DM) and inclusion body myositis (IBM). Dermatomyositis is associated with a highly characteristic heliotrope rash and Gottron papules. The presence of inclusion bodies on muscle biopsy is the defining feature of IBM. In association with other connective tissue diseases, myositis is typically seen in systemic lupus erythematosus (SLE), rheumatoid arthritis (RA), Sjögren syndrome, and progressive systemic sclerosis (scleroderma). Autoantibodies are infrequent in cancer-associated myositis and IBM. Anti-synthetases (eg, anti-Jo-1, anti-PL-7, etc) are the most common autoantibody found and are associated with a high frequency of pulmonary fibrosis. Anti-SRP is found mainly in PM (rather than DM) patients and is associated with a high frequency of cardiac involvement, DR5, and a very poor prognosis. Anti-Mi-2 is associated almost exclusively with DM and tends to have a good prognosis.

- **Myasthenia gravis** presents as muscle weakness and fatigue, with typical signs such as ptosis or diplopia, and fatiguable muscle weakness on physical examination. The diagnosis is supported by: (1) the characteristic EMG finding of progressive decrement in muscle action potential on repetitive stimulation, (2) a Tensilon test showing a dramatic response to cholinesterase inhibitor, and (3) characteristic autoantibodies. Treatment involves thymectomy, particularly in patients less than 60 years old, immunosuppression (eg, prednisone), and in selected cases plasma exchange and intravenous immunoglobulins. There are five clinical types of MG: early-onset, late-onset, thymoma-associated, ocular, and seronegative. Early-onset MG affects primarily females under 40 who tend to have thymic follicular hyperplasia; whereas late-onset MG affects predominantly males over 40 with no thymic pathology. Thymoma-associated MG has no age or sex predilection. Antibodies to the muscle acetylcholine receptor (AChR) are present in 75%-95% of patients with MG, and false positives are extremely rare. Particularly in thymoma-associated disease, antibodies to skeletal muscle components (ryanodine receptor and titin) can be found. Recently, antibodies to MuSK have been found in a proportion of patients with AChR-antibody negative ("seronegative") MG. MuSK is a tyrosine kinase that is restricted to the neuromuscular junction, and antibodies to MuSK appear to define a steroid-refractory form of MG seen in younger females with frequent bulbar manifestations T5.6.

- Sjögren syndrome may be primary, or it can be associated with other systemic autoimmune diseases (secondary SS), particularly rheumatoid arthritis (RA) and systemic lupus erythematosus (SLE). Anti-Ro and anti-La antibodies are characteristic of SS. The presence of either anti-Ro or anti-La has a sensitivity and specificity of around 95%. While anti-Ro antibodies are seen in both primary and secondary SS, anti-La is largely confined to primary SS. Neither antibody is useful to follow disease activity.

T5.6
Myasthenia Gravis Testing

Type	Anti-AchR	Anti-Titin	Anti-MuSK
Early-onset	+	–	–
Late-onset	+	+	–
Thymoma-associated	+	+	–
Ocular	+/–	–	–
Seronegative	–	–	+/–

Laboratory diagnosis of anaphylaxis

- Serum (or plasma) levels of tryptase are recommended in laboratory diagnosis of anaphylaxis (and systemic mastocytosis). Tryptase may be measured as total tryptase or mature tryptase. Total tryptase levels generally reflect the mast cell burden within the body (as in mastocytosis), while mature tryptase more closely reflects mast cell degranulation. Serum tryptase levels peak about 60–90 minutes after the onset of anaphylaxis and persist for several hours.

- Plasma histamine levels peak more quickly than tryptase, at about 10 minutes after the onset of anaphylaxis. Levels return to normal within an hour. The urinary histamine, however, may be elevated for 24 hours.

- While the tryptase and histamine are helpful tests, the laboratory can be of great help in excluding conditions that mimic anaphylaxis. For example, carcinoid syndrome can be excluded by measuring urinary HIAA, serum serotonin, and other analytes. A peculiar form of histamine poisoning (scombroidosis) may result from ingestion of spoiled fish and can clinically resemble anaphylaxis. It is due to the production of histamine by bacteria within the fish. An elevated histamine, without elevated tryptase, and perhaps a history of several people affected together, point to this diagnosis. Other unusual conditions that can mimic anaphylaxis and be distinguished through laboratory testing include hereditary angioedema (C1q deficiency), urticarial vasculitis, pheochromocytoma, and hyperimmunoglobulin E (Job) syndrome.

Bibliography

Aghamohammadi A, Farhoudi A, Moin M, Rezaei N, Kouhi A, Pourpak Z, Yaseri N, Movahedi M, Gharagozlou M, Zandieh F, Yazadni F, Arshi S, Zadeh I, Ghazi B, Mahmoudi M, Tahaei S, Isaeian A. Clinical and immunological features of 65 Iranian patients with common variable immunodeficiency. *Clin Diagn Lab Immunol* 2005; 12:825-832.

Anderlini P, Korbling M, Dale D, Gratwohl A, Schmitz N, Stroncek D, Howe C, Leitman S, Horowitz M, Gluckman E, Rowley S, Przepiorka D, Champlin R. Allogeneic blood stem cell transplantation: considerations for donors. *Blood* 1997; 90:903

Barrett DJ, Lee CG, Ammann AJ, Ayoub EM. IgG and IgM pneumococcal polysaccharide antibody responses in infants. *Pediatr Res* 1984; 18:1067-1071.

Baumgart KW, Britton WJ, Kemp A, et al. The spectrum of primary immunodeficiency disorders in Australia. *J Allergy Clin Immunol* 1997; 100:415-423.

Bork K, Meng G, Staubach P, Hardt J. Hereditary angioedema: new findings concerning symptoms, affected organs, and course. *Am J Med* 2006; 119:267-274.

Bork K, Barnstedt SE, Koch P, Traupe H. Hereditary angioedema with normal C1-inhibitor activity in women. *Lancet* 2000; 356:213-217.

Bourne HC, Weston S, Prasad M, Edkins E, Benson EM. Identification of WASP mutations in 10 Australian families with Wiskott-Aldrich syndrome and X-linked thrombocytopenia. *Pathology* 2004; 36(3):262-264.

Buckley RH. Primary immunodeficiency diseases due to defects in lymphocytes. *N Engl J Med* 2000; 343:1313-1324.

Carlucci F, Tabucchi A, Aiuti A, Rosi F, Floccari F, Pagani R, Marinello E. Capillary electrophoresis in diagnosis and monitoring of adenosine deaminase deficiency. *Clin Chem* 2003; 49:1830-1838.

Cunningham-Rundles C, Bodian C. Common variable immunodeficiency: clinical and immunological features of 248 patients. *Clin Immunol* 1999; 92:34-48.

Cunningham-Rundles C. Hematologic complications of primary immune deficiencies. *Blood Rev* 2002; 16:61-64.

Davidson A, Diamond B. Autoimmune diseases. *N Engl J Med* 2001; 345:340-350.

Delves PJ, Roitt IM. The immune system: first of two parts. *N Engl J Med* 2000; 343;1:37-49.

Derry J, Kerns J, Weinberg K. *WASP* gene mutations in Wiskott-Aldrich syndrome and X-linked thrombocytopenia. *Hum Mol Genet* 1995; 4:1127-1135.

Devriendt K, Kim AS, Mathijs G, Frints SGM, Schwartz M, Van den Oord JJ, Verhoef GEG, Boogaerts MA, Fryns J-P, You D, Rosen MK, Vandenberghe P. Constitutively activating mutation in WASP causes X-linked severe congenital neutropenia. *Nature Genetics* 2001; 27:313-317.

Dickey W, Hughes DF, McMillan SA. Disappearance of endomysial antibodies in treated celiac disease does not indicate histological recovery. *Am J Gastroenterol* 2000; 95:712-714.

Eiermann TH, van Bekkum DW, Vriesendorp HM, Machida U, Kami M, Hirai H, Bolan CD, Leitman SF, Sasazuki T, Juji T, Kodera Y, Aversa F, Martelli MF, Reisner Y. Hematopoietic stem-cell transplantation for acute leukemia. *N Engl J Med* 1999; 340(10):809-812.

Farrell RF, Kelly CP. Celiac sprue. *New Engl J Med* 2002; 346:180-188.

Fleisher TA. Evaluation of suspected immunodeficiency. *MLO* 2003; February:10-21.

Gennery AR, Cant AJ. Diagnosis of severe combined immunodeficiency. *J Clin Pathol* 2001; 54:191-195.

Germenis AE, Yiannaki EE, Zachou K, Roka V, Barbanis S, Liaskos C, Adam K, Kapsoritakis AN, Potamianos S, Dalekos GN. Prevalence and clinical significance of immunoglobulin A antibodies against tissue transglutaminase in patients with diverse chronic liver diseases. *Clin Diagn Lab Immunol* 2005; 12:941-948.

Gonzalez-Gay MA, Lopez-Diaz MJ, Barros S, Garcia-Porrua C, Sanchez-Andrade A, Paz-Carreira J, Martin J, Llorca J. Giant cell arteritis laboratory tests at the time of diagnosis in a series of 240 patients. *Medicine* 2005; 84(5):277-290.

Bibliography

Hamano H, Kawa S, Horiuchi A, Unno H, Furuya N, Akamatsu T, Fukushima M, Nikaido T, Nakayama K, Usuda N, Kiyosawa K. High serum IgG4 concentrations in patients with sclerosing pancreatitis. *N Engl J Med* 2001; 344:732-738.

Hong R. The DiGeorge anomaly (CATCH 22, DiGeorge/velocardiofacial syndrome). *Semin Hematol* 1998; 35:282-290.

Illoh OC. Current applications of flow cytometry in the diagnosis of primary immunodeficiency diseases. *Arch Pathol Lab Med* 2004; 128:23-31.

Imai K, Morio T, Zhu Y, Jin Y, Itoh S, Kajiwara M, Yata J, Mizutani S, Ochs HD, Nonoyama S. Clinical course of patients with *WASP* gene mutations. *Blood* 2004;103(2):456-464.

Imai K, Nonayama S, Ochs HD. *WASP* (Wiskott-Aldrich Syndrome Protein) gene mutations and phenotype. *Curr Opin All Clin Immunol* 2003; 3:427-436.

Jin Y, Mazza C, Christie JR, Giliani S, Fiorini M, Mella M, Gandellini F, Stewart DM, Zhu Q, Nelson DL, Notarangelo LD, Ochs HD. Mutations of the Wiskott-Aldrich Syndrome Protein (WASP): hotspots, effect on transcription, and translation and phenotype/genotype correlation. *Blood* 2004; 104(13):4010-4019.

Kamisawa T, Okamoto A, Funata N. Clinicopathologic features of autoimmune pancreatitis in relation to elevation of serum IgG4. *Pancreas* 2005; 31(1):28-31.

Kamradt T, Mitchison NA. Tolerance and autoimmunity. *N Engl J Med* 2001; 344:655-664.

Kavanaugh A, Tomar R, Reveille J, Solomon DH, Homburger HA. Guidelines for clinical use of the antinuclear antibody test and tests for specific autoantibodies to nuclear antigens. *Arch Pathol Lab Med* 2000; 124:71-82.

Kitagawa S, Zen Y, Harada K, Sasaki M, Sato Y, Minato H, Watanabe K, Kurumaya H, Katayanagi K, Masuda S, Niwa H, Tsuneyama K, Saito K, Haratake J, Takagawa K, Nakanuma Y. Abundant IgG4-positive plasma cell infiltration characterizes chronic sclerosing sialadenitis (Kuttner's tumor). *Am J Surg Pathol* 2005; 29:783-791.

Lekstrom-Himes JA, Gallin JI. Primary immunodeficiency diseases due to defects in phagocytes. *N Engl J Med* 2000; 343:1703-1714.

Levine JS, Branch DW, Rauch J. The antiphospholipid syndrome. *N Engl J Med* 2002; 346:752-763.

Lieberman P. Anaphylaxis. *Med Clin N Am* 2006; 90:77-95.

Lobo PI, Spencer C, Gorman J, Pirsch G. Critical appraisal of complement dependent microlymphocytotoxicity assay for detecting donor-specific alloantibody pretransplant—importance of indirect immunofluorescence as a superior alternative. *Human Immunol* 1981; 2(1):55-64.

Lutskiy MI, Rosen FS, Remold-O'Donnell E. Genotype-proteotype linkage in the Wiskott-Aldrich syndrome. *J Immunol* 2005; 175(2):1329-1336.

Mackay IR, Rosen FS. The immune system: first of two parts. *N Engl J Med* 2000; 343:37-49.

Mackay IR, Rosen FS. The immune system: second of two parts. *N Engl J Med* 2000; 343:108-117.

Mackay IR, Rosen FS. Immunodeficiency diseases caused by defects in phagocytosis. *N Engl J Med* 2000; 343:1703-1714.

McMillan SA, Dickey W, Douglas JP, Hughes DF. Transthyretin values correlate with mucosal recovery in patients with coeliac disease taking a gluten free diet. *J Clin Pathol* 2001; 54:783-786.

Moder KG. Use and interpretation of rheumatologic tests: a guide for clinicians. *Mayo Clin Proc* 1996; 71:391-396.

Notohara K, Burgart L, Lawrence J, Yadav D, Chari S, Smyrk TC. Idiopathic chronic pancreatitis with periductal lymphoplasmacytic infiltration: clinicopathologic features of 35 cases. *Am J Surg Pathol* 2003; 27(8):1119-1127.

Picard C, Puel A, Bustamante J, Ku C, Casanova J. Primary immunodeficienies associated with pneumococcal disease. *Curr Opin All Clin Immunol* 2003; 3:451-459.

Sanders DB, El-Salem K, Massey JM, McConville J, Vincent A. Clinical aspects of MuSK antibody positive seronegative MG. *Neurology* 2003; 60:1978-1980.

Bibliography

Sarkar K, Miller FW. Autoantibodies as predictive and diagnostic markers of idiopathic inflammatory myopathies. *Autoimmunity* 2004; 37(4):291-294.

Sategna-Guidetti C, Grossa S, Bruno M, et al. Reliability of immunologic markers of celiac sprue in assessment of mucosal recovery after gluten withdrawal. *J Clin Gastroenterol* 1996; 23:101-104.

Schwartz LB. Diagnostic value of tryptase in anaphylaxis and mastocytosis. *Immunol Allergy Clin N Am* 2006; 26:451-463.

Schwartz RS. Diversity of the immune repertoire and immunoregulation. *N Engl J Med* 348:1017-1026.

Soliotis FC, Moutsopoulos HM. Sjögren's syndrome. *Autoimmunity* 2004; 37(4):305-307.

Specks U, Homburger HA. Anti-neutrophil cytoplasmic antibodies. *Mayo Clin Proc* 1994; 69:1197-1198.

Thiele DL. Autoimmune hepatitis. *Clin Liver Dis* 2005; 9:635-646.

Thomas R. Celiac disease. *Adolesc Med Clin* 2004; 15(1):91-103.

Tursi A, Brandimarte G, Giorgetti GM. Lack of usefulness of anti-transglutaminase antibodies in assessing histologic recovery after gluten-free diet in celiac disease. *J Clin Gastroenterol* 2003; 37:387-391.

Vergani D, Mieli-Vergani G. Autoimmune hepatitis and sclerosing cholangitis. *Autoimmunity* 2004; 37(4):329-332.

Vincent A, Rothwell P. Myasthenia gravis. *Autoimmunity* 2004; 37(4):317-319.

Walport MJ. Complement—first of two parts. *N Engl J Med* 2001; 344:1058-1066.

Walport MJ. Complement—second of two parts. *N Engl J Med* 2001; 344:1140-1144.

Weiler CR, Bankers-Fulbright JL. Common variable immunodeficiency: test indications and interpretations. *Mayo Clin Proc* 2005; 80(9):1187-1200.

Zen Y, Kasahara Y, Horita K, Miyayama S, Miura S, Kitagawa S, Nakanuma Y. Inflammatory pseudotumor of the breast in a patient with a high serum IgG4 level: histologic similarity to sclerosing pancreatitis. *Am J Surg Pathol* 2005; 29:275-278.

Zhu Q, Watanabe C, Liu T, Hollenbaugh, Blaese RM, Kanner SB, Aruffo A, Ochs HD. Wiskott-Alrich syndrome/X-linked thrombocytopenia: *WASP* gene mutations, protein expression, and phenotype. *Blood* 1997; 90:2680-2689.

Chapter 7

Molecular Methods

Molecular Methods

Cytogenetics

Karyotyping (classical cytogenetics) is the visualization of the chromosomes of cells, grown in culture and arrested in metaphase, obtained from a clinical sample. Banding methods are utilized to visualize the chromosomes. Cytogenetic analysis requires viable, fresh tissue.

- For cell culture, the cells may be resuspended from the specimen and attached directly to the surface of a coverslip (the in-situ method) or cultured in a flask. In either case, cultures are subsequently selected, the harvested cells subjected to a hypotonic solution (to separate the chromosomes), and fixed. The cells are treated to enhance banding, stained, and then mounted on a slide. When chromosomally abnormal cells are found, the first question is whether the abnormalities arose in culture (a common artifact). The ability to distinguish true mosaicism from artifact increases with the number of cells studied (in true mosaicism, one expects to find the same abnormality in more than one cell).

- Banding methods exploit A-T and G-C rich areas to provide staining contrast. Banding patterns are highly reproducible, and the banding pattern of each chromosome is unique. The expected bands are numbered. With experience, a cytogeneticist can distinguish like-sized normal chromosomes from one another and visually detect subtle chromosomal abnormalities.

Fluorescence in situ hybridization (FISH) is sometimes called molecular cytogenetics.

- FISH can be performed on direct clinical samples—fresh tissue, frozen tissue, cytologic preparations, paraffin-embedded tissue—and viable cells are not required. It is unique among molecular techniques, because it involves direct microscopy. The visualized intranuclear signal may be chromogenic (CISH) or fluorescent (FISH). Since cells in any phase of the cell cycle may be evaluated (metaphase cells not required), this technique has also been referred to as interphase cytogenetics.

- FISH uses labeled DNA oligonucleotide probes designed to be complementary to DNA regions of interest. There are three types of probes used

commonly: allele-specific probes that adhere to a specific target DNA sequence, centromeric probes (identify a particular chromosome by its centromere), and painting probes (identify an entire chromosome).

- FISH is a highly sensitive and specific way to assess the status of a gene; that is, whether it has been rearranged, deleted, or duplicated.

  □ In comparison with PCR, FISH is in one respect less sensitive: the alteration in question must be large to be detected (but not as large as necessary for conventional cytogenetics), and FISH probes are typically 30 Kb or more in size. FISH cannot detect small (point) mutations and is best viewed as sensitive to alterations intermediate in size between those detectable by cytogenetics and those detectable by PCR.

  □ However, PCR is less sensitive than FISH in another respect: some rearrangements occur in sufficiently variable ways that a primer capable of detecting some rearrangements will not detect others (eg, FISH is much better than PCR for detecting the *BCL1* rearrangement of mantle cell lymphoma). PCR is dependent upon the choice of primers and therefore capable of failing to amplify an easily visible anomaly. *Given the use of an appropriate primer or set of primers,* however, it is safe to say that PCR is significantly more sensitive than FISH, capable of detecting one affected cell per million.

  □ For detecting translocations, combination probes are utilized that hybridize to the opposite sides of the translocation breakpoints. There are two main strategies employed: break-apart probes and fusion probes. With break-apart probes, the germline form of the gene produces a single signal of one color; a translocation separates the two probes, generating two signals of different colors. With fusion probes, the opposite is true.

- Probes for a constant portion of a chromosome (eg, the centromere) can be used to detect aneuploidy. For example, a probe for chromosome 12 can be used to screen for trisomy 12 in CLL.

- Like immunohistochemistry, there are several artifacts that can affect FISH interpretation.

- □ Truncation artifact refers simply to the sectioning through of a nucleus such that not all of its chromosomal material is present in the section being evaluated. This can lead to a falsely negative signal.

- □ Aneuploidy and polyploidy, if present in the neoplastic cells, can lead to apparent duplications.

- □ Autofluorescence is similar to endogenous enzymatic activity in immunohistochemistry, and like immunohistochemistry has morphologically different features than a true positive signal. In immunohistochemistry, a blocking step is critical, while in FISH, filters are used to block these signals.

- Spectral karyotyping (spectral karyotype imaging—SKI) is a term that refers to the application of 23 sets of different chromosome-specific painting probes of 23 different "colors" (fluorescent spectra). This can be used as a form of cytogenetic study.

Polymerase Chain Reaction (PCR)

PCR amplification begins with primers—DNA sequences complimentary to those that flank the genomic DNA region of interest. The genomic sequence that one wishes to amplify may be an entire gene or a portion of a gene that is often mutated in a disease-causing allele (a genomic 'hot spot'). The sample DNA, primers, and excess nucleotide (A, T, G, and C) triphosphates (dNTPs) are incubated together in the presence of a heat-stable DNA polymerase obtained from the *Thermas aquaticus* bacterium (*Taq* polymerase) and carried through numerous hot then cold (denaturation, replication, then annealing) cycles so that amplification can take place. The reaction products then subjected to electrophoresis on agarose gels and visualized under UV light. Alternatively, the reaction products may be sequenced. Lastly, they may be hybridized with allele-specific oligonucleotide (ASO) or reverse dot blot hybridization.

There are now numerous variations on the fundamental PCR method:

- Nested PCR is a highly sensitive qualitative assay, in which an initial amplification product (amplicon) is subjected to a second round of PCR using a new set of primers intrinsic to the first. The major disadvantage of nested PCR is the high rate of contamination that can occur.

- Competitive PCR (cPCR) is a broad term to encompass PCR techniques that are quantitative by way of comparison with a known standard. While the quantity of PCR reaction product is theoretically proportional to the starting quantity, there are too many confounding variables for this assessment to be made directly. The basic concept underlying cPCR is the simultaneous amplification, within the same reaction chamber, of two templates having similar size with the same primers. The starting amount of one of the templates is known and, after amplification, products from both templates are compared. These assays are used, for example, to quantify HIV-1 and HCV RNA.

- Real-time PCR can produce either qualitative or quantitative results. Also called homogeneous or kinetic PCR, real-time PCR refers to methods in which reaction product detection occurs simultaneously with target amplification. These methods require special thermal cyclers with optics capable of monitoring small amounts of fluorescence. The PCR product may be detected with fluorescent dyes that bind double-stranded DNA (relatively nonspecific) or fluorescent hybridization probes.

- Reverse transcriptase PCR (RT-PCR) is used when RNA is studied. RNA is first converted to complementary DNA (cDNA) using reverse transcriptase (RT). The cDNA can then be subjected to standard PCR.

- Allele-specific oligonucleotides (ASO) is a technique in which synthetic oligonucleotides, 15 to 18 bases in length (ASOs) are manufactured. The ASOs are designed to be complimentary to and capable of hybridizing with a sample of DNA only if a particular sequence is present. ASOs can be used following amplification to generate dot-blots.

- Multiplex PCR makes use of two or more primers within the same reaction mix. Such a reaction is capable of simultaneously detecting a number of different sequences. This modification is used, for example, in molecular microbiology (eg, multiple agents can be looked for in a sample).

- Transcription-based amplification is a term that encompasses transcription-mediated amplification (TMA) and nucleic acid sequence-based amplification (NASBA). These are isothermal amplification techniques (no thermal cycler) that convert RNA into DNA and then

Molecular Methods>Important Terms and Concepts

- Inversions (inv) result from two breaks occurring on a single arm with inversion of the reading frame. Inversions may be paracentric (spares centromere) or pericentric (involves centromere); eg, inv(9)(q21q31) is paracentric.

- Duplication (dup) is the presence of an extra segment of DNA, usually resulting in redundant copies of a gene or portion of a gene.

- Derivative (der) is an abnormal chromosome formed from portions of two or more chromosomes

Mendelian disorders are those that result from alterations (mutations) in a single gene and therefore are transmitted in simple (Mendelian) patterns.

- Autosomal dominant (AD) disorders are ones in which the disease is manifested in those with only one copy of the disease-causing allele (manifested in heterozygotes). AD disorders are characterized by a family pedigree that shows a vertical inheritance pattern; that is, the disorder is passed from generation to generation. Both males and females are affected, and phenotypically normal individuals do not pass the disorder to their offspring. A child with one affected parent has a 50% chance of being affected.

- Autosomal recessive (AR) disorders are ones in which the disease is manifested only in those with two copies of the disease-causing allele (homozygotes). AR disor-

ders display what is called horizontal transmission; that is, they affect several members within a generation but not the parents (and not the following generation). Both males and females are affected. A child of two carrier parents has a 25% chance of being affected.

- X-linked recessive disorders characterized by a pedigree that has skipped generations, with males affected solely or males are affected more often than females. Daughters of affected males are obligate carriers, and male offspring of affected males are completely spared. Male offspring of carrier moms have a 50% chance of being affected. X-linked dominant inheritance is quite rare T7.1.

- Calculating allele (gene) frequencies

  □ For every gene locus there is at least one allele. For most gene loci there are two major alleles. For some gene loci, such as the hemoglobin beta chain gene, there are several alleles, and for others, such as some of the HLA loci, there are numerous alleles.

  □ The frequency of all the alleles for a gene can be determined by working backward from the observed phenotypes, using the Hardy-Weinberg equation. In this equation p is the frequency of homozygotes for the first allele, pq is the frequency of heterozygotes, and q is the frequency for homozygotes for the second allele. The sum of all the gene frequencies at a locus must equal 1.

T7.1
Inheritance of Several Mendelian Disorders

Autosomal recessive: Recessive disorders, which are mostly enzyme deficiencies, tend to be those that impair the affected individual's ability to reproduce or reach the age of reproduction.	Alpha-1-antitrypsin deficiency, Wilson disease, hemochromatosis, cystic fibrosis, infantile polycystic kidney disease, congenital adrenal hyperplasias, phenylketonuria (PKU)
X-linked dominant	Hypophosphatemic rickets, incontinentia pigmenti type 1
X-linked recessive: Like autosomal recessives, these tend to impair reproductive potential.	Hemophilia A (factor VIII deficiency), hemophilia B (factor IX deficiency), Duchenne muscular dystrophy, chronic granulomatous disease, Fragile X syndrome, glucose-6-phosphate dehydrogenase deficiency, Bruton agammaglobulinemia, Lesch-Nyhan syndrome, color blindness, Duncan disease (X-linked immunoproliferative disorder), Mencke syndrome
Autosomal dominant: the rest	Huntington disease, Peutz-Jegher syndrome, protein C deficiency, Osler-Weber-Rendu (hereditary hemorrhagic telangiectasia), adult polycystic kidney disease, neurofibromatosis 1 & 2, familial hypercholesterolemia, osteogenesis imperfecta, familial adenomatous polyposis, myotonic muscular dystrophy, tuberous sclerosis, hereditary spherocytosis, von Willebrand disease, Marfan syndrome

7: Molecular Methods

Molecular Methods>Important Terms and Concepts I
Applications of Molecular Methods in Tumor Pathology>Demonstration of Lymphoid Clonality; Demonstration of Gene Rearrangements

$$p2 + 2pq + q2 = 1$$

- Pedigrees are commonly used to illustrate a genetic disease within a family. By looking at a pedigree, you can tell how the disease is inherited and make predictions about whether offspring will be affected.

Mutations are alterations in the nucleotide sequence of a gene. Mutations are classified as:

- Missense mutations are those that alter a codon so that a different amino acid is encoded in the ultimate protein.

- Silent mutations alter a codon without changing the encoded amino acid.

- Nonsense mutations are those that change a codon into a translation stop codon.

- Messenger RNA (mRNA) splice site point mutations corrupt a true mRNA splice site, or create a novel one.

Applications of Molecular Methods in Tumor Pathology

Demonstration of Lymphoid Clonality

Molecular assays are occasionally required to demonstrate clonality, through the demonstration of clonal Ig or TCR gene rearrangements. Gene-rearrangement assays cannot generally stand alone as evidence for clonality. Clonal populations can be found in reactive lymphoid proliferations, and they may be missed in neoplastic proliferations.

- Either Southern blot analysis or PCR may be used for this purpose, each capable of finding a clone as small as 1% of all cells present.

- The immunoglobulin heavy chain (IgH) gene is the preferred target for evaluating B-cell processes, and for T-cell processes, either the T-cell receptor β (TCR β) gene or TCRγ gene may be targeted. Note that while the vast majority of T-cell neoplasms express αβ T-cell receptors, the γ and δ chains rearrange first in T-cell development; thus clonal γ gene rearrangements may serve as the basis for diagnosing an αβ-expressing T-cell lymphoma. The TCR β gene is the usual target

of Southern blot analysis, while PCR assays often look at TCR γ.

In the Southern blot analysis (SBA), a probe that is labeled and complimentary to segments of either the IgH or TCR gene of interest is hybridized to a DNA sample that has been digested with restriction-endonucleases. The presence of new bands of different size indicate clones. These bands must be seen in at least two restriction enzymes for the result to be unequivocally positive.

PCR assays detect a smaller proportion of clonal rearrangements than SBA and, in this respect, is less sensitive than SBA. Since PCR relies upon primers which may or may not actually bind to an amplify the segments of interest, some clonal rearrangements may be missed entirely. Overall, PCR can detect about 85% of all rearrangements identified by SBA. However, for a given rearrangement that is detectable by either PCR or SBA, PCR requires fewer cells than SBA for a positive result. In this respect, PCR is more sensitive than SBA. Thus, a negative PCR does not fully exclude a neoplasm, but if the PCR was previously positive, a negative PCR does essentially exclude minimal residual disease.

Demonstration of Gene Rearrangements

Molecular methods can be used to detect specific rearrangements that serve the dual purpose of confirming the neoplastic nature of a proliferation and classifying it. This is the case in many hematolymphoid neoplasms and some solid tumors (particularly soft tissue and glial neoplasms). The same rearrangements serve later as sensitive markers of minimal residual disease (MRD).

Conventional cytogenetics can be used for this purpose, but fresh viable tissue is required, and rearrangements must be relatively large to be detected.

- While it is true that other molecular methods (PCR, FISH) are more sensitive for these rearrangements, these methods detect only the anomaly that is looked for or anticipated. They may miss other abnormalities which may point to another diagnosis or impact the prognosis.

7: Molecular Methods

Applications of Molecular Methods in Tumor Pathology>Demonstration of Gene Rearrangements;
Hereditary Cancer and Tumor Syndromes

- For example, in CML it is important to document the Philadelphia chromosome. While cytogenetic studies can detect a great number of these, the most sensitive test for this is PCR. Furthermore, cytogenetic studies are too insensitive to detect minimal residual disease (MRD), for which PCR is an excellent test. However, the presence of additional abnormalities, which define disease progression, are missed by PCR. Thus, initial testing for CML should include both cytogenetics and PCR.

- In cytogenetic terms, a clone is defined as 2 or more cells within a sample having the same chromosomal anomaly. A subclone is a second population (2 or more cells) that has the original chromosome anomaly plus one or more additional anomalies.

So-called molecular cytogenetics (FISH) is very useful for this purpose, particularly when the number of tumor cells is large.

PCR can detect a much smaller number of tumor cells in a mixed population, permitting sensitive diagnosis of minimal residual (MRD). Most MRD assays currently are based upon real-time quantitative PCR.

Hereditary Cancer and Tumor Syndromes

Hereditary cancer and tumor syndromes may be suspected based upon (1) tumor type (eg, medullary thyroid carcinoma), (2) unusually young age at presentation, (2) a characteristic histologic appearance (eg, colon and breast). Many hereditary cancer syndromes can be identified through the demonstration of specific *germline* mutations. That is, the disease-causing mutations is found in all somatic cells, not just the tumor cells.

Hereditary nonpolyposis colorectal carcinoma (HNPCC, Lynch syndrome)

- HNPCC is an autosomal dominant syndrome associated with a 60-80% lifetime risk of colorectal carcinoma in which affected persons have germline mutations that result in defective mismatch repair. Defective mismatch repair is a cause of microsatellite instability (MSI). It is estimated that about 5% of colorectal carcinomas are due to HNPCC. There are two types of HNPCC: Lynch syndrome I (colon cancer), and Lynch syndrome II (colon, endometrial, and ovarian cancer). Additional tumors to which Lynch

syndrome is predisposed include small intestinal adenocarcinoma, pancreaticobiliary adenocarcinoma, gastric adenocarcinoma, and urothelial carcinoma. Related syndromes are Muir-Torre (sebaceous neoplasms and colon cancer) and Turcot (brain tumors and colon cancer).

- HNPCC is due to germline (present in all somatic cells) mutations in one of the DNA mismatch repair genes: MLH1 (40% of cases), MSH2 (40%), MSH6 (10%), PMS2 (5%), MSH3, PMS1, and MLH3.

- These germline mutations are not the only way to get an MSI-associated tumor, however. Approximately 15% of sporadic colorectal and gastric cancers display MSI. These cases appear to be due to a hypermethylation, present in only the tumor DNA, of the promoter for MLH1. Thus, MSI alone is not diagnostic of HNPCC. Furthermore, while diagnosing HNPCC is important (for genetic counseling and future surveillance for new primary tumors) it is the presence of MSI (with or without HNPCC) that impacts the clinicopathologic features of the tumor.

- Microsatellite instability (MSI) testing is performed by extracting DNA from paraffin-embedded neoplastic and nonneoplastic tissue. PCR, using a set of primers, is used to amplify 5 specific microsatellite regions. These are BAT25, BAT26 (both of which are regions of mononucleotide repeats), D2S123, D5S346, and D17S250 (regions of dinucleotide repeats). These regions from the tumor are compared to those from nonneoplastic tissue for differences to assess for differences in length, indicative of MSI. Tumors are classified as MSI-high (MSI-H) when differences are present in 2 or more markers, MSI-low (MSI-L) when present in 1 marker, and microsatellite stable (MSS) when all markers are unchanged.

- Another approach is to perform immunohistochemical staining on neoplastic and nonneoplastic tissue for MLH1, MSH2, and MSH6 protein expression. IHC appears to have good sensitivity (>90%) and specificity (nearly 100%) for MSI.

- If a tumor is deemed to have MSI by one of these studies, this implies that the patient may have HNPCC, and testing for mutations is indicated.

- Regardless of whether the patient has HNPCC, MSI-high tumors have a different biology than non-MSI-high tumors.

  □ They tend to be located in the right colon.

  □ They are poorly differentiated and often arranged in trabeculae. They tend to have mucinous (colloid) differentiation and a component of signet ring cells.

  □ They tend to have prominent tumor-infiltrating lymphocytes (TIL) and a peri-tumoral 'Crohn's-like' nodular lymphoid infiltrate.

  □ They often have a pushing tumor margin and may appear well-circumsribed. Because of this and some of the other features listed, the tumors have been described as medullary-like (referring to medullary breast carcinoma).

  □ In HNPCC, the patients are younger than in sporadic MSI-high tumors. Furthermore, HNPCC tumors are more likely to be tubular adenoma-associated; while sporadic MSI-high tumors are more often serrated adenoma-associated.

- To help guide testing for HNPCC, the Amsterdam criteria were established and later modified (Amsterdam II). Slightly more liberal Bethesda guidelines have also been published. MSI testing and IHC are considered screening tests, and DNA-based testing for germline mutations is still considered the gold standard.**T7.2**

T7.2
Molecular Genetics of HNPCC

Gene Symbol	Chromosomal Locus
MLH1	3p21.3
MSH2	2p22
MSH6	2p16
PMS2	7p22

Familial Adenomatous Polyposis (FAP)

- FAP is characterized by carpeting of the colon with hundreds of adenomatous polyps by age 20, and adenocarcinoma by age 50. It is associated with about 1% of all cases of colorectal carcinoma. In FAP, there is also an increased incidence of gastric polyps (fundic gland polyps, especially) and small intestinal polyps (adenomas) with a slightly increased risk of small bowel adenocarcinoma, ampullary adenocarcinoma, thyroid cancer, and desmoids. If FAP is recognized, prophylactic colectomy in young adulthood is indicated.

- FAP is inherited in an autosomal dominant manner and is caused by mutations in the *APC* gene. As many as 30% represent a new mutation.

von Hippel-Lindau disease

- von Hippel–Lindau (vHL) is an autosomal dominant disease in which patients are at high risk for numerous tumor types: hemangioblastomas (cerebellar, cerebral, or retinal), pheochromocytoma, renal cell carcinoma (clear cell type), pancreatic cysts, islet cell tumors, cystadenomas (epididymal, ovarian), and/or tumors of the endolymphatic sac of the inner ear.

- vHL is due to a germline mutation in the *VHL* gene, a tumor suppressor gene found at 3p25-26. Deletion or other alteration of 3p is also extremely common in sporadic clear cell type renal cell carcinoma.

- Renal cell carcinomas in vHL tend to present in young patients (mean 37 years) and to be multifocal and bilateral. They have exclusively clear cell histology, but they are somewhat more indolent than sporadic tumors (metastasize only when quite large).

Tuberous Sclerosis

- Tuberous sclerosis is an autosomal dominant syndrome that is characterized by numerous, mostly benign, tumors: angiofibromas (adenoma sebaceum) of the skin, periungual fibromas, shagreen patches, hypopigmented macules, cardiac rhabdomyomas, pulmonary lymphangioleiomyomatosis (LAM), subependymal giant cell astrocytomas (SEGA), and renal angiomyolipomas (AML). There is an increased risk of renal neoplasms, including clear cell type renal cell carcinoma and oncocytomas.

- Tuberous sclerosis is caused by mutations in either the *TSC1* gene (9q34—hamartin protein) or the *TSC2* gene (16p13.3—tuberin protein).

BRCA1 and BRCA2

- In families harboring germline *BRCA1* and *BRCA2* mutations, there are often two or more generations of women with premenopausal breast cancer, sometimes bilateral, and sometimes associated with epithelial ovarian malignancy. There appears to also be increased risk of cancer in the pancreas, uterus, and prostate. In fact, it appears that a variant mutation in BRCA is the cause of familial pancreatic cancer.

- About 5% of all women with breast cancer and 25% of Ashkenazi Jewish women with breast cancer can be found to have a BRCA mutation. While the lifetime incidence of breast cancer in women is about 10%, the lifetime risk in *BRCA1* or *BRCA2* is about 70%.

- *BRCA1* and *BRCA2* are tumor suppressor genes. They encode proteins that mediate the DNA repair process. More than 2000 different mutations have been identified in *BRCA1* and *BRCA2*. Three of these appear with high frequency in persons of Ashkenazi Jewish descent, together accounting for over 90% of the BRCA mutations in this population: a two-base pair deletion in codon 23 (185delAG) of *BRCA1*, a 5382insC mutation in *BRCA1*, and a 6174delT mutation of *BRCA2*.

- BRCA-associated breast cancers have a high rate of medullary-type histology. Even those without this appearance tend to have a high grade and tend to be ER/PR negative.

Multiple Endocrine Neoplasia Type 1 (MEN1)

- *MEN1* manifests as parathyroid adenomas, pituitary adenomas, and pancreatic islet cell tumors. Other sites within the GI tract may give rise to endocrine tumors. Nonendocrine lesions associated with MEN1 include facial angiofibromas, collagenomas, lipomas, and meningiomas.

- The *MEN1* gene is found on chromosome 11q13 where it encodes the protein menin. Direct sequence analysis is capable of identifying germline MEN1 gene mutations in about 90% of families with MEN1. Persons with so-called simplex cases (MEN1 devel-

oping sporadically in a single person, without apparent inheritance), the mutation is found in about 60%. Among those with a single MEN1-associated tumor, the germline mutation is rare. In this latter regard, a key distinction must be made: a germline mutation is one present in all cells in the body (all somatic cells); a somatic mutation is one found only in the lesional cells. Somatic *MEN1* mutations are found in 15%-20% of sporadic parathyroid adenomas, islet cell tumors, and gastrinomas.

- Specific germline mutations in the *MEN1* gene can give rise to familial isolated hyperparathyroidism (FIHP).

Multiple Endocrine Neoplasia Type 2 (MEN2, Sipple syndrome)

The *RET* gene is found on 10q. MEN2A is due to mutations affecting exons 10-11 of the *RET* gene, most often affecting a particular cysteine residue (634 Cys). FMTC mutations usually also affect cysteine residues, particularly 609, 611, 618, and 620 Cys. MEN2B is most often due to a mutation affecting exon 16, encoding the tyrosine kinase domain. Targeted mutation analysis as well as sequence analysis are clinically available.

Interestingly, about 20% of cases of Hirschsprung disease are due to germline mutations in *RET*. In addition, about 40% of sporadic papillary thyroid carcinomas have somatic mutations in *RET*.

- There are three subtypes of MEN2—MEN 2A, familial medullary thyroid carcinoma (FMTC), and MEN 2B—all imparting a high risk for medullary thyroid carcinoma, all autosomal dominant, and all due to a RET gene mutation. MEN2a is characterized by medullary thyroid carcinoma plus pheochromocytoma and parathyroid adenoma. MEN2b is characterized by medullary thyroid carcinoma plus pheochromocytoma, mucosal neuromas, ganglioneuromatous intestinal polyps, and Marfanoid body habitus. FMTC has only medullary thyroid carcinoma.

- The *RET* gene is associated with all three forms of MEN2. Mutations in *RET* are found in >95% of affected individuals. In MEN2a, mutations tend to be found in exons 10 or 11, often at locations affecting cysteine residues. MEN2b is found to have a single point mutation in codon 918 (within the tyrosine kinase domain) in most cases. Most mutations responsible for disease can be found with either targeted mutation analysis, direct sequencing of 'hot spot' exons (10-16) or full gene sequencing.

- While the histology of medullary thyroid carcinomas is not particularly distinctive in these syndromes, the appearance of the background thyroid is: C-cell hyperplasia and numerous small foci of medullary carcinoma.

Carney Complex

- Carney complex (LAMB syndrome, NAME syndrome) is characterized by the formation of multiple tumors, most of them benign. Cutaneous lentigines (simple lentigos) are the most common presenting finding, located on the face (particularly the oral and conjunctival mucosa), vagina, and penis. Blue nevi, particularly the cellular blue nevus, are also common. Cardiac myxomas occur frequently, at a young age, and may affect any chamber. Myxomas arise at other sites as well, including the breast, female genital tract, and skin (especially on the eyelid and external ear). Endocrine tumors arise, particularly follicular adenomas of the thyroid, pituitary adenomas (GH-secreting), and the so-called primary pigmented nodular adrenocortical disease (PPNAD) of the adrenal gland. The latter is a form of multiodular hyperplasia of the adrenal cortex and causes Cushing syndrome. Large-cell calcifying Sertoli cell tumors arise in most affected males. Note that this unusual tumor is also seen in Peutz-Jeghers syndrome; however, the SCTAT of Peutz-Jeghers is not seen in females with Carney complex. Psammomatous melanotic schwannoma, rare as a sporadic tumor, is common in the Carney complex. Note that, though similarly named, the Carney Triad is an entirely different syndrome (triad of gastric GIST, pulmonary chondroma, and extra-adrenal paraganglioma).

- About half of cases are due to mutations in the *PRKAR1A* gene, located on 17q24, which encodes a regulatory subunit of cAMP-dependent protein kinase. In the remaining cases, a specific gene has not been implicated, but a locus at 2p16 appears promising. Direct sequence analysis for the *PRKAR1A* gene is clinically available.

Cowden Syndrome and other PTEN-related disorders

- The *PTEN* gene is located at 10q23 and encodes the phosphatidylinositol-3,4,5-trisphosphate 3-phosphatase (PTEN). Direct sequence analysis is available for detecting *PTEN* gene mutations. Disorders associated with mutations in the *PTEN* gene share a tendency to develop hamartomatous lesions and include Cowden syndrome, Bannayan-Riley-Ruvalcaba syndrome, and Proteus syndrome.

- Hamartomatous intestinal polyps, multiple lipomas, fibromas, GU malformations, and multiple mucocutaneous lesions (facial trichilemmomas, papillomas, palmoplantar keratoses, and palmoplantar hyperkeratotic pits) characterize Cowden syndrome. Microcephaly and mental retardation are common, and it is strongly associated with cerebellar dysplastic gangliocytoma (Lhermitte-Duclos), which is considered pathognomonic. Those with Cowden syndrome have an increased risk of malignancy, especially of the breast, thyroid (follicular carcinoma), colon, and endometrium.

- Bannayan-Riley-Ruvalcaba syndrome is characterized by high birth weight with macrocephaly, mental retardation, myopathy, joint hypermobility, pectus excavatum, scoliosis, hamartomatous intestinal polyps, lipomas, and pigmented macules of the glans penis.

- Proteus syndrome is has highly variable manifestations, due to overgrowths confined to several organs or tissue types. It is said to affect individuals in a mosaic distribution; ie, some organs or tissues heavily affected, others entirely spared. Some examples include connective tissue nevi (considered pathognomonic), asymmetric limb growth, skull hyperostosis, megaspondylodysplasia of the vertebrae, or visceral overgrowth (especially spleen and thymus).

Juvenile Polyposis

Juvenile polyposis is an autosomal dominant disorder in which two genes have thus far been implicated: *BMPR1A* (10q22.3) and *SMAD4* (18q21.1). Direct sequence analysis is clinically available to detect mutations in these genes. However, these combined account for slightly fewer than half of cases. A small subset of patients have mutations in the PTEN gene (causative of Cowden and Bannayan-Riley-Ruvalcaba syndromes) and in fact have juvenile polyps as part of one of those syndromes. Juvenile polyposis syndrome manifests as a tendency to develop juvenile polyps in the stomach, small and large intestine, and an increased risk of gastrointestinal malignancy. The juvenile polyp is a particular histologic type of polyp (the name does not refer to age of onset) with a smooth outer contour, cystically dilated mucus-filled glands having nonadenomatous epithelium, and a dense nonmuscular collagenous stroma permeated by inflammatory cells. Most affected individuals have some polyps by the age of 20, but the number of polyps developed over a lifetime is highly variable, ranging from 1 to over 100. The lifetime risk of malignancy ranges from 9% to 50%, and most of these are colorectal adenocarcinomas.

Peutz-Jeghers Syndrome (PJS)

Peutz-Jeghers syndrome (PJS) is an autosomal dominant disorder with mucocutaneous pigmentation and a specific type of hamartomatous polyp. The polyps arise in greatest numbers in the small intestine, especially the jejunum, but also occur in the stomach and colon. They first arise around age 10. Lined by mucinous mucosa, their characteristic feature is a stroma of thin complexly branching muscle bundles with an arborizing appearance. Mucocutaneous hyperpigmentation begins in early childhood with dark blue or brown macules around the mouth, eyes, nostrils, perianal area, and sometimes the fingers. Females are at risk for the sex cord tumor with annular tubules (SCTAT) of the ovaries and adenoma malignum of the cervix. Males are at risk for calcifying Sertoli cell tumors of the testes. There is a >90% lifetime risk of malignancy, with a risk of 50% by age 65. The relative risk is highest for cancers of the GI tract and breast. Mutations in the *STK11* gene (chromosome 19p) underlie about 75% of cases.

The Birt-Hogg-Dubé Syndrome

The Birt-Hogg-Dubé syndrome is an autosomal dominant disorder characterized by three cardinal features: fibrofolliculomas, pneumothorax, and renal tumors. Renal tumors actually develop in only about 15%-20% of cases, but they tend to be multifocal, bilateral, and have features of combined oncocytoma and chromophobe carcinoma. Birt-Hogg-Dubé is due to mutations in the *BHD* gene (chromosome 17p11.2—encoding folliculin).

Neurofibromatosis Type 1 (von Recklinghausen disease, NF1)

Neurofibromatosis type 1 (von Recklinghausen disease, NF1) is an autosomal dominant disease (but about half are due to new mutations) that presents with multiple café au lait spots and intertriginous (groin, axilla) freckling. Neurofibromas may not be seen until adulthood, and the less common plexiform neurofibroma is considered pathognomonic. Ocular Lisch nodules are fairly common but innocuous. Inconsistent features include optic gliomas, vertebral dysplasia, scoliosis, bone cortical thinning, pseudarthrosis, mental retardation, pulmonic stenosis, NF1 vasculopathy with associated hypertension, leukemia, and malignant peripheral nerve sheath tumors. Hyperintense lesions, seen on T2-weighted imaging and often called 'unidentified bright objects,' may be seen in the optic tracts, basal ganglia, brainstem, cerebellum, or cortex. They are usually inconsequential clinically and seen primarily in childhood, disappearing into adulthood. A Noonan syndrome appearance is seen in about 12% of individuals with NF1. Many women with NF1 experience a rapid increase in the number and size of neurofibromas during pregnancy. NF1 is due to mutations in the *NF1* gene (17q11.2—encoding neurofibromin). Half of affected individuals have NF1 as the result of a de novo *NF1* mutation. Several molecular assays are clinically available. These include cytogenetic testing (detects about 1% of cases that are due to a structural chromosomal rearrangement), FISH testing (detects about 5% of cases that are due to a total gene deletion), protein truncation testing (detects about 80%), and direct sequence analysis (90%).

Neurofibromatosis Type 2 (bilateral acoustic neuromas, NF2)

Neurofibromatosis Type 2 (bilateral acoustic neuromas, NF2) is an autosomal dominant condition, but about 1/3 are due to new mutations (simplex cases). Much about the nomenclature of this syndrome is confusing: NF2 is characterized by bilateral vestibular nerve (not acoustic nerve) schwannomas (neither neurofibromas nor neuromas occur), and it has almost no relationship to NF1. The disease first manifests around the age of 20, and nearly all affected individuals have bilateral vestibular schwannomas by the age of 30. They are at increased risk for schwannomas of other nerves, meningiomas, ependymomas, and astrocytomas. Many develop posterior subcapsular lens opacities. Mutations in the NF2 gene (22q—encodes merlin) are the cause of NF2. Direct sequence analysis is clinically available, capable of detecting about 90% of causative mutations.

Molecular Basis and Diagnosis of Specific Neoplasms

Hematolymphoid Neoplasms—see Chapter 4

Solid Tumors

- ■ Renal Cell Carcinoma

  - □ Conventional clear cell renal cell carcinoma is most often associated with deletion of portions of the short arm of chromosome 3. Three particular loci are disproportionately affected: 3p14, 3p25.3 (the location of the *vHL* gene), and 3p21.3. While present in the vast majority of tumors, del (3p) is the sole abnormality in only about 15% of cases. Additional anomalies at 14q, 9p, 8p, and 6q are common; in fact, it appears that 3p is necessary for initial tumorigenesis, but the additional anomalies contribute to tumor aggressiveness. For example, loss of 14q or 9p correlates with higher stage and a worse prognosis.

  - □ Papillary renal cell carcinomas are associated with loss of the Y chromosome (in males) and gains of (trisomy of) 7p, 17p, 12, and 16.

  - □ Chromophobe carcinomas display complex cytogenetics, with multiple anomalies (mainly losses) of Y, 1, 2, 6, 10, 13, 17, and 21.

  - □ Renal carcinomas associated with Xp11.2 translocations, most commonly in the form of t(X;1) and t(X;17), are a subset of renal carcinomas that most commonly affect young patients. These rearrangements involve the *TFE3* gene—the same gene that is involved in the *ASPL–TFE3* gene fusion of t(X;17) in alveolar soft part sarcoma (ASPS)—and multiple partners. The most common result is the *PRCC-TFE3* fusion. The *PRCC-TFE3* fusion tumors arise usually before the age of 30 years. The tumor has a distinctive appearance with alveolar (nested) and papillary architecture, clear cells, and psammoma bodies. A thick, calcified capsule is seen in some cases. They are characteristically negative for EMA (a marker uniformly positive in conventional clear cell carcinoma) but positive for CD10. The *ASPL–TFE3* renal cell carcinomas characteristically present at advanced stage but, like ASPS, follow an indolent course marked by very late relapses/metastases.

  - □ Renal cell carcinomas with t(6:11)(p11.2;q12) involve the *TFEB* gene which is closely related in function to the *TFE3* gene. The resulting tumor is essentially identical to Xp11.2 tumors.

- ■ Breast Carcinoma

  - □ The Her-2/neu (c-erbB-2) protein is a transmembrane glycoprotein in the epidermal growth factor receptor (EGFR) family. While it is expressed in a variety of normal epithelia, including breast ductal epithelium, it is found to be over-expressed in some invasive breast cancers. This over-expression has been associated with: (1) poor outcome, independent of other prognostic markers, (2) high nuclear grade (3) good response to Adriamycin-based adjuvant chemotherapy, (4) a poor response to tamoxifen, independent of ER/PR status, and (5) good response to anti-Her-2/neu antibody (trastuzumab, Herceptin).

  - □ Over-expression of *Her-2/neu* gene is usually a result of gene amplification (multiple copies of the gene).

  - □ Many laboratories use immunohistochemistry to test for *Her2/neu* amplification. In assessing *HER-2/neu* expression, only membranous staining is considered. Expression is usually reported as 0 to 3+, depending upon the proportion of cells displaying strong circumferential membranous staining. Scores of 0 and 1+ are considered negative. 3+ is considered positive. These scores correlate well with direct (FISH) gene testing, except in the borderline (2+) cases. In cases demonstrating 2+ staining for Her2/neu by immunohistochemistry, FISH analysis is indicated.

  - □ FISH may be used as either the primary means of her-2 assessment, or as a reflex test in 2+ cases. Using a centromeric chromosome 17 probe (eg, with a green label) in combination with an allele-specific probe for the *Her-2/neu* oncogene (eg, with an orange label) one can determine whether the gene is amplified. Visualization of 2 green and 2 orange signals is expected in a nonamplified cell (a ratio of 1:1). In cells with Her-2/neu amplification, 4 or more orange signals are visualized in nuclei showing 2 green signals (a ratio of 2:1 or more).

399

■ Gliomas

□ Due to their frequent unresectability, radiotherapy and chemotherapy are entertained as therapeutic modalities for gliomas. Predicting response to these modalities has traditionally been based upon accurate morphologic tumor classification, since oligodendrogliomas respond much more favorably to treatment with chemotherapy and are associated with a much better prognosis.

□ While routine histology can reliably distinguish a large number of oligodendrogliomas from astrocytomas; there remains a considerable number with indeterminate morphologic features. Several immunohistochemical markers—GFAP, Leu7, p53—have failed to demonstrate reliable discrimination.

□ Genetic markers have shown the greatest potential to date. There are genetic alterations that occur with equal frequency in astrocytomas and oligodendrogliomas, usually with devolution to a higher grade, including loss of 9p21 (*p16/CDKN2A*) and losses involving chromosome 10 (*PTEN/DMBT1*). These markers may provide prognostic information but do not aid in the distinction of oligodendrogliomas from astrocytomas. The genetic markers with the greatest power in this regard are the combined loss of genetic material from chromosomes 1p and 19q. The loss of either of these is more common in oligodendrogliomas, and their combined loss is highly specific (but only about 60-80% sensitive). Furthermore, other tumors often confused with oligodendrogliomas—the dysembryoblastic neuroectodermal tumor (DNET), protoplasmic astrocytoma, and central neurocytoma—lack 1p/19q losses.

□ Perhaps distinct from and more important than the question of oligodendrogliomas versus astrocytoma, the combined loss of 1p and 19q identifies a set of tumors with enhanced chemosensitivity and prolonged survival. The combined loss of 1p and 19q occurs in 1-10% of clear-cut astrocytomas, and this is of unclear significance at this time.

□ Poor prognostic factors in gliomas include: retention of 1p and 19q, del(16p), LOH 10q, and *EGFR* amplification. Amplification of the *EGFR* gene is found in about half of glioblastomas (rarely in lower grade astrocytomas and oligodendrogliomas) and may be useful in correctly categorizing small cell astrocytomas, which have *EGFR* amplification and chromosome 10 losses but intact chromosomes 1p and 19q.

□ In assessing the status of 1p and 19q, either loss of-heterozygosity (LOH), fluorescence in situ hybridization (FISH), or comparative genomic hybridization (CGH) may be used with equal efficacy.

■ Retinoblastoma

□ The *RB1* gene is associated with the development of retinoblastoma. About 70% of *RB1* mutations are in the form of point mutations. These are only detectable by direct sequence analysis. Larger deletions of all or part of the *RB1* gene may be identified by FISH. Hypermethylation is found in about 10% of cases, detectable by methylation analysis, particularly of the promoter region.

□ About 5%-7% of children with retinoblastoma harbor a germline chromosome deletion, detectable by cytogenetics, involving chromosome 13q14. The incidence is higher for patients with bilateral retinoblastoma. About another 10% have no detectable deletion but have a family history of retinoblastoma. The remaining cases appear to be sporadic cases.

□ Individuals with germline *RB1* mutations are at increased risk of developing tumors outside the eye, including: pineal gland tumors, PNET, and osteosarcomas. These secondary tumors usually present in late childhood or adulthood.

■ Meningioma

□ Monosomy of chromosome 22 is the most common abnormality found in meningiomas. The key region appears to be 22q12.2 where the *NF2* gene is located. Recall that meningioma is one of the features of the NF2 syndrome (caused by germline *NF2* mutations); about half of sporadic meningiomas have NF2 anomalies.

□ Merlin is the protein encoded by the *NF2* gene. Merlin is found in the cell membrane where its function is to mediate cell-cell contact and cell contact inhibition. It is thought that CD44, one of the merlin ligands, is a signal for the cessation of growth.

❑ Certain histologic features have shown moderate correlation with aggressive behavior (recurrence and progression). The term 'anaplastic meningioma' has been applied to such tumors. The mitotic rate is perhaps the strongest single feature. Others, in combination, portend a high rate of recurrence: the presence of true cerebral invasion, high cellularity, small cell growth, prominent nucleoli, sheet-like growth, and necrosis. In addition, particular histologic subtypes are felt to have a higher rate of progression: clear cell, chordoid, rhabdoid, and papillary. Lastly, a high proportion of cells with MIB-1 (Ki-67) immunostaining is associated with recurrence.

❑ 22q12.2 deletions are thought to be a key early step in development of many meningiomas. However, progression seems to involve other alterations; anaplastic meningiomas show frequent losses of (eg, 1p, 9p, and others) as well as gains (eg, 1q, 9q, and others). In fact, del 1p is the second most common chromosomal abnormality in meningiomas. Deletion of 9p21 is another common finding and is associated with shortened survival.

■ Ewing/PNET

❑ Ewing/PNET (Ewing family of tumors) encompasses several entities previously considered distinct, including Ewing sarcoma, PNET, Askin tumor, and others. These tumors share numerous histologic and immunohistochemical traits in addition to molecular rearrangements that result in *FLI1/EWS* fusion transcripts.

❑ The most common structural rearrangement leading to this fusion is t(11;22)(q24;q12). The *EWS* gene is found on 22q12, and the FLI1 gene is on 11q24. The precise location of fusion differs from case to case, but most commonly it is formed between exon 7 of *EWS* and exon 6 of *FLI1* (termed the type 1 fusion). The type 1 fusion is associated with a relatively favorable prognosis. Some cases have instead a t(21;22) translocation, involving *EWS* and *ERG*, or rarely a t(7;22) or t(17;22).

■ Intra-abdominal desmoplastic small round cell tumor (IADSRCT) has a similar but unique translocation: t(11;22)(p13;q12) which results in the fusion of the *EWS* gene to the Wilms tumor gene (*WT1*) on 11p13.

■ Clear cell sarcoma (malignant melanoma of soft parts) is another *EWS*-associated tumor. It is consistently associated with the t(12;22)(q13;q12) translocation which produces the *EWS-ATF1* fusion gene.

■ Neuroblastoma

❑ Amplification of the *MYCN* proto-oncogene is found in 20%-30% of neuroblastomas and is a marker of aggressive clinical behavior. Abnormalities of 17q23-qter are present in >50% of cases, deletion of 1p36 is present in 30%-40%, and deletion of 11q23 in 40%-50%.

❑ Beyond those broad generalizations, the molecular basis of neuroblastoma is extremely complex. The amplification of *MYCN* appears to be central to disease progression and may occur in a variety of ways—amplification, duplication, and segmental chromosome gain. Cytogenetically, amplification may be observable as chromosomal abnormalities such as homogeneously staining regions (HSRs) or double minutes, but these are often remote from native location of *MYCN* (2p). The degree of *MYCN* amplification is generally >10-fold in neuroblastoma, and it may be as high as 500-fold. FISH is the best way to identify *MYCN* duplication, which most often occurs at or near 2p. Segmental chromosome gains are felt to result from the manner of structural rearrangements in places like 17q and 1p.

❑ The DNA content (ploidy) of the tumor has been shown to correlate with outcome, particularly in infants. Those with hyperdiploid tumors (DNA index greater than 1.0) have a more favorable outcome (similar to what is seen in acute lymphoblastic lymphoma).

❑ The 1p deletion is associated with poor prognosis.

7: Molecular Methods

Applications of Molecular Methods in Tumor Pathology>Molecular Basis and Diagnosis of Specific Neoplasms I
Applications of Molecular Methods in Nonneoplastic Disease>Diagnosis of Mendelian disorders

- Wilms tumor

  □ *WT1* is a tumor suppressor gene located at 11p13.
    The WAGR syndrome (Wilms tumor, aniridia,
    genitourinary anomalies, retardation) is caused by a
    large germline 11p13 deletion that encompasses the
    PAX6 gene (causing aniridia) and the *WT1* gene.
    Germline mutations in *WT1* are also present in the
    Denys-Drash syndrome. Sporadic Wilms tumors
    have *WT1* mutations, but in almost all such cases,
    these are present only in tumor tissue (somatic
    mutations).

  □ *WT2* is a gene located at 11p15. The Beckwith-
    Wiedemann syndrome is caused by germline
    mutations in *WT2*. Manifestations iclude high
    birth weight, macroglossia, organomegaly,
    hemihypertrophy (asymmetric growth), neonatal
    hypoglycemia, and increased risk of embryonal
    tumors, especially Wilms tumor and
    hepatoblastoma. Additional features are anterior
    ear creases or pits, abdominal wall defects,
    adrenocortical cytomegaly, and renal anomalies
    (renal medullary dysplasia, nephrocalcinosis,
    medullary sponge kidney, and nephromegaly). In
    utero there is polyhydramnios, a long umbilical
    cord, an enlarged placenta, and often a premature
    delivery. Beckwith-Weidemann syndrome is due to
    numerous defects that lead to abnormal
    transcription of genes in 11p15.5. This normally is
    an imprinted domain (one that is chemically
    modified depending upon whether inherited from
    the mother or from the father). Structural
    anomalies at 11p15 can be detected by cytogenetics
    in only about 1% of cases and by FISH in 1%-2%.
    Methylation assays may detect many more. Paternal
    uniparental disomy for 11p15 is observed by
    methylation analysis in 10%-20%.

- Rhabdomyosarcoma occurs as one of several subtypes,
  only one of which has a recurring chromosomal
  anomaly: the alveolar rhabdomyosarcoma with
  t(2;13)(q35;q14). This translocation results in the
  apposition of the *PAX3* gene (2q35) and the *FKHR*
  gene (13q14). A significant minority of cases have been
  found instead to have a t(1;13)(p36;q14) translocation
  involving the *PAX7* gene.

- Synovial sarcoma is consistently associated with the
  t(X;18)(p11;q11) translocation, resulting in the fusion
  of the *SYT* gene (18q11) with either the *SSX1* or *SSX2*
  gene (Xp11). There is some evidence that the *SSX1*
  fusion is associated with biphasic histology and *SSX2*
  with monophasic histology.

Applications of Molecular Studies in Nonneoplastic Disease (T7.3)

Diagnosis of Mendelian Disorders

In diseases caused by gene deletions, failure to amplify
the gene by PCR or failure to hybridize the gene (by
ASO or dot-blot) is consistent with the presence of the
disease (the absence of the gene). This principal is
applied to the molecular diagnosis of α-thalassemia, for
example, which is often caused by large gene deletions.
It is not applicable to most cases of β-thalassemia, however, which is usually due to a point mutation.

For diseases that are regularly caused by the same mutation (eg, sickle cell anemia), so-called direct mutation
analysis may be applied. Direct mutation analysis refers
to such methods as Southern blot analysis or ASO.
Sometimes these are applied after DNA amplification
by PCR.

For diseases caused by a large number of different mutations in one gene, the situation becomes more complex.
Alternatives include the use of PCR primers for several
of the more common mutations, complete gene
sequencing, and linkage analysis. Such methods are considered forms of indirect mutation analysis.

For diseases caused by unknown gene mutations, linkage analysis is usually applied. Linkage analysis can also
be used to identify carrier status. Linkage analysis
exploits DNA polymorphisms—inconsequential differences in DNA sequences that exist among individuals.
DNA polymorphisms result in differing restriction fragment lengths when DNA from one person to the next is
subjected to digestion by restriction endonucleases, separated by electrophoresis, and visualized (Southern
blot). Thus, DNA polymorphisms are responsible for
restriction fragment length polymorphisms (RFLPs).
One hopes that members of an affected family will show
differing RFLPs such that family members with disease
have a fragment that is absent in those without disease
(ie, there is an 'informative marker'). The utility of a
marker (and the specificity of the assay) is limited by
meiotic crossing-over. When a marker is closely linked
to the unknown disease-causing locus, the specificity is
better, but it is never 100%. Despite these caveats, linkage analysis provides a diagnosis in many cases where a
specific mutation has not been identified or too many
possible mutations in a known gene (eg, hemophilia A,
hemophilia B, β-thalassemia, Huntingtons).

T7.3
Genetic Features of Various Nonneoplastic Diseases

Disease	Molecular defect	Genes	Notes
Acue myelogenous leukemia (AML)	t(8;21)(q22;q22)	ETO/AMLI	M2 morphology; good prognosis
	inv(16)/t(16;16)	CBFB/MYHII	M4 morphology; good prognosis, CNS infiltration
	t(15;17)(q22;q21)	PML/RARα	APML morphology; good response to ATRA, DIC common
	t(11;17)(q23.1;q21)	PLZF/RARα	Variant APML, poor response to ATRA
	11q23	MLL	Poor prognosis; high risk of CNS involvement; post-topoisomerase II therapy
	t(1;22)(p13;q13)	OTT/MAL	Infantile AML-M7 subtype
5q– MDS	5q–		Good prognosis; elderly women, with macrocytic anemia and thrombocytosis
Therapy-related MDS and AML	Inv(16), t(15/17)	CBFβ, RARα	
Chronic myelogenous leukemia (CML)	t(9;22)(q34;q11.2)	BCR/ABL	
	t(9;22) +	ASS	Poor prognosis
	t(9;22) + Ph, +8, +19, i(17q), del(9q)		Indicates transition to blast phase
B-precursor ALL	Hyperdiploidy >54 chromosomes		Good prognosis
	t(12;21)	TEL/AMLIL	Good prognosis
	t(4;11)(q21;q23)	MLL	Neonates and infants, poor prognosis
	t(1;19)		
	t(9;22) (q34;q11.2)	BCR/ABL	Poor prognosis
Burkitt lymphoma	t(8;14), t(8;22), t(2;8)	cMyc/IgH; cMyc/Igλ; cMyc/Igκ	
Follicular lymphoma (FL)	t(14;18)(q32;q21)	BCL2/IgH	
Mantle cell lymphoma (MCL)	t(11;14)(q13;q32)	BCL1/IgH	
MALT	t(11;18)(q21;q21)	MLT/API2	
Myeloma	Hyperdiploidy		Good prognosis
	t(11;14)(q13;q32)	CCNDI/IgH	Most common
	Del13, t(4;14), t(14;16)		Poor prognosis
	t(8;14)	cMyc/IgH	
ALCL	t(2;5)(p23;q35)	ALK/NPM	Good prognosis
Ewing/PNET	t(11;22)(q24;q12)	FLI1/EWS	
	t(21;22)(q22;q21)	ERG/EWS	
Neuroblastoma	del(1p), +17	n-MYC	
Alveolar rhabdomyosarcoma	t(2;13)(q37;q14)	PAX3/FKHR	
	t(1;13)(p36;q14)	PAX7/FKHR	
Desmoplastic small round cell tumor	t(11;22)(p13;q12)	EWS/WT1	
Alveolar soft part sarcoma	t(X;17)	ASPL/TFE3	
Dermatofibrosarcoma protuberans, giant cell fibroblastoma	t(17;22)	COL1A1/PDGF	
Infantile fibrosarcoma, congenital mesoblastic nephroma	t(12;15)(p12;q25),+11,+17,+20	ETV6/NTRK3	
Myxoid chondrosarcoma	t(9;22)(q22;q12)	CHN/EWS	

T7.3 continued			
Disease	**Molecular defect**	**Genes**	**Notes**
Liposarcoma	t(12;16)(q13;p11)	FUS/CHOP	
Clear cell sarcoma	t(12;22)(q13;q12)	ATFI/EWS	
Synovial sarcoma	t(X;18)(p11;q11)	SSX1/SYT, SSX2/SYT	SSX1—biphasic, SSX2—monophasic
Oligodendroglioma	del(1p36), del(19q13.3)		
Meningioma	−22 or del(22q11.2)	NF2	Del 1p or 14q—anaplastic
Clear cell RCC	del(3p)	VHL	
Papillary RCC	Loss of Y, +7, +17, t(X;1)		
Translocation RCC	t(X;1)	PRCC/TFE3	
	t(X;17)	ASPSCR1/TFE3	

Prenatal Diagnosis

Samples

- Amniocentesis is usually performed in the second trimester but may be performed as early as 13-14 weeks. The procedure is relatively safe but carries a risk of fetal loss. The procedure appears to carry a risk of fetal loss that is about 1% over baseline. CVS and amniocentesis can provide essentially the same information—chromosomal status, enzyme levels, and mutation status—but measurement of AFP requires amniocentesis.

- Chorionic villus sampling (CVS) allows prenatal diagnosis in the first trimester. The risk of fetal death is roughly the same as or slightly greater than amniocentesis.

- Fetal blood sampling can be performed by percutaneous umbilical blood sampling (PUBS), also called cordocentesis. Fetal blood can be used in hematologic diagnosis as well, to evaluate hemolytic disease of the newborn (HDN) or clotting factor deficiencies. PUBS can be performed from about 18 weeks onward. The risk of fetal loss is somewhat high, possibly as high as 3%. For cytogenetic studies, it is necessary to ensure that fetal and not maternal blood has been sampled.

- Cystic hygromas are often quite large and associated with oligohydramnios; thus, it may occasionally be easier to obtain cystic hygromal fluid than amniotic fluid. Cystic hygromas are associated with 45 X (Turner syndrome) most commonly, but they are also associated with trisomy 21, trisomy 18, and several Mendelian disorders.

- Like cystic hygromas, bladders can become quite large in utero. This is often the result of a congenital genitourinary anomaly (posterior urethral valve) and is, like cystic hygroma, usually associated with oligohydramnios. This makes the urine a more approachable specimen for cytogenetic studies. The danger in this circumstance is the so-called oligohydramnio sequence, a group of anatomic lesions that result from oligohydramnios, most importantly including pulmonary hypoplasia and death. If there is intervention, in the simple form of a vesico-amniotic shunt, these consequences are avoidable. This may not be undertaken without evidence of normal cytogenetics, and urine can provide acceptable cytogenetic studies in >95% of cases.

- A fetal skin biopsy may be performed for the prenatal diagnosis of primary skin or systemic disorders. Some have advocated the use of skin biopsies to clarify questions of mosaicism.

Indications

- Diagnosis of cytogenetic disorders can be performed from any of these samples. The most common indication for prenatal cytogenetic studies is advanced maternal age. The incidence of trisomy 21, trisomy 13, trisomy 18, 47XXX, and 47XXY all increase with maternal age. Generally, prenatal diagnosis is offered to all women who will be over 35 at the time of delivery. The risk for a 35-year-old woman is 1 in 270 for bearing a Down syndrome fetus at the time of amniocentesis; note that the risk is actually somewhat lower for delivering a Down syndrome baby, since these pregnancies have a higher-than-normal risk of fetal demise.

For women under the age of 35, the results of prenatal maternal serum screening tests (triple screen or quad screen) are used to guide detection efforts. Women who have given birth to a child with a cytogenetic disorder are at increased risk for a second affected child—eg, the recurrence risk for trisomy 21 is about 1 percent. In some cases, one of the parents is found to harbor a balanced translocation, imparting a very high risk of affected offspring. Chromosome abnormalities account for approximately half of all spontaneous pregnancy losses, and recurrent spontaneous abortion is one possible indication for prenatal cytogenetic studies (or studies on an abortus). While classical cytogenetic studies may be performed, FISH panels are commonly available for the most likely anomalies: aneuploidies of 21, 13, 18, X and Y.

- Diagnosis of Mendelian disorders can usually be performed from one of these samples. Sometimes enzymatic assays are utilized to make these diagnoses (eg, metabolic disorders), sometimes hematologic parameters are used (hemoglobinopathies, clotting factor deficiencies), and at other times a metabolic by-product can be used (eg, 17α-hydroxyprogesterone in the 21-hydroxylase deficiency form of congenital adrenal hyperplasia). Increasingly, direct DNA methods are being applied, especially if the enzyme defect is not manifested in amniotic fluid (eg, phenylketonuria).

Methods

- Conventional cytogenetics can be used to diagnose structural chromosomal anomalies. There are several potential limitations, including failure of cells to grow, maternal contamination, and mosaicism. Sometimes chromosomal anomalies actually arise in cells during cell culture; often, this finding is present in only one of several clones and is easily recognized as pseudomosaicism. True mosaicism is extremely rare and the diagnosis depends upon finding the same anomaly in more than one clone. Sometimes PUBS must be performed to confirm this suspicion.

- FISH (molecular cytogenetics) can be performed using chromosome-specific probes for the most common anomalies (21, 13, 18, X, Y) to provide rapid turn around time.

- Direct DNA analysis (usually Southern blot or PCR) can be used to assay for known mutations which underlie Mendelian disorders.

- Linkage analysis (see prior discussion).

Molecular Basis and Molecular Diagnosis of Specific Nonneoplastic Diseases

Disorders of Coagulation and Thrombosis—see Chapter 5

Hematologic Disorders—see Chapter 4

Neurologic and Muscular Diseases

- Central neurodegenerative diseases (Alzheimer disease, Parkinson disease, and Huntington disease) can be sporadic or familial.

  □ Alzheimer disease is the most common cause of dementia in the United States, with an incidence of 5%-10% in persons over 70 and 15%-20% in persons over 85. About 25% of cases are familial, some with early onset and others with usual (late) onset.

  □ About 5% of all cases of Alzheimer disease have an early onset (<60 years), and about half of these are familial or so-called early-onset familial Alzheimer disease (EOFAD). EOFAD has been associated with mutations in three genes—PSEN1, APP, and PSEN2. PSEN1 is found at 14q24 and encodes presenilin 1. The APP gene is located on 21q21 and encodes amyloid β A4 protein. PSEN2 is on 1q and encodes presenilin 2.

  □ There is an association of usual (late) onset Alzheimer disease with the E4 allele at the APOE gene locus at 19q13.2; however, there is not 100% correlation.

  □ About 1% of all cases of Alzheimer disease are associated with Down syndrome. Essentially everybody with trisomy 21 (Down syndrome) develops Alzheimer disease if they live beyond the age of 40. This is believed to be due to over-expression of the APP gene on chromosome 21.

□ Skeletal muscle biopsy findings are somewhat characteristic, showing variable fiber size and scattered hyper-eosinophilic small rounded fibers. Immunohistochemical staining (or Western blot) for dystrophin is negative. A mosaic pattern of staining is described in female carriers.

□ Targeted mutation analysis with multiplex PCR is available for finding a limited number of exon deletions that are responsible for about 65% of DMD, BMD, and dystrophin-associated cardiomyopathy. About 5% of BMD and DMD are due to DNA duplications within the *DMD* gene, and these can be detected by Southern blot and quantitative PCR. Direct sequence analysis can be used to detect the 30%-35% of cases that are due to point mutations.

■ Other inherited skeletal muscle disorders

□ Inclusion body myositis (IBM) is unusual for a primary myopathic process in that it presents with distal muscle weakness. Many cases display autosomal recessive inheritance, and others occur as spontaneous new mutations. IBM classically presents in young adulthood with weakness of the anterior tibialis muscle, resulting in gait difficulties due to foot drop, progressing to hand weakness and thigh muscle weakness. Characteristically, the quadriceps muscle is spared. Likewise, in the upper extremity, the triceps is usually spared. The CPK is modestly elevated, 2-4× normal. The muscle biopsy shows characteristic rimmed vacuoles and filamentous inclusions. The vacuoles are rimmed by basophilic granular material on H&E-stained sections and purple-red granular material on trichrome-stained sections. Note that rimmed vacuoles are seen only in frozen muscle biopsy tissue. Tissue fixed in glutaraldehyde or formalin does not show vacuoles. With electron microscopy the vacuoles are found to contain whorls of membranous material. Inclusion body myositis is caused by mutations in the *GNE* gene, on 9p, that encodes the enzyme UDP-N-acetylglucosamine 2-epimerase/ N-acetylmannosamine kinase. In persons of Middle-Eastern (especially Iranian) Jewish descent, the disease is due almost exclusively to a single mutation for which targeted mutation analysis is clinically available.

□ Nemaline rod myopathy refers to a group of myopathies united by the finding of nemaline rods on muscle biopsy. Inheritance is autosomal dominant, autosomal recessive, or sporadic (simplex). The muscle biopsy shows rod-like inclusions (nemaline bodies) in the cytoplasm (sarcoplasm) of skeletal muscle fibers. The rods are easily visible in trichrome-stained sections but not seen in H&E-stained sections. The rods contain the same lattice-like structure as the Z-discs, appear to be in continuity with them, and are composed of Z-disc proteins such as a-actinin. Rods are not specific for nemaline rod myopathy. They may sometimes be seen in other inherited and acquired myopathies. Several gene mutations may give rise to nemaline rod myopathy, including *ACTA1* (1q42: actin), NEB (2q22: nebulin), *TNNT1* (19q: troponin T), and *TPM3* (1q: tropomyosin).

□ Myotonic muscular dystrophy (Steinert disease) is an autosomal recessive trinucleotide repeat disorder, unusual in that it affects both skeletal and smooth muscle as well as having effects upon the eyes, cardiac conduction system, endocrine system, and central nervous system. The other unusual feature is that skeletal muscle, while weak, is persistently contracted (myotonic). Smooth muscle effects are noted mainly in terms of bowel dysmotility. The serum CPK is mildly elevated. Muscle biopsy is nonspecific but markedly abnormal, with rows of internalized nuclei, ring fibers, and type I fiber atrophy. Molecular testing in the form of targeted mutation analysis is clinically available to determine the number of CTG repeats in the *DMPK* gene (19q). Unaffected persons have up to 35 CTG repeats, and premutation alleles have up to 49. Disease-associated alleles have >50 repeats. Generally speaking, the greater the number of repeats, the more severe the disease; for example, those with congenital-onset disease often have >2000 repeats.

□ Malignant hyperthermia (MH) may be triggered by inhalational anesthesia (halothane, isoflurane, etc.) and succinylcholine. There is a very high mortality (70%) without treatment. Since its recognition, the mortality has been reduced to about 5% with improved monitoring (particularly for hypercarbia during general anesthesia) and the use of dantrolene. The onset of MH is heralded by hypercarbia, a physiologic reaction to systemic lactic acidosis. Laboratory findings in MH include an increased PCO_2, metabolic (lactic) acidosis, hyperkalemia, increased creatine kinase, myoglobin in blood and urine, and abnormal coagulation tests. Untreated MH leads to rhabdomyolysis, hyperkalemia, myoglobinuria, DIC, congestive heart failure, bowel ischemia, and compartment syndrome. Treatment includes discontinuation of the anesthetic agent and administration of dantrolene sodium, with supportive measures for hyperthermia, acidosis, hyperkalemia, and myoglobinuria. Patients with known susceptibility to MH can be safely administered regional anesthesia (spinal, epidural, or nerve block) or general anesthesia with nontriggering agents (barbiturates, benzodiazepines, opioids, propofol, ketamine, nitrous oxide, and nondepolarizing neuromuscular blockers). Underlying MH is an abnormally uncontrolled release of calcium from the sarcoplasmic reticulum of skeletal muscle, resulting in muscle contraction, ATP consumption, and increased anaerobic metabolism. *The calcium channel—RYR1—located in the membrane of the sarcoplasmic reticulum is defective in MH,* displaying prolonged channel opening when exposed to triggering agents and inhibition of this effect by Dantrolene. There are two main tests for MH susceptibility: a muscle contracture test and a genetic test. The caffeine-halothane contracture test has a sensitivity of >95%, with a specificity of only about 80%. This test involves removing a segment of skeletal muscle and, while the specimen is still fresh, determining its contractile properties when exposed to halothane and caffeine. Given the high sensitivity, a negative contracture test goes a long way towards excluding MH susceptibility, but the test is not widely available and some have questioned its reproducibility. Genetic testing for *RYR1* mutations has recently become available. The difficulty is that more than 60 mutations in *RYR1* have been found to be associated with MH susceptibility, most of which are private (confined to a particular kindred). Tests currently available are capable of screening for 17 of the most common mutations, but this permits for a sensitivity of only about 25%.

Disorders Principally Cardiovascular

■ Brugada syndrome is associated with a high risk of ventricular arrhythmias. It may present with electrocardiographic (ECG) abnormalities, cardiac rhythm disturbances, or sudden cardiac death (sudden unexpected nocturnal death syndrome). The incidence is higher in males. While most cases are found in adulthood, the syndrome may present as sudden infant death syndrome (SIDS). The Brugada syndrome may be diagnosed either by characteristic ECG findings or by molecular testing. The *SCN5A* gene, on 3p21, encodes the α subunit of the sodium channel. Mutations in this gene are the cause of about ¼ of cases, the remaining cases having as yet undetermined causes. Direct sequencing analysis is clinically available for this gene. Interestingly, mutations in *SCN5A* are also responsible for one type of the long QT syndrome (LQT type 3—Romano-Ward Syndrome). It appears that Brugada syndrome is most prevalent in Southeast Asia, where the prevalence may reach 5 per 10,000 inhabitants, and where the term "sudden unexpected nocturnal death syndrome" originated.

■ Arrhythmogenic right ventricular dysplasia (ARVD, Uhl anomaly) is an autosomal dominant disorder characterized by cardiac conduction disturbances in association with the histologic findings of fatty and fibrous replacement of the right ventricular wall. Three genes have been associated with ARVD: *RYR2* (ARVD2), on 1q, encodes the cardiac ryanodine receptor protein; *DSP* (ARVD8), on 6p, encodes desmoplakin; and *PKP2* (ARVD9), also on 6p, encodes plakophilin-2, a component of the desmosome. The clinical diagnosis of ARVD often begins with echocardiogram, ECG and 24-hour Holter monitoring, followed by formal invasive electrophysiological (EP) testing and possible right ventricular endomyocardial biopsy. Molecular genetic testing is available in the form of direct sequence analysis of the *RYR2, DSP,* and *PKP2* genes.

7: Molecular Methods

Applications of Molecular Methods in Nonneoplastic Disease>Molecular Basis and Molecular Diagnosis of Specific Nonneoplastic Diseases

- Long QT syndromes

  □ The Romano-Ward syndrome is the most common form of inherited long QT syndrome, with autosomal dominant inheritance and an estimated prevalence of 1:7000. Affected persons are prone to develop ventricular tachyarrhythmias, including the type of ventricular tachycardia known as *torsade de pointes,* and sudden cardiac death. The diagnosis can be made with relative confidence when there is a prolonged QT interval, particularly when a familial autosomal dominant pattern can be established, in the *absence* of sensorineural hearing loss (to suggest Jervell and Lange-Nielsen syndrome). Molecular testing is clinically available for the known underlying genes.

  □ Jervell and Lange-Nielsen syndrome, in contrast, is autosomal recessive and associated with bilateral sensorineural hearing loss. JLNS classically presents as a child with *hearing loss* who experiences syncopal episodes during periods of stress, often resulting in sudden cardiac death at a young age. Two genes are known to be associated with JLNS: *KCNQ1* (90%) and *KCNE1* (10%). Direct sequence analysis is clinically available for these genes. The *KCNQ1* gene is found at 11p15.5 and encodes a voltage gated transmembrane potassium channel protein. The *KCNE1* gene is found at 21q22 and encodes a similar protein.

Disorders Principally Immunologic—see Chapter 6

Disorders Principally Gastrointestinal and Hepatic

- **Medium-chain acyl-coenzyme A dehydrogenase (MCAD) deficiency**

  □ When a child presents with hepatic failure and is found on biopsy (or autopsy) to have widespread microvesicular steatosis, the diagnosis of idiopathic Reye syndrome is suggested. However, cases previously classified as Reye syndrome are increasingly found to have underlying metabolic defects which account for the findings, including respiratory chain disorders, disorders of fatty acid oxidation (the most common being MCAD deficiency), and carnitine transport disorders.

□ Medium-chain acyl-coenzyme A dehydrogenase (MCAD) is responsible for the first step in mitochondrial oxidation of CoA esters of medium-chain fatty acids. This begins the enzymes involved in mitochondrial fatty acid β-oxidation, leading to ketogenesis, which is the major source of fuel during fasting periods, once hepatic glycogen stores are depleted.

□ Some patients with MCAD deficiency present in the neonatal period, and neonatal presentations appear to be more common in breast-fed babies. The largest group comes to clinical attention during post-neonatal infancy or early childhood as a result of hypoglycemia (*without ketosis*) in association with a period of fasting or increased metabolic demands (a transient viral infection, for example can produce both). In a typical clinical scenario, a previously healthy child presents with hypoketotic hypoglycemia, vomiting, lethargy, hepatomegaly and elevated liver enzymes. These episodes may be fatal. Some cases do not present until adulthood, at which time the manifestations may be cardiac. The prognosis is excellent once the diagnosis is established and frequent feedings are instituted to avoid any prolonged period of fasting; thus, MCAD deficiency appears to be an excellent candidate for neonatal screening.

□ Autopsies in patients who die of MCAD deficiency show primarily fatty infiltration (microvesicular fat), mainly within the liver and heart.

□ MCAD deficiency is most prevalent in Caucasians, especially those of Northern European descent. The estimated disease frequency is between 1 in 5000 and 1 in 15,000. The gene (carrier) frequency is between 1 in 50 and 1 in 100.

□ MCAD deficiency is caused by mutations in the *ACADM* gene on chromosome 1p. The K304E (985A to G) mutation is by far the most common mutation; however, this is present in only about half of cases. If molecular diagnosis is desired, then targeted mutation analysis for this gene is the first step. If this is negative, gene sequencing is the only good way to detect a mutation.

□ The screening test for MCAD deficiency is tandem mass spectrometry for detection of acylcarnitines in blood. This test is now being applied in newborn screening programs.

7: Molecular Methods

Applications of Molecular Methods in Nonneoplastic Disease>Molecular Basis and Molecular Diagnosis of Specific Nonneoplastic Diseases

■ Cystic fibrosis (CF)

□ The *CFTR* gene encodes the cystic fibrosis transmembrane regulator (CFTR), a transmembrane protein that serves as a regulated chloride channel. When mutations occur, the resulting epithelial ion channel abnormality results in multisystem disease affecting the upper and lower aerodigestive tract, hepatobiliary system, gastrointestinal tract, and male reproductive tract.

□ CF occurs in approximately 1/2000 live births in Caucasians and about 1/17,000 live births in African-Americans. CF is inherited as an autosomal recessive trait. Cystic fibrosis is the most common autosomal recessive disease affecting Caucasians, the gene frequency in whom is about 1:20.

□ Due to the variable clinical severity and manifestations, CF must be considered in the differential diagnosis of several clinical presentations T7.4. CF is a cause of chronic lung disease and pancreatic exocrine deficiency in children. It is also responsible for many cases of salt depletion, sinusitis, rectal prolapse, and pancreatitis. The pathologist should raise the possibility of CF whenever a nasal polyp is received from a child as a surgical specimen. CF may present as failure to thrive and occasionally as cirrhosis or other forms of hepatic dysfunction. Congenital bilateral absence of vas deferens (CBAVD) occurs in isolation, without multisystem disease, in some males. The patients present with azoospermia with nonpalpable vas deferens. Mutation analysis confirms the diagnosis.

□ Mutations in the *CFTR* gene, on 7q31.2, are the cause of CF. Over 1000 such mutations have been described. The presently recommended 23-mutation targeted mutation analysis panel is capable of detecting about 90% of cases overall; however, due to population differences, the detection rate is lower in Hispanics and African-Americans. Direct sequence analysis is capable of detecting >98% of mutations. The most common disease-causing mutation is δF508 (present in approximately 70% of affected individuals). The δF508 mutation lacks a phenylalanine (F) residue at position 508. The mutation results in a protein that, though functional, is rapidly degraded. About 5%-10% of *CFTR* mutations are due to premature truncation, and

these are particularly common in Ashkenazi Jews. The W1282X mutation, a truncating mutation, occurs in 60% of the Ashkenazi Jews with CF. The CF transmembrane regulator (CFTR) is expressed largely on the surface of epithelial cells of airways, the gastrointestinal tract, sweat glands, and genitourinary system.

□ The severity of lung disease cannot be predicted by genotype. This suggests other inherited or environmental contributions to disease progression. For example, the MPO activity within circulating neutrophils varies in CF patients, and the activity correlates with the FEV1/FVC.

□ The diagnosis of CF can be established in a patient with suggestive clinical features, with one of the following: molecular testing that confirms homozygosity or compound heterozygosity for *CFTR* gene mutations, two consecutive abnormal pilocarpine iontophoresis sweat chloride tests, or an abnormal transepithelial nasal potential difference (NPD) measurement.

□ Many states have implemented newborn screening for CF. The method commonly employed for this is an immunoreactive trypsinogen (IRT) assay, performed on blood spots. IRT levels are elevated in cystic fibrosis. This finding must be confirmed by

---

T7.4

Most Common Presentations of Cystic Fibrosis (in Order of Decreasing Frequency)

Recurrent pneumonia and/or bronchiectasis

Unexplained malnutrition or failure to thrive

Meconium ileus

Hyponatremia, especially with hypochloremia and metabolic alkalosis

Rectal prolapse

Unexplained chronic diarrhea

Refractory sinusitis or asthma

Nasal polyps in childhood

Chronic, recurrent, pancreatitis

Hepatic disease (focal biliary obstruction)

Male infertility

another modality. The utility of immunoreactive trypsinogen declines after the first several months of life, and it appears to be less sensitive in newborns with a meconium ileus. The test should not be used after about 2 months of age.

☐ The sweat test uses pilocarpine iontophoresis. Sweat is collected and analyzed for chloride content. Positive results should be confirmed with a repeat test, and negative tests should be repeated if suspicion is high. More than 60 mEq/L of chloride in sweat is considered diagnostic of CF in the appropriate setting. Values between 40 and 60 mEq/L are suggestive of CF. False positive tests may be produced by: adrenal insufficiency, ectodermal dysplasia, nephrogenic diabetes insipidus, glucose-6-phosphatase deficiency, hypothyroidism, hypoparathyroidism, mucopolysaccharidoses, fucosidosis, and malnutrition.

☐ Increased potential (voltage) differences across nasal epithelium has been used to confirm the diagnosis in patients with borderline sweat tests.

☐ Measurement of immunoreactive serum trypsinogen can be used to distinguish CF from other causes of pancreatitis. The test is unreliable before the age of 7 years.

☐ Pulmonary infection in childhood that is due to either *S aureus, B cepacia* or *P aeruginosa* is strong presumptive evidence of CF. In particular, mucoid forms of *Pseudomonas* are considered diagnostic of CF. **T7.5**

■ Hereditary hemorrhagic telangiectasia (Osler-Weber-Rendu disease) is an autosomal dominant condition characterized by recurrent bleeding due to arteriovenous malformations (AVMs). Common presentations include recurrent spontaneous nose bleeds (usually presenting in the second decade) numerous mucocutaneous telangiectasias (arising in the 3rd decade), and GI bleeds (4th to 5th decade). AVMs may be found in the brain, lung, or liver. Osler-Weber-Rendu may be due to mutations in either the *ENG* gene or the *ACVRL1* gene. *ENG* is found at 9q34 and encodes endoglin. *ACVRL1* is found at 12q and encodes a serine/threonine protein kinase receptor. About 80% of all disease-causing mutations can be detected by direct sequence analysis, with another 10% detected by duplication/deletion analysis.

■ **Hereditary hemochromatosis (HH)**

☐ HH is an autosomal recessive disease and the most common inherited genetic defect in persons of northern European ancestry. The prevalence is approximately 1:200-1:300 in the United States. There is a lower prevalence among American Hispanics (0.27 per 1000), African-Americans (0.14 per 1000), and Asian-Americans (<0.001 per 1000).

☐ The vast majority of cases are due to one of two point mutations of the *HFE* gene on chromosome 6p21.3. Most (60-90%) affected individuals are homozygous for the C282Y (845A) mutation, and the remaining cases are due to compound heterozygosity for C282Y and the H63D (187G) mutation. There is a less common group of non-HFE-related cases **T7.6**. Hemochromatosis displays overall low

T7.5
Most Common *CFTR* Gene Mutations

Mutation	Frequency in Affected Persons
δF508	66.0%
G542X	2.4%
G551D	1.6%
N1303K	1.3%
W1282X	1.2%
R553X	0.7%

T7.6
Most Common Hemochromatosis Gene Mutations

Gene	Location	Disease
HFE (most common variants: C282Y, H63D, S65C)	6p21.3	Hereditary hemochromatosis
HFE2 (hemojuvlin)	1q21	Juvenile hemochromatosis A
HAMP (hepcidin)	19q13	Juvenile hemochromatosis B
TFR2 (transferrin receptor)	7q22	Hemochromatosis type 3
FTH1 (ferritin heavy chain)	11q13	Familial iron overload

7: Molecular Methods

Applications of Molecular Methods in Nonneoplastic Disease>Molecular Basis and Molecular Diagnosis of Specific Nonneoplastic Diseases

penetrance. Disease likelihood is greatest for those homozygous for C282Y, but even in these individuals the development of clinically significant hemochromatosis (penetrance) is relatively low. Slightly less severe but still capable of fully manifesting hemochromatosis are compound heterozygotes for C282Y/H63D. Homozygotes for H63D are not commonly affected. Simple heterozygotes for either C282Y or H63D are generally healthy, with the following caveats: many have abnormal iron studies reflecting some degree of iron overload; and there is a greater likelihood of progression in other forms of hepatic injury, such as steatohepatitis. Women are half as likely as men to develop complications of hemochromatosis.

☐ Screening for HH involves serum iron studies, especially iron, transferrin, and ferritin. A transferrin saturation ≥ 45% has a sensitivity of >95%. The serum iron is elevated, and the ferritin is elevated. The liver biopsy displays increased hepatocellular iron histologically, particularly when stained with Prussian blue, with the greatest deposition in periportal hepatocytes. Semi-quantitative iron grading (0-4+ scale) correlates extremely well with hepatic iron quantitation, especially at the extremes (0-1+ and 4+). Hepatic iron can be measured quantitatively and expressed either as the hepatic iron concentration (micromoles of iron per gram of dry liver weight) or as the hepatic iron index (hepatic iron concentration divided by age in years). A normal hepatic iron index is < 1.1. Definitive diagnosis requires genetic testing which is now widely available.

☐ Iron accumulation causes damage to the liver (usually pauci-inflammatory fibrosis progressing to cirrhosis), pancreas (fibrosis with impairment of islet cell function leading to diabetes), skin (bronzing secondary to increased melanin), heart (dilated or restrictive cardiomyopathy), and pituitary gland (hypogonadotrophic hypogonadism leading to infertility—not much direct impact on the gonads). It has been suggested that increased iron may lead to oxidative damage to DNA and an increased cancer risk. Case-control studies have reported associations between *HFE* mutations and several cancers.

■ **Wilson disease** (hepatolenticular degeneration)

☐ Wilson disease is an autosomal recessive disorder which occurs with a frequency of about 1 in 30,000. It is caused by a mutation of the *ATP7B* gene on chromosome 13 involved in copper transport.

☐ Wilson disease may present in one of three ways: liver disease, neuropsychiatric disease, or hemolysis. WD usually presents in childhood. Typical patients are in adolescence or early adulthood at the time of presentation. It is important to think of the possibility of Wilson disease when examining a liver biopsy from somebody in this age range. Hepatitis due to Wilson disease often presents acutely with jaundice and abdominal pain, but it may present with chronic hepatitis. Sometimes this is discovered only incidentally through abnormal liver function tests. Often coincident with hepatitis is a nonimmune *hemolytic anemia*. Kayser-Fleischer rings often develop in association with neurologic disease. The neurologic manifestations are protean and may include movement disorders (dysarthria, tremors, rigidity, bradykinesia, and abnormal gait) and psychosis.

☐ The liver biopsy shows glycogenated nuclei, steatosis, and inflammation that may mimic the pattern of chronic viral hepatitis. Fibrosis ultimately leads to cirrhosis. Unlike liver iron stains, hepatic copper stains are somewhat unreliable in comparison with formal hepatic copper quantitation (which is considered the gold standard). Furthermore, the finding of stainable copper is highly nonspecific and may be seen in steatohepatitis and cholestasis.

☐ The plasma ceruloplasmin may serve as a screening test. Low levels are found in Wilson disease, but they may also be found in malnutrition, protein loss, liver disease from other causes. Ceruloplasmin may be falsely normal in pregnancy, estrogen therapy, acute phase reactions. In fully established Wilson disease, the serum copper is elevated; however, at various stages, the copper may be low, normal, or high. The urinary copper excretion is usually elevated as is the hepatic copper which can be quantified by liver biopsy.

7: Molecular Methods

Applications of Molecular Methods in Nonneoplastic Disease>Molecular Basis and Molecular Diagnosis of Specific Nonneoplastic Diseases

■ Alpha 1 antitrypsin (AAT) deficiency

□ AAT is an autosomal recessive disease. Most normal people are homozygous for the M allele of the *SER-PINA1* (PI) gene on chromosome 14q31-32.3 (denoted genotype PiMM). About 10% of the normal Caucasian population is heterozygous for M and some other allele, of which there are about 75. Most people with clinical AAT deficiency are homozygous for the Z allele (PiZZ). The Z allele has a frequency in the US population of about 1%-2%. In Europe, the allele frequency is highest in the North (5% in Scandinavians) and lowest in the South (1% of Italians). The second most common disease-associated allele, S, has the opposite distribution: 10% in Southern Europe, 5% in the north **T7.7**.

□ AAT deficiency presents as neonatal hepatitis in a significant portion of patients. Others are spared this complication and may present later with early-onset emphysema, cirrhosis, hepatocellular carcinoma, or panniculitis. There appears to be an increased incidence of Wegener granulomatosis and other vasculitides. In contrast to usual-type emphysema which is centro-acinar and upper lobe-predominant, AAT-associated emphysema has panacinar histopathology and basilar predominance.

□ The alleles are named according to the electrophoretic mobility of the encoded protein; fastest variants are A, slowest Z. Many cases of AAT deficiency are picked up incidentally on SPEP, when a quantitative decrease in the α1 region is measured. The α1 band looks abnormal as well, losing its normally peaked morphology and appearing flattened or blunted. Occasionally, a heterozygote is noted on electrophoresis due to the presence of two peaks; many of these have no quantitative deficiency of AAT.

■ Alagille syndrome

□ Alagille syndrome (arteriohepatic dysplasia, syndromic paucity of bile ducts) is most likely to come to the attention of a pathologist when a liver biopsy, performed for evaluation of cholestasis, shows a *noninflammatory paucity of interlobular bile ducts* (increased portal tract:bile duct ratio). The number of bile ducts is normal in infants with Alagille syndrome and progressively diminishes thereafter (hence the alternate designation—the disappearing bile duct syndrome). The clinical manifestations include autosomal dominant inheritance (although half are new mutations), cholestasis, cardiac defects (pulmonary stenosis), posterior embryotoxon of the eye, a characteristic form of dysmorphic facial features, and butterfly vertebrae. The prevalence of Alagille syndrome has been estimated to be 1 in 70,000 live births

□ Alagille syndrome is nearly always due to a mutation in the *JAG1* gene, located on 20p12. About half of these are inherited mutations and half de novo. A small percentage of patients with this syndrome have instead a mutation in the *NOTCH2* gene. *JAG1* encodes a protein that serves as a cell-surface ligand for Notch transmembrane receptors. Interestingly, *NOTCH1* mutations (translocations)

T7.7
Alleles Related to AAT Deficiency

Genotype	Prevalence	α-1 antitrypsin (mmol/L)	α-1 antitrypsin (mg/dL)	Risk of emphysema
MM	90%	20-53	150-350	Not increased
MS	6%	18-52	125-300	Not increased
MZ	5%	15-33	100-200	Not increased
SS	<1%	15-33	100-200	Not increased
SZ	<1%	8-16	75-120	High
ZZ	<1%	2-7	20-50	Very high

are found in T-ALLs, and *NOTCH3* mutations cause cerebral autosomal dominant arteriopathy with subcortical infarcts and leukoencephalopathy (CADASIL). While the diagnosis of Alagille syndrome is based largely upon clinical findings, mutations can be found in the *JAG1* gene in the vast majority of cases by direct gene sequencing. A FISH assay for microdeletions in *JAG1* detects <10% of cases.

■ **Hirschsprung disease**

□ Hirschsprung disease is aganglionosis of a segment of the colon that always includes the distal rectum and a variable length proximal to and contiguous with the rectum. Most cases are restricted to the rectosigmoid and considered short-segment Hirschsprung disease. In about 15%, the aganglionosis extends proximal to the sigmoid (long-segment Hirschsprung disease). Rare cases (<5%) involve the entire colon (total colonic aganglionosis). Short-segment disease is four times more common in males than in females; however, the numbers are essentially equal for long-segment Hirschsprung disease.

□ Hirschsprung disease usually presents as failure to pass meconium (meconium ileus) within the first 48 hours of neonatal life. Those with very short affected segments may be capable of passing meconium, and will present somewhat later with constipation or other evidence of altered bowel motility. Of course, other common causes of meconium ileus must be considered, including cystic fibrosis, intestinal atresia, imperforate anus, intestinal neuronal dysplasia, et cetera. The diagnosis is usually made histologically by finding an absence of ganglion cells, with associated axonal hypertrophy, in a biopsy taken >2 cm from the dentate line.

□ A structural chromosomal abnormality is present in about 12% of individuals with Hirschsprung disease, most commonly trisomy 21. This is peculiar, since the genes known to cause Hirschsprung disease are not found on 21. These include the *RET* gene (10q11.2), *GDNF* gene (5p), *EDNRB* gene (13q), and *EDN3* gene (20q). In addition, the Hirschsprung phenotype is often a component of another syndrome: NF1, MEN2A, Waardenburg syndrome, congenital central hypoventilation (Haddad) syndrome, familial dysautonomia (Riley-Day) syndrome, and Smith-Lemli-Opitz syndrome.

Disorders Principally Endocrine

■ **Congenital adrenal hyperplasia**

□ Congenital adrenal hyperplasia (CAH) is caused by a group of autosomal recessive enzyme defects, each representing one of the enzymes involved in the biosynthesis of cortisol from cholesterol. The two most commonly implicated enzymes are 21-hydroxylase and 11-hydroxylase (others are 20,22-hydroxylase, 3-hydroxysteroid-dehydrogenase, and 17-hydroxylase). The estimated incidence ranges from 1 in 10,000 to 1 in 25,000.

□ *21-hydroxylase deficiency* is responsible for about 90% of cases. The range of clinical severity can best be understood based upon three principles. First, mild enzyme deficiency affects mainly the quantity of cortisol, while severe deficiency impairs both cortisol and mineralocorticoid (aldosterone) production. Only severe enzyme deficiencies result in the salt-wasting form of disease. Second, the most profound consequences of hypocortisolism for the developing fetus is not the paucity of cortisol itself but rather the very high ACTH that drives the build-up of androgens (and other cortisol precursors such as 17-hydroxyprogesterone). Third, males and females have differing reactions to androgen. Thus, there are several potential presentations: a female who is virilized at birth; a female who becomes virilized during infancy or shortly thereafter; a female with precocious puberty; a male with pseudoprecocious puberty (the appearance of puberty in the external genitalia); a male or female infant with salt-losing crisis (similar to an Addisonian crisis).

□ 17-hydroxyprogesterone (17-OHP) is elevated in all forms of CAH; this forms the basis for diagnosis in many cases. 17-OHP can be measured by immunoassay which can be performed on dried blood spots for neonatal screening. Since some neonates may present in the first days of life with an adrenal insufficiency crisis, early knowledge of the diagnosis can be extremely beneficial. While an elevated serum 17-OHP is indicative of 21-hydroxylase deficiency, a concomitant elevation in plasma renin activity (PRA) is consistent with the salt-wasting form of the disease.

□ Molecular testing of the *CYP21A2* (6p21) gene is usually confirmatory. Directed mutation analysis for a set of common mutations can detect >90% of abnormal alleles. Direct sequence analysis, to detect unusual mutations, is also clinically available.

■ **Androgen insensitivity syndrome** (testicular feminization)

□ Androgen insensitivity syndrome (AIS) often presents at birth in genotypic male (XY) infants with evidence of feminization of the external genitalia. Milder forms of insensitivity may present as abnormal secondary sexual development at puberty or simply as infertility. Often a mass is detected in the inguinal canal, representing undescended testes.

□ AIS is due to mutations in the *AR* (androgen receptor) gene on Xq11-12. Direct sequence analysis detects nearly all cases.

Disorders Principally Renal

■ **Inherited nephritic syndromes** (collagen IV-related nephropathies).

□ There is a spectrum of disease associated with derangements in collagen type IV, ranging from Alport syndrome to thin basement membrane disease.

□ Alport syndrome may be XLR (80%), AR (15%), or AD (5%). In the most common X-linked recessive form, males manifest the full syndrome, and female carriers experience largely asymptomatic hematuria. The Alport syndrome manifests as glomerulonephritis progressing to end-stage renal disease, sensorineural hearing loss, and ocular lesions (corneal, lens, and macular lesions). The simplest way of making the diagnosis is through examination of skin or renal biopsies. Immunohistochemical staining of skin for the α5 chain of type IV collagen [α5(IV)] shows a complete absence of staining in the epidermal basement membrane; female carriers for XLR Alport show discontinuous staining for α5(IV). Immunohistochemical staining of kidney for the α3, α4, and α5 chains of type IV collagen shows complete absence of staining in glomerular and tubular basement membranes. Neither of these tests are perfect, with normal staining seen in up to 20%

of cases. Electron microscopy shows a disrupted and abnormally inhomogeneous lamina densa that entraps rounded electron-dense bodies. EM may show scalloping of the epithelial aspect of the glomerular basement membrane.

□ Thin basement membrane disease shows normal staining for α3, α4, and α5 chains. Electron microscopy displays the diffuse uniform thinning of glomerular basement membranes. It manifests as persistent hematuria, without proteinuria or progression to renal failure.

□ Three genes—*COL4A3, COL4A4,* and *COL4A5*—have been associated with the collagen IV-related nephropathies. XLR Alport syndrome is due to mutations in *COL4A5*, on Xq22.3, which encodes the α5 chain of type IV collagen. AR and AD cases are due to mutations in *COL4A3* and *COL4A4,* both on 2q36-q37, encoding the α3 and α4 chains of type IV collage, respectively. Direct sequence analysis is available for these genes.

□ Alport syndrome with diffuse leiomyomatosis is an association for which several reports now exist. This appears to result from large deletions that span the adjacent *COL4A5* and *COL4A6* genes.

■ **Inherited polycystic kidney diseases**

□ In autosomal recessive polycystic kidney disease (ARPKD), also called infantile polycystic kidney disease, oligohydramnios is often the first manifestation. Echogenic cysts can be detected on prenatal ultrasound. Hypertension and respiratory distress are often present at birth, the latter a result of pulmonary hypoplasia as part of the oligohydramnios sequence. At birth, the kidneys are enlarged (palpable) by radially oriented 'cysts' composed of ectatic collecting ducts, but they retain their reniform shape. The large rounded macrocysts of ADPKD are not seen. More than half progress to end-stage renal disease, usually within the first decade of life. Hepatic involvement is present to some degree in nearly all cases, but this becomes problematic only in those who survive into adulthood. The morphologic features are those of typical biliary plate malformations: ectatic portal bile ducts, circumferential proliferation of ductules, and periportal fibrosis. Mutations in the *PKHD1* gene (6p) are responsible for ARPKD.

☐ Glomerulocystic kidney disease (GCKD) is a rare disorder that also presents in the neonatal period with large palpable flank masses. It may be very difficult to distinguish, clinically and radiographically, from ARPKD; however, it appears to be related genotypically more to ADPKD. Microscopic examination shows dilation of Bowman capsule and renal dysplasia.

☐ Cystic renal dysplasia (multicystic dysplastic kidney) is a non-Mendelian disorder that arises sporadically and may result from in utero obstruction. Kidneys are distinctly nonreniform in shape and contain a mixture of cartilage, cystic structures, and mesenchymal cells. Sometimes the disease affects only a segment of the kidney, but usually the entire kidney is involved, and occasionally it is bilateral. This is a fairly common cause of flank masses in infants.

☐ Nephronophthisis (juvenile nephronophthisis, medullary sponge kidney, medullary cystic kidney disease) is an autosomal recessive condition in which cysts arise at the corticomedullary junction. Various genotypic forms of the disease exist, leading to phenotypes that differ mainly in age at presentation. The NPHP1 gene, on 2q, is mutated in juvenile-onset forms of the disease. These present in children as a renal tubular defect (Fanconi syndrome, impaired renal concentrating capacity, polyuria, polydipsia), sometimes in association with extra-renal anomalies (hepatic fibrosis, retinal degeneration). The NPHP2 and NPHP3 genes are mutated in adult-onset disease. Adult onset cases have a similar presentation, without the extrarenal features.

☐ Autosomal dominant polycystic kidney disease (ADPKD), also called adult polycystic kidney disease, is the most common of the inherited polycystic disorders, with an estimated prevalence at birth of 1 in 500. Penetrance is essentially 100%, with most cases presenting in the 4th-5th decades. Hypertension is ubiquitous in this condition, resulting from a reduction in renal blood flow, and may be the initial manifestation. Pre-symptomatically, the kidneys display an impaired concentrating capacity (isosthenuria). Flank pain is a common complaint, and sorting out the specific cause can be challenging: cyst hemorrhage, cyst infection, intracystic tumor, and renal stones are in the differ-

ential. The prevalence of renal stones in ADPKD is 20%, usually in the form of calcium oxalate or urate. About half have end-stage renal disease by the age of 60. In the kidneys, cysts arise from multiple parts of the nephron, are cortical and medullary, and highly variable in size. Grossly, the kidneys are enlarged, with at least vague retention of the basic reniform shape. There has been debate regarding an increased susceptibility to renal cell carcinoma (the only cystic disease unequivocally associated with an increased risk is that associated with long-term dialysis), but when tumors occur they occur at younger-than-usual age, are often multicentric or bilateral, and are very hard to detect. The liver is involved in 75% of cases (polycystic liver disease). Pancreatic cysts are identified in about 10%, intracranial berry aneurysms in 10%-20%, and mitral valve prolapse in up to 25%. Other associations are seminal vesicle cysts, arachnoid cysts, and dilation of the aortic root. In 85% of those with ADPKD, the cause is a mutation in PKD1 (16p13). PKD1 is located immediately adjacent to the TSC2 gene of tuberous sclerosis, and 'contiguous gene' syndromes with overlapping features of ADPKD and TS have been reported. The remaining 15% have mutations in PKD2 (4q). PKD1 and 2 encode polycystins 1 and 2, respectively. Direct sequence analysis is clinically available for these genes. Usually the diagnosis can be confirmed with imaging studies alone, for which specific criteria exist; however, these findings are not fully penetrant until about the age of 30, so molecular testing may be needed if earlier diagnosis is desired. ADPKD is relatively common,

Metabolic Diseases

■ Metabolic diseases are usually enzyme disorders that are recessively inherited. Fabry, Lesch-Nyhan, and Hunter diseases are X-linked recessive (XLR).

■ All states currently require newborn screening for metabolic disorders; although the details differ. All states currently require screening for phenylketonuria (PKU) and congenital hypothyroidism. Nearly all states require testing for galactosemia and sickle cell disease. Many mandate testing for biotinidase deficiency, homocystinuria, maple syrup urine disease, cystic fibrosis, and/or congenital adrenal hyperplasia. Testing is typically performed by elution of dried blood spots from heel sticks placed upon filter paper (Guthrie) cards.

7: Molecular Methods

Applications of Molecular Methods in Nonneoplastic Disease>Molecular Basis and Molecular Diagnosis of Specific Nonneoplastic Diseases

- When not detected through neonatal screening, a metabolic disease should be considered in the differential diagnosis of an infant or child manifesting nonspecific clinical features, especially when they include such things as lethargy, dehydration, acidosis, vomiting, ammonemia, hypoglycemia, seizures, dysmorphic features and/or hepatosplenomegaly.
Many appear normal at birth.

- **Phenylketonuria** (PKU) is an extremely common genetic abnormality, with a gene frequency of 1 in 50 and disease prevalence of 1 in 15,000 live births. It is caused by an autosomal recessive deficiency of the enzyme phenylalanine hydroxylase, which is normally responsible for the conversion of phenylalanine to tyrosine. When deficient individuals ingest protein (or the artificial sweetener asparatame), phenylalanine accumulates in the blood, spilling over into the urine and cerebrospinal fluid. This results in progressive mental retardation, seizures, and an acid odor. However, if detected and treated (diet restriction), affected individuals are entirely normal. While it appears that diet control may not be very necessary after childhood, it is crucial during pregnancy. PKU in pregnant women can lead to miscarriage, intrauterine growth retardation, mental retardation, and congenital heart defects even though the fetus has normal phenylalanine hydroxylase activity.

- **Galactosemia** is an autosomal recessive disorder with an incidence of about 1 in 60,000. The most common enzyme responsible for galactosemia is galactose-1-phosphate uridyl transferase (GALT). Others are galactokinase and ridine-diphosphategalactose-4-epimerase. Affected infants cannot metabolize galactose (found in breast milk, standard formula, and cow milk), and in the first two weeks of life begin to display vomiting and elevated liver function tests. They are at particular risk for neonatal *E. coli* sepsis. Eventually they develop chronic liver disease, mental retardation, cataracts, and failure to thrive. A milk-free diet is the recommended treatment.

- **Biotinidase deficiency** results in a multi-enzyme defect, as biotinidase is an enzyme that liberates the enzyme cofactor biotin from its bound form. This autosomal recessive disorder has a prevalence of about 1 in 60,000 births. Symptoms begin to develop around 3-6 months of age

- **Tay-Sachs disease** (GM2 gangliosidosis) is an autosomal recessive disorder that results from deficiency of hexosaminidase A. A biochemical assay is available for this enzyme. For Ashkenazi Jewish individuals, DNA analysis for Tay-Sachs is also available. The deficiency results in lysosomal accumulation of a glycosphingolipid (GM2 ganglioside), leading to a progressive neurodegenerative disease and death, usually by the age of four years. Characteristic features of Tay-Sachs disease emerge in the first year of life and include weakness, motor apraxia, decreased attentiveness, increased startle response, and a cherry-red spot on the macula (may also be seen in GM1 gangliosidosis, galactosialidosis, Niemann-Pick disease, Sandhoff disease, and Gaucher). The liver and spleen have normal size. The affected gene is the *HEXA* gene on 15q. Targeted mutation analysis is clinically available, which screens for the most common disease-causing alleles. While the sensitivity of this assay is quite high in the Ashkenazi Jewish population, it is fairly low in the non-Jewish population.

- **Zellweger syndrome** is the prototype peroxisomal disorder. Traditionally, three phenotypes have been distinguished: classic Zellweger syndrome, neonatal adrenoleukodystrophy, and infantile Refsum disease. Classic Zellweger syndrome describes the most severe phenotype and is characterized by neonatal hypotonia, poor feeding, seizures, hepatic dysfunction, liver cysts, characteristic facial dysmorphism (flattened facies, abnormally large anterior fontanelle, broad nasal bridge), and chondrodysplasia punctata. When the presentation is that of neonatal adrenoleukodystrophy or Refsum disease, manifestations may develop later in such ways as developmental delays or hearing loss. Biochemical assays are available to determine plasma levels of very long chain fatty acids (VLCFA). While numerous genes have been implicated, *PEX1* mutations are responsible for about 70% of cases. *PEX1* is located at 7q21 and encodes peroxisome biogenesis factor 1 **T7.8**.

- **Gaucher disease** (glucocerebrosidase deficiency, glucosylceramidase deficiency) manifests in three different syndromes. Type 1 (nonneuronopathic), the most common type, is notable for the absence of central nervous system involvement. It presents with bone involvement, hepatosplenomegaly, and blood cytopenias. Types 2 and 3 are characterized by neurologic disease, with type 2 presenting early (<2 years) and progressing rapidly and type 3 presenting somewhat later and progressing quite slowly. Mutations in the

GBA gene, on 1q, that encodes glucosylceramidase, underlie all forms of Gaucher disease. A biochemical assay is available for assessing the activity of glucosylceramidase. Targeted mutation analysis is clinically available for the more common *GBA* mutations. These detect about 90% of cases in the Ashkenazi Jewish population and about 60% in the non-Jewish population. Direct sequence analysis is also clinically available.

■ Organic adidemias and urea cycle disorders **T7.9** are a group of autosomal recessive disorders that share a tendency to produce hyperammonemia.

   □ Ammonia is produced normally within hepatocytes from the catabolism of amino acids through the urea cycle. Ammonia is normally combined with aspartate to form the less toxic urea. Common causes of hyperammonemia in children include urea cycle disorders, organic acidemias, and hepatic dysfunction (which may itself be caused by other metabolic diseases). At high concentrations, ammonia is a neurotoxin, capable of producing clinical manifestations including lethargy, vomiting, asterixis, coma, and death.

   □ Organic acidemias are autosomal recessive disorders causing an abnormal urinary excretion of non-amino acid organic acids. Most are due to a defective enzyme in the pathway for amino acid catabolism. Affected individuals are normal at birth, but

(in most cases) shortly thereafter develop vomiting, poor feeding, and progressive neurologic deterioration. In other cases, the disease may present later—still usually in childhood—with neurologic dysfunction, Reye syndrome, or recurrent ketoacidosis. Laboratory findings usually include metabolic acidosis with increased anion gap (due to unmeasured organic acid), ketosis (due to β-hydroxybutyrate and acetoacetate), hyperammonemia, hypoglycemia, neutropenia, and abnormal LFTs. A urine organic acid analysis (GC/MS) will disclose the abnormal presence of specific organic acids, as will plasma amino acid analysis. Biochemical assays are also available for the activity of specific enzymes. Organic aciduria may also be seen in biotinidase deficiency, MCAD deficiency, mevalonic aciduria, and mitochondrial diseases.

   □ In urea cycle disorders, newborns with a complete deficiency appear initially normal but soon develop lethargy, anorexia, vomiting, seizures, and coma. In milder urea cycle enzyme deficiencies, symptoms may arise only when there is an illness or other stress. In such instances, an elevated plasma ammonia concentration, with a normal anion gap and normal serum glucose, is suggestive of a urea cycle enzyme deficiency. Protein catabolism results in the generation of ammonia (NH_4), a by-product with which the urea cycle is uniquely capable of dispensing. Deficiency of urea cycle enzymes, particularly those active early in the cycle—Carbamyl phosphate synthetase I (CPSI), Ornithine transcarbamylase (OTC), Argininosuccinic acid synthetase (ASS), Argininosuccinic acid lyase (ASL), Arginase (ARG), N-acetyl glutamate synthetase (NAGS)—results in the accumulation of ammonia. A measurement of plasma amino acids can help to support the diagnosis of a urea cycle disorder; however, definitive diagnosis depends upon a measurement of enzyme activity. Presently, molecular testing is only available for OTC deficiency.

T7.8
Organic Acidemias

Disease	Notes
Maple syrup urine disease (MSUD), branched-chain ketoacid dehydrogenase deficiency	Accumulation of branched-chain amino acids; Maple syrup odor
Propionic acidemia, propionyl CoA carboxylase deficiency	Neutropenia
Methylmalonic acidemia (MMA), methylmalonyl CoA mutase deficiency	Neutropenia
Isovaleric acidemia	Sweaty feet odor
3-methylcrotony-l-CoA carboxylase deficiency	Hypoglycemia
3-hydroxy-3-methylglutaryl-CoA (HMG-CoA) lyase deficiency	Reye syndrome, hypoglycemia
Ketothiolase deficiency	Hypoglycemia
Glutaricacidemia type I	Basal ganglia injury with movement disorder
Multiple carboxylase deficiency	

T 7.9
Urea Cycle Disorders

Carbamyl phosphate synthetase deficiency

Ornithine transcarbamylase (OTC) deficiency

Arginosuccinic acid synthetase deficiency

Arginsocuccinase deficiency

Arginase deficiency

T7.10
Inherited Metabolic Disorders

	Disease	Genetics/Enzyme	Accumulation	Comments	
Sphingolipidoses	Gaucher	AR (1q21) glucocerebrosi-dase	Glucocerebrosides in macrophages, marrow, spleen, liver, neurons (types II/III only)	Type I: most common (80%), nonneuronopathic, Ashkenazi Jews	Affected individuals manifest HSM, pancytopenias, and bone deformity (Ehrlenmeyer flask deformity). Types II/III: neurologic manifestations
				Type II: neuronopathic, lethal in infancy	
				Type III: neuronopathic, intermediate severity	
	Niemann-Pick	AR sphingomyelinase	Sphingomyelin in macrophages, marrow, liver, spleen, lungs, CNS	Type A: most common, neuronopathic	
				EM: myelin-like zebra bodies	
				Vacuolated lymphocytes in peripheral blood.	
	Fabry	XLR α-galactosidase (acid maltase)	Glycolipids in endothelium, smooth musicle, myocardium, ganglia, macrophages	Angiokeratomas	
				Renal dysfunction	
				EM: whorled inclusions	
	Tay-Sachs	AR (chromosome 15) hexosaminidase A	GM$_2$ gangliosides in neurons, retina, liver, spleen	Affected are normal at birth, develop neurologic symptoms by 6 months	
				Macular cherry-red spot	
				Vacuolated lymphocytes in peripheral blood	
				EM: whorled inclusions	
Muco-polysaccharidoses	Hurler	AR α-L-iduronidase	Mucopolysaccharides (dermatan, heparan, keratan, or chrondroitin sulfate) in marrow, blood vessels, spleen, liver, brain, heart valves, urine	Death ≤ 10 years, usually due to involvement of cardiac valves.	
				Atherosclerotic vascular lesions	
	Hunter	XLR iduronidase-2-sulfatase		Alder-Reilly anomaly in peripheral blood	
				EM: myelin-like zebra bodies	
Amino Acid Disorders	Alkoptonuria	AR homogentisic oxidase	Homogentisic acid in connective tissues (cartilage), urine, heart	Severe degenerative joint disease	
				Cardiac failure	
				Black urine	
	PKU	AR phenylalanine hydroxylase	Phenylalanine in blood, brain	Severe mental retardation and seizures	
				'Mousy' odor	
				Screening test: a drop of blood is placed on filter paper. Confirmatory test: plasma is placed in a green-top tube. Guthrie test: bacterial inhibition test	
	Tyrosinemia	AR		Very high incidence in Quebec	
				Very high risk for hepatocellular carcinoma	
	Cystinosis	AR defective renal tubular epithelial membrane protein	Cystine in blood & urine	Fanconi renal syndrome & renal failure	
				Renal calculi due to cystine crystals	
				Defective transmembrane protein is the cellular transmembrane transporter for cystine	
	Cystinuria	AR defective renal tubular epithelial membrane protein	Cystine, ornithine, lysine, and arginine in urine	Relatively benign clinically except for renal calculi due to cystine crystals	
				The defective renal tubular protein is the transmembrane transporter for cystine, ornithine, lysine, and arginine.	
	Homocystinuria	AR defective cystathionine synthetase	Homocysteine and methionine	Marfanoid changes (lens dislocation and body habitus), livedo reticularis, mental retardation, premature atherosclerosis, and arteriovenous thromboses	
Carbohydrate Disorders	Galactosemia	AR galactose-1-uridyl transferase (systemic disease) or Galactokinase (cataracts only)	Galactose in liver, brain, lenses	Clinical manifestations appear when the child is fed lactose and include: liver failure, proximal renal tubular dysfunction (Fanconi syndrome), and eventual mental retardation, steatosis, cirrhosis, and cataracts	
				High risk for *E coli* septicemia	
				Screen: serum galactose levels	
	Hereditary fructose intolerance	AR fructose-1,6-phosphatase			

- **Krabbe disease** (galactocerebrosidase deficiency, galactosylceramidase deficiency, globoid cell leukodystrophy) is an autosomal recessive disease in which most affected individuals present during infancy with neurologic symptoms (developmental delay, irritability) and progress to severe impairment and death by age 2. Some present later and progress more slowly; in later onset forms, vision loss is often an initial manifestation. Developmental regression follows, leading eventually to incapacitation and death, at a highly variable rate. While the disease is found worldwide, there have been no reported cases in persons of Jewish ancestry, and there is a notably high incidence in some Moslem groups. A biochemical assay is available for the affected enzyme—galactocerebrosidase. The underlying defect is a mutation in the GALC gene on 14q31, which encodes this enzyme.

- **Lesch-Nyhan syndrome** is an X-linked recessive disorder in which persistent hyperuricemia leads to neurologic dysfunction. A developmental delay becomes evident by 1 year of age, and walking is rarely achieved. By 2-3 years of age, extrapyramidal symptoms (choreoathetosis, etc) and self-mutilating behavior (biting, head-banging) occur. Deposition of urate leads to renal stones and sometimes gout. Megaloblastic anemia (with normal levels of folate and B$_{12}$) is common. Since Lesch-Nyhan is a disease of urate overproduction, affected individuals are found to have an increased urinary urate:creatinine ratio. The serum urate itself is not always elevated, due to adequate urinary excretion. An assay for the deficient enzyme—hypoxanthine-guanine phosphoribosyltransferase (HGPRT)—is clinically available. Molecular testing of the *HPRT1* gene, found at Xq26-27.2 and encoding HGPRT, is also available. The overproduction of urate can be controlled with allopurinol; however, urate control appears to have no effect on neurologic symptoms.

- **Fabry disease** has its onset in childhood, adolescence, or early adulthood in the form of pain in the distal extremities, angiokeratomas of the skin, hypohydrosis, corneal and lenticular opacities, and eventual death from either renal failure, cardiovascular disease, or cerebrovascular disease. The disease displays X-linked recessive inheritance and results from deficient α-galactosidase, which leads to lysosomal accumulation of globotriaosylceramide. A biochemical assay for α-galactosidase activity is available. Fully affected males have <1% activity; however, some males with limited variants of the disease have >1% activity. While many female carriers demonstrate decreased enzyme activity, most do not. Molecular assays are available in the form of direct sequence analysis of the GLA gene on Xq22.

- **Cystinosis** results in rickets, small stature, corneal deposits, and renal Fanconi syndrome (a defect of the proximal tubule in which there is urinary loss of electrolytes, glucose, and amino acids). In the severe form, the disease presents in the first year of life, eventually leading to renal failure by the age of 10 years. Milder forms present later, and in a form of the disease known as nonnephropathic cystinosis, only ocular manifestations are seen. Slit lamp examination of the cornea shows typical cystine crystals. This manifests clinically as photophobia. Mutations in the CTNS gene, found at 17p13, cause cystinosis. Histopathologic examination of bone marrow, cornea, kidney, and other tissues displays cystine crystals—hexagonal and birefringent—as does microscopic examination of urine.

Structural and Numerical Chromosomal Disorders

- Spontaneous abortions are associated with chromosomal anomalies in about 50% of cases; whereas, only about 0.5% of live born infants have them. The three most common abnormalities to be found in a spontaneous abortus are: monosomy X (45,X), triploidy (eg 69, XXY), and trisomy 16 (eg, 47, XX,+16). Among live births, trisomy 21 is the most common disorder.

- **Down syndrome** (trisomy 21) is found on the karyotype in >95% of individuals with Down syndrome. About 4% have unbalanced translocations (most commonly t(14;21)), which is important because it indicates that one of the parents harbors an unbalanced translocation that can be passed to additional offspring. Most of the remaining 1% are mosaics. Down syndrome affects about 1/700 newborns per year. The incidence increases with maternal age: in mothers < 20 years of age, the incidence is about 1 in 2000. Since most births occur to young women, however, >80% of Down syndrome babies are born to mothers younger than 35. The extra chromosome 21 is maternally derived.

- In **Patau syndrome** (trisomy 13), few survive beyond 1 year of age. The incidence is approximately 1/5000 live births and increases with maternal age.

- **Edward syndrome** (trisomy 18) has an incidence of approximately 1/3000 live births and increases with maternal age. Few survive beyond 1 year of age.

- **Turner syndrome** (monosomy X, 45X) occurs with an incidence of about 1 in 2500 live female births. Interestingly, while 45, X is the most common chromosomal finding detected in spontaneous abortions, most of those born alive live into adulthood. It is estimated that 99% of 45, X conceptions abort spontaneously.

421

Many present as neonates with lymphedema, predominantly on the dorsum of the hands, feet, and neck. Other findings include a webbed neck, broad chest, widely spaced inverted nipples, short stature, and a low hairline on the back of the neck. Coarctation of the aorta and bicuspid aortic valve are common cardiac anomalies. Hypertension frequently occurs even in the absence of coarctation. Ovaries, which are normal in utero, are progressively depleted of ova and end up as fibrous streaks of tissue. Intelligence is usually normal.

☐ **Noonan syndrome** was once referred to as "male Turner syndrome," because there are a great number of morphologic similarities. However, Noonan syndrome affects an equal number of females and males and is now known to be molecularly distinct. Key differences are that in Turner syndrome, of course, an easily detectable cytogenetic anomaly is present, renal anomalies are common, intelligence is usually normal, and left-sided heart defects predominate. In Noonan syndrome, short stature, abnormal-appearing chest, and webbed neck give rise to a superficial resemblance to Turner syndrome. However, the associated congenital heart disease is right-sided, including most commonly pulmonic stenosis. Lymphatic malformations are also common. Prolonged coagulation times are frequently observed, due to a wide range of defects (vWD phenotypes, factor V deficiency, factor VIII deficiency, et cetera). Mental retardation is seen in a significant minority. A characteristic facial dysmorphism includes low-set ears, blue-green irides, and hypertelorism. The incidence of Noonan syndrome is estimated to be about 1 in 1000, making it among the more common inherited syndromes. It is inherited in an AD manner, but many cases are sporadic, due to de novo mutations. Noonan syndrome is caused by mutations in either the *PTPN11* gene (12q) or the *KRAS* gene (12p). Direct sequence analysis is clinically available for these loci. *PTPN11* has also been implicated in some examples of LEOPARD syndrome and juvenile myelomonocytic leukemia (JMML).

■ **Klinefelter syndrome** (47,XXY) has an incidence of about 1 in 1000 live male births. Most survive to adulthood. Affected boys tend to be tall, with disproportionately long arms and legs. They have hypogonadism, and some develop gynecomastia. Most have a mild mental retardation. Some may come to clinical attention only through evaluation for infertility. The testicular biopsy shows hyalinized atrophic, nonspermatogenic seminiferous tubules.

■ **Microdeletion/microduplication syndromes** (contiguous gene syndromes) are a group of disorders that share a common molecular basis: the loss or gain of a portion of chromosome that is small by cytogenetic standards but large enough to affect multiple genes. They can usually be diagnosed by high-resolution cytogenetic studies or FISH. Prader-Willi and Angelman syndromes are diagnosed by parent-of-origin (methylation) studies.

☐ **Angelman syndrome** and **Prader-Willi syndrome** have vastly different clinical manifestations but result from the same deletion of 15q11.2. Imprinting forms the basis for most of these phenotypic differences and refers to the preferential inactivation of an allele based upon the parent of origin. The most common way for a cell to turn genes off, and the way that it is accomplished at 15q11.2, is hypermethylation (an example of an epigenetic phenomenon). If one allele is inactivated and the other is missing, then the cell has no 15q11.2 to transcribe. About 15% of Angleman and Prader-Willi syndrome result from uniparental disomy. Uniparental disomy occurs when part or all of a chromosome comes from just one parent. This arises as a result of nondisjunction during meiosis such that one gamete gets both homologs and the other gamete gets neither. Prader-Willi syndrome is due to a microdeletion in the paternally derived 15q11.2 or uniparental (maternal) disomy. Rare cases have an abnormality in the imprinting (methylation) process. Angelman syndrome is usually due to a microdeletion in the maternally derived chromosome 15q11.2 or, less commonly, uniparental (paternal) disomy. Rarely, it is due to an abnormality in the imprinting (methylation) process. 5-10% of Angelman syndrome patients have a point mutation in the *UBE3A* gene, located within the critical 15q11.2 region. *UBE3A* encodes the E6-AP ubiquitin ligase protein **T7.11**.

Chromosomal Breakage (Trinucleotide repeat, Chromosomal Instability) Syndromes

■ Most of these disorders are due to the expansion of a repeated sequence of three nucleotides (trinucleotide repeat) in the coding or noncoding sequence of a given gene. These trinucleotide repeat regions are present in the normal gene, polymorphic in length throughout the population, but within a range that is short enough to be stable. When expanded beyond a certain length, they become unstable. Others are due to defective repair of spontaneous chromosomal breakage. The diagnosis was

Applications of Molecular Methods in Nonneoplastic Disease>Molecular Basis and Molecular Diagnosis of Specific Nonneoplastic Diseases

T7.11
Microdeletion/Microduplication Syndromes

Syndrome	Deletion	Manifestations
DiGeorge syndrome, Catch 22 syndrome, CHARGE sequence, Velo-Cardio-Facial syndrome	22q11.2	Thymic aplasia/hypoplasia (immunodeficiency), parathyroid aplasia/hypoplasia (hypocalcemia, tetany), abnormal facial features, mental retardation, conotruncal cardiac anomalies
Crit-du-chat	5p15.2	Abnormal (cat) cry, microcephaly, mental retardation
Kallman	Xp22.3	Anosmia, hypogonadism
Prader-Willi	15q11.2 (paternal)	Hyperphagia, obesity, hypogonadism, mild mental retardation
Angelman	15q11.2 (maternal)	Hyperactivity, inappropriate laughter, aphasia, ataxia, mental retardation, seizures
Smith-Magenis syndrome	17p11.2	Moderate mental retardation, prominent forehead, flat, broad midface, self-mutilating behavior, disturbed REM sleep
Williams syndrome	7q11.23	Elfin-like facies, abnormal dentation, growth deficiency, heart malformations, infantile hypercalcemia, mental retardation
Wolf Syndrome	4p deletion	Intrauterine growth retardation, heart malformations, microcephaly, cleft lip and palate, broad nasal root, severe mental retardation
Miller-Dieker syndrome	17p13	Microcephaly, type I lissencephaly, heart malformations, renal malformations, seizures, prominent forehead, vertical furrowing of brow
CHARGE Sequence	22q11.2	Colomba, heart malformations, choanal atresia, genital hypoplasia, deafness, mental retardation

traditionally based upon demonstration of chromosome breakage (fragility) in culture. A unique feature of trinucleotide repeat expansions is that they tend to expand more with each successive generation; thus, they phenotypically display either greater severity or younger age at onset in offspring (anticipation).

- **Fragile X syndrome** (FRAX A) is an X-linked disorder with an incidence of 1 in 4000 males. While mental retardation is a common feature, the physical appearance is variable. Most have large head size, prominent ears, prominent jaw, and macro-orchidism. The underlying molecular defect is an expansion of a CGG trinucleotide repeat in the region of the *FMR1* gene on Xq27.3. Alleles with 6-53 CGG repeats are considered to be normal, while those with 54 to 200 repeats are considered permutations. Greater than 200 repeats are associated with the fragile X syndrome. Such expansions lead to methylation and inactivation of the *FMR1* gene. Rare cases of FRAX A are due to mutations actually within the *FMR1* gene. The molecular diagnosis may be made by Southern blot or methylation analysis. In the past, a modified form of cytogenetics was used to make the diagnosis of fragile X, in which chromosome fragility could be enhanced by growth in thymidine deprivation culture.

- **Friedreich ataxia** is an autosomal recessive disorder in which affected individuals suffer deterioration of the spinal dorsal root ganglia, posterior columns, corticospinal tracts, and spinocerebellar tracts. This manifests initially with gait ataxia, usually no later than the age of 20, with eventual limb ataxia and dysarthria. There is loss of deep tendon reflexes, impaired proprioception, and decreased pain and temperature sensation. A minority display optic atrophy or sensorineural hearing loss. About 60% develop a hypertrophic cardiomyopathy. Friedreich ataxia is caused by a GAA trinucleotide expansion in the *FRDA* gene (9q13). Those with fully manifested Friedreich ataxia display homozygosity for pathologic trinucleotide GAA expansion, with >500 repeats. Premutation alleles are considered to be those up to 65 repeats (with those between 66 and 500 capable of going either way). The expansion size correlates with age of onset and disease severity. There is a direct correlation between the length of the trinucleotide expansion and the thickness of the interventricular septum. What is unique about Friedreich ataxia is that, unlike other trinucleotide repeat disorders, anticipation is not observed. This is because two copies of an abnormal allele must be inherited in order for the disease to occur; thus, the disease is not directly transmitted from one generation to the next.

- **Xeroderma pigmentosa** (DeSanctis-Cacchione syndrome, XP) is characterized by profound photosensitivity and a markedly increased risk of cutaneous and

Applications of Molecular Methods in Nonneoplastic Disease>Molecular Basis and Molecular Diagnosis of Specific Nonneoplastic Diseases

ocular neoplasms. In childhood, most affected individuals manifest severe sunburns, extensive freckling of sun-exposed skin (freckling under two years of age is unusual in normal children), dry skin, poikiloderma, and telangiectasias. A first skin cancer often develops by the age of 10. Ocular exposure to the sun results in severe keratitis with eventual corneal opacification, loss of eyelashes, and eyelid atrophy with ectropion. Some experience sensorineural hearing loss and cognitive impairment. Chromosomal breakage is enhanced by in vitro exposure to UV light. The basic defect is failure to specifically repair UV-induced DNA damage. In cytogenetic preparations, cultures must be exposed to UV light to bring out the defect. The incidence is highest in Japan. While mutations in several genes are known to underlie XP—especially *XPA* (9q22) and *XPC* (3p), both encoding DNA repair proteins—molecular testing is not presently available on a clinical basis.

- **Ataxia telangiectasia** (A-T) is an autosomal recessive disease that results in progressive neurological impairment (cerebellar degeneration) and variable immunodeficiency (deficiency of cell mediated immunity and a degree of immunoglobulin, usually IgA, deficiency). Other characteristic features of A-T are thymic hypoplasia, high serum a fetoprotein (AFP) concentrations, growth retardation, and telangiectasias (especially of the bulbar conjunctiva). Lastly, patients have an increased sensitivity to ionizing radiation and a great tendency to develop cancer, especially hematolymphoid neoplasms. Approximately 0.5% of the population carries a mutation in the responsible *ATM* gene. Classic A-T results from the presence of two truncating *ATM* mutations, leading to total loss of the encoded *ATM* protein kinase. By unknown mechanisms, this protein kinase is instrumental in protecting cells from degeneration. The diagnosis of A-T can be confirmed by identification of both *ATM* mutations, but this can be difficult and time-consuming. Documenting increased chromosomal radiosensitivity and/or absence of the *ATM* protiein are much simpler procedures. More slowly-progressive or mild variants of A-T result from less deleterious mutations in the *ATM* gene wherein *ATM* protein kinase activity is somewhat preserved.

- **Bloom syndrome** is an autosomal recessive disorder characterized by short stature, narrow face with beaked nose, telangiectasias, chronic infections, and susceptibility to acute leukemia. Bloom syndrome is due to a mutation in the *BLM* gene, on 15q26.1, encoding a DNA helicase. It is characterized by growth retardation, a photosensitive erythematous skin lesion (usually on the face), recurrent respiratory infections, the development of bronchiectasis, diabetes mellitus, and eventual death from early-developing malignant neoplasms. The characteristic skin lesions are absent at birth and develop during the first year of life, following sun exposure, most commonly as a butterfly-pattern facial lesion. Café-au-lait spots and areas of hypopigmentation are common. The immunodeficiency in Bloom syndrome is one of hypogammaglobulinemia, leading to repeated episodes of otitis media and bacterial pneumonia. Cancer occurs with great frequency and at a very young age, most commonly in the form of a hematolymphoid neoplasm; however, epithelial neoplasms (especially colorectal, cutaneous, and pulmonary malignancies) are very common as well. The syndrome may be diagnosed by demonstrating a greatly increased frequency of sister chromatid exchanges (SCEs) in cytogenetic cultures exposed to bromodeoxyuridine (BUDR). Even in cultures not exposed, there is a notably increased number of chromosomal breaks, chromatid gaps, and chromosomal rearrangements. In addition, testing for mutations in the *BLM* gene is clinically available. If the ethnicity of the affected individual is known, targeted mutation analysis can be employed; in Ashkenazi Jewish persons, Bloom syndrome is nearly always due to a particular mutation known as BLMASH, whose frequency is about 1% in that population.

- **Nijmegen breakage syndrome** (Berlin syndrome, Seemanova syndrome) is an autosomal recessive chromosomal breakage syndrome characterized by short stature, microcephaly, mental retardation, premature ovarian failure, immunodefiency, and an increased risk for malignancy. A characteristic dysmorphic appearance is often present: sloping forehead, prominent nasal root, large ears, and upwardly slanting palpebral fissures. The vast majority of Nimmegen syndrome-associated malignancies are B-cell lymphomas. Recurrent sinopulmonary infections are a common problem. Laboratory testing discloses hypo- or agammaglobulinemia and in some cases decreased CD3+/CD4+ T cell subsets. Chromosomal instability may be noted in cytogenetic cultures. Mutations in the *NBS1* gene (8q21—encoding nibrin) underlie all known cases.

- **Fanconi anemia** is an autosomal recessive disease characterized by a set of characteristic dysmorphic features, aplastic anemia, and an increased risk of malignancy. The physical findings include short stature, café-au-lait spots, hypopigmentation, thumb and forearm malformations, ocular anomalies, renal anomalies, and sensorineural hearing loss; however, up to 40% of those with FA have no physical anomalies. Within the first decade, there is progressive marrow insufficiency leading to aplastic anemia. Most malignancies are hematolymphoid, but up to ¼ are solid tumors. As in all chromosomal breakage syndromes, cells in cytogenetic culture may show an increased rate of spontaneous chromosomal damage. However, FA breakage is specifically enhanced by DNA cross-linking agents (diepoxybutane or mitomycin C). Molecular testing is complicated by the fact that multiple genes may be causative, including the *FANCA* (>60% of FA), *FANCC* (10%), and others. In Ashkenazi Jewish individuals testing is more practical, since a single gene—*FANCC*—is usually involved.

Mitochondrial disease is a term that refers to a group of disorders unified by a basis in mutations of genes that encode mitochondrial proteins, especially proteins in the respiratory chain. They will then affect most profoundly those tissues that rely heavily or exclusively on oxidative metabolism. The actual underlying mutation may be in either nuclear or mitochondrial DNA. This results in a heterogeneous group of disorders that usually affect the neuromuscular system at some level, tending to produce such manifestations as ophthalmoplegia, ptosis, retinopathy, optic atrophy, skeletal myopathy, cardiomyopathy, sensorineural deafness, and encephalopathy. Note that while the cells of normal individuals contain a single clone of mitochondria (with identical genomes, inherited from the mother, a condition known as homoplasmy), persons with mitochondrial diseases often, but not always, harbor a dual population of mitochondria—one normal and one containing the mutation (heteroplasmy). Varying proportions of these populations may account for the clinical variability noted in this set of diseases. Those mitochondrial diseases that are due to mutations in nuclear DNA tend to present in childhood, while those due to mutations in mitochondrial DNA often present later. Mitochondrial diseases should be considered in the differential whenever there is an unexplained multi-level neuromuscular disorder. Screening tests that should be abnormal in mitochondrial diseases include plasma or CSF lactic acid, ketones, acylcarnitines, and urinary organic acids. If these are abnormal, one should next consider muscle biopsy. The muscle biopsy classically contains ragged red fibers (trichrome stain). The succinate dehydrogenase stain, in addition to highlighting the muscle fibers, shows stronger than usual staining in blood vessels, due

to an abundance of mitochondria. Ultrastructural examination shows characteristic (parking-lot) inclusions.

- **Kearns-Sayre syndrome** has the following features: presentation before the age of 20, pigmentary (salt and pepper) retinopathy, external ophthalmoplegia, elevated CSF protein, cerebellar ataxia, cardiac conduction block, sensorineural hearing loss, myopathy, diabetes mellitus, and hypoparathyroidism. Large mitochondrial DNA deletions are the basis for Kearns-Sayre syndrome, Pearson syndrome, and progressive external ophthalmoplegia (PEA). Duplication/deletion analysis by Southern blot is clinically available for these diagnoses. Pearson syndrome presents in childhood and is uniformly fatal. Its manifestations include sideroblastic anemia, progressing to pancytopenia, and pancreatic exocrine insufficiency. Chronic progressive external ophthalmoplegia (CPEO) manifests primarily as external ophthalmoplegia, ptosis, and a mild myopathy.

- **Mitochondrial encephalopathy with lactic acidosis and stroke-like episodes** (MELAS) presents in childhood, between 2-10 years of age. It is characterized by stroke-like neurologic deficits (transient hemiparesis or cortical blindness), seizures, diabetes mellitus, cardiomyopathy, sensorineural hearing loss, pigmentary retinopathy, cerebellar ataxia, and lactic acidosis. MELAS is caused by mutations in the *MT-TL1* gene, which is located within the mitochondrial DNA and encodes tRNA^{Leu}. Interstingly, during stroke-like episodes, the brain MRI shows lesions inconsistent with a vascular distribution. The basal ganglia often show calcifications. Since a single mutation—an A to G substitution at nucleotide 3243 (A3243G)—is responsible for >80% of cases, this disease lends itself to targeted mutation analysis.

- **Myoclonic epilepsy with ragged red fibers** (MERRF) manifests as seizures, myoclonus, cerebellar ataxia, dementia, optic atrophy, sensorineural hearing loss, cardiomyopathy, and multiple lipomas. Myoclonus is usually the first sign. Like MELAS, a single mutation is responsible for >80% of cases—an A to G substitution at nucleotide 8344 (A8344G)—in the mitochondrial MT-TK gene which encodes tRNA^{Lys}. Targeted mutation analysis for this and 2-3 other mutations can detect >90% of cases.

- **Leber hereditary optic neuropathy** presents in young adults, mainly males, with visual failure.

- **Mitochondrial neurogastrointestinal encephalopathy** (MGNIE)

Bibliography

Aaltonen LA, Salovaara R, Kristo P, Canzian F, Hemminki A, Peltomaki P, Chadwick RB, Kaariainen H, Eskelinen M, Jarvinen H, Mecklin JP, de la Chapelle A. Incidence of hereditary nonpolyposis colorectal cancer and the feasibility of molecular screening for the disease. *N Engl J Med* 1998; 338:1481-1487.

Abrahamov A, Elstein D, Gross-Tsur V, Farber B, Glaser Y, Hadas-Halpern I, Ronen S, Tafakjdi M, Horowitz M, Zimran A. Gaucher's disease variant characterised by progressive calcification of heart valves and unique genotype. *Lancet* 1995; 346:1000-1003.

Ackerman MJ, Siu BL, Sturner WQ, Tester DJ, Valdivia CR, Makielski JC, Towbin JA. Postmortem molecular analysis of SCN5A defects in sudden infant death syndrome. *JAMA* 2001;286:2264-2269.

Ahmad F, Li D, Karibe A, Gonzalez O, Tapscott T, Hill R, Weilbaecher D, Blackie P, Furey M, Gardner M, Bachinski LL, Roberts R Localization of a gene responsible for arrhythmogenic right ventricular dysplasia to chromosome 3p23. *Circulation* 1998; 98:2791-2795.

Allen DB, Hoffman GL, Fitzpatrick P, Laessig R, Maby S, Slyper A (1997) Improved precision of newborn screening for congenital adrenal hyperplasia using weight-adjusted criteria for 17-hydroxyprogesterone levels. *J Pediatr* 1997;130:128-133.

Amir G, Ron N Pulmonary pathology in Gaucher's disease. *Hum Pathol* 1999;30:666-670.

Amos CI, Keitheri-Cheteri MB, Sabripour M, Wei C, McGarrity TJ, Seldin MF, Nations L, Lynch PM, Fidder HH, Friedman E, Frazier ML. Genotype-phenotype correlations in Peutz-Jeghers syndrome. *J Med Genet* 2004; 41:327-333.

Anderson SL, Coli R, Daly IW, Kichula EA, Rork MJ, Volpi SA, Ekstein J, Rubin BY. Familial dysautonomia is caused by mutations of the IKAP gene. *Am J Hum Genet* 2001; 68:753-758.

Ando Y, Nakamura M, Araki S. Transthyretin-related familial amyloidotic polyneuropathy. *Arch Neurol* 2005; 62:1057-1062.

Andresen BS, Bross P, Udvari S, Kirk J, Gray G, Kmoch S, Chamoles N, Knudsen I, Winter V, Wilcken B, Yokota I, Hart K, Packman S, Harpey JP, Saudubray JM, Hale DE, Bolund L, Kolvraa S, Gregersen N. The molecular basis of medium-chain acyl-CoA dehydrogenase (MCAD) deficiency in compound heterozygous patients: is there correlation between genotype and phenotype? *Hum Mol Genet* 1997; 6:695-707.

Anikster Y, Lacbawan F, Brantly M, Gochuico BL, Avila NA, Travis W, Gahl WA. Pulmonary dysfunction in adults with nephropathic cystinosis. *Chest* 2001; 119:394-401.

Anikster Y, Shotelersuk V, Gahl WA. CTNS mutations in patients with cystinosis. *Hum Mutat* 1999; 14:454-458.

Antonarakis SE, Rossiter JP, Young M, Horst J, de Moerloose P, Sommer SS, Ketterling RP, Kazazian HH Jr, Négrier C, Vinciguerra C, Gitschier J, Goossens M, Girodon E, Ghanem N, Plassa F, Lavergne JM, Vidaud M, Costa JM, Laurian Y, Lin SW, Lin SR, Shen MC, Lillicrap D, Taylor SA, Windsor S, Valleix SV, Nafa K, Sultan Y, Delpech M, Vnencak-Jones CL, Phillips JA 3rd, Ljung RC, Koumbarelis E, Gialeraki A, Mandalaki T, Jenkins PV, Collins PW, Pasi KJ, Goodeve A, Peake I, Preston FE, Schwartz M, Scheibel E, Ingerslev J, Cooper DN, Millar DS, Kakkar VV, Giannelli F, Naylor JA, Tizzano EF, Baiget M, Domenech M, Altisent C, Tusell J, Beneyto M, Lorenzo JI, Gaucher C, Mazurier C, Peerlinck K, Matthijs G, Cassiman JJ, Vermylen J, Mori PG, Acquila M, Caprino D, Inaba H. Factor VIII Gene Inversions in Severe Hemophilia A: Results of an International Consortium Study. *Blood* 1995; 86 (6): 2206-2212.

Antonescu CR, Tschernyavsky SJ, Woodruff JM, Jungbluth AA, Brennan FM, Ladanyi M. Molecular Diagnosis of Clear Cell Sarcoma:. *J Mol Diag* 2002; 4:44–52.

Antzelevitch C, Brugada P, Brugada J, Brugada R, Towbin JA, Nademanee K Brugada syndrome. 1992-2002:a historical perspective. *J Am Coll Cardiol* 2003; 41:1665-1671.

Anwar R, Miloszewski KJ. Factor XIII Deficiency. *Br J Haematol* 1999; 107(3): 468-484.

Bibliography

Argani P, Antonescu CR, Couturier J, Fournet J, Sciot R, Debiec-Rychter M, Hutchinson B, Reuter VE, Boccon-Gibod L, Timmons C, Hafez N, Ladanyi M. PRCC-TFE3 Renal Carcinomas Morphologic, Immunohistochemical, Ultrastructural, and Molecular Analysis of an Entity Associated With the t(X,1)(p11.2;q21) *Am J Surg Pathol* 2002; 26(12): 1553–1566.

Argov Z, Eisenberg I, Grabov-Nardini G, Sadeh M, Wirguin I, Soffer D, Mitrani-Rosenbaum S Hereditary inclusion body myopathy: The Middle Eastern genetic cluster. *Neurology* 2003; 60:1519-1523.

Arico M, Imashuku S, Clementi R, Hibi S, Teramura T, Danesino C, Haber DA, Nichols KE. Hemophagocytic lymphohistiocytosis due to germline mutations in SH2D1A, the X-linked lymphoproliferative disease gene. *Blood* 2001;97:1131-1133.

Asakai R, Chung DW, Davie EW, Seligsohn U. Factor XI Deficiency in Ashkenazi Jews in Israel. *N Engl J Med* 1991; 325(3): 153-158.

Aylward EH, Sparks BF, Field KM, Yallapragada V, Shpritz BD, Rosenblatt A, Brandt J, Gourley LM, Liang K, Zhou H, Margolis RL, Ross CA. Onset and rate of striatal atrophy in preclinical Huntington disease. *Neurology* 2004; 63:66-72.

Bacon BR, Powell LW, Adams PC, Kresina TF, Hoofnagle JH. Molecular medicine and hemochromatosis: at the crossroads. *Gastroenterology* 1999; 116:193-207.

Bagnall RD, Waseem N, Green PM, Giannelli F. Recurrent inversion breaking intron 1 of the factor VIII gene is a frequent cause of severe hemophilia A. *Blood* 2002; 99:168-174.

Barragan-Campos HM, Vallee JN, Lo D, Barrera-Ramirez CF, Argote-Greene M, Sanchez-Guerrero J, Estanol B, Guillevin R, Chiras J. Brain magnetic resonance imaging findings in patients with mitochondrial cytopathies. *Arch Neurol* 2005; 62:737-742.

Barbeau JM, Goforth J, Caliendo AM, Nolte FS. Performance characteristics of a quantitative TaqMan hepatitis C virus RNA analyte-specific reagent. *J Clin Microbiol* 2004; 42:3739-3746.

Barness LA. An Approach to the Diagnosis of Metabolic Diseases. *Fetal and Pediatric Pathology* 2004; 23:3-10.

Baser ME, Friedman JM, Evans DG. Increasing the specificity of diagnostic criteria for schwannomatosis. *Neurology* 2006; 66:730-732.

Beggs AH. Dystrophinopathy, the expanding phenotype. Dystrophin abnormalities in X-linked dilated cardiomyopathy. *Circulation* 1997; 95:2344-2347.

Belz MM, Fick-Brosnahan GM, Hughes RL, Rubinstein D, Chapman AB, Johnson AM, McFann KK, Kaehny WD, Gabow PA. Recurrence of intracranial aneurysms in autosomal-dominant polycystic kidney disease. *Kidney Int* 2003; 63:1824-1830.

Bennett MJ, Rinaldo P, Millington DS, Tanaka K, Yokota I, Coates PM. Medium-chain acyl-CoA dehydrogenase deficiency: postmortem diagnosis in a case of sudden infant death and neonatal diagnosis of an affected sibling. *Pediatr Pathol* 1991; 11:889-895.

Bernard R, Boyer A, Negre P, Malzac P, Latour P, Vandenberghe A, Philip N, Levy N. Prenatal detection of the 17p11.2 duplication in Charcot-Marie-Tooth disease type 1A: necessity of a multidisciplinary approach for heterogeneous disorders. *Eur J Hum Genet* 2002; 10:297-302.

Beutler E, Beutler L, West C. Mutations in the gene encoding cytosolic beta-glucosidase in Gaucher disease. *J Lab Clin Med* 2004;144:65-68.

Bhala A, Willi SM, Rinaldo P, Bennett MJ, Schmidt-Sommerfeld E, Hale DE. Clinical and biochemical characterization of short-chain acyl-coenzyme A dehydrogenase deficiency. *J Pediatr* 1995; 126:910-915.

Bisceglia M, Galliani CA, Senger C, Stallone C, Sessa A. Renal cystic diseases. *Adv Anat Pathol* 2006;13(1):26-56.

Boardman LA. Heritable colorectal cancer syndromes: recognition and preventive management. *Gastroenterol Clin North Am* 2002;31:1107-1131.

Boardman LA, Thibodeau SN, Schaid DJ, Lindor NM, McDonnell SK, Burgart LJ, Ahlquist DA, Podratz KC, Pittelkow M, Hartmann LC. Increased risk for cancer in patients with the Peutz-Jeghers syndrome. *Ann Intern Med* 1998; 128:896-899.

Bibliography

Boerger LM, Morris PC, Thurnau GR, Esmon CT, Comp PC. Oral contraceptives and gender affect protein S status. *Blood* 1987; 69(2): 692-694.

Boerkoel CF, Takashima H, Garcia CA, Olney RK, Johnson J, Berry K, Russo P, Kennedy S, Teebi AS, Scavina M, Williams LL, Mancias P, Butler IJ, Krajewski K, Shy M, Lupski JR. Charcot-Marie-Tooth disease and related neuropathies: mutation distribution and genotype-phenotype correlation. *Ann Neurol* 2002; 51:190-201.

Bolton-Maggs PH. Factor XI Deficiency and its management. *Haemophilia* 2000; 6 (Suppl 1): 100-109.

Bolton-Maggs PH and Pasi KJ. Haemophilias A and B. *Lancet* 2003;361:1801-1809.

Boot RG, Verhoek M, de Fost M, Hollak CE, Maas M, Bleijlevens B, van Breemen MJ, van Meurs M, Boven LA, Laman JD, Moran MT, Cox TM, Aerts JM. Marked elevation of the chemokine CCL18/PARC in Gaucher disease: a novel surrogate marker for assessing therapeutic intervention. *Blood* 2004;103:33-39.

Boushey CJ, Beresford SAA, Omenn GS, Motulsky AG. A quantitative assessment of plasma homocysteine as a risk factor for vascular disease. *JAMA* 1995; 274:1049-1057.

Bouzourene H, Taminelli L, Chaubert P, Monnerat C, Seelentag W, Sandmeier D, Andrejevic S, Matter M, Bosman F, Benhattar J. A cost-effective algorithm for hereditary nonpolyposis colorectal cancer detection. *Am J Clin Pathol* 2006; 125:823-831.

Bowen DJ. Haemophilia A and haemophilia B: molecular insights. *J Clin Pathol: Mol Pathol* 2002; 55:127–144.

Boye E, Mollet G, Forestier L, Cohen-Solal L, Heidet L, Cochat P, Grunfeld JP, Palcoux JB, Gubler MC, Antignac C. Determination of the genomic structure of the COL4A4 gene and of novel mutations causing autosomal recessive Alport syndrome. *Am J Hum Genet* 1998; 63:1329-1340.

Brock PR, de Zegher F, Casteels-Van Daele M, Vanderschueren-Lodeweyckx M. Malignant disease in Bloom's syndrome children treated with growth hormone. *Lancet* 1991;337:1345-1346.

Brussino A, Gellera C, Saluto A, Mariotti C, Arduino C, Castellotti B, Camerlingo M, de Angelis V, Orsi L, Tosca P, Migone N, Taroni F, Brusco A. FMR1 gene premutation is a frequent genetic cause of late-onset sporadic cerebellar ataxia. *Neurology* 2005; 64:145-147.

Bulaj ZJ, Griffen LM, Jorde LB, Edwards CQ, Kushner JP. Clinical and biochemical abnormalities in people heterozygous for hemochromatosis. *N Engl J Med* 1996; 335:1799-1805.

Burt MJ, George PM, Upton JD, Collett JA, Frampton CM, Chapman TM, Walmsley TA, Chapman BA. The significance of haemochromatosis gene mutations in the general population: implications for screening. *Gut* 1998. 43:830-836.

Buxbaum JN and Tagoe CE. The genetics of the amyloidoses. *Annu Rev Med* 2000; 51:543-569.

Buzza M, Dagher H, Wang YY, Wilson D, Babon JJ, Cotton RG, Savige J. Mutations in the COL4A4 gene in thin basement membrane disease. *Kidney Int* 2003; 63:447-453.

Caldas C, Carneiro F, Lynch HT, et. Al. Familial Gastric Cancer: Overview and Guidelines for Management. *J Med Genet* 1999; 36:873-880.

Calonge N, and the U.S. Preventive Services Task Force. Screening for hemochromatosis: recommendation statement. *Ann Intern Med* 2006;145:204-208.

Cao A, Saba L, Galanello R, Rosatelli MC. Molecular diagnosis and carrier screening for beta thalassemia. *JAMA* 1997; 278:1273-1277.

Carney JA, Young WF. Primary pigmented nodular adrenocortical disease and its associated conditions. *Endocrinologist* 1992;2:6-21.

Cataldo KA, Jalal SM, Law ME, Ansell SM, Inwards DJ, Fine M, Arber DA, Pulford KA, Strickler JG. Detection of t(2;5) in anaplastic large cell lymphoma: Comparison of immunohistochemical studies, FISH, and RT-PCR in paraffin-embedded tissue. *Am J Surg Pathol* 1999;23:1386-1392.

Chabriat H, Levy C, Taillia H, Iba-Zizen MT, Vahedi K, Joutel A, Tournier-Lasserve E, Bousser MG. Patterns of MRI lesions in CADASIL. *Neurology* 1998;51:452-457.

Bibliography

Chabriat H, Mrissa R, Levy C, Vahedi K, Taillia H, Iba-Zizen MT, Joutel A, Tournier-Lasserve E, Bousser MG. Brain stem MRI signal abnormalities in CADASIL. *Stroke* 1999; 30:457-459.

Chabriat H, Vahedi K, Iba-Zizen MT, Joutel A, Nibbio A, Nagy TG, Krebs MO, Julien J, Dubois B, Ducrocq X. Clinical spectrum of CADASIL: a study of 7 families. Cerebral autosomal dominant arteriopathy with subcortical infarcts and leukoencephalopathy. *Lancet* 1995; 346:934-939.

Chace DH, DiPerna JC, Mitchell BL, Sgroi B, Hofman LF, Naylor EW. Electrospray tandem mass spectrometry for analysis of acylcarnitines in dried postmortem blood specimens collected at autopsy from infants with unexplained cause of death. *Clin Chem* 2001; 47:1166-1182.

Chang CC, Gould SJ. Phenotype-genotype relationships in complementation group 3 of the peroxisome-biogenesis disorders. *Am J Hum Genet* 1998;63:1294-1306.

Chang CC, Lee WH, Moser H, Valle D, Gould SJ. Isolation of the human PEX12 gene, mutated in group 3 of the peroxisome biogenesis disorders. *Nat Genet* 1997;15:385-388.

Charlton A, Blair V, Shaw D, Parry S Guilford P, Martin IG. Hereditary diffuse gastric cancer: predominance of multiple foci of signet ring carcinoma in distal stomach and transitional zone. *Gut* 2004;53:814-820.

Charrow J, Esplin JA, Gribble TJ, Kaplan P, Kolodny EH, Pastores GM, Scott CR, Wappner RS, Weinreb NJ, Wisch JS. Gaucher disease: recommendations on diagnosis, evaluation, and monitoring. *Arch Intern Med* 1998;158:1754-1760.

Cheadle JP, Reeve MP, Sampson JR, Kwiatkowski DJ. Molecular genetic advances in tuberous sclerosis. *Hum Genet* 2000;107(2):97-114.

Chen Q, Zhang D, Gingell RL, Moss AJ, Napolitano C, Priori SG, Schwartz PJ, Kehoe E, Robinson JL, Schulze-Bahr E, Wang Q, Towbin JA. Homozygous deletion in KVLQT1 associated with Jervell and Lange-Nielsen syndrome. *Circulation* 1999; 99:1344-1347.

Chinnery PF, DiMauro S, Shanske S, Schon EA, Zeviani M, Mariotti C, Carrara F, Lombes A, Laforet P, Ogier H, Jaksch M, Lochmuller H, Horvath R, Deschauer M, Thorburn DR, Bindoff LA, Poulton J, Taylor RW, Matthews JN, Turnbull DM. Risk of developing a mitochondrial DNA deletion disorder. *Lancet* 2004; 364:592-596.

Chmiel JF, Drumm ML, Konstan MW, Ferkol TW, Kercsmar CM. Pitfall in the use of genetic analysis as the sole diagnostic criterion for cystic fibrosis. *Pediatrics* 1999; 103:823-826.

Clarke R, Daly L, Robinson K. Hyperhomocysteinemia: an independent risk factor for vascular disease. *N Eng J Med* 1991; 324:1149-1155.

Clericuzio CL, Chen E, McNeil DE, O'Connor T, Zackai EH, Medne L, Tomlinson G, DeBaun M. Serum alpha-fetoprotein screening for hepatoblastoma in children with Beckwith-Wiedemann syndrome or isolated hemihyperplasia. *J Pediatr* 2003;143:270-272.

Cohen D, Zhou M. Molecular genetics of familial renal cell carcinoma Syndromes. *Clin Lab Med* 2005; 25:259–277.

Cohn JA, Friedman KJ, Noone PG, Knowles MR, Silverman LM, Jowell PS. Relation between mutations of the cystic fibrosis gene and idiopathic pancreatitis. *N Engl J Med* 1998; 339:653-658.

Collins CS, Gould SJ. Identification of a common PEX1 mutatin in Zellweger syndrome. *Hum Mutat* 1999; 14:45-53.

Colliton RP, Bason L, Lu FM, Piccoli DA, Krantz ID, Spinner NB. Mutation analysis of Jagged1 (JAG1) in Alagille syndrome patients. *Hum Mutat* 2001;17:151-152.

Cook JR, Shekhter-Levin S, Swerdlow SH. Utility of routine classical cytogenetic studies in the evaluation of suspected lymphomas: results of 279 consecutive lymph node/extranodal tissue biopsies. *Am J Clin Pathol* 2004;121:826-835.

Comp PC, Thurnau GR, Welsh J, Esmon CT. Functional and immunologic protein s levels are decreased during pregnancy. *Blood* 1986; 68(4): 881-885.

Bibliography

Concannon P. ATM heterozygosity and cancer risk. *Nat Genet* 2002; 32:89-90.

Dabora SL, Jozwiak S, Franz DN, Roberts PS, Nieto A, Chung J, Choy YS, Reeve MP, Thiele E, Egelhoff JC, Kasprzyk-Obara J, Domanska-Pakiela D, Kwiatkowski DJ. Mutational analysis in a cohort of 224 tuberous sclerosis patients indicates increased severity of TSC2, compared with TSC1, disease in multiple organs. *Am J Hum Genet* 2001. 68:64-80.

Danek A, Rubio JP, Rampoldi L, Ho M, Dobson-Stone C, Tison F, Symmans WA, Oechsner M, Kalckreuth W, Watt JM, Corbett AJ, Hamdalla HH, Marshall AG, Sutton I, Dotti MT, Malandrini A, Walker RH, Daniels G, Monaco AP. McLeod neuroacanthocytosis: genotype and phenotype. *Ann Neurol* 2001; 50:755-764.

Danek A, Uttner I, Vogl T, Tatsch K, Witt TN. Cerebral involvement in McLeod syndrome. *Neurology* 1994; 44:117-120.

Darin N, Oldfors A, Moslemi AR, Holme E, Tulinius M. The incidence of mitochondrial encephalomyopathies in childhood: clinical features and morphological, biochemical, and DNA anbormalities. *Ann Neurol* 2001; 49:377-383

De Alava E, Kawai A, Healey JH, et al. EWS-FLI1 fusion transcript structure is an independent determinant of prognosis in Ewing's sarcoma. *J Clin Oncol* 1998;16(4):1248–1455.

De Avala E, Panizo A, Antonescu CR, et al. Association of EWS-FLI1 type 1 fusion with lower proliferative rate in Ewing's sarcoma. *Am J Pathol* 2000;156:849– 55.

De Gobbi M, Roetto A, Piperno A, Mariani R, Alberti F, Papanikolaou G, Politou M, Lockitch G, Girelli D, Fargion S, Cox TM, Gasparini P, Cazzola M, Camaschella C. Natural history of juvenile haemochromatosis. *Br J Haematol* 2002; 117:973-979.

Delattre O, Zucman J, Melot T, et al. The Ewing family of tumors: a subgroup of small-round cell tumors defined by specific chimeric transcripts. *N Engl J Med* 1994;331:294-299.

De Moerloose P, Reber G, Perrier A, Perneger T, Bounameaux H. Prevalence of factor V Leiden and prothrombin G20210A mutations in unselected patients with venous thromboembolism. *Br J Haematol* 2000; 110(1): 125-129.

Derks TGJ, Reijngoud D, Waterham HR, Gerver WM, Van Den Berg MP, Sauer PJJ, Smit GPA. The natural history of medium-chain Acyl CoA dehydrogenase deficiency in the netherlands: clinical presentation and outcome. *J Pediatr* 2006;148:665-670.

DeSanjose S, Leone M, Berez V, et al. Prevalence of BRCA1 and BRCA2 germline mutations in young breast cancer patients: a population-based study. *Int J Cancer* 2003;106(4):588–593.

Desnick RJ, Brady R, Barranger J, Collins AJ, Germain DP, Goldman M, Grabowski G, Packman S, Wilcox WR. Fabry disease, an under-recognized multisystemic disorder: expert recommendations for diagnosis, management, and enzyme replacement therapy. *Ann Intern Med* 2003;138:338-346.

De Stefano V, Martinelli I, Mannucci PM, Paciaroni K, Chiusolo P, Casorelli I, Rossi E, Leone G. The risk of recurrent deep venous thrombosis among heterozygous carriers of both factor V Leiden and the G20210A prothrombin mutation. *N Engl J Med* 2000; 342(3): 214-215.

Die-Smulders CE, Howeler CJ, Thijs C, Mirandolle JF, Anten HB, Smeets HJ, Chandler KE, Geraedts JP. Age and causes of death in adult-onset myotonic dystrophy. *Brain* 1998; 121:1557-1563.

DiMauro S and Schon EA Mitochondrial DNA mutations in human disease. *Am J Med Genet* 2001; 106:18-26.

Dichgans M, Herzog J, Gasser T. NOTCH3 mutation involving three cysteine residues in a family with typical CADASIL. *Neurology* 2001; 57:1714-1717.

Dogulu CF, Tsilou E, Rubin B, Fitzgibbon EJ, Kaiser-Kupper MI, Rennert OM, Gahl WA. Idiopathic intracranial hypertension in cystinosis. *J Pediatr* 2004; 145:673-678.

Bibliography

Döhner H, Stilgenbauer S, Benner A, Leupolt E, Kröber A, Bullinger L, Döhner K, Bentz M, Lichter P. Genomic aberrations and survival in chronic lymphocytic leukemia. *N Engl J Med* 2000;343:1910-1916.

Dome JS, Coppes MJ. Recent advances in Wilms tumor genetics. *Curr Opin Pediatr* 2002;14:5-12.

Dorak MT, Burnett AK, Worwood M. HFE gene mutations in susceptibility to childhood leukemia: HuGE review. *Genetics in Medicine* 2005; 7(3):159-168.

Dork T, Dworniczak B, Aulehla-Scholz C, Wieczorek D, Bohm I, Mayerova A, Seydewitz HH, Nieschlag E, Meschede D, Horst J, Pander HJ, Sperling H, Ratjen F, Passarge E, Schmidtke J, Stuhrmann M. Distinct spectrum of CFTR mutation in congenital absence of vas deferens. *Hum Genet* 1997;100:365-377.

Dossenbach-Glaninger A, Hopmeier P. Coagulation factor XI: a database of mutations and polymorphisms associated with factor XI deficiency. *Blood Coagul Fibrinolysis* 2005; 16(4): 231-238.

Duan J, Nilsson L, Lambert B. Structural and functional analysis of mutations at the human hypoxanthine phosphoribosyl transferase (HPRT1) locus. *Hum Mutat* 2004; 23:599-611.

Everman DB, Shuman C, Dzolganovski B, O'riordan MA, Weksberg R, Robin NH. Serum alpha-fetoprotein levels in Beckwith-Wiedemann syndrome. *J Pediatr* 2000; 137:123-127.

Giardiello FM, Brensinger JD, Tersmette AC, Goodman SN, Petersen GM, Booker SV, Cruz-Correa M, Offerhaus JA. Very high risk of cancer in familial Peutz-Jeghers syndrome. *Gastroenterology* 2000;119:1447-1453.

Facon T, Avet-Loiseau H, Guillerm G, Moreau P, Geneviève F, Zandecki M, Laï JL, Leleu X, Jouet JP, Bauters F, Harousseau JL, Bataille R, Mary JY. Intergroupe Francophone du Myélome. Chromosome 13 abnormalities identified by FISH analysis and serum beta2-microglobulin roduce a powerful myeloma staging system for patients receiving high-dose therapy. *Blood* 2001;97:1566-1571.

Fakharzadeh SS, Kazazian Jr HH. Correlation Between Factor VIII Genotype and Inhibitor Development in Hemophilia A. *Semin Thromb Hemost* 2000; 26:167-171.

Furie B, Greene E, Furie BC. Syndrome of acquired factor X deficiency and systemic amyloidosis in vivo studies of the metabolic fate of factor X. *N Engl J Med* 1977; 297(2):81-85

Garner HP, Phillips JR, Herron JG, Severson SJ, Milla CE, Regelmann WE. Peroxidase Activity Within Circulating Neutrophils Correlates With Pulmonary Phenotype In Cystic Fibrosis. *J Lab Clin Med* 2004;144:127-133.

Gascoyne RD, Aoun P, Wu D, Chhanabhai M, Skinnider BF, Greiner TC, Morris SW, Connors JM, Vose JM, Viswanatha DS, Coldman A, Weisenburger DD Prognostic significance of anaplastic lymphoma kinase (ALK) protein expression in adults with anaplastic large cell lymphoma. *Blood* 1999;93:3913-3921.

Gatel A, Cacoub P, Piette JC. AL amyloidosis combined with acquired factor v deficiency. *Ann Int Med*1998; 128 (7): 604-605.

George DJ, Kaelin WG Jr. The von Hippel-Lindau protein, vascular endothelial growth factor, and kidney cancer. *N Engl J Med* 2003;349:419–421.

Gharehbaghi-Schnell EB, Finsterer J, Korschineck I, Mamoli B, Binder BR. Genotype-phenotype correlation in myotonic dystrophy. *Clin Genet* 1998; 53:20-26.

Gill JC. Diagnosis and treatment of von Willebrand disease. *Hematol Oncol Clin N Am* 2004; 18:1277–1299.

Grady WM. Genetic testing for high-risk colon cancer patients. *Gastroenterology* 2003;124:1574–1594.

Gregg RG, Simantel A, Farrell PM, Koscik R, Kosorok MR, Laxova A, Laessig R, Hoffman G, Hassemer D, Mischler EH, Splaingard M. Newborn screening for cystic fibrosis in Wisconsin: comparison of biochemical and molecular methods. *Pediatrics* 1997;99:819-824.

Griffin JH, Evatt B, Wideman C, Fernandez JA. Anticoagulant protein C pathway defective in the majority of thrombophilic patients. *Blood* 1993; 82:1989-1994.

431

Bibliography

Grody WW. Cystic fibrosis: Molecular diagnosis, population screening, and public policy. *Arch Pathol Lab Med* 1999; 123:1041-1046.

Gubler MC, Knebelmann B, Beziau A, Broyer M, Pirson Y, Haddoum F, Kleppel MM, Antignac C. Autosomal recessive Alport syndrome: immunohistochemical study of type IV collagen chain distribution. *Kidney Int* 1995; 47:1142-1147.

Gupta M, Djalilvand A, Brat DJ. Clarifying the diffuse gliomas: an update on the morphologic features and markers that discriminate oligodendroglioma from astrocytoma. *Am J Clin Pathol* 2005;124:755-768.

Gutmann DH, Aylsworth A, Carey JC, Korf B, Marks J, Pyeritz RE, Rubenstein A, Viskochil D. The diagnostic evaluation and multidisciplinary management of neurofibromatosis 1 and neurofibromatosis 2. *JAMA* 1997; 278:51-57.

Harrison C. The detection and significance of chromosomal abnormalities in childhood acute lymphoblastic leukemia. *Blood Rev* 2001;15:49.

Herrmann FH, Auerswald G, Ruiz-Saez A, Navarrete M, Pollmann H, Lopaciuk S, Batorova A, Wulff K. Factor X Deficiency: Clinical manifestation of 102 subjects from Europe and Latin America with mutations in the factor 10 gene. *Haemophilia* 2006; 12(5): 479-489.

Herrmann FH, Wulff K, Auberger K, Aumann V, Bergmann F, Bergmann K, Bratanoff E, Franke D, Grundeis M, Kreuz W, Lenk H, Losonczy H, Maak B, Marx G, Mauz-Körholz C, Pollmann H, Serban M, Sutor A, Syrbe G, Vogel G, Weinstock N, Wenzel E, Wolf K. Molecular biology and clinical manifestation of hereditary factor VII deficiency. *Semin Thromb Hemost* 2000; 26(4): 393-400.

Hjalmar V, Kimby E, Matutes E, et al. Trisomy 12 and lymphoplasmacytoid lymphocytes in chronic leukemia B-cell disorders. *Haematologica* 1998;83:602-608.

Insinga RP, Laessig RH, Hoffman GL. Newborn screening with tandem mass spectrometry: examining its cost-effectiveness in the Wisconsin Newborn Screening Panel. *J Pediatr* 2002; 141:524-531.

Irons M. Use of subtelomeric fluorescence in situ hybridization in cytogenetic diagnosis. *Curr Opin Pediatr* 2003; 15:594-597.

Johansson B, Fioretos T, Mitelman F. Cytogenetic and molecular genetic evolution of chronic myeloid leukemia. *Acta Haematol* 2002;107:76-81.

Johnson C, Butler SM, Konstan MW, Morgan W, Wohl ME. Factors influencing outcomes in cystic fibrosis: a center-based analysis. *Chest* 2003;123:20-27.

Jorquera JI, Montoro JM, Fernández MA, Aznar JA. Modified test for activated protein c resistance [letter]. *Lancet* 1994; 344:1162-1163.

Jover R, Payá A, Alenda C, Poveda MJ, Peiró G, Aranda I, Pérez-Mateo M. Defective mismatch-repair colorectal cancer: clinicopathologic characteristics and usefulness of immunohistochemical analysis for diagnosis. *Am J Clin Pathol* 2004;122:389-394.

Kanter WR, Eldridge R, Fabricant R, Allen JC, Koerber T. Central neurofibromatosis with bilateral acoustic neuroma: genetic, clinical and biochemical distinctions from peripheral neurofibromatosis. *Neurology* 1980; 30:851-859.

Kapiotis S, Quehenberger P, Jilma B, Handler S, Pabinger-Fasching I, Mannhalter C, Speiser W. Improved characteristics of APC-resistance assay: coatest APC resistance by predilution of samples with factor V deficient plasma. *Am J Clin Pathol* 1996; 106(5): 588-593.

Kashtan CE. Diagnosis of Alport syndrome. *Kidney Int* 2004;66:1290-1291.

Kattar MM, Grignon DJ, Wallis T, Haas GP, Sakr WA, Pontes JE, Visscher DW. Clinicopathologic and interphase cytogenetic analysis of papillary (chromophilic) renal cell carcinoma. *Mod Pathol* 1997;10:1143-1150.

Kawai A, Woodruff J, Healey JH, et al: SYT-SSX gene fusion as a determinant of morphology and prognosis in synovial sarcoma. *N Engl J Med* 1998;338:153-158.

Kelley TW, Tubbs RR, Prayson RA. Molecular diagnostic techniques for the clinical evaluation of gliomas. *Diagn Mol Pathol* 2005; 14:1–8.

Bibliography

Ketter R, Henn W, Niedermayer I, Steilen-Gimbel H, König J, Zang KD, Steudel WI. Predictive value of progression-associated chromosomal aberrations for the prognosis of meningiomas: a retrospective study of 198 cases. *J Neurosurg* 2001;95:601-607.

Kovacs G. Molecular differential pathology of renal cell tumours. *Histopathology* 1993;22:1–8.

Kratz CP, Niemeyer CM, Castleberry RP, Cetin M, Bergstrasser E, Emanuel PD, Hasle H, Kardos G, Klein C, Kojima S, Stary J, Trebo M, Zecca M, Gelb BD, Tartaglia M, Loh ML. The mutational spectrum of PTPN11 in juvenile myelomonocytic leukemia and Noonan syndrome/myeloproliferative disease. *Blood* 2005;106:2183-2185.

Kricka LJ. Nucleic acid detection technologies—labels, strategies, and formats. *Clin Chem* 1999; 45:453-458.

Lae ME, Roche PC, Jin L, Lloyd RV, Nascimento AG. Desmoplastic small round cell tumor: a clinicopathologic, immunohistochemical, and molecular study of 32 tumors. *Am J Surg Pathol* 2002; 26(7): 823–835.

Lazar A, Abruzzo LV, Pollock RE, Lee S, Czerniak B. Molecular Diagnosis of sarcomas: chromosomal translocations in sarcomas. *Arch Pathol Lab Med* 2006;130:1199–1207.

LeGrys VA. Sweat testing for the diagnosis of cystic fibrosis: practical considerations. *J Pediatr* 1996; 129:892-897.

LeGrys VA. Common errors in sweat testing reporting for cystic fibrosis. *Lab Med* 2002; 33:55-60.

LeGrys VA. Sweat testing for cystic fibrosis. *Lab Med* 2001; 32:750-755.

LeGrys VA. Assessment of sweat-testing practices for the diagnosis of cystic fibrosis. *Arch Pathol Lab Med* 2001; 125:1420-1424.

Leroyer C, Mercier B, Escoffre M, Ferec C, Mottier D. Factor V Leiden prevalence in venous thromboembolism patients. *Chest* 1997; 111(6): 1603-1606.

Litman RS, Rosenberg H. Malignant hyperthermia: update on susceptibility testing. *JAMA* 2005;293:2918-2924.

Liu H, Ye H, Ruskone-Fourmestraux A, De Jong D, Pileri S, Thiede C, Lavergne A, Boot H, Caletti G, Wündisch T, Molina T, Taal BG, Elena S, Thomas T, Zinzani PL, Neubauer A, Stolte M, Hamoudi RA, Dogan A, Isaacson PG, Du MQ. t(11;18) is a marker for all stage gastric MALT lymphomas that will not respond to *H pylori* eradication. *Gastroenterology* 2002;1286-1294.

Loke J, MacLennan DH. Malignant hyperthermia and central core disease: disorders of calcium release channels. *Am J Med* 1998;104:470-486.

Louis DN, Holland EC, Cairncross JG. Glioma classification: a molecular reappraisal. *Am J Pathol* 2001; 159(3): 779-785.

Lynch HT, de la Chapelle A. Hereditary colorectal cancer. *N Engl J Med* 2003; 348:919-932.

Mariani G, Herrmann FH, Dolce A, Batorova A, Etro D, Peyvandi F, Wulff K, Schved JF, Auerswald G, Ingerslev J, Bernardi F. Clinical phenotypes and factor VII genotype in congenital factor VII deficiency. *Thromb Haemost* 2005; 93(3): 481-487.

Martinez A, Fullwood P, Kondo K, et al: Role of chromosome 3p12-p21 tumor suppressor genes in clear renal cell carcinoma: analysis of VHL dependent and VHL independent pathways to tumorigenesis. *Mod Pathol* 2000;53:137.

McCarth y TV, Quane KA, Lynch PJ. Ryanodine receptor mutations in malignant hyperthermia and central core disease. *Hum Mutat* 2000; 15:410-417.

McDermid HE, Morrow BE. Genomic disorders on 22q11. *Am J Hum Genet* 2002; 70:1077-1088.

McGarrity TJ, Wagner Baker MJ, Ruggiero FM, Thiboutot DM, Hampel H, Zhou XP, Eng C. GI polyposis and glycogenic acanthosis of the esophagus associated with PTEN mutation positive Cowden syndrome in the absence of cutaneous manifestations. *Am J Gastroenterol* 2003; 98:1429-1434.

McGarrity TJ, Kulin HE, Zaino RJ. Peutz-Jeghers syndrome. *Am J Gastroenterol* 2000; 95:596-604.

Bibliography

McGarrity TJ, Peiffer LP, Amos CI, Frazier ML, Ward MG, Howett MK. Overexpression of cyclooxygenase 2 in hamartomatous polyps of Peutz-Jeghers syndrome. *Am J Gastroenterol* 2003; 98:671-678.

McKone EF, Emerson SS, Edwards KL, Aitken ML (2003) Effect of genotype on phenotype and mortality in cystic fibrosis: a retrospective cohort study. *Lancet* 2003; 361:1671-1676.

Medeiros LJ, Carr J. Overview of the role of molecular methods in the diagnosis of malignant lymphomas. *Arch Pathol Lab Med* 1999; 123:1189-1207.

Messiaen LM, Callens T, Mortier G, Beysen D, Vandenbroucke I, Van Roy N, Speleman F, Paepe AD. Exhaustive mutation analysis of the NF1 gene allows identification of 95% of mutations and reveals a high frequency of unusual splicing defects. *Hum Mutat* 2000; 15:541-555.

Mikkola H, Palotie A. Gene defects in congenital factor XIII deficiency. *Semin Thromb Hemost* 1996; 22(5): 393-398.

Neumann HP, Bender BU, Berger DP, et al. Prevalence, morphology and biology of renal cell carcinoma in von Hippel-Lindau disease compared to sporadic renal cell carcinoma. *J Urol* 1998;160:1248-1254.

Newman EA, Mulholland MW. Prophylactic gastrectomy for hereditary diffuse gastric cancer syndrome. *J Am Coll Surg* 2006;202:602-617.

Noll WW. Utility of RET mutation analysis in multiple endocrine neoplasia type 2. *Arch Pathol Lab Med* 1999; 123:1047-1049.

Ohgaki H, Kleihues P. Population-based studies on incidence, survival rates, and genetic alterations in astrocytic and oligodendroglial gliomas. *J Neuropathol Exp Neurol* 2005; 64(6): 479-489.

Perez EA, Roche PC, Jenkins RB, Reynolds CA, Halling KC, Ingle JN, Wold LE. HER2 testing in patients with breast cancer: poor correlation between weak positivity by immunohistochemistry and gene amplification by fluorescence in situ hybridization. *Mayo Clin Proc* 2002;77:148-154.

Pratt G. Molecular aspects of multiple myeloma. *Mol Pathol* 2002;55:273–283.

Pui CH. Acute lymphoblastic leukemia in children. *Curr Opin Oncol* 2000;12:3.

Raimondi SC, Chang MN, Ravindranath Y, Behm FG, Gresik MV, Steuber CP, Weinstein HJ, Carroll AJ. Chromosomal abnormalities in 478 children with acute myelod leukemia: Clinical characteristics and treatment outcome in a cooperative Pediatric Oncology Group study-POG 8821. *Blood* 1999;94:3707-3716.

Riemenschneider MJ, Perry A, Reifenberger G. Histological classification and molecular genetics of Meningiomas. *Lancet Neurol* 2006; 5:1045–1054.

Riley RD, Heney D, Jones DR, Sutton AJ, Lambert PC, Abrams KR, Young B, Wailoo AJ, Burchill SA. A systematic review of molecular and biological tumor markers in neuroblastoma. *Clinical Cancer Research* 2004; 10:4-12.

Rowe SM, Miller S, Sorscher EJ. Cystic fibrosis. *NEJM* 2005; 352:1992-2001

Roelse J, Koopman R, Büller H, Berends F, ten Cate JW, Mertens K, van Mourik JA. Association of idiopathic venous thromboembolism with single point-mutation at Arg506 of factor V. *Lancet* 1994; 343:1535-1539.

Rosenstein BJ and Cutting GR. The diagnosis of cystic fibrosis: a consensus statement. Cystic Fibrosis Foundation Consensus Panel. *J Pediatr* 1998; 132:589-595.

Rucker JC, Shapiro BE, Han YH, Kumar AN, Garbutt S, Keller EL, Leigh RJ. Neuro-ophthalmology of late-onset Tay-Sachs disease (LOTS). *Neurology* 2004; 63:1918-1926.

Ruggieri M and Huson SM. The clinical and diagnostic implications of mosaicism in the neurofibromatoses. *Neurology* 2001;56:1433-1443.

Rustgi AK. Hereditary gastrointestinal polyposis and non-polyposis syndromes. *N Engl J Med* 1994;331:1694-702.

Bibliography

Schloesser M, Zeerleder S, Lutze G, Halbmayer WM, Hofferbert S, Hinney B, Koestering H, Lämmle B, Pindur G, Thies K, Köhler M, Engel W. Mutations in the human factor XII gene. *Blood* 1997; 90(10):3967-3977.

Schrager CA, Schneider D, Gruener AC, Tsou HC, Peacocke M. Clinical and pathological features of breast disease in Cowden's syndrome: an underrecognized syndrome with an increased risk of breast cancer. *Hum Pathol* 1998; 29:47-53.

Schwab M, Westermann F, Hero B, Berthold F. Neuroblastoma: biology and molecular and chromosomal pathology. *Lancet Oncol* 2003; 4:472–480.

Shia J, Klimstra DS, Nafa K, Offit K, Guillem JG, Markowitz AJ, Gerald JG, Ellis NA. Value of immunohistochemical detection of DNA mismatch repair proteins in predicting germline mutation in hereditary colorectal neoplasms. *Am J Surg Pathol* 2005;29:96–104.

Sperfeld AD, Hein C, Schroder JM, Ludolph AC, Hanemann CO. Occurrence and characterization of peripheral nerve involvement in neurofibromatosis type 2. *Brain* 2002; 125:996-1004.

Stratakis CA, Bertherat J, Carney JA. Mutation of perinatal myosin heavy chain. *N Engl J Med* 2004;351:2556-2258.

Stoller JK, Aboussouan LS. Alpha-1-antitrypsin deficiency. *Lancet* 2005; 365:2225–2236.

Svensson PJ, Dahlback B. Resistance to activated protein C as a basis for venous thrombosis. *N Engl J Med* 1994; 330:517-522.

Tada K, Shiraishi S, Kamiryo T, Nakamura H, Hirano H, Kuratsu J, Kochi M, Saya H, Ushio Y. Analysis of loss of heterozygosity chromosome 10 in patients with malignant astrocytic tumors: Correlation with patient age and survival. *J Neurosurg* 2001;95:651-659.

Tartaglia M, Martinelli S, Cazzaniga G, Cordeddu V, Iavarone I, Spinelli M, Palmi C, Carta C, Pession A, Arico M, Masera G, Basso G, Sorcini M, Gelb BD, Biondi A. Genetic evidence for lineage-related and differentiation stage-related contribution of somatic PTPN11 mutations to leukemogenesis in childhood acute leukemia. *Blood* 2004;104:307-313.

Taylor AMR, Byrd PJ. Molecular pathology of ataxia telangiectasia. *J Clin Pathol* 2005; 58:1009–1015

Theodoropoulos DS, Krasnewich D, Kaiser-Kupfer MI, Gahl WA. Classic nephropathic cystinosis as an adult disease. *JAMA* 1993; 270:2200-2204.

Tiebosch AT, Frederik PM, van Breda Vriesman PJ, Mooy JM, van Rie H, van de Wiel TW, Wolters J, Zeppenfeldt E. Thin-basement-membrane nephropathy in adults with persistent hematuria. *N Engl J Med* 1989; 320:14-18.

Trueworthy R, Shuster J, Look T, et al. Ploidy of lymphoblasts is the strongest predictor of treatment outcome in B progenitor cell ALL of childhood: A Pediatric Oncology Group study. *J Clin Oncol* 1992;10:606–613.

Tsilchorozidou T, Menko FH, Lalloo F, Kidd A, De Silva R, Thomas H, Smith P, Malcolmson A, Dore J, Madan K, Brown A, Yovos JG, Tsaligopoulos M, Vogiatzis N, Baser ME, Wallace AJ, Evans DG. Constitutional rearrangements of chromosome 22 as a cause of neurofibromatosis 2. *J Med Genet* 2004; 41:529-534.

Uprichard J, Perry DJ. Factor X deficiency. *Blood Rev* 2002; 16(2): 97-110.

Venditti LN, Venditti CP, Berry GT, Kaplan PB, Kaye EM, Glick H, Stanley CA. Newborn screening by tandem mass spectrometry for medium-chain Acyl-CoA dehydrogenase deficiency: a cost-effectiveness analysis. *Pediatrics* 2003; 112:1005-1015.

Viskochil D, White R, Cawthon R. The neurofibromatosis type 1 gene. *Annu Rev Neurosci* 1993;16:183-205.

Wang X, Moylan B, Leopold DA, Kim J, Rubenstein RC, Togias A, Proud D, Zeitlin PL, Cutting GR. Mutation in the gene responsible for cystic fibrosis and predisposition to chronic rhinosinusitis in the general population. *JAMA* 2000;284:1814-1819.

Young RH, Welch WR, Dickersin GR, Scully RE. Ovarian sex cord tumor with annular tubules: review of 74 cases including 27 with Peutz-Jeghers syndrome and four with adenoma malignum of the cervix. *Cancer* 1982; 50:1384-1402.

Bibliography

Young S, Gooneratne S, Straus FH, Zeller WP, Bulun SE, Rosenthal IM. Feminizing Sertoli cell tumors in boys with Peutz-Jeghers syndrome. Am J *Surg Pathol* 1995;19:50-58.

Zenker M, Buheitel G, Rauch R, Koenig R, Bosse K, Kress W, Tietze HU, Doerr HG, Hofbeck M, Singer H, Reis A, Rauch A. Genotype-phenotype correlations in Noonan syndrome. *J Pediatr* 2004;144:368-374.

Zhou X, Hampel H, Thiele H, Gorlin RJ, Hennekam RC, Parisi M, Winter RM, Eng C. Association of germline mutation in the PTEN tumour suppressor gene and Proteus and Proteus-like syndromes. *Lancet* 2001;358:210-211.

Zytkovicz TH, Fitzgerald EF, Marsden D, Larson CA, Shih VE, Johnson DM, Strauss AW, Comeau AM, Eaton RB, Grady GF. Tandem mass spectrometric analysis for amino, organic, and fatty acid disorders in newborn dried blood spots: a two-year summary from the New England Newborn Screening Program. *Clin Chem* 2001; 47:1945-1955.

Chapter 8

Laboratory Statistics and Quality Control

Interpretation of Laboratory Values

Definitions

Gaussian distribution: a distribution of datapoints that is arranged symmetrically around the mean with most values closest to the center. Since this distribution is describable by a mathematical equation, it is considered parametric. Random testing of a population often results in a Gaussian normal distribution. In this ideal distribution, 68% of the population falls within –1 SD and +1 SD, 95.5% falls within –2 SD and +2 SD, and 99.7% fall within –3 SD and +3 SD **F8.1**.

Mean and standard deviation: Mean is the arithmetic average of a set of data points. The mean is calculated as the sum of the individual values divided by the number of values. The standard deviation (SD) is also a calculation of an average (mean): it is the average distance of an individual value from the mean.

$$Mean = \sum x_i / n = \bar{x}$$

$$SD = \sqrt{\sum (x_i - mean)^2 / (n - 1)}$$

Median: the middle value of a range of values.

Mode: the most frequently occurring value in a range of values.

Accuracy: the extent to which a test result approximates the "true" value. Most often the "true" value is considered to be that obtained by the definitive method or the reference method. A definitive method is the one that uses the highest quality instrumentation available. Reference methods utilize materials more widely available and have been validated by a definitive method. Accuracy has no numerical value.

Precision: reproducibility of a test result. It is affected by the random variability inherent in processes. The within-run precision is a function of analyte concentration: low concentrations usually have the least precision. Within-run precision for most analytes should run between 1-10%. Between-run precision (day-to-day precision) is affected by changing environmental conditions, and changing technologists (operator bias). Generally precision is expressed in terms of the **coefficient of variation(CV)**. The CV describes the standard deviation as a percentage of the mean. Note that, since the CV is a function of the mean, it refers to the precision at a particular analyte concentration. Generally, CV increases as the analyte increases. Thus, one can assess test performance at critical cut-off values, if desired.

$$CV = SD/mean \times 100$$

Clinical sensitivity: the ability of the test to detect disease when present, or positivity in the presence of disease **F8.2**. Distinguished from analytical sensitivity (see below)

$$Sens = TP/(TP + FN)$$

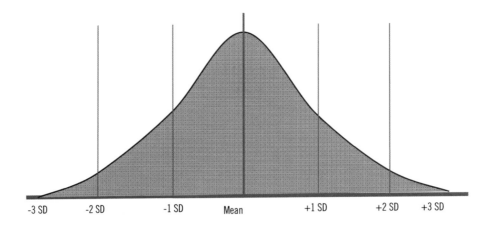

-3 SD   -2 SD   -1 SD   Mean   +1 SD   +2 SD   +3 SD

F8.1 Gaussian normal distrubution

Interpretation of Laboratory Values>Definitions

Specificity: the ability of the test to detect only the disease sought, or its negativity in the absence of disease **F8.2**.

	disease	no disease
positive test	true positive (TP)	false positive (FP)
negative test	false negative (FN)	true negative (TN)

F8.2 Punnett Square

$$Spec = TN/(TN + FP)$$

Positive predictive value (PPV): the percent of positive results that actually indicate disease **F8.2**. That is, if the test is positive, the likelihood that the individual has the disease. The negative predictive value is the probability of no disease when the test is negative.

$$PPV = TP/(TP + FP)$$

$$NPV = TN/(TN + FN)$$

The effect of disease prevalence on predictive value: the *pretest probability* affects the performance of a test. One of the most powerful estimates of pretest probability is the *prevalence* of the disease in the population. Note that sensitivity and specificity are not mathematically influenced by prevalence, but positive and negative predictive values are. The practical consequence of this effect is that when disease prevalence is low, the PPV of a test declines (and the NPV increases). The converse is also true.

Relative risk: the risk of an outcome 'y' in the presence of condition 'x' as compared to the population.

$$Relative\ risk = \frac{\#\ with\ X\ who\ develop\ Y\ /\ \#\ with\ X}{\#\ in\ population\ who\ develop\ Y\ /\ \#\ in\ population}$$

Scales: Tests may give results on scales that are nominal, interval, or ordinal. An interval scale is one that gives discrete numbers that have their usual mathematical meaning (eg, the sodium). An ordinal scale is one that gives a number with an assigned value (eg, the urine dipstick protein: 1+ to 4+). A nominal test is one that gives a category (positive, negative).

Receiver operating characteristic (ROC) curves: An ROC curve is used to answer the question: how does a test perform, particularly at different cut-off values.

An ROC curve is generated by: (1) placing sensitivity (true positive rate) on the y axis and 1-specificity (false positive rate) on the x axis; (2) plotting the sensitivity & specificity of different cut-offs on the graph; (3) drawing a curve along the dots.

Thus, the ROC curve displays a test's sensitivity over a range of false-positive rates. One can also derive quantitative measures of accuracy, such as the area under the ROC curve.

Despite the fact that it is stated as such throughout the literature, a diagnostic test does not have only one sensitivity or specificity, but many, depending upon the cut-off used. For any given test, one can always identify a cut-off (decision threshold, decision level) value and state a diagnostic sensitivity and specificity at that point. However, ROC plots provide a view of the whole spectrum of sensitivities and specificities, and this provides the most informative basis for comparisons between tests.

Each point on the ROC plot represents a sensitivity/specificity pair corresponding to a particular cut-off (decision level). A test with perfect discrimination would have an ROC plot that passes through the upper left corner, a point where sensitivity is 1.0 (100%, perfect sensitivity) and the false-positive rate is 0 (specificity is 1.0). A test with no ability to discriminate would have an ROC plot that is a 45° diagonal line from the lower left corner to the upper right corner. Most actual tests fall in between these two extremes, with tests having plots that most closely approach the upper left corner deemed most accurate.

In the ROC curve **F8.3**, an imaginary diagonal line with a slope of 1 beginning at the intercepts represents a test with no discrimination. Any curve above this line represents a test that performs better than chance. The greater the area under the curve, the better the test is performing.

Looking at the ROC curve, it should be clear why selecting a low cut-off results in high sensitivity but low specificity. A high cut-off will do the opposite. The cut-off selected depends on what you would like the test to do. For example, a screening test would require high sensitivity (with low specificity), while a confirmatory test would demand high specificity.

Reference Intervals

In order to determine the likelihood that disease is present, test results are typically compared to values obtained from healthy individuals; the range of such results is termed the reference interval, while the high and low ends of the interval are termed the upper and lower reference limits, respectively.

Most laboratories publish a single reference interval for most laboratory tests, defined as the central 95% (± 2 SD) of results obtained from healthy persons. In many cases, there are recognized factors that can affect the results of tests without indicating the presence of disease, particularly when only a single reference interval is used. The necessary result of this practice is that about 5% of test results performed on completely normal and healthy subjects will fall outside 2 SD and be flagged as abnormal. For example, if 20 analytes are measured in a

healthy subject, it is likely that 1 (5%) of those results will be abnormal. The above approach has been termed parametric, and this works when the population studied is roughly Gaussian. When the population, instead, is skewed, a nonparametric apporach may be taken.

For some tests, reference limits are defined by health outcomes; examples include currently used reference limits for cholesterol and fasting glucose. Use of outcome-based reference limits also requires a high degree of standardization of measurement between laboratories to assure that results from all laboratories have a similar relationship to the upper reference limit.

Quality Control

CLIA regulations stipulate 4 categories of lab tests: waived tests, provider performed microscopy (PPM), moderate complexity, and high complexity. Each category has different requirements. CLIA standards are enforced by the Health Care Finance Administration (HCFA).

- Waived testing has the least regulation: follow the manufacturers' directions and/or follow good laboratory practices (run & document controls before reporting results). Waived tests include such things as: dipstick urinalysis, fecal occult blood, urine pregnancy tests, home glucose tests, clinic *H. pylori* tests, etc.

- Provider performed microscopy (PPM). Providers must follow good laboratory practices. PPM tests include

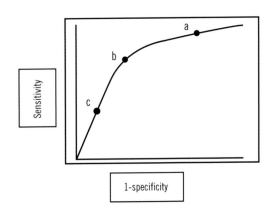

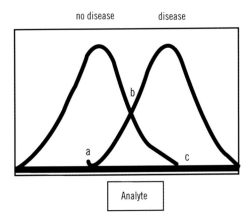

F8.3 On the left is a typical ROC curve with three arbitrarily selected points, a-c, labeled. On the right is a representation of two theoretical populations with the same points, a-c, labeled. It can be seen that if 'a' is the selected cut-off, the test will have high sensitivity (all people with disease would be detected), but low specificity (a good number of people without disease test positive). If 'c' were selected, the opposite would apply. Point 'b' is an 'ideal' cutoff, but , of course, this depends on what you want the test to accomplish.

such thing as: wet mounts, KOH preps, ferning tests, nasal smears for leukocytes, etc.

- Moderate complexity tests include most tests in the typical laboratory. In performing these tests, laboratorians are required to: have an SOP, follow manufacturer's directions, perform and document calibration and controls (see below), perform and document corrective actions when QC is out.

- High complexity tests are tests that are primarily tests developed within the laboratory. Regulatory requirements are essentially those for moderate complexity testing plus specific requirements regarding establishing the validity of the procedure.

Control specimens: these are most often samples provided by an outside source, usually the manufacturer of an instrument. They are designed to target values at or near the cut-off values; there are usually two controls for each test: a 'low' QC reagent and a 'high' QC reagent.

When a new control sample is received in the lab, it is reconstituted and run on the instrument in question several times. The results from these several test runs are used to calculate a mean and standard deviation (SD). Based on these, a **Levey-Jennings** chart is created **F8.4**. Only one Levey-Jennings chart is illustrated, but usually you will have two, one for a high control and one for the low control.

After these initial steps, the controls are run at intervals—with each run, once each day, etc, depending on the type of test and its frequency. The result obtained when the control is tested is plotted on the Levey-Jennings chart. If the control sample result falls within 2 SD of the mean, then the run is considered 'in control,' and the results of patient samples can be reported. If, however, the control sample result falls outside 2 SD of the mean, then the Levey-Jennings chart is interpreted in terms of Westgard's rules. Based on this interpretation, the run is determined to be 'in control' or 'out of control.' The results of 'out of control' runs should not generally be reported.

The Westgard Rules

1:3s rule: is 1 value ± 3 SD from the mean?

2:2s rule: are 2 consecutive values located >2 SD on the same side of the mean?

R:4s rule: are 2 values within the same run located >4 SD from each other?

4:1s rule: are 4 consecutive values located >1 SD on the same side of the mean?

10:mean rule: are 10 consecutive values on the same side of the mean?

Addressing 'out of control' tests

- Sometimes it is tempting to hope that an 'out of control' value will go away by repeating the assay of the control or by trying another control. This practice may only delay finding a potentially important problem and is not recommended.

- Determine the type of error. Out of control runs may be due to random or systematic errors. Often, the different types of errors lead to violations of different Westgard rules. Rules that address widening distributions of results (1_{3s} and R_{4s}) are sensitive to random error. Rules that address drifts and shifts (2_{2s}, 4_{1s} and 10_X) are sensitive to systematic error.

- The type of error points towards the source of error. Systematic errors may be due to changes in reagent lot, changes in calibrator lot, improper preparation of reagent/calibrator reagents, deterioration of reagents over time, mechanical pipette problems, temperature changes, gradual deterioration of the light source, etc. Random errors may be due to bubbles in reagents, bubbles in the lines, incomplete mixing of reagents, fluctuating temperature, fluctuating electrical supply, and intertech variation.

- Correct any defects you identify and document resolution of the problem (retest the controls). Don't forget to repeat testing on samples from the original out of control run. All these remedial actions must be documented.

Proficiency Testing

Under CLIA '88, each lab must enroll in a proficiency testing program, for each area in which it performs testing, administered by an agency approved by the Department of Health and Human Services.

The Westgard Rules>Proficiency Testing

Day	Interpretation	
2	Accept run.	Control value <2 SD. Run is in control.
3	Accept run.	Control value <2 SD. Run is in control
4	Accept run.	Control value <2 SD. Run is in control
5	Accept run.	Control value >2 SD. No rules violated. Run is in control.
6	Reject run.	Control value >2 SD. 2:2s rule violated.
7	Accept run.	Control value <2 SD. Run is in control.
8	Reject run.	Control value >2 SD. 1:3s rule violated.
9	Accept run.	Control value <2 SD. Run is in control.
10	Accept run.	Control value <2 SD. Run is in control.
11	Accept run.	Control value <2 SD. Run is in control.
12	Accept run.	Control value >2 SD. No rules violated. Run is in control.
13	Reject run.	Control value >2 SD. 2:2s (and 10:mean) rule violated.
14	Accept run.	Control value <2 SD. Run is in control.
15	Accept run.	Control value <2 SD. Run is in control.
16	Accept run.	Control value >2 SD. No rules violated. Run is in control.
17	Accept run.	Control value <2 SD. Run is in control.
18	Reject run.	Control value >2 SD. 4:1s rule violated.

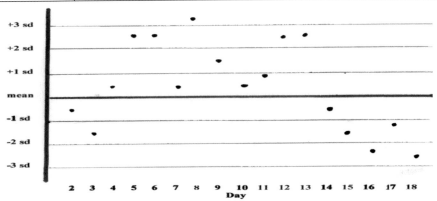

F8.4 Levey-Jennings chart

In proficiency testing programs such as that administered by the College of American Pathologists (CAP), participants receive survey specimens several times per year. They perform the indicated assays, treating the survey sample as they would any other sample, and report their results to CAP.

CAP compiles the data and calculates the mean and SD from all the results sent in by labs using the same methodology (the peer group). In compliance with CLIA, participants are graded as acceptable (<2 SD), needs improvement (<2-3 SD) or unacceptable (>3 SD). For this determination, CAP calculates a **standard deviation index (SDI)** for each participant.

$$SDI = \frac{\text{lab's result} - \text{mean for peer group}}{\text{SD for peer group}}$$

The lab is surveyed three times per year in batches of 5 samples. The lab must achieve acceptable results in >4/5 (80%) to be satisfactory. According to CLIA '88, a satisfactory result is necessary for lab accreditation.

The "1/3" rule: your lab has a good chance of passing if your lab's SD for the surveyed analyte is <33% of the SD allowed. Eg, if the SD allowed is 4 and your lab's SD is 1, then you will probably pass.

Analytical Correlation

This refers to the method by which a new assay is compared to an existing assay. In a correlation study, multiple samples are obtained and run on both assays. The resulting data are plotted **F8.5**.

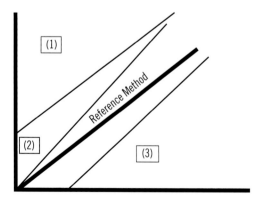

F8.5 Correlation study: (1) constant bias, (2) proportional bias, and (3) mixed.

Ideal correlation exists when the slopes are close to 1, the intercepts close to 0. The correlation study can expose various kinds of analytical variability:

- **Systematic variability** (analytical bias):

  □ A constant (offset) bias exists when the slope is similar but the intercepts are different

  □ A proportional bias exists when the slope differs significantly

  □ Both biases may coexist

- **Random variability:** exists when the points are randomly placed and a line cannot be drawn. Random variability that increases with increasing analyte concentration often points to a pipetting problem. Random variability that is constant in magnitude may point to a turbidometric error.

Analytical Sensitivity

Analytical sensitivity differs from the clinical sensitivity described above. It refers to the lowest analyte concentration detectable by the test.

Assays where analytic sensitivity is very important: TSH, troponin, d-dimer, CRP, microalbumin, hCG.

The analytical sensitivity can be determined by repeated assays on samples that contain no analyte. The mean and SD of the results are figured, and the analytical sensitivity is equal to the mean +3 SD.

Linearity

Just as analytical sensitivity addresses the problems of low analyte concentrations, the linearity addresses the problem of high analyte concentrations.

Samples with high concentrations are used to assess linearity. The samples are serially diluted and assayed. The results are plotted against the known dilutions and these two lines are drawn. The resulting graph is interpreted similarly to a correlation study. The point at which correlation becomes poor is the limit of linearity.

8: Laboratory Statistics and Quality Control

The Westgard Rules>Interference | Preanalytic Variables>Physiologic Variables Affecting Blood Samples; Collection Parameters

Interference

Interference studies address the problem of interfering substances in an assay. For example, hyperbilirubinemia and hyperlipidemia are known to interfere with several assays.

Interferences are often responsible for a constant bias.

Heterophile antibody interference is a major problem in immunoassay-based testing. Human heterophile antibodies may interfere with immunoassays by binding to the animal antibodies used in the assay. Knowing how to detect heterophile antibody interference and how to avoid it are of paramount importance. Typically, the possibility of this sort of interference comes by way of a clinician phoning about an inexplicable laboratory result. Once there is suspicion of such interference, if the sample is still available, one can make serial dilutions of the sample. Heterophile antibody interference does not change linearly with dilution; whereas, a true result will. Numerous strategies have been evaluated that are aimed at avoiding heterophile antibody interference. These include removal of immunoglobulins from a sample (eg, with PEG), modification of assay antibodies (in ways similar to those used in monoclonal antibody therapies) to make them less prone to react with heterophile antibodies, and the use of buffers to reduce interference.

Another sort of 'interference' is the so-called solvent exclusion effect. This term refers to a falsely low analyte concentration that results from a higher than normal 'solid phase.' Each blood sample has a solid phase and an aqueous phase. An 'indirect ISE' instrument measures, for example, a sodium concentration within the aqueous phase and calculates the sodium concentration for the entire volume of blood. When the solid phase is increased as, for example, in lipemia and high-levels or paraprotein (myeloma effect), the apparent sodium concentration artifactually goes down. This artifact is not a problem for 'direct ISE' analyzers, but the vast majority of labs use indirect ISE analyzers.

Preanalytic Variables

Physiologic Variables Affecting Blood Samples

Age has a profound effect on expected lab results for various analytes. In particular, neonates can be expected to have noticeably different white cell differential than adults, with a relative increase in mononuclear cells. Adolescent children can have alarmingly high alkaline phosphatase, up to 5 times the upper limit of normal for adults. In the elderly, a long list of changes occur, including decreased creatinine clearance, decreased glucose tolerance, increased releasing hormones (TRH, ACTH), and increased lipids.

Sex: Among other differences, males can be expected to have an increased CK and LDL cholesterol.

Food intake: After meals, glucose concentration may be abnormally elevated or depressed, and it is never as reliable as in the fasting state. Triglycerides increase for 8 to 12 hours after a meal. Other analytes, such as gastrin and insulin, are also increased. Bilirubin is decreased following a meal. Fasting, so long as it is not prolonged, imparts a sort of steady state and is the best state in which to measure most analytes; however, it should be noted that prolonged fasting can alter several analytes as well, including elevated ketones, elevated bilirubin, decreased albumin, decreased potassium, and decreased magnesium.

Exercise increases the serum concentration of CK, LDH, and AST. In addition, exercise induces neutrophil demargination, resulting in apparent neutrophilia.

Pregnancy has a profound effect on many analytes (see Chapter 1, p 34)

Intraindividual variation: Some analytes show marked differences within an individual from one time of collection to another. Analytes notorious for this are: PSA, triglycerides, AST, serum cortisol, bilirubin, and urate.

Collection Parameters

Effect of posture: When a patient goes from the supine to the sitting or standing position, the increased hydrostatic pressure forces water out of the circulation and into the interstitial fluid. Small molecules such as electrolytes can easily follow the water, but larger molecules such as proteins, substances largely bound to proteins, and formed elements (blood cells) cannot. Thus, when sitting, the concentration of these 3 types of substances goes up relative to supine. The change is in the range of 5% to 15%.

Time of day: Many analytes vary throughout the day. Most notably, serum cortisol has wide diurnal variation, peaking around 6 to 8 am, and should be measured at the same time every day in every patient.

Tourniquets, though useful, create an artificially hemo-concentrated and anaerobic region of the body after prolonged (>1 to 3 minutes) application. Such effects are made worse with fist clenching or if the tourniquet is released during blood collection.

Order of draw: In order to maximize the integrity of samples obtained by venipuncture, it is important to draw tubes in a particular order. Ideally, cultures are drawn first (to reduce the likelihood of contamination), followed by tubes with no additive (eg, red top tubes), followed by coagulation tests (to reduce activation of coagulation and contamination by additives), next serum separator tubes, and last tubes with additives (heparin, EDTA).

Errors in Laboratory Medicine

Errors in laboratory medicine may be thought of as analytical (what happens in the assay), preanalytical (what happens before the assay), and postanalytical.

Examples of preanalytic errors include inappropriate test selection, incorrect patient identification, inappropriate timing of specimen collection, and sample defects (hemolysis, aged samples, clotted samples, and low-quantity samples).

Analytic errors include systematic and random error. Systematic errors are influenced by constant bias, proportional bias, reagent carryover, and sample carryover. Random error is influenced mainly by interferences and technologist factors.

Postanalytic error may take the form of delayed reporting, errors within reports (transcription and proofreading errors), misreading or incorrectly hearing the report, misunderstanding the information, and incorrect response to the information.

While pathologists pay great attention to the analytic phase, it appears that the largest proportion of errors occur in the pre- and postanalytic phases.

Formulas and Units

Unit	Definition
1 IU	micromol/minute
1 Katal	mol/second
1 IU	16.67 nanokatals
micro (µ)	10^{-6}
nano	10^{-9}
pico	10^{-12}
femto	10^{-15}

T8.1

Blood Collection Tubes

Tube	Additive	Used for
Red	None	Serum chemistry, blood bank, and serology
Green	Heparin	Plasma chemistry
Blue	Citrate	Coagulation tests. Note: A 1:9 ratio of anticoagulant:blood is ideal. Higher ratios lead to increased coagulation times, affecting the aPTT>PT. For polycythemic patients with Hct>60%, the PT and PTT can be prolonged due to decreased effective plasma
Black	Buffered sodium citrate	ESR
Lavender (purple)	EDTA	Cell counts
Yellow	Citrate & dextrose (ACD)	Blood bank tests, HLA typing
Gray	Sodium fluoride	Glucose

Reticulocyte Proliferation Index (RPI)

$$RPI = \text{reticulocytes (\%)} \times \text{Hct}/45 \times 1/\text{MI}$$

Hct = hematocrit, MI = maturation index

Hct	MI
45	1
35	1.5
25	2.0
15	2.5

FOR REFERENCE

Index to start on following page

Index

Note: **f** refers to figures, **t** refers to tables.

M